To Charlotte & Conn[illegible]

with Admiration and

Gratitude for your

support and encouragement

[illegible signature]

May 91

EYE Trauma

Mosby Year Book
Dedicated to Publishing Excellence

Editor: Kimberly Kist
Assistant Editor: Penny Rudolph
Project Manager: Linda J. Daly
Designer: Laura Steube
Cover Design: Laurel L. Cook

Printed in the United States of America

Mosby–Year Book, Inc.
11830 Westline Industrial Drive
St. Louis, MO 63146

Library of Congress Cataloging-in-Publication Data

Eye trauma / edited by Bradford J. Shingleton, Peter S. Hersh, Kenneth R. Kenyon ; associate editors, Trexler M. Topping, John J. Woog ; with 596 illustrations, 70 in color.
p. cm.
Includes bibliographical references.
Includes index.
ISBN 0-8016-5820-9
1. Eye—Wounds and injuries. I. Shingleton, Bradford J. II. Hersh, Peter S. III. Kenyon, Kenneth R.
[DNLM: 1. Eye Injuries. 2. Eye Injuries, Penetrating. WW525 E97]
RE831.E94 1991
617.7′13—dc20
DNLM/DLC
for Library of Congress

90-13371
CIP

GW/MY/MY 9 8 7 6 5 4 3 2 1

EYE Trauma

Edited by:

BRADFORD J. SHINGLETON, MD, FACS

Associate Surgeon in Ophthalmology and
Former Director, Eye Emergency Service
Massachusetts Eye and Ear Infirmary
Clinical Instructor of Ophthalmology
Harvard Medical School
Boston, Massachusetts

PETER S. HERSH, MD

Assistant Professor of Ophthalmology
Albert Einstein College of Medicine
Chairman of Ophthalmology
Bronx-Lebanon Hospital Center
Cornea Consultation Service
Montefiore Medical Center
New York, New York

KENNETH R. KENYON, MD, FACS

Surgeon in Ophthalmology and
Former Director, Cornea Service
Massachusetts Eye and Ear Infirmary
Associate Professor of Ophthalmology
Harvard Medical School
Senior Scientist
Eye Research Institute of Retina Foundation
Boston, Massachusetts

Associate Editors

TREXLER M. TOPPING, MD, FACS
Posterior Segment Trauma

JOHN J. WOOG, MD
Orbital and Adnexal Trauma

Laurel L. Cook, Illustrator
With 596 illustrations, 70 in color

Mosby Year Book

St. Louis Baltimore Boston Chicago London Philadelphia Sydney Toronto

Contributors

NEIL M. BRESSLER, M.D.

Associate Professor of Ophthalmology
The Wilmer Ophthalmological Institute
The Johns Hopkins University School of Medicine
Baltimore, Maryland

SUSAN B. BRESSLER, M.D.

Associate Professor of Ophthalmology
The Wilmer Ophthalmological Institute
The Johns Hopkins University School of Medicine
Baltimore, Maryland

SERGE DE BUSTROS, M.D.

Associate Professor of Ophthalmology
The Wilmer Ophthalmological Institute
The Johns Hopkins University School of Medicine
Baltimore, Maryland

J. DOUGLAS CAMERON, M.D.

Associate Professor of Ophthalmology
Associate Professor of Laboratory Medicine and Pathology
University of Minnesota
Hennepin County Medical Center
Minneapolis, Minnesota

DAVID G. CAMPBELL, M.D.

Professor of Ophthalmology
Dartmouth-Hitchcock Medical Center
Hanover, New Hampshire

D. JACKSON COLEMAN, M.D.

Professor and Chairman
Department of Ophthalmology
New York Hospital
Cornell Medical Center
New York, New York

DONALD J. D'AMICO, M.D.

Director
Diabetic Retinopathy Unit
Massachusetts Eye and Ear Infirmary
Associate Professor of Ophthalmology
Harvard Medical School
Boston, Massachusetts

RICHARD K. DORTZBACH, M.D.

Clinical Professor of Ophthalmology
University of Wisconsin Medical School
Madison, Wisconsin

ROBERT M. ELLSWORTH, M.D.

Professor of Ophthalmology and Director
Ophthalmic Oncology Center
New York Hospital
Cornell Medical Center
New York, New York

ARTHUR T. GLOVER, M.D.

Clinical Instructor
Department of Ophthalmology
University of California, Davis
Sacramento, California

RUSSELL S. GONNERING, M.D., F.A.C.S.

Assistant Clinical Professor
Department of Ophthalmology
University of Wisconsin
Madison, Wisconsin

M. BOWES HAMILL, M.D.

Assistant Professor of Ophthalmology
Cullen Eye Institute
Baylor College of Medicine
Houston, Texas

THOMAS R. HEDGES III, M.D.

Associate Professor
Department of Ophthalmology and Neurology
Tufts University
New England Medical Center
Boston, Massachusetts

PETER S. HERSH, M.D.

Chairman of Ophthalmology
Bronx-Lebanon Hospital Center
Cornea Consultation Service
Montefiore Medical Center
New York, New York

DOUG HOLMES, M.D.

Clinical Instructor in Ophthalmology
Oregon Health Sciences University
Portland, Oregon

DARREN L. HOOVER, M.D.

Clinical Instructor
Department of Ophthalmology
University of Pittsburgh
School of Medicine
Children's Hospital of Pittsburgh
Pittsburgh, Pennsylvania

W. JACKSON ILIFF, M.D.

Associate Professor of Ophthalmology
The Wilmer Ophthalmological Institute
The Johns Hopkins University School of Medicine
Baltimore, Maryland

JOHN A. IRVINE, M.D.

Assistant Professor of Ophthalmology
Doheny Eye Institute
University of Southern California School of Medicine
Los Angeles, California

KENNETH R. KENYON, M.D., F.A.C.S.

Surgeon in Ophthalmology
Former Director
Cornea Service
Massachusetts Eye and Ear Infirmary
Associate Professor of Ophthalmology
Harvard Medical School
Senior Scientist
Eye Research Institute of Retina Foundation
Boston, Massachusetts

JEMSHED A. KHAN, M.D.

Director of Oculoplastic Surgery
Department of Ophthalmology
Kansas University Medical Center
Kansas City, Kansas

TERESA P. KUNZWILER, R.N.

Nurse Manager
Emergency Department
Massachusetts Eye and Ear Infirmary
Boston, Massachusetts

JAN KYLSTRA, M.D.

Assistant Professor of Ophthalmology
University of North Carolina School of Medicine
Chapel Hill, North Carolina

BRADLEY N. LEMKE, M.D., F.A.C.S.

Assistant Clinical Professor of Ophthalmology
University of Wisconsin
Madison, Wisconsin

SIMMONS LESSELL, M.D.

Professor of Ophthalmology
Harvard Medical School
Director
Neuro-Ophthalmology Service
Massachusetts Eye and Ear Infirmary
Boston, Massachusetts

MARC R. LEVIN, M.D.

Clinical Fellow in Ophthalmology
Harvard Medical School
Retina Service
Massachusetts Eye and Ear Infirmary
Boston, Massachusetts

DAVID B. LYON, M.D.

Clinical Instructor
Department of Ophthalmology
University of Wisconsin Medical School
Madison, Wisconsin

COLIN MA, M.D.

Clinical Instructor in Ophthalmology
Doheny Eye Institute
University of Southern California School of Medicine
Los Angeles, California

CLINTON D. MCCORD, JR., M.D.

Director of Ophthalmic Plastic and Reconstructive Surgery
Emory University
Professor of Ophthalmology
Associate Professor of Plastic Surgery
Emory School of Medicine
Atlanta, Georgia

KATHRYN E. MCGOLDRICK, M.D.

Associate Professor of Anesthesiology
Yale University School of Medicine
New Haven, Connecticut

MARK J. RONDEAU

Research Associate in Ophthalmology
The New York Hospital
Cornell Medical Center
New York, New York

J. JAMES ROWSEY, M.D.

Clinical Professor of Ophthalmology
University of Oklahoma College of Medicine
Director
Cornea Services
Dean A. McGee Eye Institute
Oklahoma City, Oklahoma

STEVEN J. RYAN, M.D.

Professor and Chairman
Doheny Eye Institute
University of Southern California School of Medicine
Los Angeles, California

OLIVER D. SCHEIN, M.D.

Assistant Professor of Ophthalmology
The Wilmer Ophthalmological Institute
The Johns Hopkins School of Medicine
Baltimore, Maryland

PHILIP A. SHELTON, M.D., J.D.

Senior Staff
Department of Ophthalmology
Hartford Hospital
Assistant Clinical Professor
University of Connecticut
School of Medicine
Hartford, Connecticut

BRADFORD J. SHINGLETON, M.D., F.A.C.S.

Associate Surgeon in Ophthalmology
Former Director
Eye Emergency Service
Massachusetts Eye and Ear Infirmary
Clinical Instructor of Ophthalmology
Harvard Medical School
Boston, Massachusetts

JOHN W. SHORE, M.D.

Assistant Professor of Ophthalmology
Harvard Medical School
Director Eye Plastic
Orbital and Ocular Trauma Services
Massachusetts Eye and Ear Infirmary
Boston, Massachusetts

WILLIAM E. SMIDDY, M.D.

Assistant Professor of Ophthalmology
University of Miami School of Medicine
Bascum Palmer Eye Institute
Miami, Florida

LOIS E. H. SMITH, M.D.

Professor and Vice Chairman
Department of Ophthalmology
Children's Hospital
Boston, Massachusetts

RONALD E. SMITH, M.D.

Professor of Ophthalmology
Doheny Eye Institute
University of Southern California School of Medicine
Los Angeles, California

WALTER J. STARK, M.D.

Professor of Ophthalmology
The Wilmer Ophthalmological Institute
The Johns Hopkins University School of Medicine
Baltimore, Maryland

GEORGE O. STASIOR, M.D.

Fellow in Ophthalmology
Division of Eye Plastic and Ocular Plastic Reconstructive Surgery
University of Wisconsin
Madison, Wisconsin

Roger F. Steinert, M.D.

Director
Cornea Consultation Service
Massachusetts Eye and Ear Infirmary
Associate Professor of Ophthalmology
Harvard Medical School
Boston, Massachusetts

Paul Sternberg, Jr., M.D.

Assistant Professor
Department of Ophthalmology
Emory University School of Medicine
Atlanta, Georgia

John T. Thompson, M.D.

Associate Professor
Department of Ophthalmology and Visual Science
Yale University
Yale/New Haven Medical Center
New Haven, Connecticut

Trexler M. Topping, M.D.

Assistant Surgeon in Ophthalmology
Massachusetts Eye and Ear Infirmary
Clinical Instructor in Ophthalmology
Harvard Medical School
Boston, Massachusetts

Paul F. Vinger, M.D.

Assistant Clinical Professor of Ophthalmology
Harvard Medical School
Boston, Massachusetts

Michael D. Wagoner, M.D.

Associate Director
Cornea Consultation Service
Massachusetts Eye and Ear Infirmary
Assistant Professor of Ophthalmology
Harvard Medical School
Boston, Massachusetts

Robert A. Weiss, M.D.

Assistant Professor of Ophthalmology
Co-Director
Ophthalmic Plastic and Reconstructive Service
New York Hospital
Cornell Medical Center
New York, New York

Christopher T. Westfall, M.D., F.A.C.S.

Lieutenant Colonel, U.S.A.F. M.C.
Fellow
Eye Plastic and Orbital Surgery Service
Massachusetts Eye and Ear Infirmary
Boston, Massachusetts

David J. Wilson, M.D.

Assistant Professor of Ophthalmology
Director
Eye Pathology Laboratory
Oregon Health Sciences University
Portland, Oregon

Raymond F. Wong, M.D.

Clinical Instructor in Ophthalmology
Doheny Eye Institute
University of Southern California School of Medicine
Los Angeles, California

John J. Woog, M.D.

Assistant Clinical Professor of Ophthalmology
Tufts University School of Medicine
Clinical Instructor in Ophthalmology
Harvard Medical School
Boston, Massachusetts

To our families

Preface

The management of eye trauma is of concern to both the beginning ophthalmology resident and the tertiary care specialist. While the mechanisms and management of ocular injury uniquely embrace the full spectrum of ophthalmology practice and investigation, eye trauma is rapidly evolving into a subspecialty of its own. Furthermore, although the body of trauma literature is rapidly expanding, there are few texts currently available that specifically address the varied aspects of eye trauma and its management. *Eye Trauma* has been specifically conceived and written to fill this void in the ophthalmology library.

This book has been designed with two major objectives. The foremost of these is to provide a broad and definitive source of information relating to ocular injury. Sections include trauma to the anterior segment, to the posterior segment, to the lids and orbit, and to the neuroophthalmic system. Moreover, the workup and preparation of the trauma patient as well as epidemiology, prevention, and medicolegal implications of treating eye injuries are reviewed. We have strived to create an all-inclusive text, but with each chapter sufficiently detailed to serve as a definitive reference on the specific subject matter. As an avenue toward this goal, the contributing authors have been chosen as experts in their fields, all bringing to their writing extensive experience in eye trauma.

Eye Trauma, furthermore, has been specifically structured and written as a ready reference to provide practical, hands-on information to the practitioner, whether in the office, emergency room, or operating suite. In this effort, numerous surgical procedures are detailed and amply illustrated with clear line drawings and photographs. We hope that this design will enable the ophthalmologist to appropriately assess the injured patient, develop an optimal therapeutic strategy, and skillfully perform the necessary surgical procedures or seek appropriate consultation.

We hope that this book will be useful to general and subspecialty ophthalmologists, ophthalmologists-in-training, and those with specific interests in eye trauma. It also should be valuable to general emergency room physicians in their day-to-day encounters with injured patients, as well as to ophthalmic nurses, technicians, and operating room personnel.

In the past, severe blunt and lacerating trauma invariably led to devastating visual loss. Recent breakthroughs in our understanding of injury mechanisms as well as advances in medical management and surgical technique, however, have dramatically improved the prognosis of eyes that heretofore would have been lost. Continued efforts by clinicians and investigators should make the prognosis for the eye trauma patient even brighter in the future. With this outlook, it is our hope that *Eye Trauma* will play a small part in increasing knowledge, expertise, and interest in this burgeoning field of ophthalmology.

We would like to gratefully acknowledge Laurel L. Cook for her outstanding illustrations and Leona Greenhill for her editorial expertise and energetic efforts in bringing this book to fruition.

Contents

Part 1 Evaluation and Surgical Preparation of the Eye Trauma Patient

1. **Clinical evaluation 3**
   History 4
   Examination 8
   Hysteria and malingering 21
   Transportation of the eye-injured patient 22
   References 23

2. **Diagnostic imaging of ocular and orbital trauma 25**
   Plain film radiography 25
   Computed tomography 28
   Ultrasound 32
   Magnetic resonance imaging 36
   References 38

3. **Preparation of the eye trauma patient for surgery 41**
   Minimizing risk of further injury 42
   Maximizing surgical success 43
   Decreasing risk to patients' health 44
   Minimizing psychic trauma 44
   Minimizing risk of legal involvement 45
   Preoperative check list 45
   References 46

4. **Anesthesia in ocular and orbital trauma 47**
   Anesthesia for ocular injuries 47
   Anesthesia for lid and orbital injuries 51
   References 53

5. **Evaluation and management strategies for the pediatric eye trauma patient 55**
   Epidemiology 55
   Examination 56
   Unique forms of childhood eye trauma 56
   Amblyopia 58
   References 59

Part 2 Anterior Segment Trauma

6. **Conjunctival and corneal injuries 63**
   Conjunctival injury 63
   Corneal injury 65
   References 77

7. **Chemical injuries 79**
   Alkali burns 80
   Acid burns 89
   Specific therapy for chemical injury 90
   References 92

8. **Iris trauma 95**
   Penetrating injury 95
   Blunt trauma 97
   Laser and surgical repair 97
   References 103

9. **Traumatic hyphema 104**
   Causes and demographics 104
   Classification 105
   Pathophysiology 105
   Evaluation of traumatic hyphema 107
   Treatment of traumatic hyphema 107
   Surgical intervention for traumatic hyphema 109
   Complications of hyphema 112
   Special considerations 113
   Clinical outcomes and prognosis 114
   References 114

10. **Traumatic glaucoma 117**
   The seven anterior rings of tissue 117
   Anterior injury associated with tissue disruption 118
   Response to tearing of tissues: inflammation and hemorrhage 120
   Glaucomas associated with blunt injury to the angle 120
   Treatment of blunt injury and IOP elevation 122
   Ghost cell glaucoma 124
   References 124

11. **Lens injuries 126**
Pathophysiology **126**
Evaluation **127**
Approaches to management **128**
Surgical treatment and considerations **130**
References **134**

12. **Pathophysiology of anterior segment wound healing 136**
Pathophysiology of corneal wound healing **137**
Pathophysiology of scleral and limbal healing **139**
Iris and angle changes after trauma **139**
Lens changes after trauma **141**
References **141**

13. **Management of corneoscleral lacerations 143**
Preoperative management **143**
Injury hierarchy and repair techniques **144**
Postoperative management **157**
References **158**

14. **Corneal laceration repair: topographic considerations and suturing techniques 159**
Effects of penetrating injury and repair on corneal astigmatism **159**
Suturing techniques **164**
References **168**

15. **Anterior segment intraocular foreign bodies 169**
Preoperative evaluation **169**
Treatment **171**
References **173**

16. **Anterior segment reconstruction following ocular trauma 175**
Preparatory and adjunctive procedures **176**
Anterior segment reconstruction techniques **176**
Results of anterior segment reconstruction **183**
References **183**

Part 3 Posterior Segment Trauma

17. **Traumatic maculopathies 187**
Commotio retinae (Berlin's edema, concussion edema) **188**
Purtscher's retinopathy **189**
Choroidal rupture **190**
Retinitis sclopetaria **192**
Traumatic macular hole **193**
References **194**

18. **Traumatic retinal tears and detachments 195**
Pathophysiology of traumatic retinal tears from blunt trauma **195**
Traumatic retinal tears: clinical setting **197**
Clinical manifestations of trauma to the eye **198**
References **202**

19. **Pathophysiology of posterior segment trauma 204**
Pathophysiology of injury **204**
Animal models **206**
Factors influencing the healing response **208**
Rationale for surgical treatment **209**
References **210**

20. **Surgical management of posterior segment injuries 212**
Management options **212**
Surgical methods **213**
References **224**

21. **Posterior segment intraocular foreign bodies 226**
Diagnosis and localization **227**
Pathophysiology of damage **227**
Management of IOFBs **229**
References **235**

22. **Prognosis and outcomes for penetrating ocular trauma 238**
Historical perspective **238**
Prognostic features **239**
References **241**

23. **Traumatic endophthalmitis 242**
Microbiology **242**
Diagnosis **243**
Antibiotic prophylaxis and therapy **246**
Traumatic fungal endophthalmitis **248**
Vitrectomy **248**
Corticosteroids **249**
Subsequent management **250**
Prognosis **250**
References **251**

24. **Sympathetic ophthalmia 253**
Incidence **253**
Clinical features **254**
Histologic features **255**
Role of the penetrating wound **255**
Etiology **255**
Differential diagnosis **256**
Treatment and prognosis **257**
References **258**

Part 4 Orbital and Adnexal Trauma

25. **Anatomy of the orbit and ocular adnexa 261**
    Soft tissue anatomy **261**
    Osteology **276**
    Orbit **280**
    References **286**

26. **Blunt trauma to orbital soft tissues 287**
    Examination **287**
    Abrasion, contusion, and crush injury **287**
    Edema **288**
    Hemorrhage **289**
    Emphysema **290**
    Ptosis **290**
    Ophthalmoplegia **290**
    Optic nerve blindness **290**
    Therapy **291**
    Surgery **292**
    References **293**

27. **Orbital fractures 295**
    Examination **295**
    Radiographic evaluation **300**
    Classification of orbital fractures **307**
    Management of orbital fractures **310**
    References **313**

28. **Eyelid burns 315**
    Epidemiology **315**
    Classification **316**
    Examination **316**
    Early management **317**
    Tarsorrhaphy **317**
    Intermediate management **318**
    Late reconstruction **322**
    References **322**

29. **Penetrating eyelid trauma 323**
    Wound healing **323**
    Clinical evaluation **324**
    Presurgical management **325**
    Surgical repair of eyelid lacerations: general considerations **326**
    Surgical repair of eyelid lacerations: specific considerations **330**
    References **332**

30. **Lacrimal system trauma 334**
    Evaluation **334**
    Anesthesia **336**
    Instrumentation **336**
    Surgery **337**
    Complications **339**
    References **340**

31. **Intraorbital foreign bodies 341**
    Fundamentals of management **341**
    Imaging modalities **343**
    Initial management **343**
    Surgical treatment **344**
    Late effects of retained intraorbital foreign bodies **345**
    References **346**

32. **Dog bite injuries 347**
    Epidemiology **347**
    History **348**
    Examination **348**
    Therapy **349**
    References **352**

33. **Enucleation and evisceration 354**
    Enucleation **355**
    Evisceration **362**
    References **366**

Part 5 Neuroophthalmic Trauma

34. **Traumatic optic neuropathy and visual system injury 371**
    General principles **371**
    Examination **372**
    Differential diagnosis **373**
    Direct optic nerve trauma **373**
    Indirect optic nerve trauma **375**
    Traumatic aneurysms of the internal carotid artery **377**
    Chiasmal trauma **377**
    Retrochiasmal visual pathway trauma **378**
    Transient cortical blindness after blunt trauma **378**
    Visual field defects after penetrating brain wounds **378**
    References **378**

35. **Trauma to the ocular motor system 380**
    Ocular motor examination in the injured patient **380**
    Orbital injury causing ocular motor dysfunction **381**
    Ocular motor nerve injuries **382**
    Pupillary disorders following trauma **386**
    Trigeminal nerve injury **386**
    Seventh nerve injury **387**
    Central disorders of eye movements following trauma **387**
    Hypoxic effects on the ocular motor system **389**
    References **389**

Part 6 Injury Prevention and Medicolegal Aspects of Eye Trauma

36. Epidemiology and prevention 395
General epidemiology of ocular injury **396**
Work-related trauma **396**
Recreation-related trauma **397**
Prevention **398**
Patients at risk **398**
Available protection **399**
References **401**

37. Medicolegal considerations 403
Basic malpractice issues **403**
Specific applications to eye trauma and emergency care **403**
General guidelines to avoid malpractice litigation **408**
References **408**

Appendix Guidelines for Tetanus Prophylaxis 409

Color plates

The following color plates appear between pp. 110 and 111.

6-1 Persistent epithelial defect and recurrent erosion, superficial keratectomy, and anterior stromal puncture.

7-1 Alkali injury, Hughes classification.

7-2 Limbal autograft transplantation.

8-1 Iridodialysis repair.

9-1 Traumatic hyphema.

10-1 Angle recession.

10-2 Traumatic cyclodialysis cleft.

10-3 Trabecular meshwork hemorrhage.

10-4 Clot protruding from torn trabecular meshwork.

11-1 Subluxated cataractous lens.

The following color plates appear between pp. 174 and 175.

13-1 Positive Seidel's test.

13-2 Corneal puncture wound sealed with cyanoacrylate tissue adhesive.

13-3 Closure of corneal puncture wound with 10-0 nylon suture.

13-4 Shoestring suture closure.

13-5 Corneal laceration with traumatic cataract.

13-6 Corneal laceration with iris incarceration and lens involvement.

13-7 Severe corneoscleral laceration.

15-1 Multiple corneal foreign bodies.

15-2 Glass intraocular foreign body in anterior segment.

16-1 Anterior segment reconstruction with placement of anterior chamber intraocular lens.

16-2 Anterior segment reconstruction with extensive iridoplasty.

16-3 Anterior segment reconstruction with goniosynechialysis.

16-4 Anterior segment reconstruction with iridodialysis repair.

The following color plates appear between pp. 206 and 207.

17-1 Commotio retinae.

17-2 Purtscher's retinopathy.

17-3 Choroidal rupture.

17-4 Choroidal rupture in an eye with angioid streaks.

17-5 Acute retinitis sclopetaria.

17-6 Retinitis sclopetaria.

17-7 Traumatic macular hole.

18-1 Traumatic retinal dialysis.

18-2 Demarcation lines of a chronic rhegmatogenous retinal detachment.

18-3 Giant retinal tear.

19-1 Pathophysiology of posterior segment penetrating injury.

The following color plates appear between pp. 334 and 335.

29-1 Canthal and eyelid laceration.

29-2 Partial avulsion of eyelid.

30-1 Canalicular laceration.

30-2 Dog bite injury.

PART 1

Evaluation and surgical preparation of the eye trauma patient

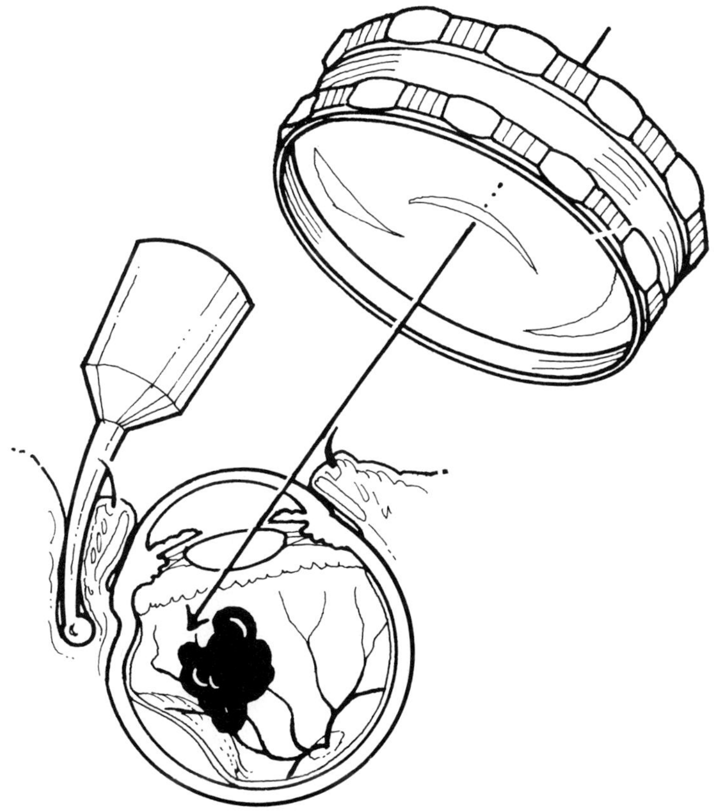

CHAPTER 1

Clinical evaluation

M. BOWES HAMILL

History
- History of the event
- Past ocular and medical history
- Prior treatment
- Specific injuries
  - Chemical injury
  - Foreign-body injury checklist
    - Gunshot wounds
  - Blunt trauma
  - Thermal burn
  - Animal bites

Examination
- Approach to the patient
- Examination technique
- External examination
  - Face and lids
  - Conjunctiva
- Visual acuity
- Pupils
- Extraocular motility
- Visual fields
- Anterior segment examination
  - Conjunctiva
  - Cornea
  - Anterior chamber
  - Iris
  - Lens
- Intraocular pressure
- Vitreous body and retina
- Optic nerve
- Special studies: ERG and VEP in the acute setting

Hysteria and malingering
- Tests for total blindness
- Tests for monocular blindness
- Visual fields and electrophysiologic testing

Transportation of the eye-injured patient
- Pretransport therapy
- Air evacuation: special considerations
  - Hypoxia
  - Decreased atmospheric pressure
  - Noise and vibration
  - Cabin humidity

References

The importance of the initial evaluation of the eye trauma patient cannot be overemphasized. Because the results of this examination determine subsequent diagnostic and therapeutic decisions, a comprehensive workup is mandatory. The initial examination may be the only time that the physician is able to observe damage to such structures as the retina and optic nerve that may later become obscured by continued hemorrhage or cataract formation. A high index of suspicion for occult injury is also critical, since injuries that initially seem to be limited may, after careful examination, be recognized as far more severe. Owing to the unique character of traumatic injuries, the examiner must adopt a logical, methodical, and thorough examination technique and be prepared for the unexpected.

The goals of the initial evaluation can be organized on four levels.

I. Complete evaluation of the eye and ocular adnexa
   A. Recognition of emergent conditions
      1. Life-threatening injuries
         a. Respiratory distress
         b. Cardiovascular compromise
         c. Massive bleeding and shock

            d. Major trauma to any organ system
        2. Emergent ocular conditions
            a. Chemical injuries
            b. Central retinal artery occlusion (CRAO)
    B. Recognition of the complete extent of ocular involvement
II. Identification of confounding factors
    A. Other associated non–life threatening injuries
        1. Bleeding
        2. CNS trauma
        3. Other injuries
    B. Concurrent medical conditions
        1. Diabetes mellitus
        2. Atherosclerotic cardiovascular disease
        3. Sickle cell hemoglobinopathy
        4. Bleeding disorders
        5. Infectious diseases
            a. Hepatitis
            b. AIDS
    C. Foreign bodies
III. Need for further testing
    A. Radiologic
    B. Ultrasonographic
    C. Electrophysiologic
    D. Hematologic/serologic
IV. Development of initial therapeutic plan

The first goal is an overall examination of the patient. This initial assessment should involve a general physical examination, and the examiner should note the presence of potentially life-threatening injuries such as respiratory distress, cardiovascular compromise, and major bleeding, the treatment of which takes precedence over *any* ocular injury. The ocular evaluation should then begin with a search for true ocular emergencies, such as chemical burns or central retinal artery occlusion (CRAO), so that appropriate emergency treatment can be started. Following this initial triage, a comprehensive examination should be performed.

The second step in the initial evaluation is identification of confounding factors that may influence diagnostic or treatment decisions. These factors include medical conditions such as diabetes mellitus, atherosclerotic cardiovascular disease, sickle cell hemoglobinopathies, and bleeding diathesis, as well as concurrent medications. Patients with potentially contagious diseases should be identified and appropriate precautions should be taken to avoid contamination and transmission. With the increasing prevalence of HIV seropositivity in emergency room patients, it is important that *all* patients evaluated for trauma be examined using appropriate precautions to prevent possible contamination of the examiner and ancillary staff.

The third step is identification of areas requiring further testing, including radiologic, ultrasonographic, and electrophysiologic studies and hematologic or serologic tests.

The fourth and final step is the consideration of all available data and the development of a therapeutic strategy. This plan should consider the extent and severity of ocular involvement and address the needs not only of the ocular injury but also of the patient on the whole. As ocular injuries often do not occur in isolation, it is important that the ophthalmologist confer with the other physicians caring for the patient so that an integrated care plan can be developed.

HISTORY

A careful history is extremely important in the evaluation of trauma. While taking the history, the practitioner should be constantly assessing the patient's risk in terms of the structures potentially involved, the degree of structural damage, and the possibility of retained foreign bodies and of occult injury. The analysis of this historical information determines to a large extent the direction and emphasis of the subsequent physical examination and ancillary studies.

Obtaining an accurate history from an injured patient is often more difficult than from a noninjured patient. For example, assault victims may seek either to minimize or to exaggerate their injuries for secondary gain. Children may be reluctant to discuss or disclose the circumstances of an injury incurred during activities that are proscribed or for which they may be punished.[1] For trauma involving children, the examiner should compare the description of the incident with the actual physical findings. A suspicion of child abuse must always be entertained (see Chapter 5), and ocular findings may be the first sign of this condition.

History of the Event

Following the determination that there are no emergent life- or sight-threatening conditions requiring immediate treatment, a complete description of the events surrounding the injury should be elicited from the patient, family members, and witnesses. This description should be in sufficient detail to provide a thorough understanding of the circumstances, such as the activity at the time of injury, the involved parties, where the incident occurred, *exactly* what happened, and how events progressed following the injury. Specific questions should be asked concerning contact lenses, spectacles, or protective eyewear, and these items should be examined for damage. The goal of this questioning is to provide the examiner with sufficient information to mentally reconstruct the injury. This permits an estimate of the potential severity of the injury and an assessment of the risk for occult ocular damage, such as retained foreign bodies, posterior globe rupture, and orbital fracture.

Past Ocular and Medical History

An understanding of any preexisting ophthalmic disease or condition is important for risk assessment in ocular injury, and therefore questions concerning past ocular and medical history are necessary at the time of initial evaluation. Previous ophthalmic surgery, even nonpenetrating procedures such as radial keratotomy, suggests an increased vulnerability of the eye to traumatic damage.[2] Patients should also be questioned about the presence of periocular appliances (e.g., scleral buckle or orbital implant) or intraocular lenses because these may become dislodged or dislocated and complicate an otherwise straightforward injury. Prior ophthalmic medical conditions may also increase the patient's risk of ocular damage following injury. For example, the glaucoma patient is at significantly increased risk for visual field compromise following even a short-duration elevation of intraocular pressure that may occur following ocular injury. The best preinjury visual acuity should also be established and specific questions asked about the presence of amblyopia or other ophthalmic conditions associated with diminished visual acuity. This is especially important in cases where litigation is likely.

The patient's past general medical history should also be assessed in every case. Any previous general medical conditions should be identified. A history of hematologic conditions, bleeding disorders, and anticoagulant medications is especially important, and any patient with a hyphema should be specifically questioned concerning the presence of sickle cell disease. Females of childbearing age should be questioned concerning the possibility of pregnancy, which may influence the choice or use of medications or other types of therapy. The examiner should also keep in mind that patients may not be entirely truthful concerning previous medical problems, such as alcohol or drug abuse or neurologic disorders such as epilepsy.[3] All medications currently being taken by the patient and any medication allergies should be identified and recorded. The patient's tetanus immunization status should be ascertained, because patients with lacerating or penetrating injuries may require tetanus prophylaxis (see Appendix).

Prior Treatment

The patient should be questioned concerning any previous treatment for the injury. A description of any self-treatment, such as the use of eye irrigants, compresses, and ocular medications, should be elicited. All medicines used should be identified and the dosage and duration of therapy recorded. This becomes especially important when prior treatment has involved antibiotics in a setting suggestive of infection, because such treatment may confound the results of microbiologic culture tests. If the patient has been treated by another physician, the name and location of that individual should be recorded so that information concerning initial findings and previous treatment may be obtained.

Patients should also be questioned about the amount and time of recent food intake. This information may affect decisions about anesthesia in patients for whom surgery will be required.

Specific Injuries

Several types of injuries deserve special attention when the patient's historical information is taken.

Chemical Injury

Chemical injuries (especially alkali burns) are true ophthalmic emergencies, and treatment should be begun simultaneously with the examination. Immediately upon determining that the patient has had a chemical injury, irrigation should be begun. The detailed history should be obtained *following* the institution of emergency treatment. Because alkalies can cause extremely rapid and serious tissue destruction, all chemical injuries should be presumed initially to be alkali injuries until proven otherwise.

Initial questioning should be directed toward establishing the type or identity of the agent(s) involved. If the patient does not know the chemical or product name, a general product description (e.g., drain cleanser, paint thinner) may provide useful information. A valuable resource for product identification is the local Poison Control Center, which maintains extensive information on a wide variety of compounds by trade name and chemical constituents, including pH and other toxic characteristics. Alternatively, direct laboratory testing of a sample of the chemical may be feasible.

Once the agent or agent type has been established, characteristics of the exposure should be determined; that is, the amount of material in contact with the eye, the duration of contact, and the physical character of the material (i.e., fluid, paste, gel, or particulate). Any prior treatment, such as lavage or irrigation, should be described. In addition, because chemical injuries to the eye are usually associated with injuries to other facial structures, special attention should be directed to inspecting the face and airway. The examining physician should keep in mind that chemical injuries may result from a variety of circumstances, including explosions, and the possible presence of a foreign body and concussive or other types of concurrent trauma must be evaluated. Chapter 7 describes the management of the chemical burned eye.

Foreign-Body Injury

The possibility of foreign bodies must be considered during the initial evaluation of any ocular injury (Fig. 1-1). When foreign bodies are present or suspected, four major characteristics should be identified: the nature of the foreign-body material, its origin (how it was produced), its probable trajectory, and the risk of microbiologic contamination. Analysis of this information allows an estimate of ocular damage and potential risks to ocular tissues (see Chapters 15, 21, and 31).

A

B

C

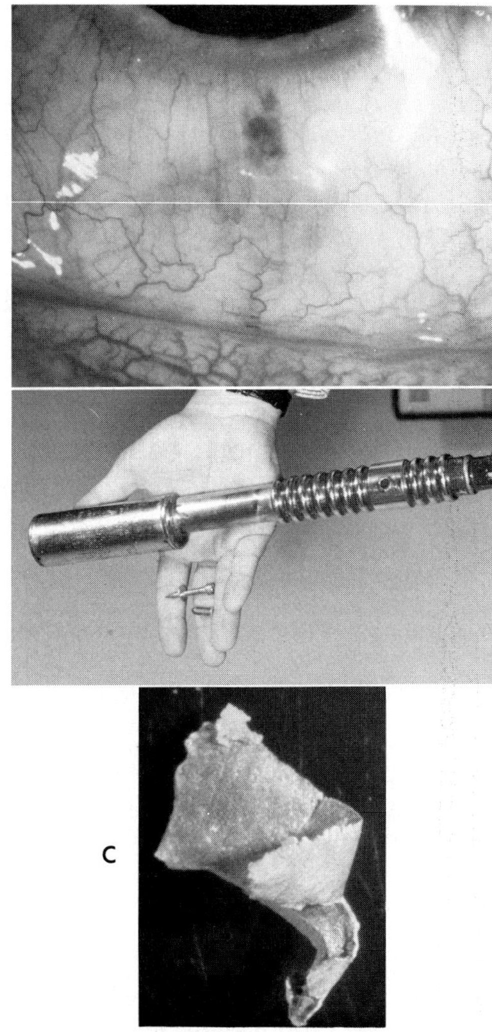

Fig. 1-1. **A,** Patient with a foreign-body injury to the left eye sustained while he was doing construction work. **B,** The patient was using an explosive cartridge type of nail driver. **C,** Foreign body removed from sclera is a fragment of brass casing.

Foreign-Body Injury Checklist

1. Source material
   Composition
   Associated activity at time of injury
2. Origin
   Size and shape
   Energy
   Temperature
3. Probable trajectory
4. Risk of microbiologic contamination

The first concern is the source and composition of the foreign body. This is critical because the composition determines the ocular toxicity (e.g., iron or copper versus glass or plastic). For this reason, the patient's activity at the time of injury should be ascertained to allow a presumptive identification of the foreign body material. If the patient was using power tools, descriptions of the tool type and design and the materials being used are frequently helpful. With an understanding of the source and setting of injury, the physical characteristics of the foreign body, including its size, speed, and kinetic energy, can be estimated. The probable trajectory can be deduced from the description of the event, characteristics of the material, and inspection of the patient. The risk of wound contamination can also be assessed once the source, size, speed, and characteristics of the foreign body are identified. From the description of the incident—with special attention to the head and eye position of the patient, the flight path of the foreign material, and any visible entrance or exit wounds—a great deal of information can be gathered and an estimate may be made about which ocular structures are involved. Should *any* doubt exist as to the presence of a foreign body, appropriate diagnostic studies should be performed to conclusively rule out this condition.

Gunshot wounds. Gunshot wounds comprise a special subset of foreign-body injuries; they are commonly seen in the urban setting. It is a common misconception that all guns inflict similar injuries, but, in fact, each type of weapon has a characteristic injury profile, and a description of the weapon involved (e.g., shotgun, handgun, or high-velocity rifle) should be obtained. Familiarity with weapon and projectile types is helpful in estimating potential damage[3] (Fig. 1-2). Shotguns characteristically produce a large number of small projectiles whose destructive power depends on the size of the shot and the distance from the gun. Handguns, on the other hand, generally fire a single projectile whose mass is dependent on the caliber of the gun. High-velocity military rifles fire a single high-speed projectile with the potential for deep tissue penetration and major injury. All types of projectiles may or may not become fragmented or deformed during passage through the tissues, depending on the angle of impact and the number of bony or solid body parts in the path. As fragmentation or deformation increases, so does tissue destruction.[3] The patient and witnesses should be questioned not only as to the weapon description, but also as to the position of the weapon and other factors, such as whether the projectile passed through glass or other material before striking the patient, which may raise the possibility that glass or other types of foreign material may be present in addition to the projectile.

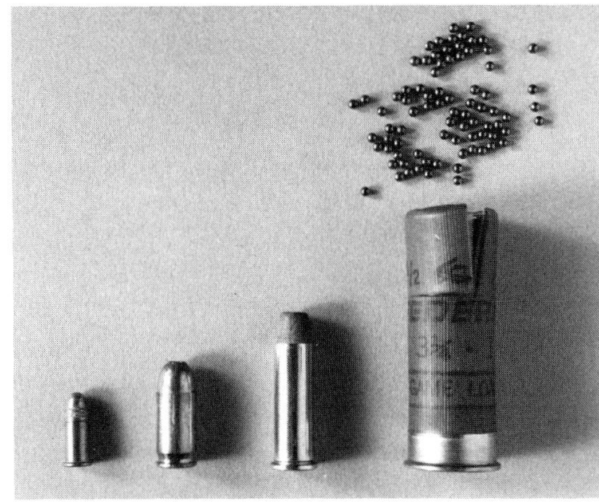

Fig. 1-2. Projectiles frequently encountered in ocular injury *(left to right)*: .22 caliber, .380 caliber, and .38 caliber bullets, and 12-gauge shotgun #7½ shot (typical bird shot; note the large number of small projectiles).

Blunt Trauma

When obtaining the history of a patient who has suffered blunt injury, questioning should be directed toward determining (1) the amount of energy transferred to the globe and orbit and (2) the physical characteristics of the object.[4] Evaluating the energy transfer involves determining the vector and quantity of the force generated by the impact and the size of the impact area. The physical characteristics of the object include density, size, and presence of sharp or cutting edges. All these characteristics are major determinants of the degree of ocular damage following blunt trauma.

In addition, the location of the impact area may be important in estimating potential damage to the orbital bony structures and visual systems.[5,6] For example, blunt trauma to the temporal brow may result in optic nerve contusion, and impact in the malar area has been associated with orbital floor fractures.[7]

Although ocular injuries following blunt trauma may occur as isolated findings, they are frequently associated with other maxillofacial injuries. If head and neck injuries are present, risk estimates can be made for associated ocular involvement. In a review of 1436 cases of maxillofacial trauma, 67% were associated with ocular injuries, and there was an increased risk of ocular damage with the presence of midfacial fractures (up to 70% of patients).[8] Ninety percent of the serious eye injuries were associated with midfacial, superorbital, or frontal sinus fractures (see also Chapter 27).

Thermal Burn

Thermal burns are an unusual type of ophthalmic injury. Questioning should reveal the temperature of the agent involved, duration of contact, and character of the agent to allow an estimate of the amount of thermal energy transmitted to the ocular tissues. The examiner should search for associated facial injuries, specifically airway involvement, because this can be life threatening (see Chapter 28).

A subgroup of thermal trauma involves electrical burns. To assist with the evaluation of this injury, the examiner should try to determine the amount of electrical energy involved (i.e., amperage and voltage of the current) and the location of entrance and exit points. Generally, electrical burns involving the eye are associated with important involvement of other tissue.

Animal Bites

Animal bites are another unusual type of ophthalmic injury that deserves specific attention. To fully assess potential ocular damage, it is important to identify the type of animal causing the injury, as well as the circumstances. Trauma subsequent to a dog bite, for example, may result in a different type of ocular damage than that following a pecking injury to the cornea.[9] The patient should also be questioned about whether the attack was spontaneous or provoked, and the animal's location should be identified to permit further testing for the presence of transmissible disease (see Chapter 32).

In summary, the initial history should establish in the examiner's mind a complete and detailed description of the traumatic event and an understanding of the patient's past medical and ocular history. The goal of this inquiry is to recognize potential occult damage, permit an accurate estimate of risk for ocular injury, and direct subsequent examination and therapeutic efforts.

EXAMINATION

The goal of the examination, in combination with the history, is to evaluate the injured eye completely so as to determine the absolute and relative position, stability, and integrity of each ocular and intraocular structure and the need for further testing and treatment. Historical information should help direct the examiner toward certain aspects of the injury, such as a foreign body or occult rupture, and as each phase of the examination is completed, findings may indicate additional areas in need of evaluation. The examination process is, therefore, a cycle, in which initial findings lead to further, more detailed evaluation. Only after all possible areas of ocular involvement are evaluated as completely as possible is the examination complete. It should, however, be appreciated that as a result of the injury the condition of the patient may require that the usual examination be altered and some aspects deferred until the condition is stabilized.

Approach to the Patient

Because of the nature of trauma, interaction with the injured patient may present special problems not generally encountered in routine office practice. Patients in an emergency setting may be frightened or in pain and thus less cooperative than usual. Trauma patients are also not uncommonly under the influence of drugs or alcohol, which may make their cooperation less than optimal. In some circumstances patients can be so combative as to preclude any but the most cursory examination. The examination of trauma patients also frequently occurs late at night when both patient and examiner are fatigued and anxious. In these situations the examiner should take sufficient time to get the patient to relax as much as possible and cooperate with the examination. It is generally counterproductive to threaten or to further frighten patients by discussing dire visual consequences in an attempt to elicit cooperation. Pediatric patients may present additional difficulties, as noted in Chapter 5.

Examination Technique

In any clinical setting involving trauma, the examiner should maintain a high index of suspicion for an occult or unsuspected injury. It is important not only to appreciate the presence of such an injury but also to prevent further damage by avoiding inappropriate examination techniques; *primum non nocere* is especially applicable to the ocular-trauma patient. For example, given a history compatible with a ruptured globe, special precautions should be taken to prevent increased intraocular pressure and extrusion of intraocular contents. These precautions dictate that no external pressure be placed on the globe. Eye shield protection is mandatory. The patient should be appropriately medicated for nausea, and vomiting should be prevented if at all possible. For patients who forcefully squeeze their lids closed, not allowing inspection of the globe, the examiner may consider the use of a lid or regional nerve block to produce lid akinesia. This technique facilitates the examination and may prevent pressure on the ruptured globe from orbicularis spasm. Under special circumstances, notably in children or uncooperative adults, the examiner should consider performing the entire examination with the patient sedated or under general anesthesia. No drops or ointments should be instilled in an eye suspected of having a rupture until this condition has been positively ruled out by examination.

Ideally, the trauma patient should be evaluated in a fully equipped eye-examination room, although this may be impractical for patients whose injuries prevent transportation. For this reason a portable emergency examination kit should be available. In addition to examination equipment, basic diagnostic and therapeutic medications and equipment should be included in the kit, as follows:

- Near reading card
- +3.00 sphere lens
- Pinhole
- Occluder
- Penlight
- Lid retractors
- Wire pediatric lid speculum
- Schiøtz tonometer
- Indirect ophthalmoscope and 20-diopter lens
- 0.5% proparacaine
- 2.5% neosynephrine
- 1% mydriacyl
- Fluorescein strips
- Rose bengal
- Cotton-tipped applicators (sterile)
- Eye pads
- Tape
- Eye shield
- Sterile ocular irrigant
- TB syringe and needles

Appropriate culture equipment and materials should be available to allow microbiologic laboratory evaluation of patients in whom an infectious process is suspected. These should include the following:

- Sterile calcium alginate swabs
- Kimura spatula
- Alcohol lamp
- Frosted etched glass slides
- Koplin jar with 95% methyl alcohol
- Blood agar plate
- Chocolate agar plate
- *Brucella* blood agar plate
- Sabouraud dextrose agar plate
- Supplemented thioglycolate broth without indicator
- Brain Heart Infusion (BHI) broth with gentamicin (50 mg/ml)
- Viral transport media

An excellent review of culture equipment, supplies, and techniques has been published by Jones, Liesegang, and Robinson.[10]

External Examination

Face and Lids

Unlike the routine examination, in which vision testing precedes the external examination, evaluation of the eye-injured patient frequently begins with the external examination. The examiner should inspect the patient carefully, looking for potentially life-threatening injuries, which should be addressed before any ocular condition. This overview should be followed by an inspection of the globe and ocular adnexa for trauma, noting the structures involved and the degree of injury.

Several external examination findings deserve specific attention. Any abnormal position of the globe relative to other bony structures should be recorded, as should the presence of subcutaneous emphysema, because these may indicate fractures of the orbital bones or sinuses, respectively. The presence of any foreign bodies should also be noted. All associated injuries to the face, head, and neck should be inspected and drawn in the record. Because one of the primary goals of the examination is to rule out occult trauma to the globe, lacerations and punc-

A

B

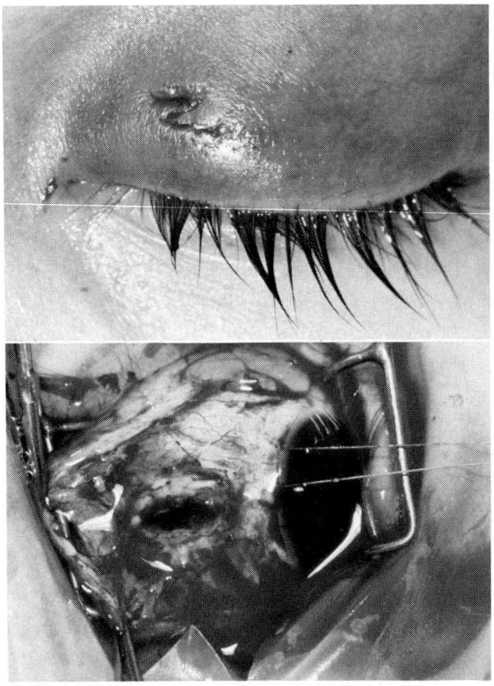

Fig. 1-3. **A,** Young female patient brought to the emergency room with a history of a cut on the upper lid. **B,** Examination revealed perforation of the globe with a retained intraocular foreign body.

ture wounds of the lids or brow should be inspected and, if appropriate, probed gently to determine their path and extent. Both active bleeding and dried blood may interfere with the satisfactory evaluation of facial injuries; therefore, bleeding should be controlled with tamponade and the tissues cleaned gently with a gauze sponge and sterile saline or hydrogen peroxide. Cleaning the surrounding skin greatly facilitates the detection and evaluation of even small wounds. After cleansing the skin, a careful search should be made for small puncture wounds. If possible, the lid should be everted and the tarsal surfaces inspected for full-thickness injuries (Fig. 1-3). The depth and extent of skin lacerations should be noted and visualization of orbital fat recorded (see Chapter 29). Lacrimal drainage system or lid margin involvement should also be noted (see Chapter 30).

In the event of suspected canalicular involvement, the lacerated ends of the canaliculus may be visible with the slit-lamp. In cases where injury is suspected but unseen, the lacerated tissues can be gently manipulated with moist cotton-tip applicators. The use of toothed for-

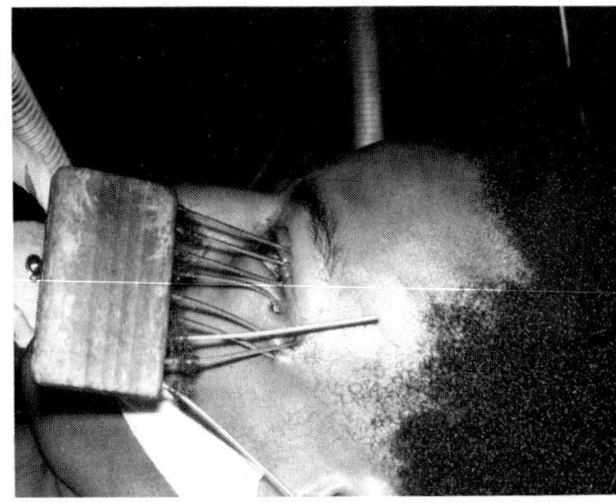

Fig. 1-4. Young male patient hit with an afro comb, which became embedded in the orbit. Large retained orbital foreign bodies should be removed only under controlled conditions, preferably in the operating room.

ceps to search for lacerations of the canaliculus at the initial inspection is to be discouraged, because these instruments can cause tissue maceration and further anatomic derangement. If outflow involvement is suspected but not visible by inspection, gentle saline irrigation through the punctum may aid in recognizing these injuries.

The presence of abnormal lid positioning should be carefully evaluated. For patients with ptosis, levator function and lid fissure size should be measured and recorded to provide a baseline for later evaluation and documentation of any spontaneous recovery.[3] If canthal structures are abnormal, the medial canthal distances should be measured and a sketch made of the observed dimensions.

The presence of particulate matter on the lids and face may alert the examiner to the possibility of a foreign-body injury and the necessity for careful inspection of the globe and intraocular contents for occult penetrating foreign bodies. If the foreign body is large and remains in the orbit (Fig. 1-4), removal should not be attempted before completion of the ophthalmic examination (see Chapter 31).

Periorbital and lid ecchymosis or hemorrhage, frequently seen with blunt injury to the eye, should also be noted. The location and character of ecchymosis may indicate underlying damage that requires further investigation. For example, fractures of the orbital roof may be associated with upper-lid hemorrhage and lateral bulbar subconjunctival hemorrhage.[11] Basal skull fractures can also be associated with periocular ecchymosis.

The orbital and facial bones should be inspected and palpated for areas of "step-off," or discontinuity, and any asymmetry should be noted (see Chapter 27). Patients with blunt injuries to the midface should be questioned concerning occlusion of the teeth, and the mouth should be inspected with the patient's jaws closed. Patients are generally very sensitive to malocclusion, which may indicate damage to the maxilla or mandible. Areas of skin anesthesia may also indicate underlying fractures. For patients with a history of trauma and sudden onset of a red eye, the examiner should auscultate the closed lids and temporal area for the presence of a bruit, which may indicate a carotid-cavernous fistula.

Conjunctiva

The conjunctiva should be examined with special attention to the inferior palpebral cul-de-sac for the presence of foreign bodies. The examiner should also evert the upper lid and inspect the superior tarsal conjunctiva and superior fornix. Areas of subconjunctival hemorrhage[12,13] or abnormal pigmentation of the bulbar conjunctiva should be documented, because they may indicate globe rupture. Lacerations or breaks in the bulbar conjunctiva should be diagrammed, and subsequent evaluation should be directed at ruling out a penetrating globe injury. Inspection of the conjunctiva and cornea should also include an inspection for the presence of contact lenses, especially in the unconscious patient.

Simultaneously with the conjunctival evaluation, the cornea should be inspected with a penlight to evaluate the epithelial surface and light reflex as well as any visible abnormalities of the anterior segment.

Visual Acuity

Following the overall inspection, the patient's visual acuity should be tested. In the emergency setting, the goal of such testing is to obtain the best objective estimate of visual function. This establishes a baseline visual acuity that is important for several reasons. If the injuries are accompanied by progressive intraocular hemorrhage, the initial visual acuity may reflect the normal status of the eye more truly than does acuity measured later, because of increasing media opacities with time. Other conditions, such as optic nerve contusion[7] and traumatic retinal angiopathy,[14] are characterized by fluctuating visual acuity, and thus an early measurement is important to detect subsequent diminution or fluctuation. The measurement of even a very poor initial visual acuity serves as a pretreatment baseline of visual function that may become important should litigation ensue. In all situations of significant trauma, work-related injury, or injury associated with assault, the ophthalmologist should evaluate visual acuity personally.

Although visual acuity testing in an emergency-room setting can be somewhat difficult, most examiners have available a near-vision card that is adequate for checking acuity. Some reading correction must be supplied by the examiner to presbyopic patients unless the patient has his or her own spectacles. A pinhole is helpful for checking distance acuity when the patient's refractive error is unknown or the patient's spectacles are not available. If a standardized vision chart is not available, several at-hand objects, such as newsprint, the hands or dial on a watch, or any nearby sign can be used to check acuity. If nonstandard testing is performed, the details of the testing methods should be documented in the record. In addition to acuity measurements, information may be forthcoming during vision testing that may indicate the need for further evaluation, such as a complaint that only the right- or left-hand side of objects is visible or that the central visual field is irregular or absent.

When visual acuity is determined as no light perception (NLP), careful confirmation and documentation of this condition by the examining ophthalmologist is of major importance. The patient should be tested several times, if at all possible by independent examiners, using the brightest light source available (usually the indirect ophthalmoscope). The finding of NLP versus bare light perception vision may have a profound impact on subsequent surgical decisions.

Pupils

Pupillary findings in the traumatized patient are extremely important because they can indicate intracranial pathology and lesions responsible for diminished vision. In an unconscious patient, the pupillary reflexes may be the only indicator of visual-system function that can be evaluated.

In addition, the shape of the pupil can provide clues about possible intraocular injury.

The pupil has a characteristic response to blunt injury. Initially the pupil shows spastic miosis, which is generally transient and may be accompanied by a spasm of accommodation. This is generally followed by traumatic mydriasis, which may be associated with loss of accommodation. The traumatic mydriatic pupil is a midposition pupil with a slightly oval contour.[15]

The pupil should be inspected for shape, location, light reaction, and any eccentricity or irregularity. A dilated pupil in the presence of a head injury is a source of concern because it may indicate increasing intracranial pressure with associated neurologic problems. There are, however, multiple causes for this condition, such as iris sphincter damage and pharmacologic mydriasis, which should also be considered when a pupil is dilated. It is important to recognize the presence of preexisting pupillary abnormalities unrelated to the injury; for this reason, the driver's-license photograph or other recent photograph of any patient with anisocoria should be examined for pupillary size and shape. Eccentric or peaked pupils are especially worrisome because they may indicate intraocular damage or scleral or corneal rupture with iris prolapse. Pupillary reactions should be measured in dim light with the patient fixing at distance; the response to direct illumination, a near target, and the presence of an afferent pupillary defect (APD) should be recorded. The presence of an APD is a finding of significance in all patients; in the trauma patient it indicates injury in the afferent pathway, which may be produced by a variety of lesions (see Chapter 34). An APD is found with optic-nerve injuries such as contusion, avulsion, and transection; with retinal injuries such as commotio retinae (Berlin's edema) and retinal detachment; and in some patients with major vitreous hemorrhage.

Extraocular Motility

Testing extraocular motility in the injured patient requires that the examiner first rule out the presence of a ruptured globe, because the force generated by the contracting extraocular muscles may cause sufficient increase in intraocular pressure to extrude intraocular contents.[1] Although posttraumatic orbital congestion alone may affect ocular motility, testing should be done in the acute setting for baseline evaluation purposes. All defects in ductions and versions should be graded on an objective scale to allow comparisons at a later date. The examiner should note the presence of any diplopia or restriction of movement of the globe and try to identify any paretic or underacting muscles. These findings may indicate conditions such as orbital wall or floor fractures, especially when associated with hypesthesia of the cheek and enophthalmos. Additionally, motility abnormalities may be secondary to injury of motor innervation, direct muscle trauma, or intraorbital injury from foreign bodies or penetrating wounds.[15]

When motility restrictions are found, forced duction testing may be of benefit, although the examiner must be sure that the globe is intact before performing this procedure. Forced duction testing enables the examiner to differentiate between restrictive and paralytic causes of apparent motor palsies. Although this test can be performed in the emergency room under topical anesthesia, forced ductions provide maximum information if performed several days after the event when some of the orbital congestion and swelling have resolved (see Chapter 27).

Visual Fields

If possible, all patients with ocular trauma should have a visual field evaluation at the time of the initial examination. A confrontation technique is appropriate in the emergency setting. This generally permits detection of significant peripheral and central defects and, in some circumstances, small abnormalities of central or peripheral vision.

Formal field testing usually requires that the patient be stable, transportable, cooperative, and able to sit up. Unless an abnormality has been noted by confrontation, or visual field documentation is necessary for diagnosis, formal testing can usually be deferred. Several types of formal field testing, however, may be of benefit in emergency or trauma patients. Tangent screen testing for neurologic deficits and factitious amblyopia (discussed later in this chapter), and Amsler grid testing for central scotoma are the most useful.

Anterior Segment Examination

Ideally, every injured patient should be examined with a slit lamp, but this may be impossible

or impractical in an emergency setting. If slit-lamp examination is not feasible, careful inspection with a penlight can be informative, especially in conjunction with magnification with a 20-diopter lens or loupe. Use of a self-retaining wire lid speculum often facilitates complete inspection of the anterior segment. Before inserting the speculum, however, the examiner should be certain that no defect in the eye wall is present. When using a lid speculum, especially in an unconscious patient, adequate corneal hydration must be maintained with artificial tears or saline drops.

The key to a successful slit-lamp or penlight examination is an orderly routine with a logical progression through anterior segment structures. The examiner should not immediately examine the site of most visible pathology, but proceed in a logical, step-by-step manner from the lid margins to the palpebral, bulbar, and tarsal conjunctiva, followed by the cornea, anterior chamber, iris, lens, and vitreous. Once the examiner is convinced of the integrity of the globe, gonioscopy may be performed if indicated. Following dilation, the crystalline lens should again be inspected by direct illumination and retroillumination.

Conjunctiva

Conjunctival examination should begin with an inspection of the lower palpebral and anterior bulbar conjunctiva, delaying eversion of the upper lid until the examiner has determined that the globe is intact. Several conjunctival findings deserve specific attention.

Subconjunctival hemorrhage is a common sequela of ocular injury. The area and extent of the hemorrhage should be recorded because, although this condition is generally benign, hemorrhage may indicate underlying scleral injury or be associated with injury elsewhere in the orbit. Conjunctival chemosis may also be a nonspecific response to trauma. Chemosis, like hemorrhage, however, can indicate underlying injury, especially if associated with subconjunctival air (sinus fractures) or subconjunctival pigment (rupture of the globe). Conjunctival abrasions can be difficult to detect by inspection, and staining with fluorescein or rose bengal highlights abraded areas so that their presence becomes immediately apparent. Conjunctival surfaces opposing an abrasion should be inspected for embedded foreign material. Conjunctival lacerations may be isolated or multiple and may indicate underlying ocular damage. For this reason it is important to explore any conjunctival laceration carefully under topical anesthesia, spreading the wound with blunt forceps or small Desmarres retractors to inspect the underlying sclera. As in abrasions, very small lacerations or puncture wounds may be difficult to detect, and staining with fluorescein or rose bengal may be helpful in recognizing them.

Foreign bodies may become embedded in either the bulbar or palpebral conjunctiva; such foreign bodies are common following explosion injuries. As with any foreign-body injury, the examiner must rule out occult perforation of the globe. If the foreign body is embedded in the conjunctiva or there is a suggestion of scleral involvement, the attachment to the sclera may be evaluated by gently moving the overlying conjunctiva with forceps to see if the foreign body is tethered to the underlying tissues. If the examiner feels that the foreign body represents a perforating injury, further assessment and removal in the operating room are indicated.

The upper lid should be everted in all situations compatible with conjunctival foreign bodies. Retained foreign material can become embedded in the conjunctiva on the upper tarsal surface and repeatedly abrade the corneal epithelium with blinking (Fig. 1-5). Therefore it is especially important to detect and remove this material to prevent further corneal injury.

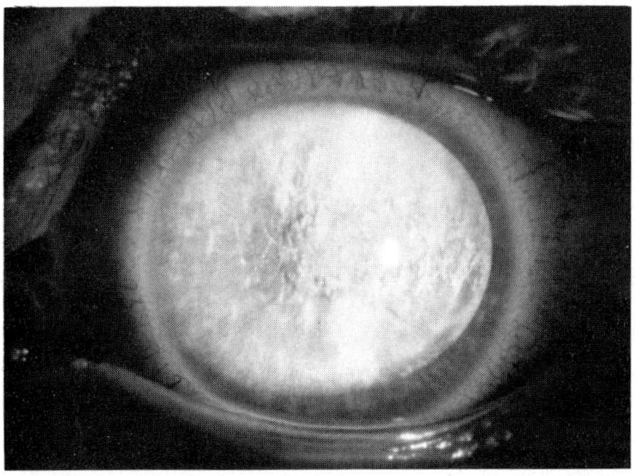

Fig. 1-5. Multiple corneal abrasions caused by foreign material retained on the upper tarsal conjunctiva.

Cornea

Slit-lamp examination of the cornea is most productive when performed in a logical, stepwise manner. The entire corneal surface and all corneal layers should be evaluated. Corneal findings in trauma may be subtle; it is necessary to use a variety of slit-lamp lighting and inspection techniques during the examination. Direct illumination is excellent for detecting foreign bodies and corneal opacities. By narrowing the beam and directing the light source obliquely, the position of a foreign body within the corneal stroma can be determined (Fig. 1-6). Similarly, the depth of a laceration or perforating injury can be estimated by using this narrow-beam, direct-illumination technique. It is extremely important to detect any corneal discontinuity or laceration, especially when associated with foreign-body injuries, because approximately 80% of intraocular foreign bodies enter the eye through the cornea.[16] Retroillumination from the iris and retina and sclerotic scatter (Fig. 1-7) are additional lighting techniques that are very helpful in the detection of subtle abnormalities. These indirect lighting techniques emphasize discontinuities in the optical properties of the tissues and thus highlight penetrating and perforating wounds. Some small transparent or translucent intrastromal foreign bodies such as glass and plastic can also best be seen by means of these techniques.

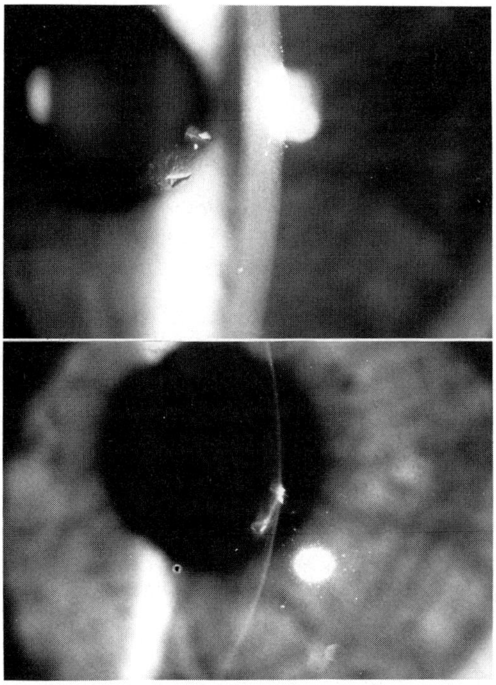

A

B

Fig. 1-6. Glass foreign material in the cornea. **A,** The location is unclear when diffusely illuminated. **B,** With narrow-beam direct illumination the fragment can be seen to be deep within the stroma.

The corneal evaluation begins with inspection of the epithelium. Any abrasion or foreign body should be carefully inspected, and the size, shape, and location should be recorded. The corneal stroma should next be examined for the presence of foreign bodies, discontinuities, and lacerations. If a laceration is noted, gentle exploration with jeweler's forceps may assist in determining the depth and extent of the injury. Seidel's testing with and without provocation (gentle pressure applied to the upper or lower bulbar conjunctiva) is also helpful in deciding whether a full-thickness corneal laceration exists. Seidel's testing is based on the phenomenon that fluorescein dye in high concentration does not fluoresce. Therefore, to perform the test, a sufficient concentration of fluorescein dye is applied to the suspect area with a dye strip or 2% fluorescein dropperette so that the pool of dye appears dark when illuminated with cobalt blue light. If a leak is present, the exiting aqueous dilutes the fluorescein to a concentration at which it will fluoresce brightly, confirming the presence of a leak (see Color Plate 13-1). If leakage of aqueous is present, the remainder of the anterior segment should be examined as gently as possible using a no-touch technique to avoid an increase in intraocular pressure; in the setting of an open globe, no topical medications should be placed in the eye for fear of access to the anterior chamber.

Foreign bodies in the cornea may lodge on the surface or within the stroma. It is important to assess the depth, location, and source of the foreign material so that the risk of removal can be weighed against the potential risk of infection, corneal toxicity, or prolonged inflammation if the foreign body is left in situ.

Other corneal findings following trauma include edema and suppuration. Generalized stromal edema is an unusual isolated finding but can occur after some toxic or chemical insults or severe concussive injury. Localized edema of the cornea secondary to regional endothelial dysfunction is much more common and is generally seen following concussive injuries, such as non-

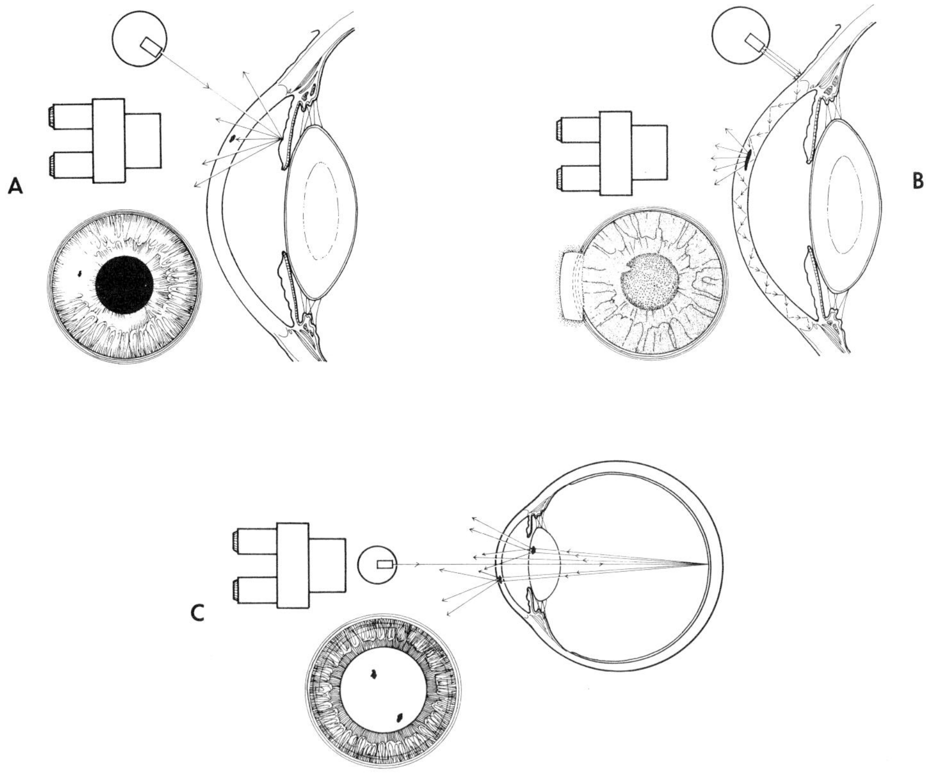

Fig. 1-7. **A,** Retroillumination from the iris. The slit-beam light source should be slightly decentered and directed obliquely onto the structures behind the object of regard. The object of regard is then backlit and stands out in relief. This is especially helpful in looking at small translucent foreign bodies within the cornea. **B,** Sclerotic scatter. This lighting technique employs the phenomenon of total internal reflection of light within the cornea. The light beam is decentered and aimed at the corneoscleral limbus. If an optical discontinuity is present within the cornea, the light is subsequently scattered and the object of regard appears brightly lit against a dimmer background. **C,** Retroillumination from the fundus. Optical discontinuities and foreign bodies are frequently well visualized against the red fundus reflex. This can be achieved in two ways: the slit beam can be decentered and directed in from off axis, or the slit beam can be centered and directed on axis through the center of the pupil to reflect from the posterior pole. The cornea and lens are viewed against the uniform red fundus reflex. Optical abnormalities in either the lens or the cornea stand out as dark irregularities against the reflex. This technique is also useful when looking for defects in the iris. A small beam sent through the center of an undilated pupil and reflected off the posterior pole allows careful inspection of the iris for transillumination defects, which may indicate underlying intraocular damage.

penetrating BB injuries. Corneal swelling, however, may also be associated with lacerating injuries of the stroma, and for this reason all areas of edema should be carefully inspected.

Injury to the epithelium and stroma can be associated with secondary infection of the cornea. If a microbial keratitis is suspected, the cornea should be scraped and materials sent for smears and microbiologic testing so that the organisms involved are identified prior to antibiotic therapy. Pending the results of laboratory studies, broad-spectrum antimicrobial therapy directed by the smear morphology and clinical impression should be initiated.

The endothelium should be inspected by direct slit beam and specular reflection techniques, with special attention to discontinuities, guttata, enlarged endothelial cells, and pseudoguttata. Pseudoguttata in the presence of overlying stromal edema may indicate a concussive endotheliopathy, and although this condition generally resolves without sequelae, the presence of blood in the anterior chamber may put these areas of endothelial damage at increased risk of localized corneal bloodstaining. For this reason, areas of concussive endothelial changes should be carefully examined and documented, and follow-up examinations should direct special attention to the stroma overlying these zones. Concussive damage to the endothelium may also be indicated by the presence of endothelial rings at the site of high-speed corneal foreign-body injuries.[17,18]

Anterior Chamber

Examination of the anterior chamber should assess the anatomy of the chamber and the contents of the space. Evaluation of the anatomy should begin with an estimation of the depth and contour of the anterior chamber across its entire height and width. Areas of localized shallowing or irregularity should be noted and drawn because they can indicate underlying problems such as choroidal detachment or hemorrhage, foreign bodies in or behind the iris, localized intumescence of the lens following rupture of the lens capsule, and iridocorneal adhesion with leakage of aqueous secondary to a corneal perforation. The chamber can be diffusely shallowed in conditions characterized by loss or misdirection of aqueous humor and in association with posterior pressure from a suprachoroidal hemorrhage. Deepening of the anterior chamber can be seen with rupture of the posterior sclera and vitreous loss.

In general, all patients with an intact globe should undergo gonioscopy, although the need for gonioscopic examination depends on the degree of ocular injury. Ideally the examination should be done with an instrument such as a Zeiss goniolens, which does not require a gel-coupling medium, therefore avoiding pressure or traction on the globe and distortion of the corneal surface. It has been suggested that bilateral simultaneous gonioscopy using a Koeppe lens and a Barkan light offers advantages over monocular gonioscopy alone by allowing rapid comparison between eyes.[19] Inspection of the angle should be directed toward recognition of iridodialyses, angle recessions, and bleeding sites. Early gonioscopy also permits inspection of the anterior chamber for foreign bodies that have migrated into the inferior angle before encapsulation or secondary hemorrhage, a situation not uncommon following injury with high-speed, low-density foreign bodies that pass through the cornea but remain in the anterior chamber. Examination with a goniolens also permits a survey of the iris surface for defects or protruding foreign bodies that may be difficult to detect with direct viewing but show up well with tangential inspection.

After an appraisal of the anatomy, the contents of the anterior chamber should be assessed. Traumatic iritis, characterized by a cell-and-flare reaction, is a frequent sequela of blunt trauma. This inflammatory response can range from the occasional cell and minimally perceptible flare to cells throughout the anterior chamber and a plasmoid aqueous with no visible cellular movement. The degree of inflammatory response in the anterior chamber should be graded and recorded so that the initial findings can be compared with subsequent examinations to document resolution or worsening of the condition. Grading of cell and flare is subjective, although the scale and degree should be consistent from examiner to examiner. Commonly this response is scored from 0 (no cell or flare) to 4+ (maximum cellular response with plasmoid aqueous).

The presence of blood in the anterior chamber should be specifically confirmed or ruled out in all cases of blunt or penetrating injury and the bleeding source identified if possible. Other abnormalities of anterior chamber contents, such as the presence of lens fragments, vitreous, or foreign bodies, should likewise be documented. Many foreign bodies that penetrate the cornea and fail to become embedded in either the iris or the lens fall to the 6 o'clock position in the angle and may be extremely difficult to see without gonioscopy. If these foreign bodies remain, they can result in progressive endothelial damage and a peculiar form of local, progressive corneal edema.

Iris

Inspection of the iris should begin with an evaluation of its overall contour and geometry. An abnormal contour may indicate local damage either to the iris itself or to structures located behind it (e.g., rupture of the lens capsule, lenticular foreign bodies, or ciliary body hemorrhage or detachment). Irregularities in the iris surface should be inspected under high magnification. In addition to inspection of the iris with direct illumination, retroillumination of the iris, with the slit beam directed through the pupil and reflected from the posterior pole, can be very helpful in detecting small holes or perforations. Any discontinuity of the iris raises the possibility of an occult penetrating injury and, with a compatible clinical history, should be taken as presumptive evidence of a perforating foreign body. Recognition of iris discontinuities can be extremely valuable in estimating the location of a foreign body because these projectiles generally travel through the globe in a straight line,[20] although they may subsequently rebound when hitting the retina or sclera.

Examination of the iris should also include an inspection of the pupil shape; any irregularities or peaking should be noted. An abnormally shaped pupil can provide information about occult injury; for example, an irregular or elliptical pupil may indicate an occult scleral perforation with peripheral iris prolapse, and peaking of the pupil may indicate vitreous prolapse into the anterior chamber. Sphincter tears and bleeding sites should also be identified and documented.

Lens

Every attempt should be made at the initial examination to evaluate the lens position, stability, clarity, and capsular integrity. The best view of the lens may be in the emergency room before significant intraocular inflammation has developed. This is especially important in situations of suspected penetrating or foreign-body injury. The lens should be examined both before and after dilation because it is helpful to locate iris defects and subsequently examine the underlying lens to confirm penetrating foreign body injuries. Evidence of dislocation or subluxation of the lens should be sought in every patient with significant head trauma. In many cases, the lens can be clearly seen to be dislocated. In other cases subtle signs, such as the presence of vitreous around the lens, may indicate a zonular rupture and lens instability. When the lens is seen to be out of its normal anatomic position, lens location, movement, and stability should be specifically evaluated and recorded. If trauma is severe, the lens may be entirely extruded from the eye, either through a scleral or corneal wound or, rarely, into the subconjunctival space via a perilimbal rupture. Extrusion of an intraocular implant is not uncommon in pseudophakic patients who have suffered blunt trauma to the anterior portion of the globe and dehiscence of their surgical wound (Fig. 1-8).

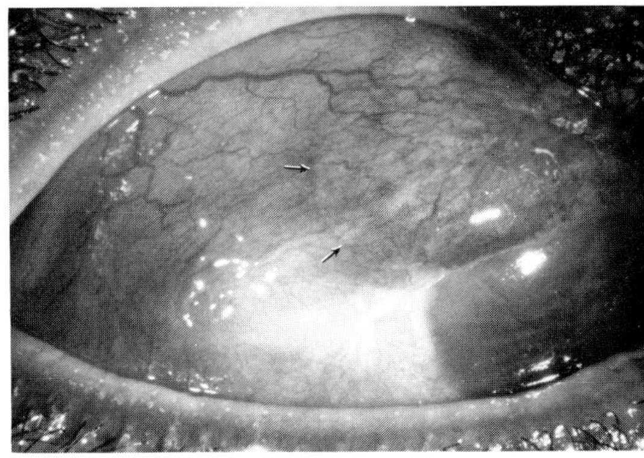

Fig. 1-8. Intraocular lens *(arrow)*, dislocated from its normal position by blunt trauma 2 years after surgery, is located subconjunctivally.

Lens clarity should be evaluated by both direct inspection and retroillumination. A variety of opacities can occur following trauma. Capsular perforation or rupture can cause regional opacification of the lens; concussive injury can result in a spectrum of changes, from subepithelial granular opacity to total opacification. Vossius' ring, or pigment deposition on the anterior capsule of the lens, indicates that significant concussive injury has occurred, although in young patients the ring may fade over time.[21]

Irregularities in light transmission through the lens will result in dark areas within the red reflex, which indicate a disruption of the crystalline lens architecture or occult perforation (Fig. 1-9). The lens capsule should be examined for discontinuities with both direct and oblique illumination. Some lens capsular breaks are obvious, but very small breaks or perforations frequently can best be seen by first locating the abnormality of the lens cortex through viewing the red retinal reflex and subsequently inspecting the capsule under moderate to high magnification with oblique illumination via a thin slit. Any free-floating fragments or flocculent lens material in the anterior chamber or vitreous should be documented. Owing to the antigenic nature of lens material, it is important to note lens disruption; if capsular discontinuities are not detected, and lens rupture goes unsuspected, the resulting inflammation may be confused with infectious endophthalmitis. The presence or absence of lens capsule rupture also has a direct impact on surgical decision-making with respect to primary reconstruction of the injured eye.

A

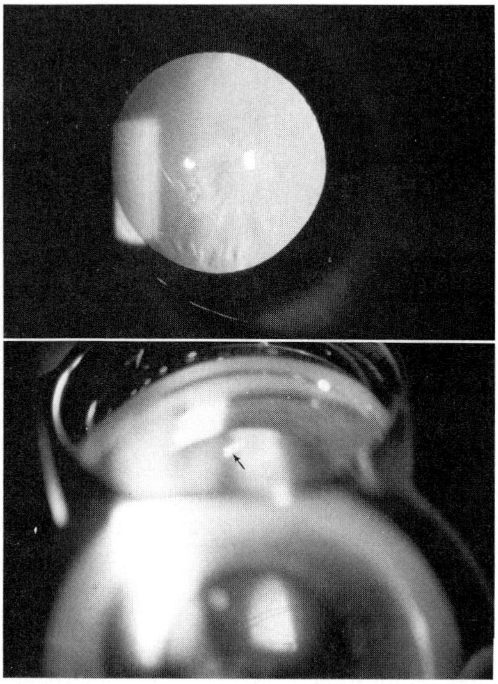

B

Fig. 1-9. **A,** Irregularities in the lens result in abnormalities of the red reflex, as in this patient with a foreign-body injury. **B,** The foreign body *(arrow)* has passed through the lens and is resting inferiorly in the anterior vitreous.

Intraocular Pressure

Intraocular pressure (IOP) can have direct prognostic and diagnostic significance in many injuries such as hyphema[22] in which early increased IOP may indicate increased risk for later complications, or in suspected rupture of the globe in which low IOP may indicate occult rupture.[23] No patient with a documented globe rupture should have the IOP checked for fear of extrusion of intraocular contents and contamination, although all patients should have an IOP measurement after determination that the globe is intact. A variety of methods are available to measure IOP, including Schiøtz tonometry, pneumotonometry, and applanation tonometry. If the patient is ambulatory and can be examined in a clinic setting, the most accurate measurements are obtained with pneumotonometry or applanation tonometry. If the patient's injuries prevent transportation, measurement of IOP by palpation, Schiøtz tonometry, or hand-held tonometry devices may be of benefit. It should be kept in mind that although low IOP may suggest occult rupture, elevated IOP does not exclude this condition.[12,13]

Vitreous Body and Retina

A careful inspection of the vitreous body, posterior pole, and peripheral retina is mandatory in all patients with eye injuries. It is extremely important that the first examiner be as thorough and careful as possible, because continued slow or secondary hemorrhage may obscure fundus details for subsequent examinations. The indirect ophthalmoscope is an excellent instrument for evaluating the posterior pole following injury because it allows a wide-field binocular examination of both the posterior pole and the peripheral retina. The direct ophthalmoscope, although allowing a higher magnification of view, is less useful in trauma because the ability to examine large areas of retina is somewhat limited. The evaluation should be directed specifically toward recognition and documentation of posterior scleral ruptures or discontinuities, foreign bodies, retinal tears or detachments, edema, hemorrhage, and vitreous opacities. Scleral depression should be attempted only when a globe rupture has been ruled out (see Chapters 17, 18, 20, and 21).

The slit lamp, when combined with a fundus contact lens or a Hruby, 78-, or 90-diopter lens, is also useful in examining the posterior pole. The introduction of noncontact lenses has greatly facilitated the slit-lamp examination of posterior structures, which can now be inspected in detail without the hazards associated with the pressure of a fundus contact lens.

All trauma patients, unless exempt for neurosurgical or other reasons, should undergo bilateral pupillary dilation for the fundus examination. Dilation is a necessary requirement for adequate examination of the retina and posterior pole of the injured eye. Dilation should be performed with caution, however, in unconscious patients and those with significant head trauma or confusion. These patients should be cleared with a neurologist before receiving mydriatic agents. Following dilation of the confused or unconscious patient, the examiner should document in the chart the time, dose, and identity of the dilating agents. It is also useful to record this information on a piece of 2-inch adhesive tape, which is then placed across the patient's forehead. This obvious documentation on more than one occasion has saved a patient from unnecessary neurosurgical intervention.

Examination of the posterior pole should begin with an inspection of the anterior, mid, and posterior vitreous. Any hemorrhage or debris within the vitreous should be noted and its position documented. Similarly, the character of any vitreous opacity or irregularity should be evaluated whether it is localized or diffuse, because both may indicate a perforating or penetrating injury or foreign body. Following concussive injury and compression of the globe, the vitreous base may detach from the pars plana, resulting in epithelium and pigment suspended in the anterior vitreous.[8] Therefore, any pigment or tissue in the vitreous should be documented. The presence of a posterior vitreous detachment should also be documented because this condition may affect the timing of subsequent surgery.

Vitreous foreign bodies should be searched for and, if present, a drawing should be made showing their position relative to other ocular structures. Tentative identification of source material should be attempted. Finally, any evidence of white-cell recruitment or purulence in the vitreous cavity should be noted and appropriate measures taken to obtain samples for culture and microbiologic analysis.

The retina and choroid may also have been damaged by direct laceration, perforation, concussive injury, or contrecoup injury. A complete inspection of the retina and choroid should, therefore, be performed in all trauma patients, from the ora to the posterior pole in all quadrants.

Edema of the retina (commotio retinae, Berlin's edema) is a distinctive response of the retina to concussive injury characterized by pale swelling and obscuration of choroidal detail. Since Berlin's edema may be associated with a significant loss of vision, the presence of visual-field defects, and an afferent pupillary defect, it is important that the affected retina be indicated on the retinal drawing so that this can be compared with other clinical findings.

Any retinal hemorrhage is noteworthy, and its location and character should be documented. Hemorrhage of the nerve fiber layer may appear as a characteristic "flame" hemorrhage, whereas intraretinal hemorrhages appear as blotches with irregular borders. Bleeding in the subretinal space is seen as a dark, homogeneous area, which may or may not exhibit layering. Subinternal limiting membrane blood may, under certain circumstances, stream into the vitreous cavity. Any site of retinal hemorrhage should be carefully inspected for the presence of a foreign body or occult rupture. This is especially important because continued hemorrhage may obscure the findings for subsequent examiners.

Tears or breaks in the retina can follow concussive or penetrating injury and should be documented in the retinal drawing. Tears appear as red, well-demarcated areas and may be associated with vitreoretinal traction. The superior nasal quadrant is the most frequently involved site, followed by the inferotemporal quadrant, so these areas should be carefully inspected.[24,25] Retinal holes, especially macular holes, can be difficult to see at the initial evaluation, although diagnosis can be facilitated with either the 90- or 78-diopter or fundus contact lens. Approximately 10% to 15% of retinal detachments are secondary to trauma,[24] so detachments should be specifically searched for in any ocular injury.

A large proportion (70%) of intraocular foreign bodies are retained in the posterior segment, and those in the retina are frequently surrounded by a halo of edema with a central plume of blood. If a foreign body appears to be embedded in the retina, the use of a magnet to test for ferrous composition is contraindicated because any movement of the foreign body may result in further retinal damage or detachment.[16]

Scleral ruptures can be seen with the indirect ophthalmoscope and should be searched for in settings compatible with this type of injury. Retinal incarceration or overlying retinal detachment should be documented and the area of scleral discontinuity carefully drawn in the record so that a directed exploration can be performed at the time of repair.

Choroidal injuries are also not uncommon, and rupture of the choroid is one of the most frequent choroidal findings in trauma. The high incidence of choroidal injury is related to the relative elasticity of the retina compared with that of Bruch's membrane.[14] Choroidal ruptures appear as a hemorrhagic linear zone with overlying retinal edema and in acute cases may be obscured by vitreous hemorrhage. Later, as the blood clears, these ruptures become sharply demarcated and take on their characteristic white color.

Optic Nerve

Injury to the optic nerve is not common, although among cranial nerves it is the third most frequently damaged by indirect injury.[7] The use of the direct ophthalmoscope, Hruby, or 90-diopter lens provides a high-magnification view of the nerve head, allowing an inspection of the disc for abnormalities such as the presence of edema, loss of margin clarity, and hemorrhages in the nerve fiber layer. Spontaneous venous pulsations of the central retinal vein can also be seen by examining the nerve with high magnification; if present, this finding suggests that the intracranial pressure is probably normal. During evaluation of the optic nerve, an estimate of the cup-to-disc ratio should be made. An increased ratio alerts the examiner to the possibility of previous glaucomatous damage and, thus, a patient more prone than normal to visual-field loss with elevated IOP. The presence of glaucoma directly affects management decisions in traumatic conditions characterized by pressure elevation such as hyphema.

The optic nerve may be traumatized directly by penetrating injuries to the orbit, and in severe trauma the nerve may be avulsed either partially or completely. In such cases examination reveals a hole in the posterior sclera at the site of the optic nerve through which retinal vessels pass posteriorly. Blunt trauma to the forehead or brow may also result in direct optic-nerve injury via contusion of the intracanalicular portion of the optic nerve.[7] In this condition the optic nerve frequently appears entirely normal immediately following contusion, and the diagnosis must be made on clinical and historical grounds.

Special Studies: ERG and VEP in the Acute Setting

One major difficulty confronting the examiner of an injured patient is the evaluation of retinal function, visual potential, or visual prognosis in eyes with opaque media. A variety of tests attempt to address these issues, among them several electrophysiologic techniques. Two potentially useful tests are the electroretinogram (ERG) and the visual evoked potential (VEP). The ERG measures the mass electrical response of the retina with the a-wave generated by the photoreceptors and the b-wave originating in the Muller cells. The VEP is an examination of the entire visual pathway and estimates function of the system as a unit. Both tests have generated intense interest as possible indicators of visual potential in severely traumatized eyes.

The ERG has been suggested as a valuable prognostic test in injuries complicated by opaque media. In a study by Jayle and Tassy[26] in 1970, patients with opaque media and an extinguished or nearly extinguished ERG following ocular trauma were uniformly left with little useful vision. Patients with a normal or near normal ERG had significantly better visual results. In a similar study of injured eyes with and without retained foreign bodies, Hirose and coworkers[27] found that although a recordable ERG and VEP did not always indicate a good prognosis, a nonrecordable ERG tended to indicate a poor visual outcome. These findings might be explained by the fact that the presence of a recordable ERG generally excludes the possibility of a total retinal detachment, whereas a nonrecordable ERG suggests that a total retinal detachment is present. Hirose concluded that the VEP did not add much useful information to the ERG alone in their patient population, because a nonrecordable VEP was generally associated with a nonrecordable ERG. Hutton and Fuller,[28] however, in a review of 194 patients undergoing vitrectomy for posterior segment injury, noted that a normal VEP provided strong support for good postoperative visual acuity and found the VEP to be the single best predictor of visual outcome.

The combination of ERG with ultrasound in traumatic injuries may be useful for interpreting an acoustic shadow when a total retinal detachment is suspected. In a study of 47 cases of vitreous opacities, total retinal detachments were undetected by ultrasound but confirmed by the ERG in 6 cases (13%).[29] However, a nonrecordable ERG does not necessarily imply the presence of a total retinal detachment. In an experimental study of a standard posterior penetrating injury with intravitreal blood injection, Mandelbaum et al.[30] found that the ERG in rhesus monkeys may decrease to nonrecordability in the absence of a retinal detachment and subsequently return to normal levels 8 to 10 weeks after the injury. Therefore, the ERG in the acute setting appears to be of little value in predicting eventual visual outcome or directing further investigations. Although a nonrecordable ERG can be taken as a poor prognostic sign, it can also be reversible.

The ERG has a more established role in cases of foreign body injury, and there is a typical progression of ERG changes associated with metallosis bulbi.[27] An ERG performed to evaluate the development of metal toxicity is most effective when the media are clear because significant media opacities may obscure the ERG findings until late in the course of the toxicity, at which time surgical removal of the foreign body may not result in significant visual improvement.[27] The electroretinogram is of no benefit in the diagnosis or management of acute foreign-body injury.

Several newer electrophysiologic testing methods have recently been developed. The visual electrical evoked potentials (VEEP) uses transcorneal electrical stimulation to generate visual evoked potentials. The source of the potentials is thought to be one of the nerve cell layers of the retina rather than the photoreceptors, and it has been reported that the VEEP can be recorded in patients with total retinal detachments.[31] At this time the role of the VEEP in evaluating the traumatized eye is limited. The main benefit seems to be support for the clinical decision to proceed with enucleation in cases of nonrecordable VEEP.[31]

In summary, although the VEP, ERG, and VEEP may have value in certain circumstances, they do not have significant advantages over a careful ophthalmic examination in the acute care setting.

HYSTERIA AND MALINGERING

In the vast majority of circumstances the patient and examining ophthalmologist are cooperative partners in the recognition and treatment of ocular injury. With some patients, however, the physician becomes aware that the symptoms are not commensurate with the objective findings. In these circumstances the examiner must be prepared to recognize and evaluate the hysterical or malingering patient. Malingering can be defined as the "willful, deliberate, and fraudulent feigning and exaggeration of symptoms of illness or injury done for the purpose of a consciously desired end."[32] Several motives are commonly found in malingering patients; for example, financial reward or the avoidance of military service. Financial incentives for malingering may be great, especially in our increasingly litigious society, and the possibility of worker's compensation or disability payments may motivate some patients to exaggerate their symptoms. These patients are typically individuals in the second or third decade, under pressure or stress associated with finances or employment, who have had some minor ocular trauma, either accidental or self-inflicted.[32] Hysterical individuals, on the other hand, are frequently described as "suggestible innocents" who fool themselves into believing they have a real ocular condition.[33] Hysterical patients are often quite calm about their conditions and present *la belle indifference*. The age range is wider for these patients than for malingerers, with the peak onset occurring in the third or fourth decade.[33]

The hysteric and the malingerer approach the examination with markedly different attitudes. The hysteric may be extremely suggestible, eager to please, an active participant who is anxiously cooperative and interested in finding out how bad his or her condition really is. The malingerer, on the other hand, has been described as suspicious, minimally cooperative, and anxious for the examination to be over. The malingerer can be very distrustful or suspicious of "new" or "unusual" tests, is consciously lying, and may be overly self-assertive and confident.[34] Malingering and hysteria frequently occur in the presence of real ocular disease, and therefore a meticulous examination is absolutely essential to rule out and assess existing pathology before the initiation of examination strategies designed to uncover the malingerer or hysteric.

A variety of tests have been developed to deal with patients with factitious amblyopia and several excellent references describe the theory and use of these strategies.[34-37] Regardless of which tests are employed, the practitioner is encouraged to remember the admonishment of Duke-Elder: "One point is important: the examiner should know thoroughly the tests he proposes to carry out, for the most important feature in such testing is rapid and sure manipulations; few succeed unless they are well prepared."[36]

Tests for these conditions fall into several categories and can be classified according to the degree of visual impairment they are designed to detect.

Tests for Total Blindness

Observation alone may provide valuable clues to the presence of sight. The truly blind individual ambulates carefully, has occasional collisions, takes short steps, has a back-leaning gait, and retains proprioception. The hysteric, however, navigates easily with only occasional reaching gestures and very few impacts with environmental obstacles. The malingerer, on the other hand, frequently collides with obstacles, has an exaggerated need for assistance, and gropes from object to object. The Schmidt-Rimpler test takes advantage of this difference.[36] When asked to hold up one hand and look at it, the blind individual looks at the location of the hand in space, whereas the malingerer will avoid looking at the area. When asked to touch fingertips of one hand to the other, the malingerer has great difficulty whereas the truly blind individual can accomplish this task without trouble.

Tests for Monocular Blindness

Monocular blindness is one of the more common complaints of the hysteric and the malingerer, and there are a variety of tests designed to prove the presence of vision. These tests include prism tests looking for refixation movement, tests using pseudoscopes to transpose images, and color confusion tests employing red-green glasses and red-green charts with duochrome filters. A type of color confusion test reported by Thompson[33] requires red-green glass spectacles and a pink felt-tip highlighting pen. When looking through the red-green glasses, only the eye behind the green glass sees the pink letters and they are perceived as black. Letters cannot be seen through the red lens. This test is quite effective. Other tests include monocular blur testing, in which both plus and minus cylinders are placed parallel in the Phoroptor and then rotated 90° to blur the "good" eye while the patient reads binocularly. In addition, high plus lenses can be placed in front of the "good" eye, and the patient can be asked to read a near target that is gradually withdrawn. The patient who continues to read at distance is then using the "bad" eye.

The mirror test is an extremely effective method for detecting whether the patient complaining of monocular blindness is incapable of vision. The seeing eye is patched and a large mirror, sufficient to fill the patient's visual field, is held in front of the "blind" eye. The mirror is then rocked gently back and forth while the examiner observes for movement of the unpatched eye. If there is vision in the eye, the patient, in an attempt to maintain fixation, will exhibit horizontal or vertical movements of the eye corresponding to the movements of the mirror.

Visual Fields and Electrophysiologic Testing

Visual field testing can be quite informative in hysterical and malingering patients. Spiral or identical tangent screen visual fields at both 1- and 2-meter testing distances generally indicate the presence of hysteria or malingering. For an accurate result, the examiner must increase the test-object's size with increasing distance. Electrophysiologic testing does not add much information to the preceding types of testing for these conditions.

TRANSPORTATION OF THE EYE-INJURED PATIENT

Transportation of the injured ophthalmic patient can present several unique problems. Before being transported, the patient should undergo a general ophthalmic examination to assess for the presence of a foreign body in the orbit or globe, an open globe, or air in the globe. A shield should be securely taped over any eye with ruptures or perforations of the sclera or cornea. If large foreign bodies are protruding from the eye or orbit, they should not be removed in the initial setting unless it can be done in a controlled manner. Any protruding objects wedged into the orbit such as knives, pencils, stakes, and so on should be stabilized by fluffy bandage material to prevent movement; the patient should be transported to a surgical facility with the foreign body in situ. It is extremely important for air in the globe to be recognized because this may have a significant impact on the selection of transportation.

Pretransport Therapy

Any patient with a serious ocular injury should have an intravenous line established to provide vascular access. If transport to the treatment facility involves a significant delay, the patient with major tissue damage, open globe, or foreign-body injuries should be given broad-spectrum prophylactic intravenous antibiotics providing gram-negative and gram-positive coverage. If infection is thought to be present, cultures of appropriate materials should be obtained before initiating antibiotic therapy. In addition, although tetanus is extremely rare following ophthalmic injuries, tetanus toxoid or tetanus immune globulin should be administered, depending on the patient's immunization status (see Appendix).

Control of nausea and vomiting is imperative in patients with rupture or laceration injuries of the eye. Antiemetic medications should be given intramuscularly or intravenously in sufficient doses to prevent vomiting, because emesis can increase IOP and cause extrusion of intraocular contents. Also, although injuries to the eye per se are not generally severely painful, the patient should be kept comfortable with appropriate pain medications.

The injured eye should be protected during transportation. If an open globe is present or suspected, pressure on the globe should be prevented by taping either a Foxx aluminum shield or some substitute rigid protective cover, such as a styrofoam cup, over the orbit. Pads or tape on the eyelid should be avoided in these circumstances. Bilateral patching is probably not warranted, because rendering a patient blind increases stress and anxiety and contributes to disorientation. No ointment or topical medication should be administered to any patient with a suspected rupture of the globe or open wound of the eye. For patients with lid lacerations, saline-moistened gauze pads can be used to keep the tissue edges fresh and prevent desiccation.

Eye-injury patients should be transported with the head of the bed elevated and vibration and patient discomfort kept to a minimum. If patients become nauseated during transport, the vehicle should be stopped if at all possible and appropriate medication given to control vomiting.

Air Evacuation: Special Considerations

Air transport of the patient with an injured eye requires special attention and planning. Several physiologic changes are induced by flight and altitude, and these must be considered for optimal safety. An excellent discussion of these factors, from which the following has been adapted, is available in an article by Colvin.[38]

Hypoxia

With the decreasing partial pressure of oxygen experienced at increasing altitude, the patient becomes hypoxic, and hypoxia subsequently causes dilation of retinal choroidal vessels, which may predispose the patient to secondary hemorrhage. Additionally, hypoxia directly causes increased IOP and decreased pupil size. It is recommended that the patient be given humidified oxygen at 6 to 8 l/min during transportation, with precautions taken to prevent pressure on the eye by the oxygen-delivery device.

Decreased Atmospheric Pressure

As aircraft altitude increases, there is a consequent decrease in atmospheric pressure, and even pressurized aircraft experience a drop in cabin pressure with sufficient altitude. Commercial pressurized aircraft flying at 30,000 feet maintain a cabin pressure equal to approximately 8000 feet of altitude. The average rate of change in commercial airliners is approximately 300 f/min.[39] This decrease in cabin pressure can result in expansion of intraocular gas in the eye, resulting in elevation of IOP. Dieckert and coworkers[39] reported that in monkeys with 0.25 cc of intraocular gas, IOP increased to almost 40 mm Hg during simulated ascents at rates comparable to those of commercial airliners. Although it is theoretically possible that under these circumstances patients with ocular trauma could experience extrusion of intraocular contents through eye wall discontinuities, it is our experience that injury per se does not result in sufficient intraocular air to cause a problem or necessitate special transport considerations. On the other hand, patients who have had repair of ocular trauma and undergone air-fluid exchange or intraocular gas injection are at significant risk for complications associated with decompression during air travel. If air travel is necessary in these cases, every effort should be made to maintain the cabin pressure at sea level or, if a pressurized aircraft is not available, to maintain altitude below 1300 meters.

Noise and Vibration

Vibration, turbulence, and acceleration forces on the eye can result in traction on intraocular tissues, and subsequent bleeding in the ocular tissues secondary to these conditions may cause further damage to the eye as well as general patient discomfort with possible vomiting. If turbulence in the flight path is a potential problem, the patient should be transported at night if possible when turbulence is generally less than during daytime.

Cabin Humidity

In most aircraft there is a significant decrease in cabin humidity compared with ground conditions. This drop in humidity may predispose to corneal exposure and desiccation of lacerated tissue edges. For this reason, if the blink response is inhibited, the eye should be kept closed, and if an open globe is present, sterile nonsaline should be used to maintain hydration.

References

1. Freeman HM: Examination of the traumatized eye. In Miller D and Stegman R, editors: Treatment of anterior segment ocular trauma, Montreal, 1986, Medicopea, 95-119.
2. Pearlstein ES et al: Ruptured globe after radial keratotomy, Am J Ophthalmol 106:755-756, 1988.

3. Fackler ML: Wound ballistics, a review of common misconceptions, JAMA 259:2730-2736, 1988.
4. Klein OG: The initial evaluation in ophthalmic injury, Otolaryngol Clin North Am 12:303-320, 1979.
5. Cherry PMH: Indirect traumatic rupture of the globe, Arch Ophthalmol 96:252-256, 1978.
6. Eagling EM: Ocular damage after blunt trauma to the eye: its relationship to the nature of the injury, Br J Ophthalmol 58:126-140, 1974.
7. Anderson RL, Panje WR, and Gross CE: Optic nerve blindness following blunt forehead trauma, Ophthalmology 89:445-455, 1982.
8. Holt JE, Holt GR, and Blodgett JM: Ocular injuries sustained during blunt facial trauma, Ophthalmology 90:14-18, 1983.
9. Gray R et al: Pecking injury of the eye, N Engl J Med 319:1021-1022, 1988 (letter).
10. Jones DB, Liesegang TJ, and Robinson NM: Laboratory diagnosis of ocular infectious, cumulative techniques and procedures in clinical microbiology, Cumitech 13, Washington, DC, 1981, American Society for Microbiology.
11. Deutsch TA and Feller DB: Paton and Goldberg's management of ocular injuries, Philadelphia, 1985, WB Saunders, 1-8.
12. Cherry PMH: Rupture of the globe, Arch Ophthalmol 88:498-507, 1972.
13. Russell SR, Olsen KR, and Folk JC: Predictors of scleral rupture and the role of vitrectomy in severe blunt ocular trauma, Am J Ophthalmol 105:253-257, 1988.
14. Archer DB et al: Traumatic retinal angiopathy—associated with wearing of car seat belts, Eye 2:650-659, 1988.
15. Duke-Elder S: System of ophthalmology, vol XIV, part 1, Mechanical injuries, St Louis, 1972, The CV Mosby Co, 90-92.
16. Coleman DJ et al: Management of intraocular foreign bodies, Ophthalmology 94:1647-1653, 1987.
17. Cibis GW, Weingeist TA, and Krachmer JH: Traumatic corneal endothelial rings, Arch Ophthalmol 96:485-488, 1978.
18. Maloney WF et al: Specular microscopy of traumatic posterior annular keratopathy, Arch Ophthalmol 97:1647-1650, 1979.
19. Simmons RJ and Kimbrough RL: Late glaucoma after trauma. In Freeman HM, editor: Ocular trauma, New York, 1979, Appleton-Century-Crofts, 169-176.
20. Davidson SI: Clinical recognition (intraocular foreign bodies), Int Ophthalmol Clin 8(1):171-179, 1968.
21. Duke-Elder S: System of ophthalmology, vol XIV, part 1, Mechanical injuries, St Louis, 1972, The CV Mosby Co, 125-127.
22. Hamill MB et al: Traumatic hyphema: a review of possible risk factors, Invest Ophthalmol Vis Sci 30(ARVO suppl):438, 1989.
23. Brown DM and Hamill MB: Preoperative assessment of occult scleral rupture, Invest Ophthalmol Vis Sci 30(ARVO suppl):439, 1989.
24. Cox MS et al: Retinal detachment due to ocular contusion, Arch Ophthalmol 76:678-685, 1966.
25. Runyan TE: Concussive and penetrating injuries of the globe and optic nerve. St Louis, 1975, The CV Mosby Co.
26. Jayle GE and Tassy AF: Prognostic value of the electroretinogram in severe recent ocular trauma, Br J Ophthalmol 54:51-58, 1970.
27. Hirose T, Miyake Y, and Hara A: Evaluation of severe ovular trauma: electroretinogram and visual evoked response. In Freeman HM, editor: Ocular trauma, New York, 1979, Appleton-Century-Crofts, 31-52.
28. Hutton WL and Fuller DG: Factors influencing final visual results in severely injured eyes, Am J Ophthalmol 97:715-722, 1984.
29. Bernard J-A et al: Interet de l'association de l'echographie et de l'electroretinographie sur sommateur dans le diagnostic du décollement du rétiné quand il existe une hemorragie du vitre, Bull Soc Ophthalmol Fr 73:1015-1023, 1973.
30. Mandelbaum S et al: Bright-flash electroretinography and vitreous hemorrhage: an experimental study in primates, Arch Ophthalmol 98:1823-1828, 1980.
31. Dorfman LJ et al: Visual electrical evoked potentials: evaluation of ocular injuries, Neurology 37:123-128, 1987.
32. Kramer KK, La Piana FG, and Appleton B: Ocular malingering and hysteria: diagnosis and management, Surv Ophthalmol 24:89-96, 1979.
33. Thompson HS: Functional visual loss, Am J Ophthalmol 100:209-213, 1985.
34. Hesterberg RC Jr and Tredici TJ: A review of ocular malingering and hysteria for the flight surgeon, Aviat Space Environ Med 54:934-936, 1983.
35. Agatston H: Ocular malingering, Arch Ophthalmol 31:223-231, 1944.
36. Duke-Elder S: System of ophthalmology, vol V, Ophthalmic optics and refraction, St Louis, 1972, The CV Mosby Co, 487-501.
37. Miller BW: A review of practical tests for ocular malingering and hysteria, Surv Ophthalmol 17:241-246, 1973.
38. Colvin J: Effective management of penetrating eye injuries in remote Australia, Med J Aust 1:329-334, 1981.
39. Dieckert JP et al: Air travel and intraocular gas, Ophthalmology 93:642-645, 1986.

CHAPTER 2

Diagnostic imaging of ocular and orbital trauma

D. JACKSON COLEMAN
MARK J. RONDEAU

Plain film radiography
Computed tomography
Ultrasound
Magnetic resonance imaging
References

Due to techniques developed within this generation of practitioners—ultrasound, computed tomography (CT), and magnetic resonance imaging (MRI)—diagnostic imaging has become an invaluable modality in the evaluation of the traumatized eye. It is indispensable when the media are opaque or when damage to the periorbital region or the presence of a foreign body is suspected. Diagnostic imaging provides the surgeon with a detailed anatomic map, allowing for a planned surgical approach.

The primary radiologic methods used in evaluating trauma are plain film radiography, CT, MRI, and ultrasonography. Each has distinct utility, but none provides all the diagnostic information needed in all cases. A combination of complementary techniques, typically CT and ultrasonography, is used to evaluate the spectrum of soft tissue and bony changes seen in eye trauma and to identify and localize radiopaque and radiolucent foreign bodies.

PLAIN FILM RADIOGRAPHY

Although plain film evaluation of the eye and orbit has been largely superseded by CT examination (because of the latter's tomographic representation of the soft tissues), it still offers advantages in depicting the shape and number of metallic foreign bodies and localizing orbital wall fractures. In some cases a negative plain film may make more expensive and invasive tests unnecessary.

The first documented cases of the successful use of plain film radiography for detecting and localizing metallic foreign bodies were published less than a year after Roentgen's demonstration of x-rays and their medical utility.[1,2] Specific plain film series for orbital trauma visualization now include use of the Caldwell projection, the Water's projection, and the lateral view, among others.[3-5] The film series will detect the presence of an intraocular, orbital, or adnexal retained foreign body if it is sufficiently radiodense. In addition, most orbital-wall and other skull fractures are well delineated by plain film series.

The ability of the plain film to outline distinctly and compress the orbit into a single viewing plane allows easy identification of radiopaque foreign bodies. Graphic examples can be seen in Figs. 2-1 through 2-6.

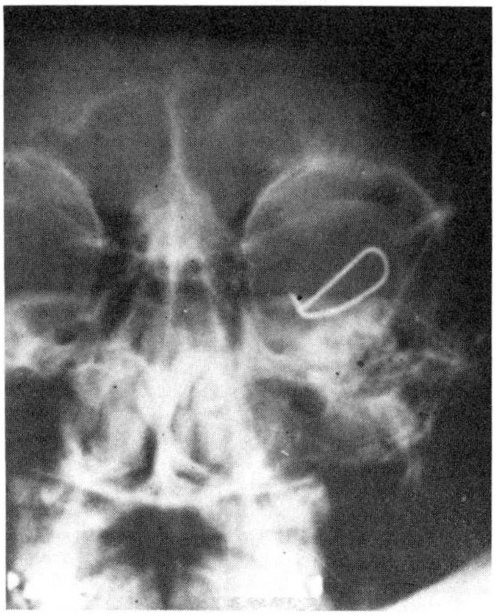

Fig. 2-1. Plain film x-ray of an intraocular broken paper clip. The shape is outlined better than with any other imaging modality, but the globe relationships are lacking. (Courtesy of Gwen Sterns, MD, Rochester, NY.)

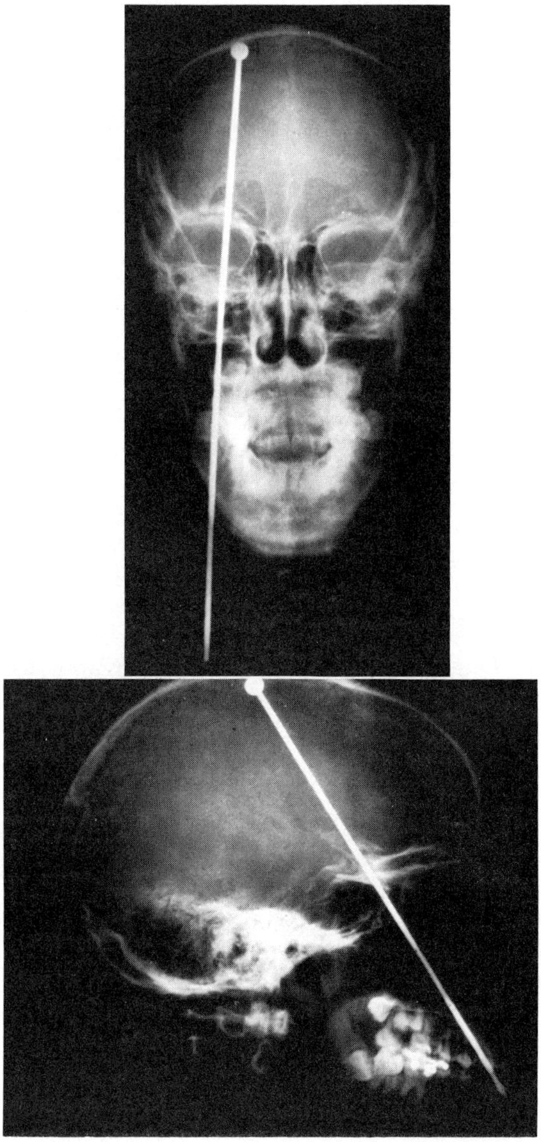

Fig. 2-2. Plain film x-rays of a car radio antenna that penetrated the orbit and cranium, demonstrating the value of x-rays in outlining the shape of the foreign body. The tip of the antenna was removed through a burr hole before the antenna was withdrawn. (Courtesy of Stephen Trokel, MD, New York, NY.)

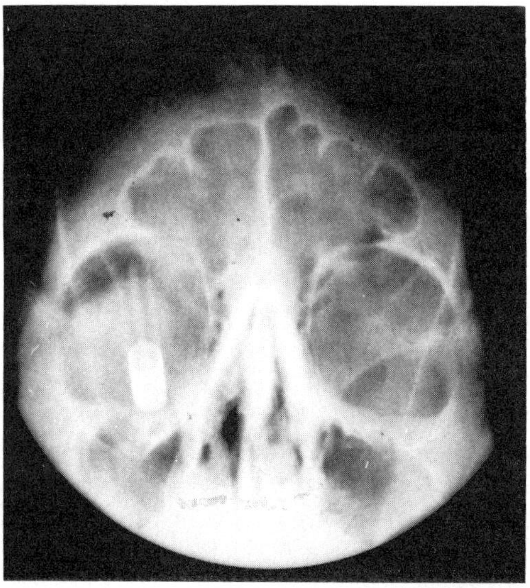

Fig. 2-3. Plain film x-ray of a pencil that penetrated the orbit. The graphite core and metal eraser holder are radiodense. (Courtesy of Stephen Trokel, MD, New York, NY.)

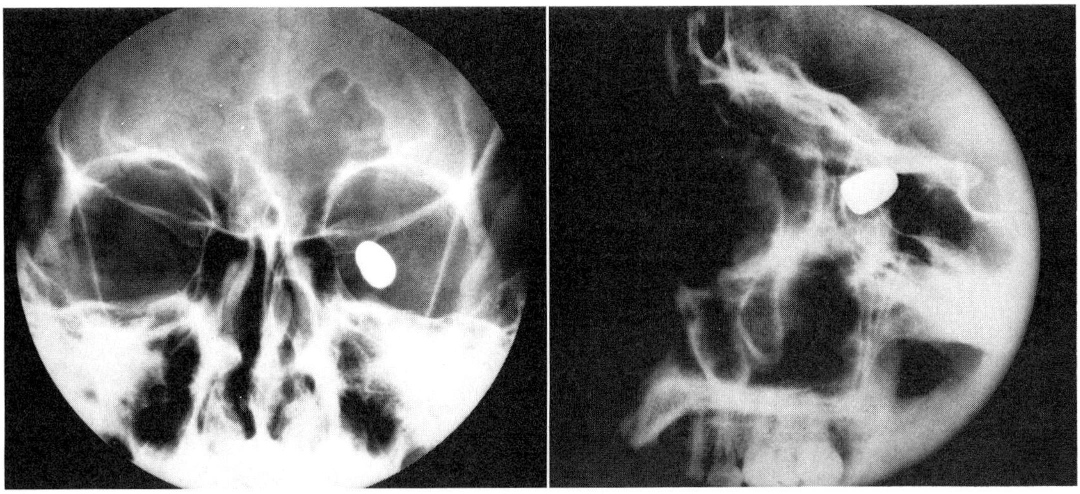

Fig. 2-4. Plain film x-rays of a bullet in the orbit that had penetrated the globe. Two perspectives show the bullet's orientation. (Courtesy of Stephen Trokel, MD, New York, NY.)

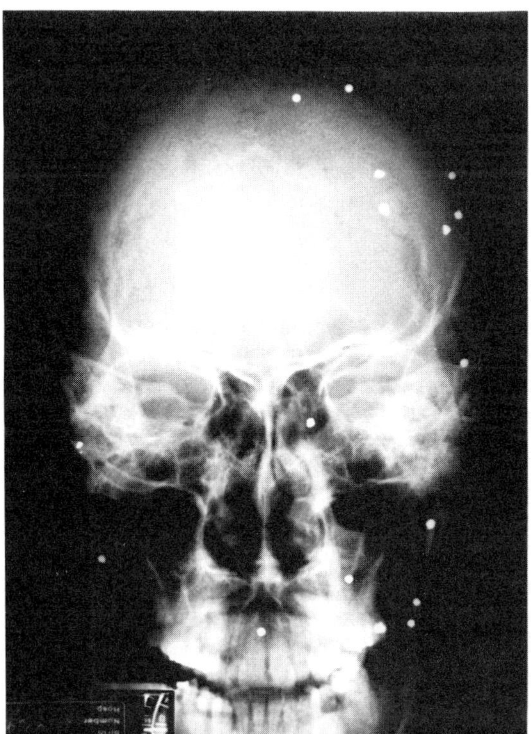

Fig. 2-5. Plain film x-ray of shotgun pellets around the face and orbit. The orbital pellet had traversed the globe. Shotgun pellets may be steel or lead. Magnetic testing can be useful, using either a similar shell supplied by the patient or family or, at surgery, a pellet from a different site. (Courtesy of Murk-Hein Heinemann, MD, New York, NY.)

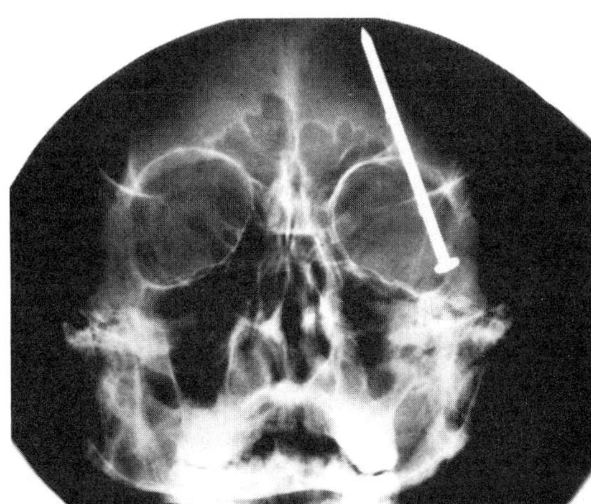

Fig. 2-6. Plain film x-ray of a nail that penetrated the orbit and cranial vault but did not puncture the globe. (Courtesy of Alan Maberley, MD, Vancouver, BC.)

Multiview plain films can provide localization for large foreign bodies and coarse localization for smaller foreign bodies. Because of the lack of soft tissue definition, however, these films cannot definitively answer the questions of interest to the ophthalmic surgeon: Is the foreign body inside or outside the eye? What is the proximity of the foreign body to the sclera? To get around this limitation in soft tissue, elaborate multiview localization schemes using radiopaque markers have been developed. They include Wessely-Comberg-Pfeiffer procedure variants, which use a contact lens with radiopaque markers in the four quadrants and an elaborate charting system[6-8]; Sweet's triangulation methods[9,10]; a number of limbal ring devices[11]; and the sub-Tenon injection of air or contrast media.[12] These techniques used alone or in combination have been very effective in the hands of skilled radiologic practitioners. One drawback to all the methods, however, has been the error induced by the assumption of a 24-mm axial length for the geometric mapping.[13] With the use of ultrasonically determined axial length, this error can be avoided and measurement mappings corrected to provide more accurate localization.[8]

Another technique, termed *bone-free* or *soft-tissue localization*, used dental film and softer (less energetic) x-rays to localize nonmetallic (hence less radiodense) foreign bodies in the anterior segment.[14] This technique was also adapted for use with radiopaque markers for geometric mapping.[13]

Although these complex localization schemes have essentially been outmoded owing to the wide availability of CT, plain films remain an excellent and cost-effective means of screening for retained foreign bodies and of evaluating orbital integrity in a variety of penetrating and blunt injuries. In the case of small metallic foreign bodies (which may be missed on a thick CT slice) or multiple tightly clustered foreign bodies (whose number and shape may be obscured by reconstruction artifacts), a plain film series can provide important diagnostic information.

COMPUTED TOMOGRAPHY

The CT scan is the standard diagnostic test for imaging the traumatized eye and orbit. Tomographic sections of the head in the axial, coronal, and sagittal planes (directly or reconstructed) at

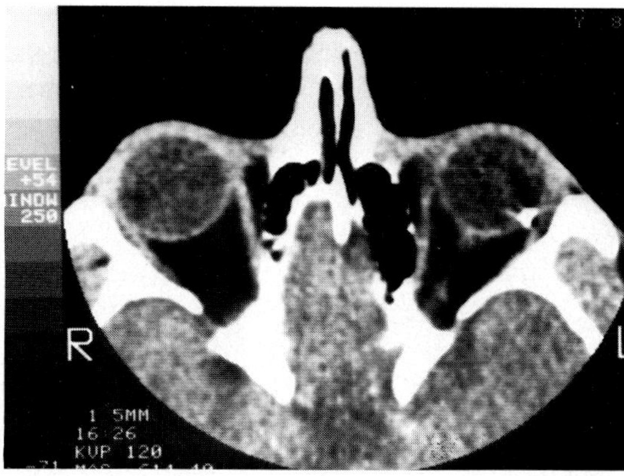

Fig. 2-7. CT scan showing a foreign body in the posterior sclera of the left globe. The ability to see the relationship of globe and foreign body is a distinct advantage of CT over plain films.

the level of the eye and orbit provide an accurate anatomic view of soft tissue and bony changes resulting from trauma. Retained foreign bodies of sufficient size and radiodensity are easily located (Fig. 2-7), and the imaging of the orbit allows detection of the exact extent of orbital wall fractures and possible incarceration of the orbital contents.

The idea of reconstructing a function or object from projections (be they ray integrals or x-ray photons) was considered at least as long ago as the first practical mathematical solution to the problem.[15] With the availability of high-speed digital computers and improved photon detector technology, the concept of tomographic reconstruction for x-ray imaging became a reality. Since the introduction of the CT to clinical medicine in 1972, the increase in speed and reduction in price of computer processors and memory, along with improvements in reconstruction algorithms and software, have led to considerable improvement in image quality and presentation. Current-generation machines allow for a slice thickness of less than 1.5 mm (down from 8 mm) and a voxel (volume/pixel) size of less than 0.5 mm^3 (down from 69 mm^3).[16]

The overall improvement in image resolution and concomitant reduction in partial volume effects allow for clinically useful multiplanar reconstruction of the standard views.[17] Multiplanar reconstruction is a data-reformatting technique for obtaining sagittal, coronal, and oblique views by mathematically manipulating the regular axial scans. Good multiplanar reconstructions with operator-determined oblique plane reconstruction are now available, along with three-dimensional block representation of the slices, on commercial scanners.[18] These methods further improve CT's ability to provide detailed images of the anatomic relationships. Beyond this block type of reconstruction, true surface and volume rendering from CT and MRI is rapidly coming into widespread clinical use, particularly for planning of maxillofacial surgery and deep brain radiotherapy.[19] With continuing increases in computer processor speeds and advances in rendering algorithms, easy-to-use three-dimensional rendering software should be available on the next generation of scanners. Rendered three-dimensional views may become the view of choice for trauma evaluation.

As with the introduction of x-ray films, the application of CT to the evaluation of the traumatized eye and orbit was almost immediate, particularly in the area of foreign-body detection.[20-22] Current-generation machines can detect metallic foreign bodies less than 1 mm in size, except for aluminum, and less radiodense objects of slightly larger size. One caveat for the clinician: Always insist on the thinnest possible slices (≤1.5 mm) through the orbits, and in the case of a suspected small foreign body, request overlapping slices.

The only drawback of CT in localization is seen when one or more foreign bodies have a sufficient attenuation coefficient and volume to cause streak and Hounsfield artifacts. These can obliterate the reproduction of individual objects and distort anatomic relationships. These artifacts are caused by local saturation of the individual projections in the area of the foreign bodies. On reconstruction, these areas, with an essentially undefined attenuation coefficient, cause the familiar flare or bloom and streaking (Figs. 2-8 and 2-9). Reconstruction algorithm modifications,[23] which can limit artifact production, are available but not widely used. The artifact problem is usually seen with metallic foreign bodies but can also be present with less radiodense substances, as seen in Fig. 2-10. CT evaluation showed three small glass fragments in the region near the ciliary body. An independent CT examination also revealed the presence of three foreign bodies. These were removed during globe repair. A confirmatory CT revealed a fourth foreign body (Fig. 2-11), which subsequently eroded forward and was removed a year later. A second confirmatory CT was performed, and no additional foreign bodies were noted (Fig. 2-12). This case not only demonstrates the localization limitations introduced by reconstruction artifacts but also raises another important point: the confirmatory CT. This should be considered in cases of retained foreign body or following complex orbital repair even if the radiation dosage for a thin-slice orbital series is nontrivial.

The other major class of injury for which the CT scan is particularly useful is the orbital frac-

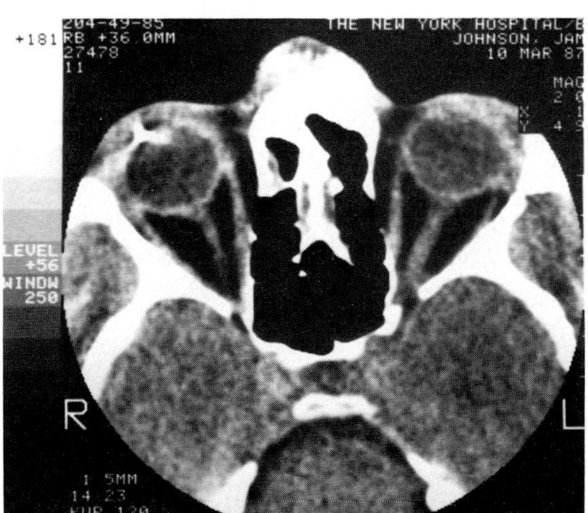

Fig. 2-8. CT scan showing a foreign body in the ciliary region of the right globe. Artifacts are produced by local saturation.

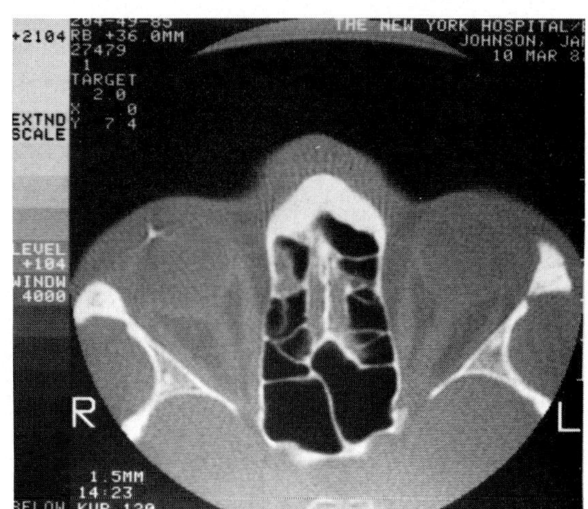

Fig. 2-9. CT scan of the foreign body shown in Fig. 2-8, with extended scale windowing to enhance the localization.

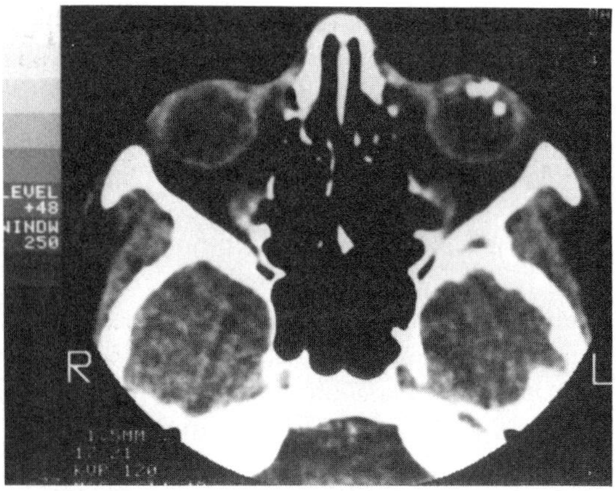

Fig. 2-10. CT scan showing three pieces of glass in the ciliary body region of the left eye. At surgery, only three glass fragments were found and removed. No other fragments were seen, but a follow-up CT scan showed a remaining occult fragment.

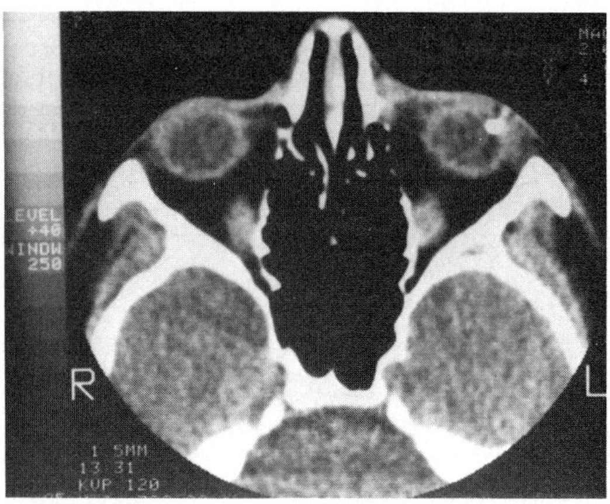

Fig. 2-11. Postoperative follow-up CT scan of eye shown in Fig. 2-10 reveals previously unrecognized glass fragment.

ture. The diagnosis and treatment of orbital fractures and the sequelae of ocular motility disturbances are described in Chapter 27. In brief, the location and extent of orbital floor, wall, roof, and rim fractures, as well as other skull fractures that may have an impact on the orbital repair, such as zygomatic arch and Le Fort fractures, are readily demonstrated.[24,25] Soft-tissue delineation is not as good as in MRI, but incarceration of orbital contents or scarring and adhesion of muscles to the orbital wall can be seen if proper slices and reconstructions are obtained. Fig. 2-13, *A* is a coronal section showing an orbital floor fracture near the region of the infraorbital canal and ethmoid sinus rupture.

In the same patient, an axial scan (Fig. 2-13, *B*) shows a cardinal sign of intraocular penetration, an air bubble in the area of the ciliary body. The attenuation coefficient of air is −1000 in Hounsfield units, so it has the lowest pixel intensity in the scan. The sharp radiolucent areas may also be seen following vitrectomy when gas-fluid exchange has been performed. Occasionally, if the CT image is windowed properly, air may also be noted in the orbit. This is usually caused by a rupture of the orbital plate of the ethmoid sinus, the fragile lamina papyracea.

A CT examination of the orbits can often identify significant nonocular findings. Such was the case with the patient shown in Fig. 2-14, who was referred for CT because of a suspected retained orbital foreign body. The scan revealed the absence of a foreign body in the orbit but also revealed occult local brain atrophy from a previous injury.

Other than the need for thin slices in orbital evaluation, specific recommendations for various types of ocular trauma are difficult to give. Certainly direct or reconstructed coronal views are important in evaluating blowout fractures, and reconstructed sagittal and oblique views may be informative in specific cases of ocular motility problems. Beyond this, consultation with the neuroradiologist and the technologist on the individual case is needed to ensure that the maximum amount of information for diagnosis and management is collected. Finally, the

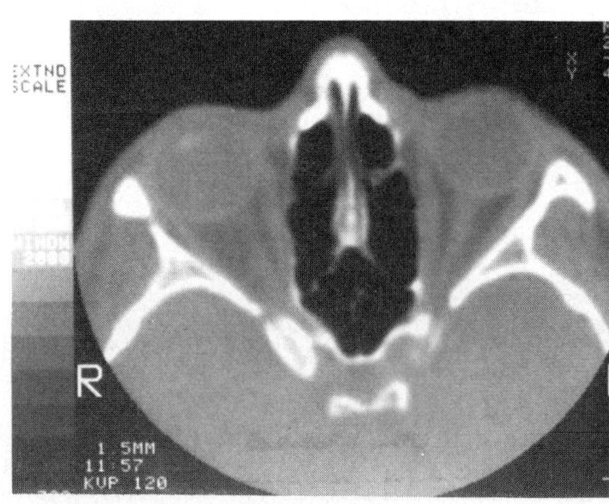

Fig. 2-12. CT scan of eye shown in Fig. 2-10, taken after second surgical procedure, confirms removal of remaining glass fragment.

A

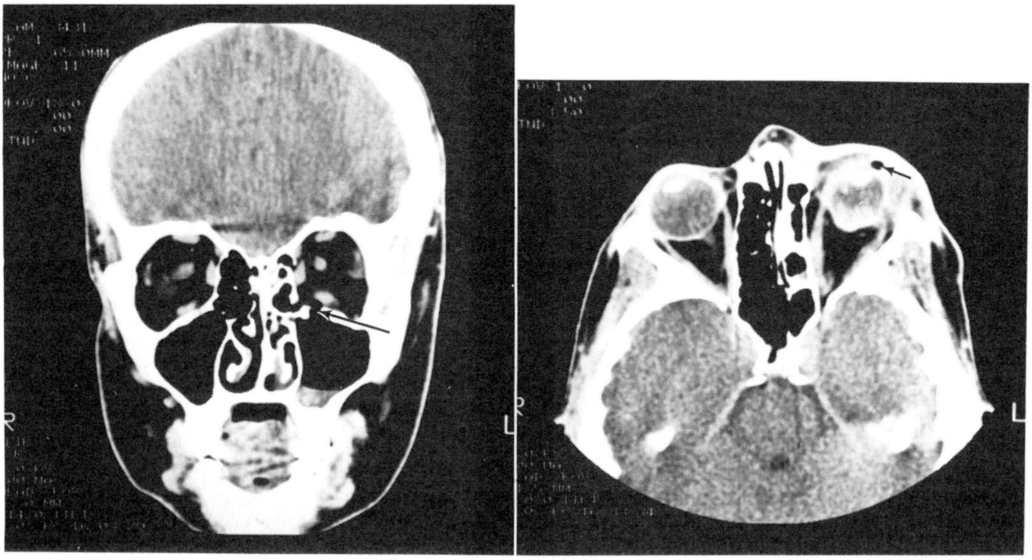

B

Fig. 2-13. **A,** CT coronal scan showing a floor fracture *(arrow)* caused by a golf-ball injury, which also ruptured the globe. Two ethmoid breaks can also be seen in this section. **B,** CT axial scan showing an air bubble *(arrow)* in a recently ruptured globe.

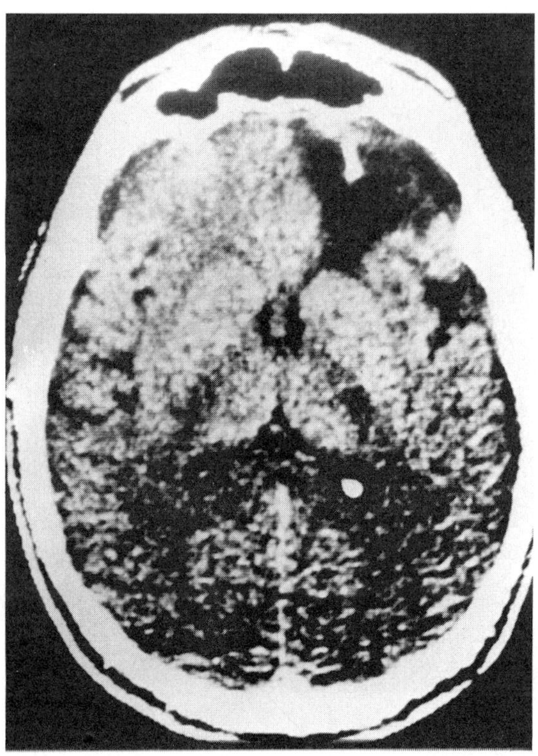

Fig. 2-14. CT scan of a suspected foreign body in the left orbit showed no orbital abnormality but did reveal atrophy of the left frontal lobe of the brain. Questioning of the patient revealed that an injury had occurred 20 years earlier when a coat hanger had penetrated the superior orbit and penetrated the brain, resulting in occult brain atrophy.

use of contrast media is not necessarily indicated in trauma evaluation, although it does enhance soft-tissue delineation in the orbit.

ULTRASOUND

Ocular ultrasound generally is used as a B-scan imaging technique for evaluating trauma, although the A-scan has a corroborative and correlative role.[26] B-scans are performed with contact or immersion techniques. The immersion technique (Fig. 2-15) is not widely used but has the important advantage of showing the anterior chamber and lens (Fig. 2-16). The lid speculum and waterbath do not put undue pressure on a possibly ruptured eye and enhance sensitivity by allowing the focal zone to be placed in the area of interest. The contact technique has the advantage of simplicity but does not permit optimal (or sometimes any) depiction of the lens and anterior chamber. This can be remedied by using a balloon stand-off of soft prophylactic latex partially filled with saline[27] (Fig. 2-17). When used with methyl cellulose and a lid speculum, this can separate the "main bang" of the transducer from the eye and allow visualization of the anterior segment. A major advantage of the balloon stand-off is that it greatly reduces pressure on the eye during the contact B-scan examination. A membrane echo may produce an artifact (Fig. 2-18), but this can be easily identified by jiggling the transducer.

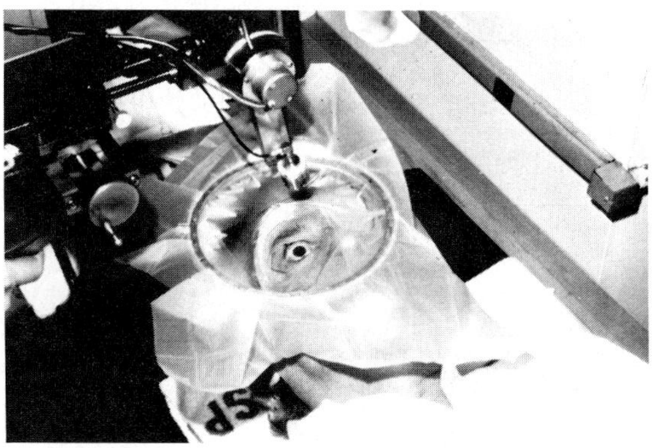

Fig. 2-15. Use of an immersion waterbath separates the transducer from the eye sufficiently to provide good definition of the anterior chamber.

Ocular ultrasound is generally performed at frequencies of 8 to 10 MHz or higher.[26] For orbital examinations or in the presence of much blood or inflammation, the use of lower frequencies (e.g., 5 MHz) may be in order to allow sufficient sensitivity for good visualization.[28,29] Although ultrasound can demonstrate the orbital soft-tissue changes quite well, it generally is limited in visualizing the apex and bone structure and offers no advantage over CT scan of the orbit. It does, however, have a considerable and unique advantage in demonstrating damage to the ocular structures.[30,31]

In planning vitreous surgery for trauma repair, four general indicators have been sug-

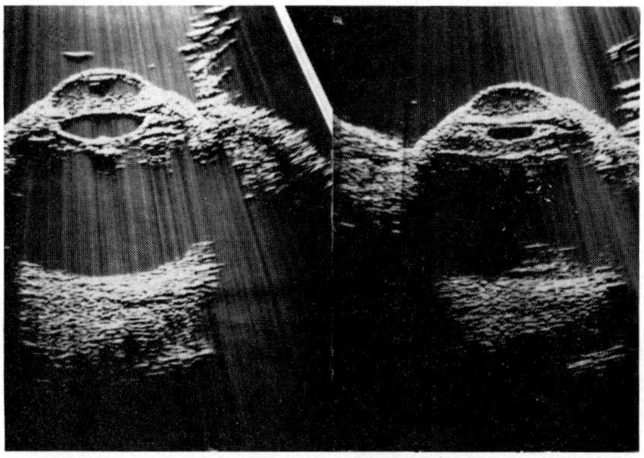

Fig. 2-16. Ultrasonogram of the anterior segment showing a hyphema and anterior vitreous hemorrhage, as well as an intact lens. This figure demonstrates the advantage of an immersion system for delineating the anterior segment.

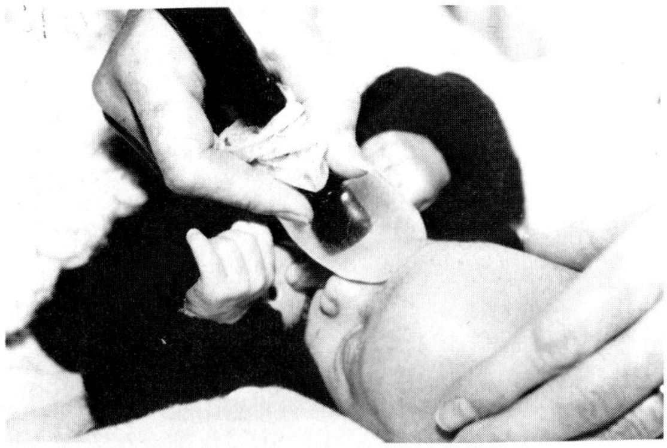

Fig. 2-17. Balloon stand-off used with a contact B-scan transducer prevents undue pressure on the eye and permits better definition of the anterior segment. (A reduplication artifact of the anterior segment curvature is often produced in midvitreous with this method; see Fig. 2-18.)

gested: lens rupture, vitreous hemorrhage with retinal detachment, retained reactive foreign body, and vitreous incarceration to the wound.[32,33] Each of these indications can be demonstrated with ultrasound.

Proceeding anteriorly to posteriorly, ultrasound can easily show hyphema (Fig. 2-19) and can usually indicate an iriododialysis. Blood surrounding the zonules outlines them well, and their integrity or lack of it can be appreciated. It is important to visualize the lens in particular to determine its position and integrity (Fig. 2-19). Lens integrity is gauged by the contour of the capsule outline (Fig. 2-20) and often by intralenticular echoes, which normally appear only in old or cataractous lenses. A dislocated lens is easily seen unless it is ruptured, in which case the remnants may be difficult to distinguish from blood.

Vitreous hemorrhage, if old or sufficiently dense, is easily seen,[31,34] but a mild recent hemorrhage may not have sufficient conglomerates of cells to be acoustically visible. One useful role of vitreous hemorrhage evaluation is in determining if the posterior "hyaloid" (the posterior limiting membrane of the vitreous) has separated from the retina. Blood along the posterior hyaloid is generally an acoustic interface of moderately good reflectance. Because the ultrasound examination is a dynamic test, if the patient moves the eye, the posterior hyaloid will sway if it is detached; this can be easily seen (Fig. 2-21).

A retinal detachment is seen as a highly reflective surface separated from the posterior ocular or chorioscleral wall. There is usually no problem in distinguishing it from a vitreous

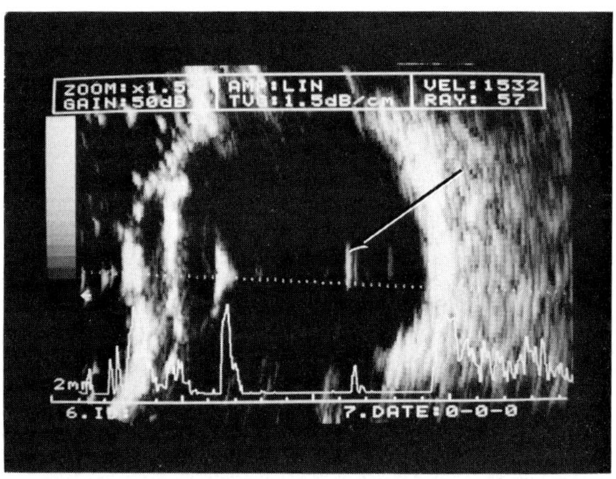

Fig. 2-18. Contact scan of an eye demonstrating the balloon stand-off with good definition of the anterior segment but a reduplication artifact *(arrow)* of the anterior segment in the vitreous.

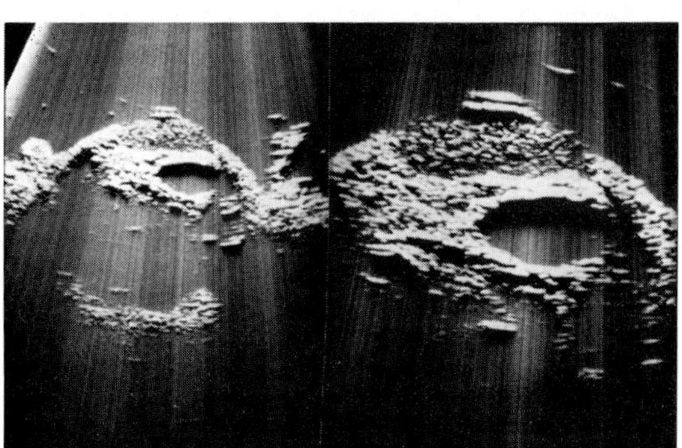

Fig. 2-19. B-scan ultrasonogram showing a hyphema and a dislocated but intact lens.

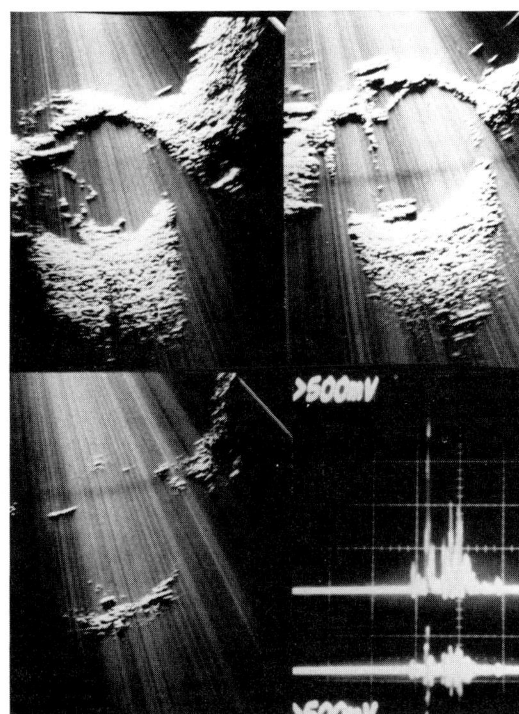

Fig. 2-20. B-scan ultrasonogram of an eye in which an intraocular foreign body is resting on the retina after having penetrated the lens. The path of the foreign body is marked by a track of blood and fibrin extending from the disrupted posterior lens capsule. Lowered gain *(lower left)* and the A-scan *(lower right)* help demonstrate the high reflectivity of the foreign body.

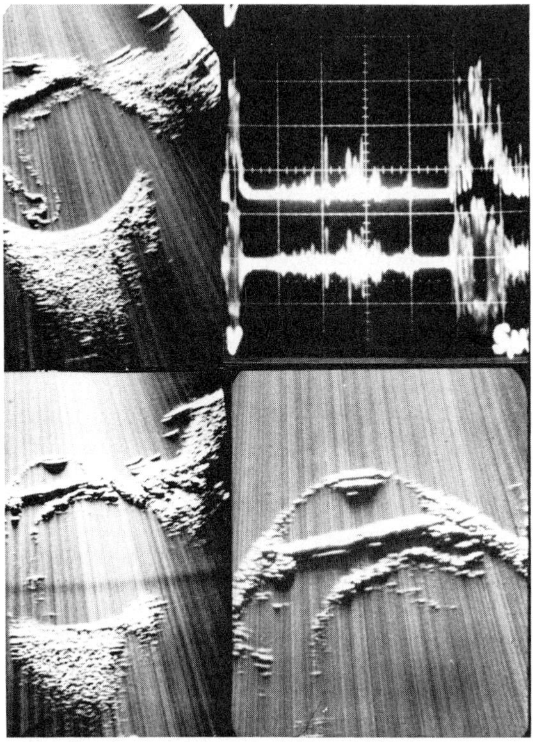

Fig. 2-21. B-scan ultrasonogram of an aphakic eye in which a hemorrhage has created an acoustic density along the posterior hyaloid face. Having the patient move the eye will allow the vitreous to sway and move away from the optic nerve, aiding in differentiating it from a detached retina and demonstrating any "tethered" or potential traction areas on the retina.

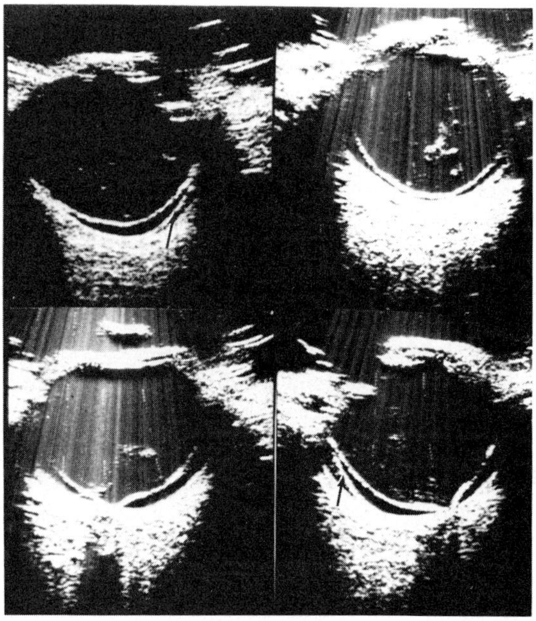

Fig. 2-22. B-scan ultrasonogram of a globe with vitreous hemorrhage, retinal detachment, and choroidal detachment (*arrow, upper left* and *lower right*). The retina and choroid have similar acoustic properties but can be differentiated by shape and attachments.

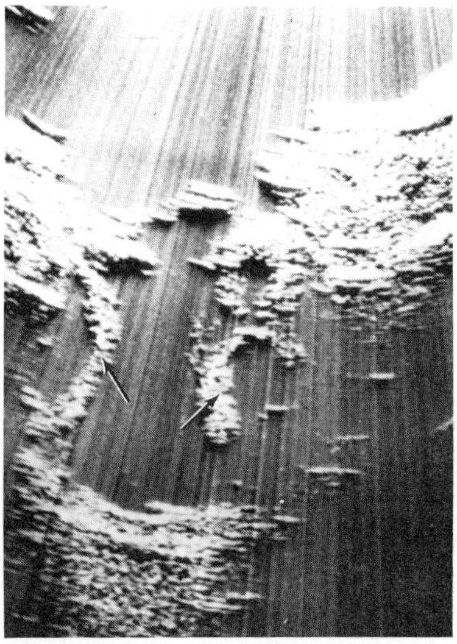

Fig. 2-23. B-scan ultrasonogram showing a traumatized globe with vitreous hemorrhage and large choroidal detachments *(arrows)* that end posteriorly at the vortex veins and extend anteriorly to the iris root.

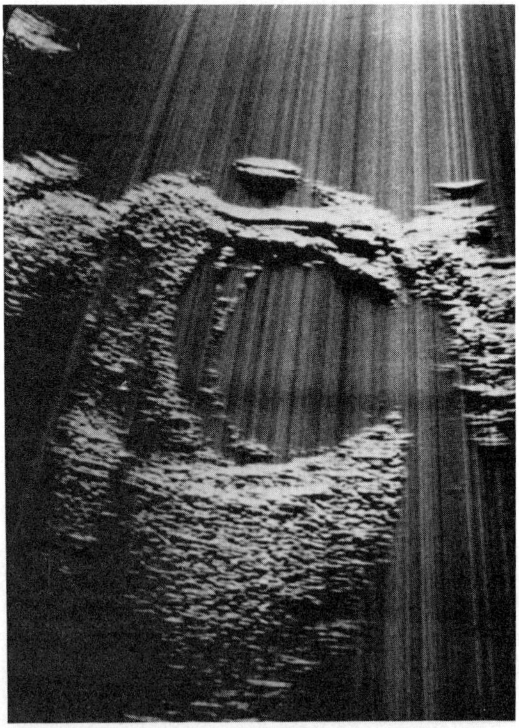

Fig. 2-24. B-scan ultrasonogram of an aphakic globe and a massive choroidal elevation that is acoustically clear. The clotted blood was easily drained from this area during surgery.

membrane, but on occasion a retinal detachment can resemble the outline of a choroidal detachment. Prime features are attachment to the optic nerve, high reflectivity along its entire course (best corroborated with the A-scan, where it should be as reflective—that is, of equal amplitude—as the posterior ocular wall), and typically a thin, uniform line on B-scan (Fig. 2-22).[35-37]

A choroidal detachment is an important diagnosis because it may alter the surgical decision about the choice of infusion technique. The vitreoretinal surface is highly reflective, as with a detached retina, but the detached structure does not extend to the optic nerve posteriorly like a retinal detachment and often, *unlike* a retinal detachment, extends anterior to the ora serrata into the ciliary body (Figs. 2-23 and 2-24). Blood can usually be seen in the suprachoroidal space and, with dynamic scanning (i.e., having the patient move the eye), can be examined for fluidity, the presence of which can be a useful presurgical observation.[34,35]

One of the main applications of ultrasound is in the *localization* of ocular foreign bodies. The CT scan and x-ray generally excel at detecting foreign bodies, but ultrasound excels at localizing the foreign body relative to the ocular coats and demonstrating the soft-tissue changes. Glass and metallic foreign bodies are very reflective and appear as bright areas on the B-scan (Fig. 2-25). The A-scan can confirm this heightened reflectance, as can slowly lowering the gain on the B-scan (Fig. 2-20). Foreign bodies have such high reflectance that they appear to absorb sound, and they often produce an anechoic zone behind them that resembles an echo-free "pointer" extending into the orbital fat—sometimes resembling an optic nerve shadow. Shotgun pellets and BBs produce an unusual ringing artifact that can extend into the anechoic zone like a comet tail (Fig. 2-26).

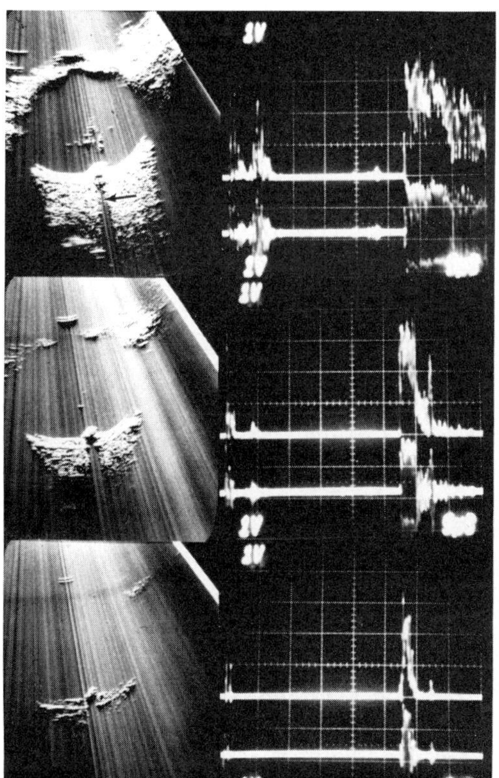

Fig. 2-25. B- and A-scan ultrasonograms of an eye with a metallic intraocular foreign body resting on the retina. An acoustic shadow *(arrow)* is created behind the foreign body, resembling a nerve shadow. The A-scans demonstrate the high reflectivity of the foreign body relative to the surrounding tissues as gain is decreased.

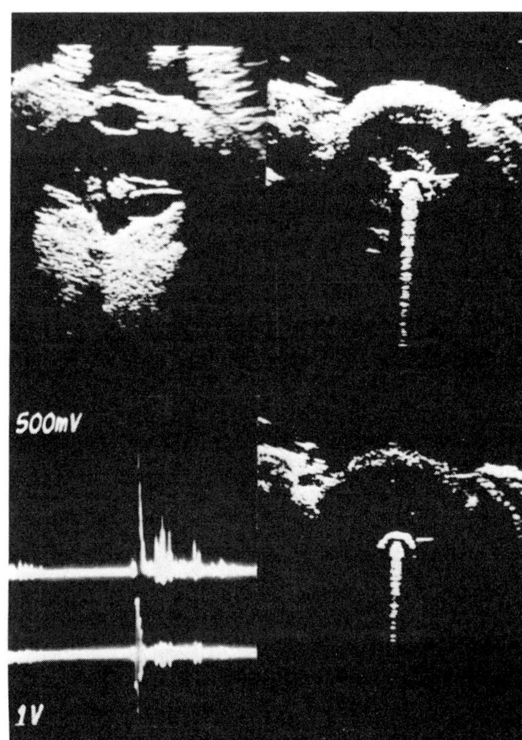

Fig. 2-26. B- and A-scan ultrasonograms of an intraocular BB demonstrating the cometlike tail of ringing artifacts produced by the BB. The A-scan shows the high initial reflectivity of the BB.

Contact ultrasound is also useful to have available in the operating room. When used with a sterile cover (such as a rubber balloon or glove with saline inside), it can be helpful in evaluating a repaired globe that could not be evaluated preoperatively because of the large size of the laceration. Preoperative or intraoperative ultrasound can assist in determining the extent of repair to be performed during the primary procedure. This may be uniquely helpful when a foreign body is still in the eye because it can show the location of the foreign body relative to the retina and even its motility when it is rocked or jiggled by a magnetic field.[36]

MAGNETIC RESONANCE IMAGING

Magnetic resonance imaging (MRI) of protons of the eye and orbit, particularly using surface coil technology,[38] provides superior tissue definition and, from an imaging point of view, would be the best technique for trauma evaluation save for the ferromagnetic nature of the majority of retained foreign bodies.[36,39,40] The potential for tissue damage from movement of a ferromagnetic foreign body in the intense field of the magnet precludes use of MRI as a screening technique,[41] even though some investigators have shown in experimental systems that only large-volume ferrous foreign bodies move in the magnetic field.[42]

If plain film, CT, and a careful history effectively preclude the possibility of a retained magnetic foreign body, MRI may be used for nonmetallic foreign-body detection and localization and ocular soft tissue and orbital imaging. In experimental series, MRI has been shown to detect a wide variety of vegetable, plastic, and glass foreign bodies in the eye, orbit, and adnexa.[43,44] With the use of surface coils, orbital imaging of concussive trauma with high resolution is also possible.[45]

The evaluation of the MR image is often considered a daunting exercise by the inexperienced, probably for two reasons: (1) several tissue parameters—proton density, proton motion, and relaxation times T1 and T2—affect MR images, rather than one, as in the case of x-ray techniques, or two, as in the case of ultrasound, and (2) these parameters are displayed in images that reflect various weights and combinations of the parameters. It is important to remember that the gray-scale encoding for a given image may be a combination of these parameters and that the pixel intensity of any given tissue in any image is relative to the general signal intensity in the image (because of autoscaling of pixel intensity) and does not represent absolute tissue values. Hence, terms such as *isointensity*, *hypointensity*, and *hyperintensity* are used to describe various differential tissue relationships.

For clinical examination, TI-weighted (short TR, short TE) and T2-weighted (long TR, long TE) spin-echo images are the most widely used, although the exact pulse repetition/echo delay (TR/TE) ratios used to obtain the weighting (contribution of the relaxation parameter to the image intensity) are not standardized. A variety of images can be obtained from H^+ MRI, including proton density–weighted images, T1 and T2 mapped images, inversion recovery sequence images, and gradient-echo images. (See texts of MRI methodology[46-48] for an in-depth exposition.) Used in combination or in a multiecho sequence, the images provide a good anatomic view of the eye and orbit and the tissue differential information needed in most cases.

The resolution and image quality in MR images depend on a complex series of system- and operator-dependent factors including signal/noise ratio, field of view, sampling matrix size, and magnetic field strength.[49] Signal/noise ratio is a function of several factors, including the number of affected protons in a sample area, which decreases proportionally when voxel size is reduced; the field intensity of the magnet; and the system's receiver characteristics. Changes in field of view also alter affected proton density and hence signal/noise ratio, which can be improved in a finite manner by signal-averaging over several sequences. This is important when using the thin-slice thicknesses needed for eye and orbit evaluation. Another system-dependent factor to consider when viewing MR images is the geometric distortion induced by the gradient fields in the magnet; in a poorly tuned system they may affect image quality significantly.

The T1-weighted sequence provides the most contrast and detail for ocular and orbital imaging. Fat, with a short T1, has the highest signal intensity. The lens capsule outline, anterior uvea, and iris plane are approximately isointense with the aqueous humor, with less signal intensity than fat. The vitreous, optic nerve, and lens body are isointense at still lower signal intensity. The recti muscles and scleral

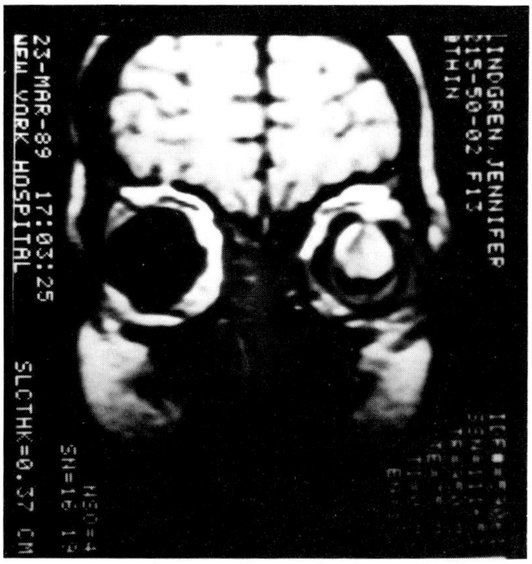

Fig. 2-27. Magnetic resonance images demonstrating typical intensity profiles of ocular and orbital tissues on *(left)* T1- and *(right)* T2-weighted images. Note the relatively high intensity of the vitreous in the T2-weighted image and the well-circumscribed orbital tumor.

and cortical bone are relatively hypointense in the image.

In the normal T2-weighted image of the eye and orbit, the vitreous and aqueous have a long T2 and the highest signal intensity if the image is sufficiently T2 weighted. The fat pad has an intermediate T2 and the next highest signal intensity. The optic nerve and muscles are isointense at a lower signal intensity. The lens appears hypointense because of a short T2 and the relative hyperintensity of the vitreous. Fig. 2-27 demonstrates T1- and T2-weighted images of a renal carcinoma metastatic to the orbit. The easiest way to distinguish between the two images, if the TR/TE numbers are not printed on the scan, is to look for the hyperintense vitreous that denotes a T2-weighted image.

Evaluation of the trauma case involves pattern recognition based on changes in ocular and orbital conformation with additional differential information provided by differing parameter-weighted images. In the eye, retinal detachment and subretinal fluid are hyperintense to the vitreous on a T1-weighted image and slightly hyperintense on a T2-weighted image.[50] The MRI appearance of vitreous or subretinal hemorrhage depends on the age of the hemorrhage (because the paramagnetic breakdown products of blood exhibit different T1 and T2 relaxation times) and on the field strength of the magnet.[51] Very fresh hemorrhage may be difficult to distinguish on MRI with both T1- and T2-weighted images. For midfield-strength magnets, as the deoxyhemoglobin converts into methemoglobin, the T1 and T2 relaxation times shorten and lengthen, respectively, causing the hemorrhage to appear intense on both T1 and T2 images. When methemoglobin converts to hemosiderin, the opposite occurs, causing hypointensity on both T1- and T2-weighted images.

In standard spin-echo images, local field inhomogeneities caused by the magnet or inherent in the tissue are not shown. For most applications this is an advantage of the spin-echo technique, allowing for a stable image. In the imaging of hemorrhage, however, it does not allow a unique physical property of hemorrhages—magnetic susceptibility–induced field inhomogeneities—to be seen. Another echo sequence, the gradient echo technique, shows local field inhomogeneities resulting from breakdown of the paramagnetic elements in blood. This technique has been used with success in intracranial hemorrhage imaging[52,53] and should be helpful in both intraocular and orbital trauma.

In the orbit, changes in the normal anatomic pattern are again the major diagnostic tool. Coronal and sagittal sections should be taken as needed. The thinnest possible slices should be obtained, as limited by scanning time, motion artifacts, and patient cooperation. There is a misconception that cortical bone is not imaged by proton MRI. This is not the case. The proton density in bone is low, so the signal intensity from bone is low, hence its dark appearance on MR images, but the tendency to consider low signal from an area as lack of definition does not mean that MRI is not useful in imaging various orbital fractures. With the hyperintensity of the orbital fat pad on proton MRI, orbital fractures are well visualized.

Soft-tissue changes in the orbit, including injury to the extraocular muscles and optic nerve, can at times be obscured by the relatively high intensity of the fat signal. In these cases, techniques such as short inversion time recovery sequences, which allow selective suppression of the signal from a tissue (in this case, orbital fat) by choosing an appropriate inversion recovery time, may be of use.[54] The muscle pattern and optic nerve configuration can be well delineated.

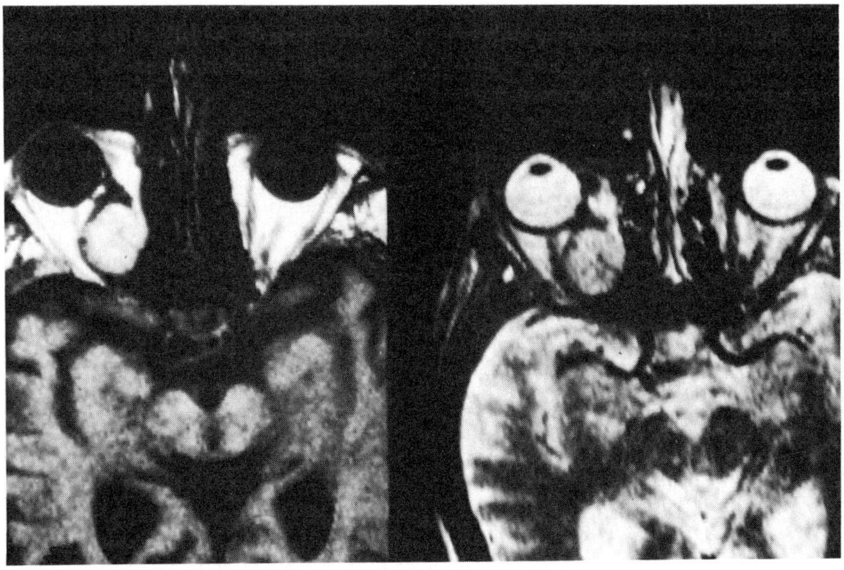

Fig. 2-28. Magnetic resonance image after repair of ruptured globe reveals intact scleral contour of silicone oil–filled eye. Silicone produces an acoustic distortion, which, like air, renders the ultrasound examination relatively useless.

In summary, MRI is less useful in trauma evaluation than the combination of CT and ultrasound for one primary reason: a magnetic foreign body, if present, could be dislodged and produce further damage to the eye. When no foreign body is present, however, MRI may have a definite utility. One advantage is in postoperative evaluation of globes into which silicone or perfluorocarbon liquid may have been injected. These compounds greatly distort the B-scan ultrasonography examination because of their low sound velocity. With T1- and T2-weighted imaging, the difference between silicone and blood is striking. A globe with choroidal blood into which silicone was injected can be inspected to permit postoperative determination of globe integrity, as in Fig. 2-28, taken after repair of a 22-mm superior scleral laceration between ora and optic nerve. In almost all cases, ocular and orbital imaging should use a surface coil if available. The increased resolution it affords in the cooperative patient can make the difference between making and missing a clinically relevant finding.

References

1. Williams C: A case of extraction of a bit of copper from the vitreous where x-rays helped to locate the metal, Trans Am Ophthalmol Soc 7:708-710, 1894-1896.
2. Clark CF: A question as to the location of a minute fragment of steel in the eye determined by roentgen rays—successful removal by the electromagnet, Trans Am Ophthalmol Soc 7:711-715, 1894-1896.
3. Zizmor Z and Noyck AM: Orbital trauma. In Newton TH and Potts DG, editors: Radiology of the skull and brain, vol 1, book 2, St Louis, 1974, The CV Mosby Co, 541-558.
4. Vignaud J, Claude C, and Mink J: Roentgen anatomy of the orbit. In Arger PH, editor: Orbital roentgenology, New York, 1977, John Wiley, 2-27.
5. Rao VM and Gonzalez CF: Plain film radiography and polytomography of the orbit. In Gonzalez CF, Becker MH, and Flanagan JC, editors: Diagnostic imaging in ophthalmology, New York, 1986, Springer-Verlag, 1-17.
6. Comberg W: Ein Hilfsgerat für mein Verfahren der Rontgenlokalisation und einige Bemerkungen über die Technik, Arch für Ophthalmol 124:665-667, 1930.
7. Pfeiffer RL: Localization of intraocular foreign bodies by means of the contact lens, Arch Ophthalmol 32:261-266, 1944.
8. Coleman DJ and Trokel SL: A protocol for B-scan and radiographic foreign body localization, Am J Ophthalmol 71:84-89, 1971.
9. Sweet WM: Improved apparatus for localizing foreign bodies in the eyeball by the Roentgen rays, Arch Roentgen Soc 14:170-176, 1909.

10. Runyan TE and Penner R: Comparison of localization of orbital foreign bodies by radiologic and ultrasonic methods, Arch Ophthalmol 81:512-517, 1969.
11. Lloyd GA: Radiology of the orbit, Philadelphia, 1975, WB Saunders, 197-210.
12. Thorpe HE: Foreign bodies in the anterior chamber angle: their management with the aid of gonioscopy, Am J Ophthalmol 61:1339-1343; 1966.
13. Duke-Elder S and MacFaul PA: Mechanical injuries. In Duke-Elder S, editor: System of ophthalmology, vol XIV, part 1, St Louis, 1972, The CV Mosby Co, 572-616.
14. Hartmann E and Gilles E: Roentgenographic diagnosis in ophthalmology, Philadelphia, 1959, JB Lippincott, 128-165.
15. Radon J: Uber die Bestimmung von Funktionen durch ihre Integralwerte langs gewisser Mannigfaltigkeiten, Ber Saechsische Akad Wiss 29:262-279, 1917.
16. Zonneveld F et al: Normal direct multiplanar CT anatomy of the orbit with correlative anatomic cryosections. In Mafee MF, editor: Imaging in ophthalmology, part 1, Philadelphia, 1987, WB Saunders, 381-407.
17. Glenn WJ: Image reconstruction and display techniques for CT scan data: thin transverse and reconstructed coronal planes, Invest Radiol 403-416, 1975.
18. Zinreich SJ: Computed tomographic three-dimensional localization and compositional evaluation of intraocular and orbital foreign bodies, Arch Ophthalmol 104:1477-1482, 1986.
19. Herman GT: Three-dimensional imaging on a CT or MR scanner, J Comput Assist Tomogr 12:450-458, 1988.
20. Kadir S, Arnow S, and Davis KR: The use of computerized tomography in the detection of intra-orbital foreign bodies, Comput Tomogr 1:151-156, 1977.
21. Kollartis C et al: Detection of orbital and intraocular foreign bodies by computerized tomography, Ophthalmologica 8(1):45-53,1977.
22. Mandelcorn MS and Brown M: Computed axial tomography localization of intra-orbital foreign body, Can J Ophthalmol 13:213-215, 1978.
23. Kalender WA, Hebel R, and Ebersberger J: Reduction of CT artifacts caused by metallic implants, Radiology 164:576-577, 1987.
24. Koornneef L and Zonneveld FW: The role of direct multiplanar high-resolution CT in the assessment and management of orbital trauma. In Mafee MF, editor: Imaging in ophthalmology, part II, Philadelphia, 1987, WB Saunders, 753-766.
25. Gilbard SM et al: Orbital blowout fractures: the prognostic significance of computed tomography, Ophthalmology 92:1523-1528, 1985.
26. Coleman DJ, Lizzi FL, and Jack RL: Ultrasonography of the eye and orbit, Philadelphia, 1977, Lea & Febiger, 376.
27. Simoni GJ and Coleman DJ: The use of contact B-scan ultrasound in the management of intraocular foreign bodies. Paper presented at the 32nd annual convention of the American Institute of Ultrasound in Medicine, New Orleans, 1987, 58.
28. Coleman DJ, Jack RL, and Franzen LA: High-resolution B-scan ultrasonography of the orbit. I. The normal orbit, Arch Ophthalmol 88:358-367, 1972.
29. Coleman DJ: Reliability of ocular and orbital diagnosis with B-scan ultrasound. II. Orbital diagnosis, Am J Ophthalmol 74:708-718, 1972.
30. Coleman DJ, Jack RL, and Franzen LA: Ultrasonography in ocular trauma, Am J Ophthalmol 75:279-288, 1973.
31. Coleman DJ and Franzen LA: Vitreous surgery: preoperative evaluation and prognostic value of ultrasonic display of vitreous, Arch Ophthalmol 92:375-381, 1974.
32. Coleman DJ: The role of vitrectomy in traumatic vitreopathy, Trans Am Acad Ophthalmol Otolaryngol 81:406-413, 1976.
33. Coleman DJ: Early vitrectomy in the management of the severely traumatized eye, Am J Ophthalmol 93:543-551, 1982.
34. Coleman DJ and Wilcox LM Jr: The choroid: its function, evaluation, and surgical management. In Transactions of the New Orleans Academy of Ophthalmology, St Louis, 1983, The CV Mosby Co, 1-24.
35. Coleman DJ, Dallow RL, and Smith ME: Immersion ultrasonography: simultaneous A-scan and B-scan, Int Ophthalmol Clin 19(4):67-102, 1979.
36. Coleman DJ et al: Management of intraocular foreign bodies, Ophthalmology 94:1647-1653, 1987.
37. Jack RL and Coleman DJ: Diagnosis of retinal detachments with B-scan ultrasonography, Can J Ophthalmol 8:10-18, 1973.
38. Schenk JF et al: Improved MR imaging of the orbit at 1.5T with surface coils, AJNR 6:193-196, 1985.
39. Percival SPB: A decade of intraocular foreign bodies, Br J Ophthalmol 56:462-468, 1972.
40. Schock JR and Adams D: Long-term visual acuity results after penetrating and perforating ocular injuries, Am J Ophthalmol 100:714-718, 1985.
41. Kelly WM et al: Ferromagnetism of intraocular foreign body causes unilateral blindness after magnetic resonance study, AJNR 7:243-245, 1986.

42. Williams S et al: Ferrous intraocular foreign bodies and magnetic resonance imaging, Am J Ophthalmol 105:398-401, 1988.
43. LoBue TD et al: Detection and localization of nonmetallic intraocular foreign bodies by magnetic resonance imaging. Arch Ophthalmol 106:260-261, 1988.
44. Wilson WB et al: Magnetic resonance imaging of nonmetallic orbital foreign bodies, Am J Ophthalmol 105:612-617, 1988.
45. Tonami H et al: Surface coil MR imaging of orbital blowout fractures: a comparison with reformatted CT, AJNR 8:445-449, 1987.
46. Partin CL et al, editors: Magnetic resonance imaging, ed 2, Philadelphia, 1988, WB Saunders.
47. Stark DD and Bradley WG, editors: Magnetic resonance imaging, St Louis, 1988, The CV Mosby Co.
48. Bushong SC: Magnetic resonance imaging: physical and biological principles, St Louis, 1988, The CV Mosby Co.
49. Wehrli FW and Kanal E: Orbital imaging: factors determining magnetic resonance imaging appearance. In Mafee MF, editor: Imaging in ophthalmology, part 1, Philadelphia, 1987, WB Saunders Co, 419-427.
50. Peyster RG et al: Intraocular tumors: evaluation with MR imaging, Radiology 168:773-779, 1988.
51. Bradley WG Jr and Schmidt PG: Effect of methemoglobin formation on the MR appearance of subarachnoid hemorrhage, Radiology 156:99-103, 1985.
52. Atlas SW et al: Intracranial hemorrhage: gradient-echo MR imaging at 1.5T, Radiology 168:803-807, 1988.
53. Seidenwurm D et al: Intracranial hemorrhagic lesions: evaluation with spin-echo and gradient-refocused MR imaging at 0.5 and 1.5T, Radiology 172:189-194, 1989.
54. Atlas SW et al: STIR MR imaging of the orbit, AJR 151:1025-1030, 1988.

CHAPTER 3

Preparation of the eye trauma patient for surgery

JAN KYLSTRA

Minimizing risk of further injury
- Mechanical factors
- Infectious factors

Maximizing surgical success
Decreasing risk to patient's health
Minimizing psychic trauma
Minimizing risk of legal involvement
Preoperative check list
References

Eye injuries present the ophthalmic surgeon with a unique set of management problems. These include the extreme variability of injury, the instability of the seriously injured eye and hence stringent time constraints, associated systemic injuries or illnesses, and medicolegal risks. Such considerations require a comprehensive and methodical approach to preoperative preparation.

Eye injuries are extremely variable and may involve every part of the eye, ocular adnexa, and orbit. The expertise needed to manage these problems potentially spans all ophthalmic subspecialties. An accurate assessment of the extent of damage before surgery is, therefore, crucial so that appropriate consultation and necessary equipment can be obtained.

Instability is the second unique problem presented by the eye trauma patient. One inadvertent sneeze, squeeze, cough, or eye rub can mean disaster. Optimal trauma management requires an attempt to stabilize and protect the eye while awaiting surgery.

A corollary of the problem of instability, and one of the hallmarks of trauma management, is time limitation. For a successful outcome, most trauma surgery must be performed shortly after injury. This makes careful presurgical preparation much more difficult. The use of a preoperative checklist can be quite helpful for surgeons who do not routinely deal with eye trauma.

Another problem faced by the eye trauma surgeon is the possible coexistence of systemic injury or preexisting illness. These systemic problems must be suspected, diagnosed, and managed promptly.

An ever-present factor in eye trauma management is the high risk to the surgeon of being involved in a subsequent legal proceeding. It is prudent, therefore, to be particularly careful in documenting examination findings and patient care, paying detailed attention to informed consent, and communicating with patient and family.

Five major goals of presurgical preparation

of the eye trauma patient are to: (1) minimize the risk of further injury while awaiting surgery, (2) maximize the chance of achieving surgical objectives, (3) minimize infectious risks and the risk to the patient's general health, (4) minimize the psychic trauma to the patient, and (5) minimize legal exposure.

MINIMIZING RISK OF FURTHER INJURY

Injured eyes can sustain further damage while awaiting surgery. Causes of further injury include mechanical factors and infectious agents. Attempts must be made to anticipate and avoid dangerous situations.

Mechanical Factors

The globe that has sustained a corneoscleral laceration is at risk of further damage due to extrusion of intraocular tissues through the wound. A number of factors, including external pressure on the eye, increased intraocular volume, and traction on already prolapsed intraocular tissue, can precipitate tissue extrusion.

A rigid eye shield diminishes the risk of external pressure on a lacerated globe (Fig. 3-1). Other steps include the following preventative measures: (1) have trained personnel accompany the patient during diagnostic x-ray studies to prevent inadvertent ocular manipulation when the shield is removed; (2) take care to minimize pressure on the globe when preparing the eye in the operating room; (3) use lid sutures or a Jaffe-type lid speculum to provide lid retraction during surgery; and (4) use general anesthesia to prevent retrobulbar hemorrhage and to prevent globe compression from the increased orbital volume caused by the anesthetic itself (see Chapter 4).

Increased intraocular volume can result from a suprachoroidal hemorrhage or simply from increased choroidal blood volume due to a Valsalva type of maneuver. To prevent this, blood pressure can be controlled through judicious use of pain medication, sedatives, or antihypertensive agents. Vomiting or coughing can be minimized by appropriate drugs. *No* pain medication or sedative should be administered until an informed consent to surgery has been obtained and documented; this includes consent to the use of general anesthesia, which often must be obtained by the anesthesiology staff.

Traction on partially prolapsed intraocular contents can be prevented by administering a facial nerve block to eliminate squeezing or blinking. The O'Brien method of injecting 2 to 3 ml of 2% lidocaine just anterior to the condyloid process of the mandible avoids the lid swelling and involuntary lid squeezing associated with the more commonly used van Lint technique (see Chapter 4).[1]

Of course, despite all these preventative measures, the eye may still suffer further damage while awaiting surgery. This is particularly

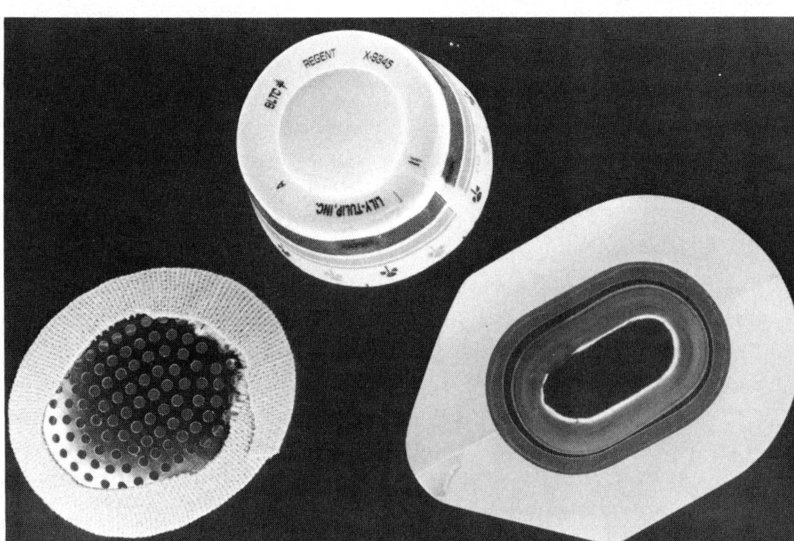

Fig. 3-1. Eye shields for protection of the lacerated eye.

true in children or mentally incompetent adults who may insert a finger under the tightest shield, thereby forcing the prolapse of intraocular contents through the wound. Thus, prompt surgical repair of the injury is necessary. Few studies have been carried out to determine the influence of surgical delay on visual outcome. One study found no difference in visual outcome as long as primary repair was carried out within 36 hours.[2] In general, however, 24 hours is a more reasonable time frame except in injuries involving children or mentally incompetent adults. These cases should be dealt with as soon as possible.

If presurgical delays are to be minimized, it is imperative that the patient have nothing to eat or drink. Most anesthesiologists are reluctant to anesthetize eye trauma patients who have consumed food or beverages within 6 hours of surgery because the risk of aspiration pneumonitis is unacceptably high.[3]

Infectious Factors

Posttraumatic endophthalmitis is a dread complication of perforating eye injury. Various studies have estimated its incidence at 2% to 7%.[4] The prognosis for eyes that develop endophthalmitis in this setting is quite poor.[5] Because of these considerations, it is prudent to treat all penetrating eye injuries with prophylactic antibiotics. Unfortunately, there have been no reports clearly showing that prophylactic antibiotic treatment is useful or that a particular regimen of intravenous, topical, or subconjunctival drugs is best. Subconjunctival injections should probably be avoided, however, since they may cause lid squeezing and could deliver concentrated drug intracamerally.

A reasonable set of guidelines for antibiotic prophylaxis must be based on knowledge of the most common pathogens, the antibiotic sensitivities of locally prevalent strains, the potential toxicity (both ocular and systemic) of various antibiotics, and the current standard of care. The most common organisms isolated from posttraumatic endophthalmitis cases are *Staphylococcus*, *Bacillus*, and *Streptococcus* species, gram-negative rods, and various fungi.[4-6] Endophthalmitis due to gram-negative bacteria and *Bacillus* species has a particularly poor prognosis. The combination of a cephalosporin (such as cefazolin) and an aminoglycoside (such as gentamicin) would theoretically cover most gram-positive and gram-negative organisms that commonly cause posttraumatic endophthalmitis. However, neither type of antibiotic is effective against *Bacillus*. The addition of clindamycin as a third antibiotic or the substitution of vancomycin for the cephalosporin might provide adequate coverage against *Bacillus*. Unfortunately, however, clindamycin carries the risk of pseudomembranous colitis, a potentially lethal disease, and vancomycin enhances the nephrotoxicity of aminoglycosides.[7] Chapter 23 presents a detailed discussion of posttraumatic endophthalmitis.

By what route and for how long should prophylactic antibiotics be administered? The conventional approach is to administer intravenous antibiotics, usually a combination of cephalosporin and aminoglycoside, starting before surgery and continuing for 3 to 5 days postoperatively. Topical antibiotics may also be used.[4-6,8,9] Until carefully controlled studies demonstrate conclusively that a particular prophylactic antibiotic regimen is superior, the following approach is reasonable. To avoid intracameral administration, use *topical antibiotic* drops when no uveal prolapse or only minimal iris prolapse is seen. Cefazolin (133 mg/ml) and gentamicin (14 mg/ml) are given every 2 hours until surgery. Always use *systemic antibiotics*. For example, cefazolin (1 g intravenously every 8 hours) and gentamicin (a 100-mg loading dose, then 80 mg intravenously every 8 hours) are given to the average healthy adult. As suggested by O'Day et al.,[10] if the injury is farm related, and especially if an intraocular foreign body is present, clindamycin (500 mg intravenously every 8 hours) may be given as well, because these patients are at higher risk for developing *Bacillus* infections.[6,10] (See Chapter 23 for detailed antibiotic protocols.)

Antibiotics are initiated in the emergency ward and as soon as the diagnosis of ruptured globe is made.

MAXIMIZING SURGICAL SUCCESS

The keys to successful surgical management of eye trauma are expertise and equipment. Few eye trauma surgeons are experienced in managing all types of ocular injuries, and few operating facilities can provide all types of equipment as well as corneal-scleral donor tissue at a moment's notice. It is of utmost importance, therefore, to anticipate the various surgical maneuvers that will be needed and to plan accordingly. Expert consultation should be obtained, if needed, before the patient is anesthetized. Special equipment should be requested before entering the operating room.

Most lacerated or ruptured eyes can be repaired by well-trained anterior-segment surgeons; however, certain injuries require special expertise. The most common situation requiring subspecialty consultation is the case of a posterior segment intraocular foreign body. Most intraocular foreign bodies should be removed at the time of primary repair. This often involves pars plana vitrectomy with or without the use of magnets (see Chapter 21). Thus, one of the most important aspects of preoperative preparation of the eye trauma patient involves ascertaining whether an intraocular foreign body is present (see Chapter 2). This determination should be made as early in the evaluation as possible because it may take considerable time to mobilize a vitreoretinal surgeon and the necessary operating room equipment.

Complicated lid and orbital injuries requiring surgical treatment should, if possible, be repaired at the time of globe repair. However, if expert consultants are not available within 24 hours, globe repair should be carried out and other definitive lid and orbital surgery deferred.

Large stellate corneal lacerations or lacerations with massive tissue loss may require patch grafting or, rarely, primary penetrating keratoplasty. This should be anticipated, and appropriate donor tissue and equipment should be arranged. Whenever complex stellate corneal lacerations are diagnosed, cyanoacrylate tissue adhesive and a bandage soft contact lens should be available in the operating room (see Chapter 13).

DECREASING RISK TO PATIENT'S HEALTH

In preparing the eye trauma patient for surgery, one must remember that life as well as vision may be threatened. This threat is due to two factors: the risk of anesthesia and the possibility of serious occult injury.

General anesthesia and, to a lesser extent, local anesthesia carry a small but definite risk of death or serious complication. This is particularly true if the patient has preexisting cardiopulmonary disease. However, unlike elective surgery, trauma surgery allows little time to optimize the patient's medical condition preoperatively. Prompt consultation with the appropriate medical specialist will decrease the risk of anesthesia and minimize any delay in carrying out the surgery.

Serious eye injuries can occur in the setting of multisystem trauma such as that caused by a motor vehicle accident or an assault. In these cases, obvious life-threatening injuries must be stabilized before eye problems are addressed, but eye trauma surgeons should always be aware of the possibility of serious occult injuries in their patients. Appropriate medical or surgical consultation is indicated if there is any suspicion of neurologic or cardiovascular problems.

Another potential life-threatening problem facing the eye trauma patient is infection with *Clostridium tetani*. Although there are no reported cases of tetanus following purely ocular injury, the current standard is to treat ocular injuries like other soft tissue injuries and administer the appropriate tetanus prophylaxis (see Appendix).[9,11]

MINIMIZING PSYCHIC TRAUMA

Blindness is among the most feared of medical catastrophes. Eye trauma, with its very real threat of loss of an eye, can be psychologically devastating. The sudden nature of trauma allows the patient no time to adjust to the reality of the situation, and adjustment is often made more difficult by feelings of guilt or denial on the part of the patient or family. The patient's fear of blindness coupled with a reluctance to accept the reality of the situation often lead the eye trauma surgeon to commit two kinds of mistakes: underemphasizing the extent of the injury and enucleating an eye before the patient has had a chance to accept the necessity of the procedure. Both of these errors can lead to an angry, depressed, and potentially litigious patient. Because they fear malpractice litigation, some clinicians may commit errors of the opposite extreme: exaggerating the severity of the injury and deferring primary enucleation in even the most irreversibly injured eyes.

In young healthy patients whose eyes can be surgically reapproximated, enucleation should be initially deferred regardless of the visual potential. The anesthesia risk in this group of patients is low, and the psychological benefit of having time to come to grips with the situation is great. On the other hand, in a sick elderly patient, severe trauma resulting in no light perception and posterior segment disruption certainly justifies primary enucleation. The anesthesia risk is too high to offset the psychological benefit of delay.

MINIMIZING RISK OF LEGAL INVOLVEMENT

Ocular trauma is associated with a high rate of litigation. In a series of 170 cases of alleged malpractice in ophthalmology, 26% were associated with trauma.[12] In Kylstra's unpublished series of 90 consecutive surgical cases of suspected globe rupture, 19% of the 78 patients who were followed for more than 1 month initiated legal proceedings.

How can the surgeon reduce the risk of being involved in a malpractice suit or voluminous legal paperwork? In eye trauma management, as in all other areas of medicine, the answer remains thorough documentation, adequate informed consent, good communication with patient and family, and discussion with consultants when needed.[12]

One should treat each patient's medical record as if it were going to be scrutinized in court. The uninjured eye should be carefully and thoroughly examined. Any evidence of ocular inflammation should be recorded in anticipation of a future claim of sympathetic ophthalmia. Photographs of the injured eye should be obtained, if possible. Foreign-body x-rays and CT scans should be performed in most cases and reviewed by a radiologist, even if there is a low probability of an intraocular foreign body.

The informed consent discussion should take place before administering pain medication or sedatives. Family members and a witness should be present if possible. The discussion should include the possibility of late-onset complications such as endophthalmitis and retinal detachment, the small possibility of sympathetic ophthalmia, and the guarded prognosis. Consent should be obtained for all measures necessary to repair the eye and might also include consent for enucleation (see Chapter 37).

PREOPERATIVE CHECK LIST

Optimal presurgical management of the eye trauma patient should proceed in a logical series of steps: (1) determine that surgery is needed; (2) stabilize the eye; (3) obtain informed consent; (4) administer pain medication and tetanus prophylaxis; (5) obtain medical and anesthesia clearance as needed; (6) organize the surgical team (including corneal, vitreoretinal, and oculoplastic specialists, as needed); and (7) request appropriate equipment. Specific steps for the preoperative preparation of the injured eye patient are presented in the following checklist.

1. Apply rigid eye shield.
2. Check NPO status.
3. Administer antiemetics as needed.
4. Administer facial nerve block as needed.
5. Begin intravenous and topical antibiotics.
6. Notify anesthesiology and operating room.
7. Obtain informed consent for surgery (including enucleation) and anesthesia.
8. Administer pain medications and sedatives as needed.
9. Administer tetanus prophylaxis
10. Perform preoperative lab tests.
11. Assess medical status and obtain consultants if needed.
12. Determine if intraocular foreign body is present, and notify retina specialist if needed.
13. Determine if other ophthalmic consultants will be needed, and notify them.
14. Arrange for special equipment in operating room
    a. *All cases:* operating microscope, standard cataract set, viscoelastics, intraocular acetylcholine, vitreous sweep, muscle hooks, appropriate sutures, disposable Wheeler knife, orbital retractor
    b. *Canalicular involvement:* silicone intubation set
    c. *Stellate corneal laceration:* tissue adhesive, donor tissue, therapeutic soft contact lens
    d. *Foreign body:* Bronson magnet, rare earth magnet, intraocular forceps
    e. *Lens involvement:* irrigation-aspiration equipment, cannulas, vitrectomy instrument, phacoemulsification unit

References

1. Frayer WC and Jacoby J: Local anesthesia. In Duane TD and Jaeger EA, editors: Clinical ophthalmology, vol 5, Philadelphia, 1988, JB Lippincott.
2. Barr CC: Prognostic factors in corneoscleral lacerations, Arch Ophthalmol 101:919-924, 1983.
3. Snow JC: Anesthesia in otolaryngology and ophthalmology, New York, 1981, Appleton-Century-Crofts.
4. Parrish CM and O'Day DM: Traumatic endophthalmitis, Int Ophthalmol Clin 27:112-119, 1987.
5. Affeldt JC et al: Microbial endophthalmitis resulting from ocular trauma, Ophthalmology 94:407-413, 1987.
6. Brinton GS et al: Posttraumatic endophthalmitis, Arch Ophthalmol 102:547-550, 1984.
7. Gilman AG et al, editors: Goodman and Gilman's the pharmacological basis of therapeutics, ed 7, New York, 1985, Macmillan.
8. Miller D and Stegman R: Treatment of penetrating anterior segment trauma. In Miller D and Stegman R, editors: Treatment of anterior segment trauma, Montreal, 1986, Medicopea International.
9. Deutsch TA and Feller DB: Paton and Goldberg's management of ocular injuries, ed 2, Philadelphia, 1985, WB Saunders.
10. O'Day DM et al: The problem of *Bacillus* species infection with special emphasis on the virulence of *Bacillus cereus*, Ophthalmology 88:833-838, 1981.
11. Advisory Committee for Immunization Practices (ACIP): Diphtheria, tetanus and pertussis: guidelines for vaccine prophylaxis and other preventive measures, MMWR 30:392-396, 401-407, 1981.
12. Bettman JW: The medicolegal implications of the management of trauma. In Freeman HM, editor: Ocular trauma, New York, 1979, Appleton-Century-Crofts.

CHAPTER 4

Anesthesia in ocular and orbital trauma

KATHRYN E. McGOLDRICK

Anesthesia for ocular injuries
- Topical
  - Indications
  - Agents
- Subconjunctival injections
  - Indications
  - Agents
  - Complications and contraindications
- Retrobulbar anesthesia and facial nerve akinesia
  - Indications
  - Techniques
  - Complications
- General anesthesia
  - Indications
  - Anesthesia management

Anesthesia for lid and orbital injuries
- Local lid blocks
  - Indications
  - Techniques
- General anesthesia for orbital injuries
  - Indications
  - Anesthesia management

References

A number of anesthesia techniques are appropriate for the eye trauma patient. This chapter will discuss the use of local anesthetics, given topically, subconjunctivally, as lid blocks, and as retrobulbar agents, and the use of general anesthesia in the setting of ocular and orbital trauma.

ANESTHESIA FOR OCULAR INJURIES

Topical

Indications

Topical anesthesia is given to facilitate ocular examination, diagnosis, and treatment. Topical anesthesia generally enables the removal of corneal foreign bodies and the exploration of conjunctival lacerations.

Agents

A variety of surface-active anesthetics are available. They all act with great rapidity and efficacy on mucosal surfaces but are relatively impotent on less permeable skin surfaces. These topical anesthetics are relatively toxic and should *not* be injected. Topical application of excessive amounts of these drugs may result in serious ocular surface problems and in systemic effects that can be life-threatening.

The currently popular topical anesthetics are tetracaine (Pontocaine), proparacaine (Ophthaine), and cocaine.

Tetracaine (Pontocaine). Solutions of 0.5% to 2% tetracaine, a derivative of para-aminobenzoic acid, may be instilled directly into the conjunctival sac. Onset of anesthesia may be noted within 15 seconds, and anesthesia lasts up to 25 minutes. Because repeated and prolonged application of tetracaine may precipitate epithelial damage and inhibit reepithelialization, topical anesthesia should never be prescribed for the patient's home use to alleviate pain from a corneal abrasion.

True allergy to tetracaine is extremely rare, although an occasional glaucoma patient may develop edematous, erythematous, pruritic lids and conjunctivitis following repeated use of topical tetracaine for tonometry.

Proparacaine (Ophthaine). Proparacaine, supplied in a 0.5% solution with additives of 0.2% chlorobutanol and 1:10,000 benzalkonium chloride, has an onset, duration, and intensity of anesthetic action similar to those of tetracaine. However, proparacaine causes less discomfort on instillation. The incidence of allergic phenomena with proparacaine is low. Patients allergic to tetracaine are not a priori allergic to proparacaine, and vice versa. The usual dose for foreign-body removal and tonometry is 1 to 2 drops of the 0.5% solution.

Cocaine. Cocaine, an ester-linked benzoic acid, was the first drug to be successfully used as a local anesthetic.[1] However, the newer synthetic topical anesthetics have largely replaced cocaine because of its corneal toxicity, sympathomimetic characteristics, and potential for abuse.

Excellent surface anesthesia is obtained by application of a 1% to 4% cocaine solution. Rate of onset is similar to that of tetracaine and proparacaine, but the duration of action of 2% cocaine is approximately 10 minutes.

A rather tenacious, but fallacious, clinical myth hypes the purportedly superior analgesic properties of cocaine.[2] As with all anesthetics, the potency of cocaine is dose related. For example, proparacaine 0.5% provides corneal and conjunctival anesthesia comparable to that of a 4% solution of cocaine, with considerably less corneal injury. Indeed, the epithelial damage produced by cocaine is significant; it is manifest by grayish corneal pits and irregularities and, not infrequently, large erosions.

Cocaine is the only local anesthetic that inherently produces vasoconstriction and shrinkage of mucous membranes. The usual maximum dose of cocaine in clinical practice for such procedures as dacryocystorhinostomy is 200 mg for a 70-kg adult, or 3 mg/kg. Although 1 g is considered to be the usual lethal dose for an adult, considerable variation exists. Furthermore, systemic reactions may appear with as little as 20 mg. It is obvious that meticulous attention must be paid to the volume used, because there is a narrow range between safety and toxicity and death.

By blocking the reuptake of endogenous norepinephrine, as well as the uptake of exogenous epinephrine, cocaine exerts an indirect sympathomimetic action. Hence, some pupillary dilation accompanies the use of ocular cocaine, although the pupil retains its ability to converge and to react to light. Meyers[3] emphasized that cocaine is contraindicated in hypertensives and in patients receiving such adrenergic-modifying drugs as guanethidine, reserpine, tricyclic antidepressants, and monoamine oxidase inhibitors. In addition, sympathomimetics such as epinephrine or phenylephrine should not be given with cocaine.

Subconjunctival Injections

Indications

Subconjunctival injections may be used to explore surface injuries requiring conjunctival incision, to remove nonperforating foreign bodies, and to allow for conjunctival suturing.

Agents

Local anesthetics used for subconjunctival injection must have a rapid onset, cause minimal tissue toxicity, and have a sufficient duration of action for the proposed procedure. Agents meeting these criteria to a greater or lesser degree include procaine (Novocaine), etidocaine (Duranest), lidocaine (Xylocaine), and bupivacaine (Marcaine); the last two are the most widely used. Procaine, available in concentrations of 0.5% to 4%, does not penetrate or diffuse well and has a rather brief duration of action.

Lidocaine may be administered in solutions of 1% to 4%; the former should be satisfactory for virtually all ophthalmic uses. Lidocaine has a rapid onset and provides reliable surgical anesthesia for 45 minutes to 1 hour. Although epinephrine is usually not added to local anesthetics injected subconjunctivally, its use will significantly prolong the duration of action of lidocaine. Not more than 4 mg/kg of lidocaine should be injected during 1 hour. Thus, for a 70-kg person, no more than 28 ml of 1% solution should be injected. A wide margin of safety should exist, since ophthalmic procedures rarely demand more than 10 to 15 ml. However, inadvertent intravenous injection or unusual patient sensitivity may markedly reduce the safe dose.

Etidocaine 1% is approximately four times as potent as lidocaine and has a rapid onset; its duration of action is approximately twice that of lidocaine.

Bupivacaine may be injected in a 0.5% or 0.75% solution. Bupivacaine may cause "burning" on injection and has a slow onset if used alone. For these reasons, bupivacaine 0.75% is commonly mixed with an equal volume of 1% lidocaine. The great advantage of bupivacaine is its lengthy duration of action, so combining bupivacaine with lidocaine allows rapid onset plus prolonged anesthesia and akinesia, exceeding 6 hours. The maximum dose of bupivacaine should not exceed 3 mg/kg. Hence, in a 70-kg adult, not more than 28 ml of 0.75% bupivacaine should be injected.

Complications and Contraindications

Great care must be exercised in the injection technique and in calculating the dose. The requisite resuscitative equipment and skilled personnel must be readily accessible whenever local anesthesia is given. Moreover, because epinephrine can produce vascular constriction and ecchymosis, it is usually not injected subconjunctivally. In addition, if a ruptured globe is suspected, subconjunctival injections should be avoided to prevent toxic intraocular doses.

Retrobulbar Anesthesia and Facial Nerve Akinesia

Indications

Retrobulbar anesthesia may be useful in ocular trauma, especially if there are contraindications to general anesthesia. Such contraindications, however, are extremely unusual. Indeed, the ophthalmologist will rarely administer retrobulbar anesthesia if a ruptured globe is suspected, since this maneuver may trigger prolapse of intraocular contents. Facial nerve akinesia produced by local injection may be indicated to permit complete ocular examination and to minimize lid compression of the globe.

Techniques

The technique of retrobulbar anesthesia will not be reviewed in this text; discussion will be restricted to useful techniques of lid akinesia in the trauma setting.

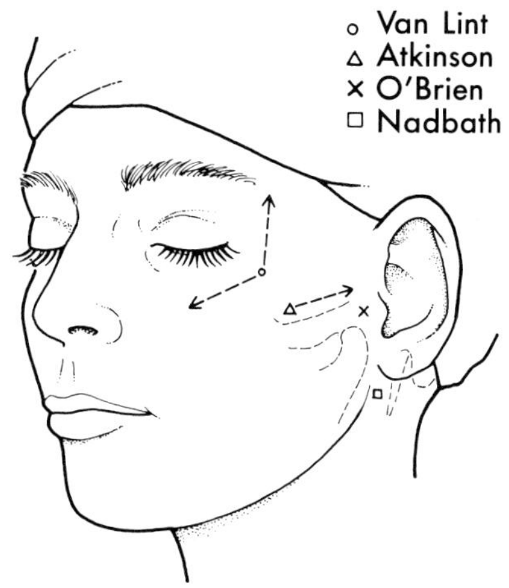

Fig. 4-1. Techniques for facial nerve akinesia.

Eyelid akinesia is obtained by blocking the branches of the facial nerve supplying the orbicularis muscle (Fig. 4-1). Since facial nerve block was first used for ophthalmic surgery by van Lint[4] in 1914, numerous methods have been described. All block the facial nerve either proximally or distally to its exit point from the skull via the stylohyoid foramen. Van Lint initially introduced the needle through facial skin, approximately 1 cm behind the intersection of a line extending temporally from the lower orbital rim and a line extending inferiorly from the temporal orbital rim to the level of the periosteum. The needle was then directed horizontally across the lower lid and the anesthetic injected as the needle was withdrawn. Without removing the needle from the skin, it was redirected along the lateral orbital rim superiorly and, again, the anesthetic solution was injected while the needle was being moved. This method effectively blocks the terminal branches of the seventh nerve.

Nadbath and Rehman[5] in the early 1960s blocked the trunk of the facial nerve as it exits the skull, below the ear. O'Brien[6] described a block in front of the tragus of the ear anesthetizing the facial nerve branches as they traverse the condyloid of the mandible.

Atkinson[7] described a technique falling midway between those of van Lint and O'Brien. The anesthetic is injected horizontally, starting at the inferior edge of the zygomatic arch, and is aimed at the pinna, taking care not to inject the facial vessels anterior to the ear. This technique affords complete block of the nerve branches to the orbicularis without blocking the branches to the lip and lower face, as happens with the methods of O'Brien and Nadbath. Moreover, it eliminates the "ballooning" of lid tissues commonly encountered with the van Lint technique.

Complications

To avoid prolapse of intraocular contents, retrobulbar blockade is contraindicated if a ruptured globe is suspected.

Potential complications associated with retrobulbar block include stimulation of the oculocardiac reflex arc, retrobulbar hemorrhage, puncture of the posterior globe resulting in retinal detachment and vitreous hemorrhage, unintentional intraocular injection, central retinal artery occlusion, penetration of the optic nerve, subdural injection, blindness, and inadvertent brain stem anesthesia.[8-17] Additionally, intravascular injection of local anesthesia by the retrobulbar or facial lid block route may cause CNS excitation followed by obtundation and cardiovascular collapse.[18,19] Although the latter complications are commonly associated with injection of local anesthetic into a vein, it is essential to appreciate that inadvertent intraarterial[20] injection may also be associated with CNS toxicity, and the amount of anesthetic involved is much less than with the IV route. As little as 1.8 ml of 2% lidocaine injected into an artery of the head or neck region can produce profound toxic reactions.[21] These reactions include virtually instantaneous seizures secondary to ophthalmic artery injection[20] with retrograde flow into the cerebral circulation.

General Anesthesia

Indications

General anesthesia is indicated for the patient with a known lacerated globe, an unknown injury requiring exploration, or multiple injuries in various sites. The eye trauma setting supplies a unique set of circumstances and dangers in anesthesia.

Anesthesia Management

Penetrating injuries include intraocular foreign bodies in the anterior and posterior chambers, the lens, or the vitreous humor, and lacerations of the sclera or cornea. Since penetrating injuries can result in extrusion of intraocular contents, a major objective of the anesthesiologist is to prevent increases in intraocular pressure (IOP), which can produce further prolapse and loss of intraocular contents. Coughing, retching, vomiting, squeezing the eyelids shut, crying, and rubbing of the eyes are extremely detrimental activities in this setting. Indeed, coughing can increase IOP as much as 50 mm Hg.

One of the most challenging situations confronting the anesthesiologist is a patient who has a penetrating eye injury and has recently eaten. It is best to wait at least 6 to 8 hours following the last oral intake before commencing surgery. However, gastric emptying and digestion are greatly impaired in a patient who is in pain and apprehensive, and the patient must still be treated as if he or she has a full stomach even if 8 hours have elapsed. It must be underscored that anesthesia management of the "open eye–full stomach" patient is controversial, and no single approach is ideal. Methods to protect against aspiration of gastric contents must be balanced against their influence on IOP.

All would agree that a rapid induction with cricoid pressure to prevent regurgitation of stomach contents and a smooth intubation must be accomplished without significant elevation of IOP. Experts disagree, however, on the best way to do this.

Antacid aspiration prophylaxis is advised. An H_2 receptor antagonist may be given to decrease gastric acid production and increase gastric pH. Additionally, metoclopramide is useful to stimulate peristalsis and facilitate gastric emptying. However, no attempt should be made to insert a nasogastric tube while the patient is awake, since such a maneuver is likely to trigger serious increases in IOP.

It is well known that nondepolarizing muscle relaxants such as curare, pancuronium, atracurium, and vecuronium relax the extraocular muscles and lower IOP. Depolarizing muscle relaxants such as succinylcholine increase IOP by about 8 mm Hg, but this modest increase is usually dissipated within 7 minutes. However, even with nondepolarizing relaxants, IOP may still increase considerably in response to laryngoscopy and intubation, especially if laryngoscopy is prolonged or attempted prematurely and intubation is difficult because of insufficient muscle relaxation or abnormal airway anatomy.

Using a barbiturate and an intubating dose of nondepolarizing muscle relaxant is often described as the method of choice for the emergency repair of a ruptured globe, since the nondepolarizing relaxant pancuronium, in a dose of 0.15 mg/kg, lowers IOP.[22] This technique has serious disadvantages, however, including the risks of aspiration and death during the relatively long time—from 75 seconds[23] to 2½ minutes[24]—that the airway is unsecured and unprotected by an endotracheal tube. Moreover, a premature attempt at intubation will produce coughing, straining, and a dramatic increase in IOP, as well as undesirable cardiovascular side effects of concern in adults with coronary artery disease. In addition, the long duration of action of pancuronium may mandate postoperative mechanical ventilation. Although newer nondepolarizing relaxants such as vecuronium and atracurium have shorter durations of action, minimal circulatory effects, and no tendency to accumulate, in equipotent doses these newer drugs have an onset of action as delayed as pancuronium's.[25,26] Attempts to reduce the time of onset of blockade have produced the priming technique (giving one tenth of an intubation dose of nondepolarizing agent, followed 4 minutes later by a full intubating dose, and then waiting 90 seconds to perform intubation) and the use of extremely high doses of nondepolarizing drugs. However, these techniques are not consistently reliable and can be associated with serious complications.

Another approach involves pretreatment with a nondepolarizing muscle relaxant followed by a barbiturate-succinylcholine sequence. However, the efficacy of pretreatment with small doses of nondepolarizing muscle relaxant to prevent succinylcholine-induced intraocular hypertension is a moot issue. Miller, Way, and Hickey,[27] using indentation tonometry, were able to prevent a succinylcholine-induced increase in IOP following pretreatment, whereas Meyers et al.,[28] using applanation tonometry, could not do so consistently. Nonetheless, in a patient with a full stomach, succinylcholine offers the important advantages of rapid onset, excellent intubating conditions, and short duration of action. Given after pretreatment with a nondepolarizing relaxant and an inducing dose of sodium thiopental (4 to 6 mg/kg), succinylcholine causes only *slight* increases in IOP above baseline.[29] Furthermore, there are no reports in the literature of loss of intraocular contents produced by a nondepolarizing pretreatment–barbiturate–succinylcholine sequence in this setting.[30,31]

Perhaps the most succinct summary of this issue is that by Baumgarten and Reynolds,[32] who wrote in 1985, "At this time, succinylcholine with precurarization probably remains the most tenable compromise in the open eye–full stomach challenge."

Once the patient has been successfully intubated, anesthesia may be maintained using an inhalational agent or the so-called balanced anesthetic technique, employing nitrous oxide, oxygen, a narcotic, and a nondepolarizing muscle relaxant. Intraoperative immobility must be ensured by monitoring the patient's muscle twitch with a peripheral nerve stimulator. Obviously, intraoperative coughing or "bucking" are to be assiduously avoided to prevent loss of intraocular contents. After the patient has been adequately anesthetized, a nasogastric tube may be introduced and suction applied to remove as much of the gastric contents as possible. Once surgery has been completed, it is essential to postpone extubation until the patient is awake and reflexes are intact. Otherwise there is a risk of periextubation aspiration.

ANESTHESIA FOR LID AND ORBITAL INJURIES

Local Lid Blocks

Indications

Local lid blocks are useful to facilitate ocular and orbital examination and in repair of lid lacerations, removal of foreign bodies, and orbital exploration.

Techniques

A variety of approaches may be used to accomplish lid anesthesia. The motor innervation to the adnexal structures is from the upper and lower zygomatic branches of the facial nerve. These branches may be blocked using the techniques described by van Lint,[4] Nadbath and Rehman,[5] O'Brien,[6] and Atkinson,[7] as discussed previously. Since the van Lint technique is closest to the lid and usually requires 6 to 10 ml of anesthetic solution, it commonly produces edema of the upper and lower lids. Indeed, tissue distension is a distinct disadvantage of direct infiltration anesthesia.

For repair of the lids after trauma, a mixture of equal parts of lidocaine (1% to 2%) with epinephrine (1:100,000 to 1:200,000) and bupiva-

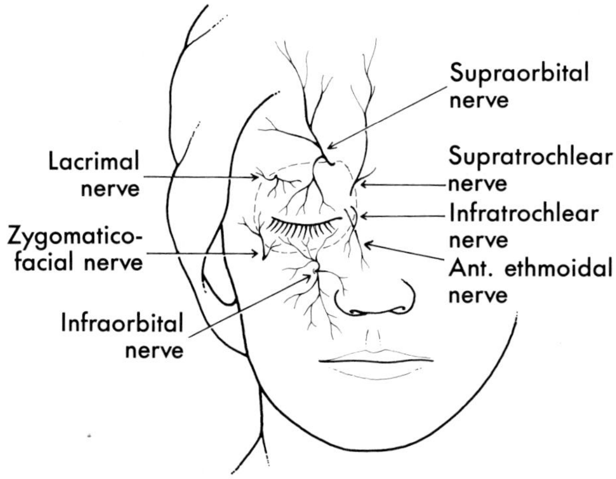

Fig. 4-2. Sensory innervation to ocular adnexal structures.

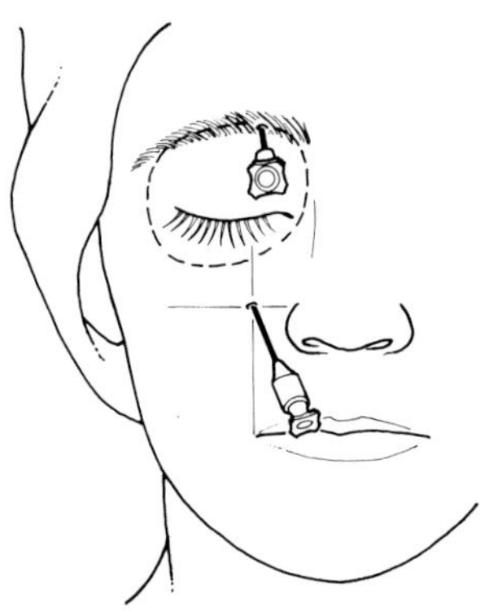

Fig. 4-3. Injection sites for sensory blockade of the supraorbital and infraorbital nerves.

caine (0.5% to 0.75%) prevents early and late pain and reduces bleeding. The improved hemostasis facilitates dissection by making it easier to follow the structural planes. However, when operating on ptotic lids, some surgeons prefer to omit the epinephrine component to avoid stimulation of Muller's muscle. This allows the surgeon to better judge the height of the lid margin as the levator muscle and aponeurosis are resected and sutured to the tarsus.[33]

Sensory innervation to the adnexal structures is entirely from the first two divisions of the trigeminal nerve. The supraorbital, supratrochlear, and lacrimal nerves are branches of the ophthalmic nerve. The infraorbital nerve branches from the maxillary nerve (Fig. 4-2).

The supraorbital nerve supplies sensory innervation to the skin and conjunctiva of the upper lid and the skin of the lower forehead. An injection of 1.0 to 1.5 ml of anesthetic solution through a skin wheal at the supraorbital notch (on the superior orbital margin approximately at the junction of the nasal one third of the superior orbital rim) will adequately supply anesthesia of this branch (Fig. 4-3). Careful aspiration should be carried out prior to injection, given the proximity of the supraorbital vessels.

The lacrimal nerve supplies the outer, upper, and lower lid skin and conjunctiva. This nerve emerges from the orbit at the junction of the lateral orbital wall and the orbital roof. It can be blocked by injecting 1 to 2 ml of anesthetic solution through a skin wheal at a depth of 2.5 cm just overlying the periosteum at the junction of the lateral wall and the orbital roof.

The infraorbital nerve supplies sensory fibers to the entire lower lid and to the medial and lateral portions of the upper lid. In addition, it innervates the lacrimal sac, side of the nose, upper lip, and zygomatic region. The infraorbital nerve emerges on the face from the infraorbital foramen, which is seen as a depression on the maxilla approximately at the midportion of the inferior orbital rim and 1.5 cm below it. The needle is inserted into the foramen, and after aspiration, approximately 2 ml of anesthetic solution is injected (Fig. 4-3).

Regional blocks of the supratrochlear and infratrochlear nerves are usually not necessary for lid surgery, but these nerves can be easily blocked by a single injection of 1 to 2 ml of anesthetic agent just anterior to the pulley of the superior oblique muscle.

General Anesthesia for Orbital Injuries

Indications

General anesthesia is required for extensive repair of orbital injuries and when the initial exploration requirements are unknown.

Anesthesia Management

A major problem with orbital injury is that it is frequently associated with fractures and serious injuries elsewhere. In addition, the associated complications can be life-threatening. Important associated injuries can include airway obstruction, skull fractures, a variety of closed head injuries, tracheobronchial rupture, myocardial and pulmonary contusions, fractured ribs, hemopneumothorax, pericardial tamponade, and ruptured liver, spleen, or diaphragm.

Airway obstruction in the setting of maxillofacial injuries can result from blood, teeth, dentures, and bony fragments in the oropharynx. These may be removed by sweeping with a gloved index finger and gently suctioning the area. Pharyngeal obstruction from bilateral mandibular fractures may result when the tongue and mandible are displaced posteriorly. This can be relieved by forward traction of the tongue or insertion of an oropharyngeal airway.

As many as 20% of Le Fort III and some Le Fort II fractures are associated with basilar skull fractures. Such fractures of the cribiform plate create a passageway from the subarachnoid space to the nasal cavity that can lead to leakage of cerebrospinal fluid (CSF), to meningitis, and to a pneumocranium from passage of air into the subarachnoid space. Physical signs of a basilar skull fracture include raccoon eyes (orbital hematomas), battle signs (retroaural hematomas), CSF rhinorrhea or otorrhea, and anosmia. Nasal intubations are contraindicated since they can result in passage of the endotracheal tube into the cranium itself. Also, if a skull fracture or CSF leak is present, a pneumocranium should be suspected, and the anesthesiologist should avoid administering nitrous oxide. In addition, cerebral edema or mass effect may be present, which may warrant hyperventilation and diuretic therapy to reduce the intracranial hypertension.

Several methods can be used to minimize operative bleeding, including infiltration with epinephrine, a head-up tilt of 15° to 30° to reduce arterial pressure at the operative site and minimize venous congestion, and controlled hypotension. The latter can be accomplished by using intravenous adrenergic or ganglionic blockers, vasodilators, or high concentrations of inhalation anesthetic agents and controlled positive-pressure ventilation. Contraindications to induced hypotension include neurologic injury, carotid occlusive or coronary artery disease, and an intrapulmonary shunt.

References

1. Koller K: On the use of cocaine to anaesthetize the eye (Translated by H Knapp). In On cocaine and its use in ophthalmic and general surgery, Arch Ophthalmol 68:31, 1962 (originally published 1884).
2. Havener WH: Ocular pharmacology, ed 5, St Louis, 1983, The CV Mosby Co, 72-119.
3. Meyers EF: Cocaine toxicity during dacryocystorhinostomy, Arch Ophthalmol 98:842-843, 1980.
4. Van Lint A: Paralysie, palpébrale temporaire provoquée dans l'operation de la cataracte, Ann Ocul 151:420-424, 1914.
5. Nadbath RP and Rehman I: Facial nerve block, Am J Ophthalmol 55:143-146, 1963.
6. O'Brien CS: Local anesthesia in ophthalmic surgery, Trans Sect Ophthalmol AMA 78:237-253, 1927.
7. Atkinson WS: Akinesia of the orbicularis, Am J Ophthalmol 36:1255-1258, 1953.
8. Beltranena HP et al: Complications of retrobulbar marcaine injection, J Clin Neuro Ophthalmol 2:159-161, 1982.
9. Rosenblatt RM, May DR, and Barsoumian K: Cardiopulmonary arrest after retrobulbar block, Am J Ophthalmol 90:425-427, 1980.
10. Hamilton RC: Brain stem anesthesia following retrobulbar blockade, Anesthesiology 63:688-690, 1985.
11. Chang JL et al: Brain stem anesthesia following retrobulbar block, Anesthesiology 61:789-790, 1984.
12. Drysdale DB: Experimental subdural retrobulbar injection of anesthetic, Ann Ophthalmol 16:716-718, 1984.
13. Lynn JG Jr and Smith RB: Intraoperative complications and their management, Int Ophthalmol Clin 13(2):149-175, 1973.

14. Ramsay RC and Knoblock WH: Ocular perforation following retrobulbar anesthesia for retinal detachment surgery, Am J Ophthalmol 86:61-64, 1978.
15. Follette JW and Locascio JA: Bilateral amaurosis following unilateral retrobulbar block, Anesthesiology 63:237-238, 1985.
16. Brookshire GL, Gleitsmann KY, and Schenk EC: Life-threatening complication of retrobulbar block, Ophthalmology 93:1476-1478, 1986.
17. Nicoll JMV et al: Central nervous system complications after 6000 retrobulbar blocks, Anesth Analg 66:1298-1302, 1987.
18. Meyers EF, Ramirez RC, and Boniu KI: Grand mal seizures after retrobulbar block, Arch Ophthalmol 96:847, 1978.
19. Beltranena HP et al: Inadvertent intravascular bupivacaine injection following retrobulbar block: report of three cases, Regional Anesthesia 6:149-151, 1981.
20. Cibis PA: General discussion. In Schepens CL and Regan CDJ, editors: Controversial aspects of the management of retinal detachment, Boston, 1965, Little, Brown, 223-233.
21. Aldrete JA et al: Reverse arterial blood flow as a pathway for central nervous system toxic responses following injection of local anesthetics, Anesth Analg 57:428-433, 1978.
22. Litwiller RW, Difazio CA, and Rushia EL: Pancuronium and intraocular pressure, Anesthesiology 42:750-752, 1975.
23. Brown EM, Krishnaprasad D, and Smiler BG: Pancuronium for rapid induction technique for tracheal intubation, Can Anaesth Soc J 26:489-491, 1979.
24. Goudsouzian NG, Liu LMP, and Cote CJ: Comparison of equipotent doses of nondepolarizing muscle relaxants in children, Anesth Analg 60:862-866, 1981.
25. Savarese JJ: New neuromuscular blocking drugs are here, Anesthesiology 55:1-3, 1981.
26. Basta SJ et al: Clinical pharmacology of atracurium besylate (BW 33A): a new nondepolarizing muscle relaxant, Anesth Analg 61:723-729, 1982.
27. Miller RD, Way WL, and Hickey RF: Inhibition of succinylcholine-induced increased intraocular pressure by nondepolarizing muscle relaxants, Anesthesiology 29:123-126, 1968.
28. Meyers EF et al: Failure of nondepolarizing neuromuscular blockers to inhibit succinylcholine-induced increased intraocular pressure—a controlled study, Anesthesiology 48:149-151, 1978.
29. Konchigeri HN, Lee YE, and Venugopal K: Effect of pancuronium on intraocular pressure changes induced by succinylcholine, Can Anaesth Soc J 26:479-481, 1979.
30. McCammon RL: Anesthesia for operations on the eye, International Anesthesia Research Society Review Course Lectures, Cleveland, 1984, 109-116.
31. Libonati MM, Leahy JJ, Ellison N: Use of succinylcholine in open eye injury, Anesthesiology 62:637-640, 1985.
32. Baumgarten RK and Reynolds WJ: Priming principle and the open eye-full stomach, Anesthesiology 63:561-562, 1985.
33. Bruce RA: Regional anesthetic techniques. In Bruce RA, McGoldrick KE, and Oppenheimer P, editors: Anesthesia for ophthalmology, Birmingham, 1982, Aesculapius, 42.

CHAPTER 5

Evaluation and management strategies for the pediatric eye trauma patient

DARREN L. HOOVER
LOIS E. H. SMITH

Epidemiology
Examination
Unique forms of childhood eye trauma
Prenatal and birth trauma
Self-inflicted eye trauma
Child abuse
Amblyopia
Critical period
Detection of amblyopia
Methods of occlusion
Guidelines for occlusion therapy
References

Ocular trauma is the leading cause of noncongenital unilateral blindness in patients under 20 years of age.[1,2] Aspects unique to the epidemiology, examination, diagnosis, and treatment of eye injuries in childhood will be considered in this chapter.

EPIDEMIOLOGY

Children and adolescents experience a disproportionate share of ocular trauma. The Israeli Ocular Injuries Study examined over 2000 patients hospitalized for ocular injuries during a 3-year period,[3] of whom 47% were under 18 years of age, with children aged 6 to 10 years the most vulnerable group (17% of the cases) followed by children aged 11 to 15 years (16%). The age-specific incidence rates of perforating eye injury in Stockholm were highest among males aged 10 to 19 years (94.3 per million person-years) and highest among females from birth to age 9 (34.1 per million person-years).[4] The male-female ratio in most studies is about 4:1.[3,5,6]

Children often sustain severe eye injuries. A 3-year survey of 278 children hospitalized for ocular trauma at Wills Eye Hospital included 100 cases of perforating injury (34.5%) and 172 cases requiring surgical treatment (61.9%).[6] In the Israeli Ocular Injuries Study, almost half of the perforating injuries and enucleations occurred in those under 18 years of age.[3] At the Wilmer Eye Institute, 43% of penetrating ocular injuries occurred in patients aged 18 years and younger.[7] Of these 159 young patients who had at least 6 months follow-up, 110 (69%) achieved a final visual acuity of 5/200 or better, and 77 (48%) achieved 20/50 or better. The type and extent of injury were thought to be more important than patient age in determining final visual outcome.

Sports equipment, stones, wooden sticks, and toys are the items most often implicated in pediatric eye trauma.[3,6] Injuries related to air-powered BB guns are particularly devastating. In 22 patients with penetrating injuries due to air-powered guns, 19 eyes were enucleated in one series; final vision in the 3 remaining eyes was worse than 5/200.[8] Inadequate adult supervision is an important contributing factor in most cases of serious childhood eye injuries (see Chapter 36).[9]

EXAMINATION

Obtaining a detailed, accurate history is the first step in evaluating pediatric eye injuries. Pertinent information regarding past medical and ophthalmic diseases and drug allergies should be elicited. Be aware that children guilty of misbehavior and adults guilty of child abuse may misrepresent the facts.

The visual acuity of each eye is measured separately. Allen picture cards, the illiterate "E" test, and Snellen letters (in ascending order of preference) are used with cooperative children. If only bedside examination is possible, a standard vision card is used to obtain a near acuity. In older children with markedly swollen eyelids, a topical anesthetic is instilled and the eyelids gently separated with Desmarres retractors to permit measurement of visual acuity. In younger children, the ability to fixate and follow objects of interest is assessed.

With patience and encouragement by the examiner, conventional examination techniques are adequate in evaluating the eyelids, orbital rims, and globes of most older children (see Chapter 1). A papoose board may be useful in restraining very young children. With assistance, slit-lamp examination is usually possible in children of all ages. Alternatively, a portable slit-lamp or loupe can be used to examine the supine patient. After fluorescein instillation, a Wood's lamp will help identify a corneal abrasion in uncooperative children.

If a ruptured globe is suspected, no diagnostic maneuvers that may further damage the eye should be attempted. A protective shield should be taped over the eye in such a way that no pressure is applied to the globe. The child should then be transported in the supine position to the operating room for examination under general anesthesia.

UNIQUE FORMS OF CHILDHOOD EYE TRAUMA

Prenatal and Birth Trauma

Amniocentesis performed during the second and third trimesters has caused damage to the anterior and posterior segments of the eye on rare occasions. Findings from five reported cases included a congenital epithelial cyst of the anterior chamber, eyelid coloboma, microphthalmos, vascularized corneal leukoma, corneal perforation, anterior chamber hyphema, filtering scleral perforation, retinal hole, axial myopia, and tractional retinal detachment.[10-14]

Ruptures in Descemet's membrane due to forceps delivery have been recognized for many years.[15] These single or multiple vertically oriented breaks are unilateral and initially associated with corneal edema. The corneal edema clears within weeks to months, but the breaks in Descemet's membrane remain visible. Marked "with-the-rule" astigmatism and axial myopia cause dense amblyopia in the affected eye. Good visual acuity can be achieved with optical correction and patching.[16] Differentiation from the Descemet's membrane breaks of congenital glaucoma (usually horizontal in orientation) is essential.

Retinal hemorrhages in the newborn infant have been recognized for more than a century. They are seen in about 20% of newborn children examined within 24 hours of birth, and most of the hemorrhages disappear within the first week.[17-19] Dense, deep retinal hemorrhages in and around the macula may persist for several weeks but clear with no apparent adverse sequelae. Birth trauma is the most likely cause of these retinal hemorrhages. Hemorrhages into the conjunctiva and orbits may also result from birth trauma.

Soft tissue swelling of the periorbital structures from obstetrical trauma is a common cause of neonatal eyelid closure.[20] Monocular axial myopia and anisometropic amblyopia may develop with prolonged eyelid closure. The exact mechanisms by which neonatal eyelid closure leads to axial myopia are uncertain.[21]

Evulsion of the eye and orbital bone fractures may also occur with a complicated birth.

Self-inflicted Eye Trauma

In retarded children with a history of head-banging or self-mutilation, serious eye injuries

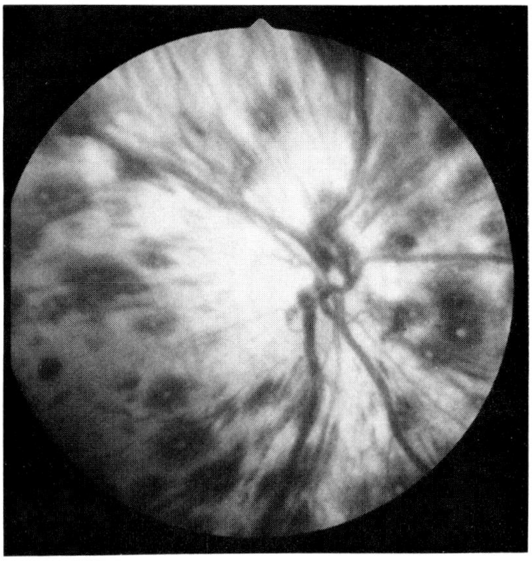

Fig. 5-1. Typical retinal hemorrhages seen in a whiplash shaken infant. (Courtesy of Joseph Giangiacomo and Roy Wilson.)

may develop; these include retinal detachment, vitreous hemorrhage, cataract, corneal laceration, and neovascular glaucoma.[22,23] Periodic examination of such children is strongly recommended. Protective helmets and spectacles may prevent permanent injury.

Child Abuse

The most recent national incidence study estimates that over 1.5 million children were abused or neglected in 1986 in the United States.[24] About one quarter of these children were physically abused. Eye abnormalities are found in about 40% of physically abused children.[25,26]

Ocular manifestations of child abuse are listed below.[25-29] The most common ophthalmic finding is extensive intraocular hemorrhages, usually associated with subdural hemorrhages (Fig. 5-1). Retinal, preretinal, and vitreal hemorrhages may precede the clinical and computerized tomography (CT) recognition of subdural hematomas; magnetic resonance imaging (MRI) is superior to CT in detecting subdural hematomas in abused children.[30,31] Visual outcomes in these cases can range from complete recovery of normal visual function to total blindness. The differential diagnosis of retinal hemorrhages in childhood includes birth trauma, bleeding disorders, acute leukemia, anemia, and sepsis. In children sustaining head trauma from causes besides physical abuse, retinal hemorrhages are extremely uncommon.[32] Battered children may occasionally have retinal and preretinal hemorrhages in the absence of intracranial hemorrhage (Purtscher retinopathy).[33] Ophthalmic findings in child abuse include the following:

1. Retina/vitreous: retinal, preretinal, and vitreous hemorrhage; retinal detachment and dialysis; chorioretinal scarring and atrophy; retinoschisis; retinal folds
2. Optic nerve: papilledema; optic atrophy
3. Lens: subluxated lens; cataract
4. Iris: traumatic mydriasis; rubeosis iridis
5. Anterior chamber: hyphema
6. Cornea: laceration; abrasion; ulcer; opacities
7. Conjunctiva: subconjunctival hemorrhage; conjunctivitis due to sexually transmitted organisms
8. Lid: laceration; periorbital edema and ecchymosis
9. Other: disconjugate eye movements; nystagmus; exotropia; esotropia; cranial nerve VI palsy; cortical blindness; proptosis

Historical and physical features of the typical battered child are as follows:[27,34]

1. Bone fractures and soft tissue injuries in different stages of resolution
2. Disproportionate soft tissue injury
3. Parent's or guardian's history incompatible with child's age and injuries
4. Multiple admissions to different hospitals
5. No new lesions occurring during hospitalization
6. Deterioration of child's academic performance and social interactions

An important subset of physically abused children is the whiplash shaken infant.[35] Repetitive violent shaking of an infant will produce massive intraocular and intracranial hemorrhages with no external signs of trauma. Blindness, mental retardation, and death are common sequelae of this syndrome.

If abuse or neglect is strongly suspected, hospitalization of the child is essential. Skeletal radiologic surveys, neuroradiologic imaging, and other medical testing can be completed as a social history is gathered and evaluated.

Laws mandating the reporting of suspected child abuse exist in all 50 states and the District of Columbia.[36] The physician need only *suspect* maltreatment to report it. If suspected child

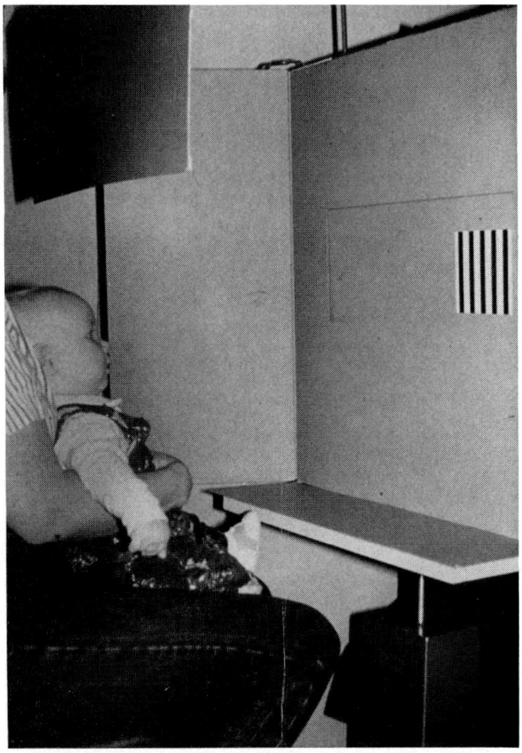

Fig. 5-2. Forced-choice preferential looking (PL) acuity card testing of an infant.

abuse is reported in accordance with the law, the physician is protected from civil and criminal liability. The responsibility for investigating reports of suspected child abuse rests with the child protective services agency in each state. Hospital social workers can facilitate the reporting of these cases to the appropriate agency.

AMBLYOPIA

The general principles of anatomic repair of eye trauma outlined in Chapter 13 apply to persons of all ages. However, to achieve a good visual outcome following pediatric eye trauma, the prevention and treatment of amblyopia must also be addressed.

Critical Period

Children up to 9 or 10 years of age are susceptible to developing amblyopia.[37] The younger the child at the time of visual deprivation, the faster and deeper amblyopia develops. However, occlusion of the good eye to treat amblyopia can be successful in children up to 10 or 11 years of age.[38] Amblyopic children less than 8 years of age have a more favorable prognosis than older children; the high failure rate among older children is more often due to a lack of treatment compliance than to age-related factors.

Detection of Amblyopia

From a practical standpoint, a difference of two lines or more on a Snellen visual acuity chart that cannot be explained by refractive error or organic causes indicates significant amblyopia. In cooperative children, amblyopia detection is straightforward using Allen picture cards, the "E" game, or Snellen letters (in ascending order of preference).

Traumatic strabismus may result from direct injury to the extraocular muscles; orbital bone damage; third, fourth, or sixth cranial nerve palsy; or a combination of these factors. The binocular fixation pattern test is used to diagnose strabismic amblyopia in children too young to cooperate with conventional visual acuity tests.[39] The habitually fixating eye is covered, and the deviating eye is forced to fixate on an object of interest in the primary position. The cover is removed, and the time required for the habitually fixating eye to resume fixation is assessed. Most nonamblyopic patients will hold fixation with the normally deviating eye up to or through the next blink; most amblyopic patients with strabismus will resume fixation with the preferred eye within 1 to 2 seconds after the cover is removed. This test is very reliable except in strabismus patients with small angles of esotropia.

Forced-choice preferential looking (PL) tests are the preferred methods of detecting nonstrabismic amblyopia in preverbal children.[40,41] These tests are based on the observation that infants and young children are more interested in looking at black-and-white striped patterns than at homogeneous gray fields. Black-and-white striped patterns equivalent to various Snellen values are presented simultaneously with a homogeneous gray card (Fig. 5-2). The acuities obtained by PL are based on the narrowest stripes that the infant can detect.

Using PL acuity cards, visual acuity determinations can be completed in 10 to 15 minutes. Although PL tests overestimate the visual acuity of amblyopic eyes compared with recognition testing (Allen cards, Snellen letters), they are a sensitive detector of differences in visual acuity between the eyes of infants and those of young children with nonstrabismic amblyopia.

Methods of Occlusion

Occlusion therapy with patching of the sound eye is the standard treatment of amblyopia. An opaque occlusive contact lens is frequently a successful alternative in patients who fail to improve with conventional patching therapy. Atropine penalization of the preferred eye is helpful only if the amblyopia is mild (20/50 or better).

Guidelines for Occlusion Therapy

Occlusion of the preferred eye during all except 1 to 2 waking hours per day is initially used in the treatment of strabismic amblyopia. This is done for 1 week per year of chronological age up to a maximum of 4 weeks before the next examination. Full-time occlusion is continued until maximal potential vision is achieved, which usually occurs within 3 to 6 months. Part-time patching during one third to one half of waking hours is then used to maintain optimal vision in the amblyopic eye. Part-time occlusion is usually required until spontaneous or surgical realignment of the eyes is achieved. For traumatic palsy of the third, fourth, or sixth cranial nerve, a minimum period of 12 months is allowed for spontaneous recovery. If the deviation is small, prisms may help align the eyes during this interval to eliminate the development of suppression and achieve binocularity. Part-time occlusion is sometimes required even after the eyes are well aligned.

Deprivation amblyopia caused by eyelid closure or monocular media opacities is usually deeper and more resistant to treatment than is strabismic amblyopia. Traumatic causes of deprivation amblyopia include complete eyelid closure, corneal laceration, anterior chamber hyphema, traumatic cataract, and vitreous hemorrhage. The younger the child at the time the underlying factor develops, the more urgent is the need to correct this factor and treat the amblyopia.

The rehabilitation of the pediatric aphakic patient deserves special attention. Without optical correction of the aphakic eye and occlusion of the phakic eye, removal of the traumatic cataract is just a surgical exercise. A daily-wear soft contact lens is the preferred mode of optical correction. The aphakic eye is overplussed by +2.00 sphere until the child is old enough to tolerate a bifocal spectacle. Contact lens fitting can almost always be accomplished in the office. Refractions are repeated about every 3 months during the first several years of life. Patching of the phakic eye is intense and prolonged in early childhood, requiring frequent vision checks. The primary goal is the restoration of optimal vision to the aphakic eye; ocular alignment and binocularity are secondary considerations.

References

1. National Society for the Prevention of Blindness. Vision problems in the US, New York, 1980, The Society.
2. Slusher MM and Keeney AH: Monocular blindness, Sight Saving Review 35:207-212, 1965.
3. Koval R et al: The Israeli Ocular Injuries Study—a nationwide collaborative study, Arch Ophthalmol 106:776-780, 1988.
4. Blomdahl S and Norell S: Perforating eye injury in the Stockholm population—an epidemiological study, Acta Ophthalmol 62:378-390, 1984.
5. Niiranen M and Raivio I: Eye injuries in children, Br J Ophthalmol 65:436-438, 1981.
6. Grin TR, Nelson LB, and Jeffers JB: Eye injuries in childhood, Pediatrics 80:13-17, 1987.
7. Sternberg P, DeJuan E, and Michels RG: Penetrating ocular injuries in young patients—initial injuries and visual results, Retina 4:5-8, 1984.
8. Sternberg P et al: Ocular BB injuries, Ophthalmology 91:1269-1277, 1984.
9. Moreira CA, Debert-Ribeiro M, and Belfort R: Epidemiological study of eye injuries in Brazilian children, Arch Ophthalmol 106:781-784, 1988.
10. Cross HE and Maumenee AE: Ocular trauma during amniocentesis, Arch Ophthalmol 90:303-304, 1973.
11. Fortin JG and Lemire J: Une complication oculaire de l'amniocentese, Can J Ophthalmol 10:511-513, 1975.
12. Merin S and Beyth Y: Uniocular congenital blindness as a complication of midtrimester amniocentesis, Am J Ophthalmol 89:299-301, 1980.
13. Isenberg SJ and Heckenlively JR: Traumatized eye with retinal damage from amniocentesis, J Pediatr Ophthalmol Strabismus 22:65-67, 1985.
14. Admoni MM and BenEzra D: Ocular trauma following amniocentesis as the cause of leukocoria, J Pediatr Ophthalmol Strabismus 25:196-197, 1988.
15. Thomson E: Discussion of birth injuries of the eye, Trans Ophthalmol Soc UK 46:13-31, 1926.
16. Angell LK, Robb RM, and Berson FG: Visual prognosis in patients with ruptures in Descemet's membrane due to forceps injuries, Arch Ophthalmol 99:2137-2139, 1981.

17. Sezen F: Retinal haemorrhages in newborn infants, Br J Ophthalmol 55:248-253, 1970.
18. Baum JD and Bulpitt CJ: Retinal and conjunctival haemorrhage in the newborn, Arch Dis Child 45:344-349, 1970.
19. Planten JT and Schaaf PC: Retinal haemorrhage in the newborn, Ophthalmologica 162:213-222, 1971.
20. Hoyt CS et al: Monocular axial myopia associated with neonatal eyelid closure in human infants, Am J Ophthalmol 91:197-200, 1981.
21. Raviola E and Wiesel TN: An animal model of myopia, N Engl J Med 312:1609-1615, 1985.
22. Spalter HF, Bemporad JR, and Sours JA: Cataracts following chronic headbanging, Arch Ophthalmol 83:182-186, 1970.
23. Noel L-P and Clarke WN: Self-inflicted ocular injuries in children, Am J Ophthalmol 94:630-633, 1982.
24. Children's Bureau, US Department of Health and Human Services, National Center on Child Abuse and Neglect: Study of national incidence and prevalence of child abuse and neglect, Washington, DC, 1988.
25. Friendly DS: Ocular manifestations of physical child abuse, Trans Am Acad Ophthalmol Otolaryngol 75:318-332, 1971.
26. Jensen AD, Smith RE, and Olson MI: Ocular clues to child abuse, J Pediatr Ophthalmol 8:270-272, 1971.
27. Harcourt B and Hopkins D: Ophthalmic manifestations of the battered-baby syndrome, Br Med J 3:398-401, 1971.
28. Greenwald MJ et al: Traumatic retinoschisis in battered babies, Ophthalmology 93:618-625, 1986.
29. Gaynon MW et al: Retinal folds in the shaken baby syndrome, Am J Ophthalmol 106:423-425, 1988.
30. Giangiacomo J et al: Sequential cranial computed tomography in infants with retinal hemorrhages, Ophthalmology 95:295-299, 1988.
31. Alexander RC, Schor DP, and Smith WL: Magnetic resonance imaging of intracranial injuries from child abuse, J Pediatr 109:975-979, 1986.
32. Eisenbrey AB: Retinal hemorrhage in the battered child, Child's Brain 5:40-44, 1979.
33. Tomasi LG and Rosman NP: Purtscher retinopathy in the battered child syndrome, Am J Dis Child 129:1335-1337, 1975.
34. Kempe CH: The battered child and the hospital, Hosp Pract 4:44-57, 1969.
35. Caffey J: The whiplash shaken infant syndrome: manual shaking by the extremities with whiplash-induced intracranial and intraocular bleedings, linked with residual permanent brain damage and mental retardation, Pediatrics 54:396-403, 1974.
36. Clearinghouse on Child Abuse and Neglect Information, US Department of Health and Human Services, National Center on Child Abuse and Neglect: Child abuse and neglect: a shared community concern, Washington, DC, August 1988.
37. Ching FC, Parks MM, and Friendly DS: Practical management of amblyopia, J Pediatr Ophthalmol Strabismus 23:12-16, 1986.
38. Oliver M et al: Compliance and results of treatment for amblyopia in children more than 8 years old, Am J Ophthalmol 102:340-345, 1986.
39. Zipf RF: Binocular fixation pattern, Arch Ophthalmol 94:401-405, 1976.
40. Fulton AB, Hansen RM, and Manning KA: Measuring visual acuity in infants, Surv Ophthalmol 25:325-332, 1981.
41. Mayer DL, Fulton AB, and Rodier D: Grating and recognition acuities of pediatric patients, Ophthalmology 91:947-953, 1984.

PART 2

Anterior segment trauma

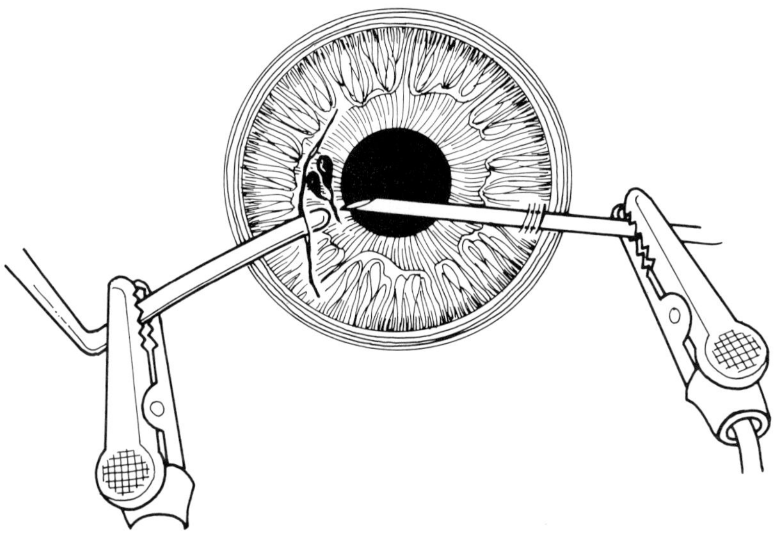

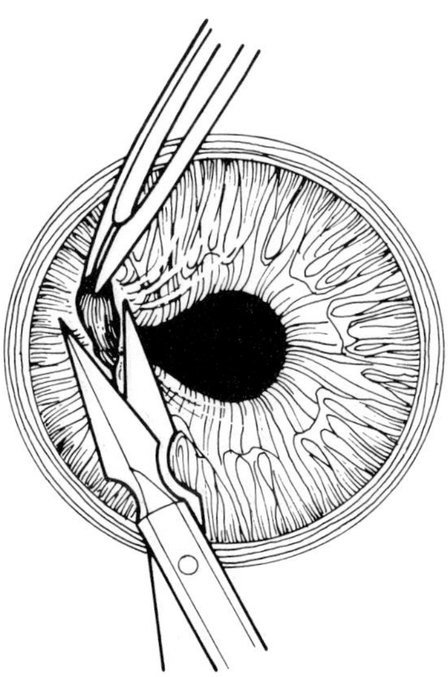

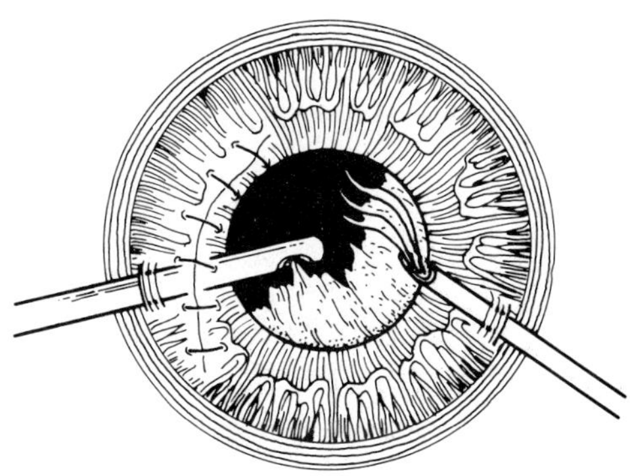

CHAPTER 6

Conjunctival and corneal injuries

KENNETH R. KENYON
MICHAEL D. WAGONER

Conjunctival injury
- Blunt trauma
- Foreign body
- Laceration

Corneal injury
- Blunt trauma
- Foreign body
- Abrasion
- Recurrent erosion, persistent epithelial defect, and noninfected stromal ulceration
  - Pathogenesis
  - Recurrent erosion
    - Diagnosis and primary therapy
    - Medical therapy
    - Surgical therapy
  - Persistent epithelial defect and noninfected stromal ulceration
    - Diagnosis and primary therapy
    - Medical therapy
    - Surgical therapy
- Infected ulceration
- Ultraviolet radiation and electrical injury

References

This chapter considers the common and often minor injuries of the cornea and conjunctiva exclusive of chemical burns (see Chapter 7) and corneal lacerations (see Chapter 13). Particular emphasis is placed upon ocular surface injuries involving the cornea, especially the difficult management problems of recurrent erosion, persistent epithelial defect, and noninfected ulceration. Since ocular surface trauma can directly cause or indirectly predispose to infectious keratitis, the principles of prophylaxis and management of microbial keratitis will also be considered.

CONJUNCTIVAL INJURY

Blunt Trauma

The conjunctiva is one component of the first line of ocular defense and is involved in many cases of blunt trauma to the eye and orbit. Thus, the clinical finding of either bleeding or air under the conjunctiva is exceedingly common. A subconjunctival hemorrhage, although alarming in appearance to the patient, is of no intrinsic consequence and is best managed with time and reassurance that the hematoma will initially spread and then, without treatment, gradually absorb over approximately 2 weeks. Conjunctival edema or chemosis is a frequent concomitant of minor trauma but may also signal a scleral rupture, retained intraorbital foreign body, or orbital fracture. Subconjunctival emphysema is distinguished by the cystic appearance of air loculated within the conjunctival stroma and by crepitus upon palpation. This finding is secondary to fracture of the periorbital sinuses, most commonly either the delicate lamina papyracea of the ethmoid sinus or the orbital floor overlying the maxillary sinus. Although each of these clinical signs may indicate only minor trauma without intraocular involvement, it is, of course, mandatory to rule out a ruptured globe or retained foreign body. The clinical examination approaches and diagnostic imaging techniques for this purpose are described in Chapters 1 and 2.

Foreign Body

Single or multiple foreign bodies embedded in the conjunctiva or cornea, common in the setting of minor occupational accidents, may also be associated with more severe trauma such as automobile accidents or explosions and may be propelled by industrial equipment, lawn mowers, and other machinery. Although nonpenetrating foreign bodies are of themselves trivial except for their irritative consequences, it is important to view them as potential indicators of a concurrent intraocular or intraorbital foreign body, especially in the classic setting of hammering or grinding metal upon metal in the absence of protective eye wear. Therefore, inspection of the entire globe for a perforating wound is mandatory, even to the extent of using imaging techniques, especially if a high-velocity injury has occurred. The examination must also include single or even double eversion of the lids to visualize and facilitate removal of foreign bodies retained on the tarsal conjunctival surface (Fig. 6-1), especially if the pattern of linear epithelial defects shows ongoing corneal abrasion with each blink and eye movement. A careful slit-lamp examination to note anterior chamber depth and inflammatory reaction, iris defects, lens clarity, and vitreous inflammation, in addition to intraocular pressure measurement and dilated ophthalmoscopy, are required to rule out a perforating injury.

Most conjunctival particulate materials will eventually be extruded spontaneously, and judicious irrigation with saline, sweeping with a cotton-tipped applicator, or removal with fine forceps, all with the aid of topical anesthesia, is effective in removing most particulate matter. A topical antibiotic ointment may then be used as infection prophylaxis and surface lubrication. Artificial tears or saline irrigations administered by the patient should also diminish irritative symptoms. In the absence either of a retained conjunctival, intraocular, or intraorbital foreign body or of increasing patient symptoms, follow-up is elective, as needed. Indeed, many inert materials can remain indefinitely within the conjunctiva without adverse reaction. A subsequent increase in irritative symptoms is most likely to represent the surfacing of a previously buried foreign body, which can then be removed.

Laceration

Conjunctival lacerations may occur in settings of injury similar to those resulting in superficial foreign bodies but also in those involving sharp projectiles, notably broken glass. The clinical

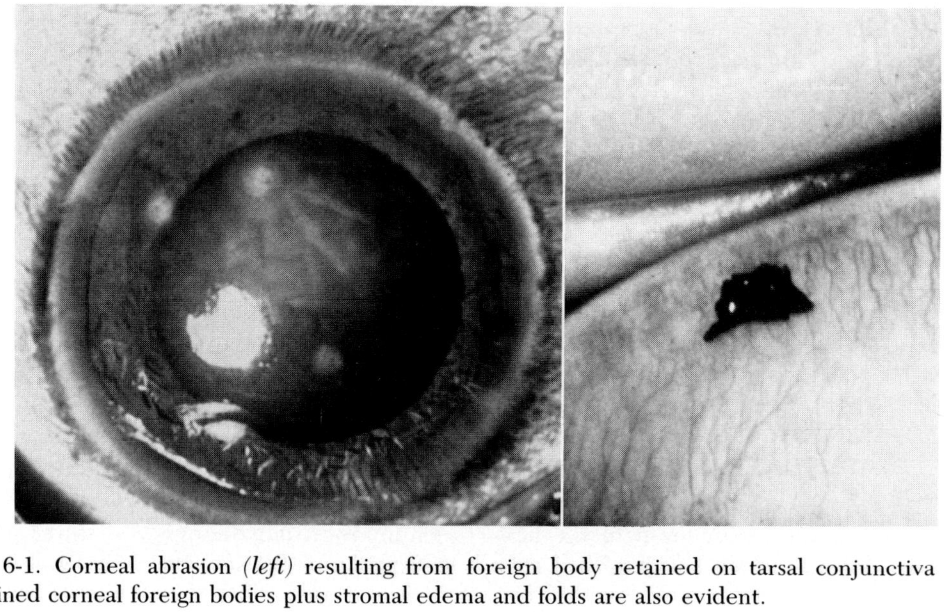

Fig. 6-1. Corneal abrasion *(left)* resulting from foreign body retained on tarsal conjunctiva *(right)*. Retained corneal foreign bodies plus stromal edema and folds are also evident.

signs may be readily evident upon external or slit-lamp examination as a conjunctival surface defect with prolapse of Tenon's tissue or orbital fat, or exposure of sclera. Subconjunctival hemorrhage is frequently present and may obscure the defect. Fluorescein staining, however, will enhance visualization of the violated conjunctival surface. As with foreign bodies, a complete history to ascertain the circumstances of injury and complete ophthalmic examination to rule out ruptured globe and intraocular foreign body are mandatory. Using topical anesthesia, the conjunctival defect must be carefully inspected to evaluate scleral integrity. Likewise, dilated ophthalmoscopy must be directed specifically toward the corresponding quadrant of injury. Depending on the extent of injury and cooperation of the patient, examination under anesthesia and diagnostic imaging techniques may be required.

In the absence of a ruptured globe or perforating injury, small conjunctival lacerations do not require surgical repair. Larger defects (greater than 1 cm) may be sutured with absorbable material, exercising care to oppose the corresponding wound margins without incarceration of Tenon's tissue within the wound and to respect the anatomic relationships of the caruncle and semilunar fold. With or without surgical intervention, antibiotic ointment and follow-up within 1 week should suffice.

CORNEAL INJURY

Blunt Trauma

Although blunt injury of insufficient force to rupture the globe can cause severe intraocular damage, its effects on the cornea are usually transient. A direct, focal, concussive blow (e.g., from a BB) causes mechanical deformation injury to the surrounding endothelium, evident as a ring of corneal edema.[1] Such localized contusion resolves with recovery of the injured cells or their replacement by adjacent endothelium. In more severe corneal contusion, ruptures of Descemet's membrane with concomitant breach of the endothelial barrier result in acute hydrops with massive stromal edema. In addition to blunt trauma, similar mechanisms account for the Descemet's membrane breaks related to forceps injury at birth, congenital glaucoma (Haab striae), keratoconus, and other peripheral degenerations. Although the decrease in vision and the acute appearance of corneal edema may be alarming, an otherwise healthy endothelium is capable of healing such defects by sliding over the area of retracted Descemet's membrane and restoring the normal endothelial pump and barrier to maintain corneal deturgescence. The residual parallel striae or fishmouth breaks in Descemet's membrane remain as historical evidence of the traumatic event but often have no effect on vision. Treatment, therefore, comprises reassurance to the patient that corneal rupture will not occur and that visual improvement will ensue, usually within 3 months. The numerous therapeutic modalities of patching, bandage soft contact lenses, topical corticosteroids, topical pressure-lowering agents, hypertonic salt preparations, and thermokeratoplasty remain of uncertain usefulness.

Specular microscopy of the corneal endothelium after blunt trauma may reveal a significant decrease in the endothelial cell population and increased cellular pleomorphism compared with the fellow eye. Corneal rupture is an uncommon consequence of blunt trauma and typically occurs only in eyes predisposed by a corneal stromal thinning disorder, such as extreme Terrien's marginal degeneration, or by prior surgery such as keratoplasty[2] or radial keratotomy (Fig. 6-2).

The presence of persistent corneal edema, especially if localized inferiorly and possibly with concomitant anterior chamber inflammatory reaction, may indicate an occult intraocular foreign body within the angle and may be visualized with gonioscopy (see Chapter 15).

Foreign Body

The same traumatic circumstances that lead to conjunctival foreign bodies are likely to involve foreign bodies lodged in the cornea. Similar clinical signs of blurred vision, photophobia, and foreign body sensation develop acutely. Biomicroscopic evidence of the retained corneal foreign body and rust ring (if the foreign body is iron-containing) are evident. If the foreign body has been present for more than 24 hours, a stromal infiltrate, usually noninfectious, is evident. However, especially in the event of vegetable foreign material, one must suspect microbial keratitis, possibly of fungal origin. Anterior chamber inflammatory reaction may be evident, usually to a mild degree and should promptly subside. Persistence of anterior cham-

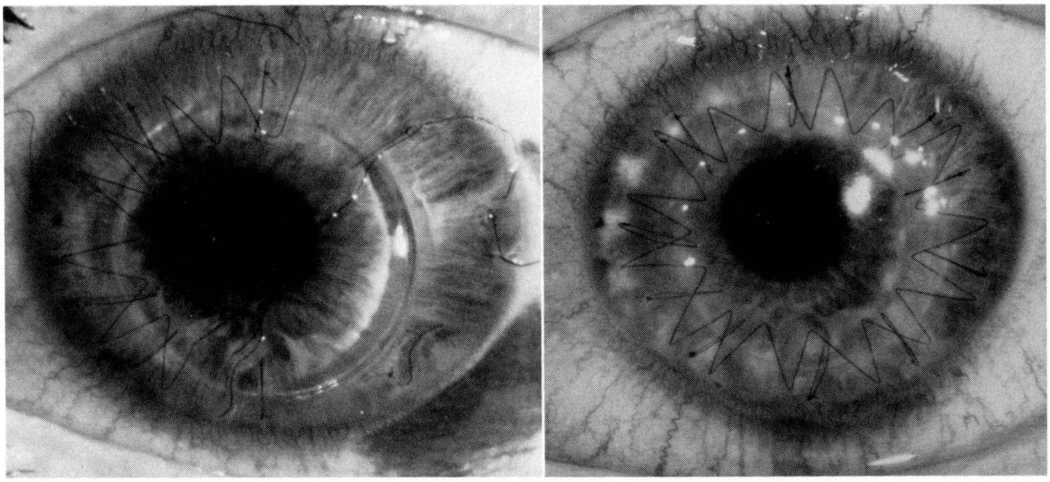

Fig. 6-2. Blunt trauma occurring 3 months postkeratoplasty causes rupture of sutures and incision with flat anterior chamber. Surgical repair without graft replacement was successful.

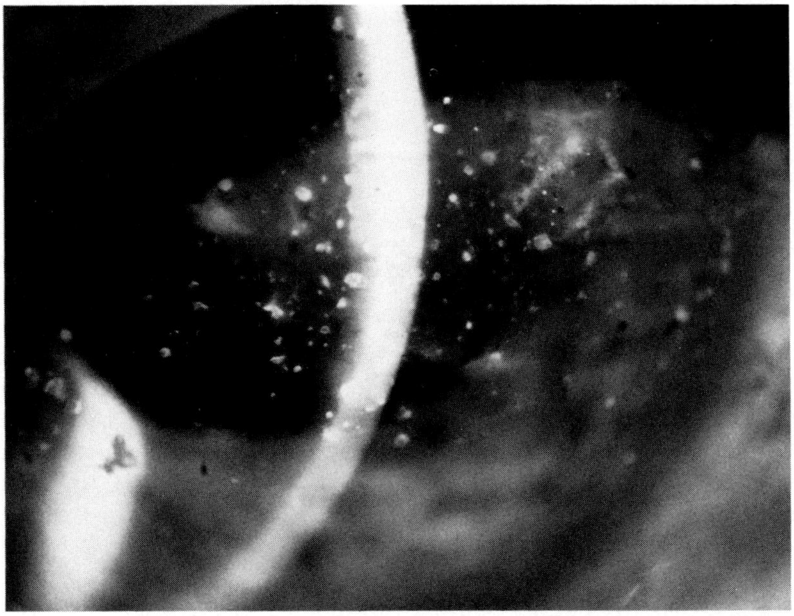

Fig. 6-3. Multiple superficial and intrastromal corneal foreign bodies following blast injury.

ber inflammation and especially hypopyon are indications of perforation and possible infectious endophthalmitis. As always, a history of the circumstances of injury with identification of the composition of the foreign material is important. Upon examination, other foreign bodies in the conjunctiva and fornices should be sought (Fig. 6-1). Finally, should any historical or examination finding suggest an occult intraocular foreign body, dilated ophthalmoscopy and possibly x-ray, B-scan ultrasound, computerized tomography (CT) scan, or magnetic resonance imaging (MRI) may be indicated.

A corneal foreign body is usually extracted using topical anesthesia at the slit lamp. Multiple superficial foreign bodies (Fig. 6-3) may be more easily removed by irrigation. Discrete, superficial foreign bodies are dislodged using a foreign-body spud or disposable 25-gauge needle under magnification. A rust ring can be re-

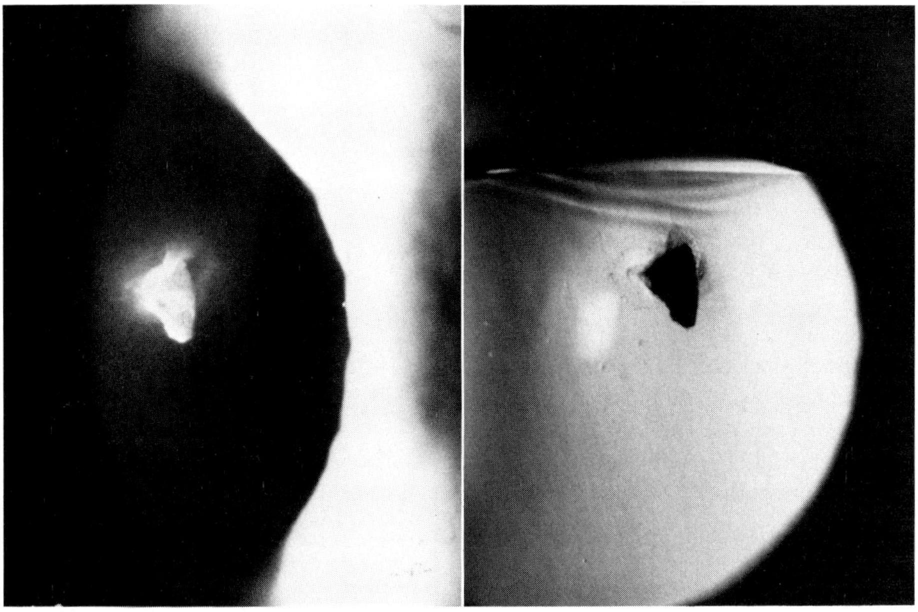

Fig. 6-4. A solitary, midstromal, metallic foreign body, shown with direct *(left)* and retroillumination *(right)*, appropriate for minor surgical removal.

moved with the foreign-body spud or a fine dental burr. Foreign bodies in the anterior or midstroma can usually be removed through the entrance wound using jeweler's forceps at the time of initial injury.

More deeply embedded foreign material or foreign bodies that have been retained for more than several days may be difficult to extract, and if there is no associated infiltrate suspicious of infection, they may be allowed to remain indefinitely or removed when spontaneously extruded at the corneal surface. Deeply embedded corneal foreign bodies must be examined carefully to determine possible perforation into the anterior chamber. Although such materials are most often remarkably noninfectious, the potential for microbial keratitis or even endophthalmitis must be carefully considered. Some deep foreign bodies may be allowed to remain or extrude spontaneously, but larger and more central foreign bodies warrant surgical removal (Fig. 6-4). If corneal penetration is suspected, a Seidel fluorescein test for aqueous leakage should be performed at the slit lamp, and occasionally a "provocative" Seidel test with cautious digital pressure on the eyelid may be required to elicit aqueous leakage in a perforating but self-sealing wound.

Although some deep foreign bodies can safely be removed at the slit lamp, they are usually better approached in the minor operating room setting where microscope magnification, more complete instrumentation, and materials such as sutures, viscoelastics, and cyanoacrylate tissue adhesive are available (see Chapter 13). To extract some deep foreign bodies, it may be necessary to enlarge the entry site with a razor blade knife. A deeply embedded corneal foreign body protruding into the anterior chamber and not removable via its entry site may be extracted via the anterior chamber using intraocular foreign-body forceps introduced through a limbal incision. With ferrous foreign bodies an appropriate magnet may be of assistance.

Following removal, the foreign body and the cornea should be cultured if any potentially infectious infiltrate is evident. A cycloplegic and a broad-spectrum antibiotic ointment with pressure patching are customary. Follow-up after 24 hours and the continued use of topical antibiotics for 3 to 5 days with additional follow-up is indicated, especially in the presence of conjunctival discharge, corneal stromal infiltrate, or substantial anterior chamber inflammatory reaction. Should the latter inflammatory signs persist, additional cultures and aggressive topical antibiotic therapy with extremely close surveillance are indicated.

Abrasion

Superficial abrasions of the corneal epithelium are caused by direct or tangential impact from a foreign body, most commonly from a fingernail, plant, paper, mascara brush, or contact lens. Because any of these objects may be microbially contaminated, the possibility for secondary infection must be borne in mind. Particular vigilance is indicated in contact lens–related abrasions, where there is a greater probability of a gram-negative organism, notably *Pseudomonas*. Such patients are exquisitely symptomatic, and the clinical diagnosis is usually evident upon biomicroscopic examination of the cornea, where an epithelial defect is most vividly appreciated with fluorescein or rose bengal stain. Although most acute abrasions display minimal stromal infiltrate or anterior chamber inflammatory reaction, these findings are particularly relevant as indicators of infection. Careful examination of the bulbar and tarsal conjunctiva with lid eversion is performed to rule out the possibility of additional foreign bodies.

Treatment consists of a topical broad-spectrum antibiotic ointment (e.g., polymyxin-bacitracin), a cycloplegic, and firm pressure patching. Follow-up examination should be performed within 24 hours to exclude the possibility of infection and monitor the progress of healing. In circumstances where a significant risk of microbial infection exists (e.g., abrasion from a tree branch or soft contact lens), an antibiotic with gram-negative activity (e.g., gentamicin or tobramycin) is added, an eye patch is withheld, and 24-hour follow-up is mandatory. Topical steroids should be avoided, especially if there is a probability that gram-negative bacteria or a fungus is the infectious agent. Once the epithelial defect has resolved, topical antibiotic ointments may be continued for an additional week as lubrication and microbial prophylaxis. Topical anesthetics should never be prescribed, because they delay wound healing and cause secondary keratitis. Contact lens wearers should abstain from lens wear for an additional week. If infection is suspected, cultures should be obtained, patching discontinued, and intensive fortified topical antibiotics (e.g., cefazolin 133 mg/ml plus gentamicin 14 mg/ml) commenced (see the box in the next column) (also see the section on infected ulceration).

FORTIFIED TOPICAL ANTIBODIES FOR MICROBIAL KERATITIS

Gentamicin/tobramycin (14 mg/ml)

- Draw up contents of 80-mg/2-ml parenteral antibiotic vial into syringe.
- With 22G or smaller needle, inject directly in 5-ml commercial aminoglycoside (3 mg/ml) bottle.
- Shelf life 1 year. Refrigeration not necessary.

Cefazolin (Kefzol, Ancef) (133 mg/ml)

- Reconstitute cefazolin 10 g with 69 ml NaCl 0.9% for injection.
- Transfer into sterile amber or opaque dropper bottles, passing through 0.45-μm filter.
- May freeze *once* for up to 12 weeks.
- Refrigerate between uses. Discard after 10 days.

Vancomycin (25 mg/ml)

- Reconstitute vancomycin 500 mg with 10 ml NaCl 0.9% for injection.
- Draw into 20-ml syringe; add saline to 20-ml total.
- Transfer into sterile amber or opaque dropper bottles, passing through 0.45-μm filter.
- May freeze *once* for up to 12 weeks.
- Refrigerate between uses. Discard after 14 days.

Protocols from the Massachusetts Eye and Ear Infirmary. Reproduced with permission.

Recurrent Erosion, Persistent Epithelial Defect, and Noninfected Stromal Ulceration

Among the effects of trauma on the ocular surface, defects of the corneal epithelium constitute a diverse group of clinical problems with significant clinical morbidity in terms of patient discomfort and visual loss. Depending upon the clinical circumstances, an epithelial erosion may become recurrent or persistent and may even progress to involve ulceration of the stroma.

Pathogenesis

The epithelial basement membrane complex, comprising the hemidesmosomes of the basal epithelial cell plasma membrane, the directly apposed extracellular collagenous basement membrane, and its attendant anchoring fibrils, is responsible for tight adhesion of the corneal epithelium to the stroma (Fig. 6-5, *A*). Consequently, any traumatic, dystrophic, or degen-

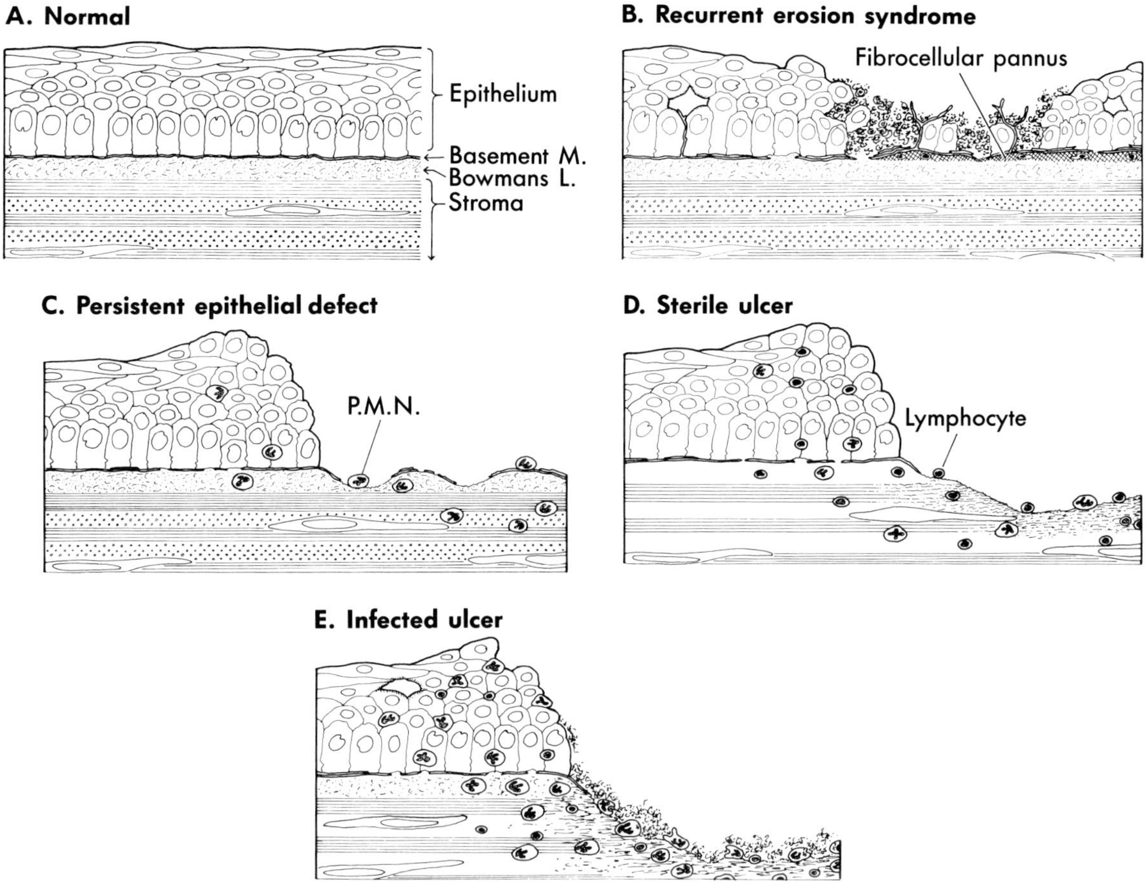

Fig. 6-5. Schematic morphology of corneal epithelial defect, erosion, and ulceration. **A,** Normal cornea displays regular epithelial layers, uniform continuous basement membrane, and Bowman's layer and stroma devoid of inflammatory cells. **B,** Recurrent epithelial erosion involves epithelial defects associated with aberrant and discontinuous basement membrane plus subepithelial fibrocellular pannus, but without Bowman's layer defect or inflammation. **C,** Persistent epithelial defect is notable for thickened and nonmotile epithelial cell layer at defect edge, defects of basement membrane and Bowman's layer, and some inflammatory cells. **D,** Sterile ulceration involves enzymatically mediated degradation of Bowman's layer and stroma, usually in the presence of acute and chronic inflammatory cells. **E,** Microbial keratitis involves more intense acute inflammatory infiltrate of epithelium and stroma in the presence of infectious microorganisms.

erative disturbance at this level can predispose to defective epithelial adhesion and repetitive breakdown of the epithelial cell layer, hence the so-called recurrent erosion syndrome (Fig. 6-5, *B*).[4] In situations where the ocular surface is further compromised by extensive epithelial damage, inflammation, denervation, tear deficiency, and stromal scarring, the problems of adhesion are compounded by a failure of epithelial mitosis and migration, resulting in a persistent defect (Fig. 6-5, *C*). Such epithelial defects frequently occur in the setting of chronic inflammation and, in fact, may be self-perpetuating since inflammatory cells inhibit epithelial wound healing. This vicious cycle of persistent epithelial defect and chronic inflammation is of further concern as it predisposes to enzymatically mediated sterile ulceration of the corneal stroma (Fig. 6-5, *D*).

An overall etiologic classification of disorders of the epithelium and basement membrane complex that result in recurrent erosion, persistent epithelial defect, or stromal ulceration is beyond the scope of this discussion. However, as an example, primary epithelial disorders such as epithelial basement membrane dystrophy (map-dot-fingerprint dystrophy) predispose to the recurrent erosion syndrome, while acquired epithelial disorders, such as neurotrophic keratitis secondary to a fifth cranial nerve palsy, may lead to persistent epithelial defects. Similarly, a primary disorder of the basement membrane complex, as in diabetes, may predispose to a persistent epithelial defect, whereas an acquired basement membrane complex disorder, most commonly following a mechanical abrasion, will produce only a recurrent corneal erosion. Following more widespread ocular surface damage, such as occurs from a chemical burn, combined epithelial and basement membrane complex disorders can precipitate both persistent epithelial defects and stromal ulceration.

Recurrent Erosion

The clinical symptoms of recurrent erosion syndrome include recurrent attacks of acute ocular pain, tearing, and redness, typically occurring during sleep or at awakening. A history of prior corneal abrasion, especially a shearing injury, as from a tree branch or fingernail scratch, can often be elicited. The clinical signs evident with slit lamp examination vary from focal superficial punctate keratitis to an area of devitalized, disadhesive epithelium to a full-thickness epithelial defect (Color Plate 6-1, *A* to *C*). Diagnosis and primary therapy, medical therapy, and surgical therapy as necessary are described in the next section and outlined in the box below.[4]

THERAPY OF RECURRENT EPITHELIAL EROSION

Diagnosis and primary therapy

- Determine etiology
- Debride devitalized tissue
- Culture as indicated

Medical therapy

- Lubricants, hypertonics, visco substances (avoid preservatives)
- Pressure patch
- Therapeutic soft contact lens (antibiotic ± cycloplegic ± steroid)
- Collagen shield

Surgical therapy

- Superficial epithelial keratectomy
- Anterior stromal puncture
- Surface cautery/diathermy

Diagnosis and primary therapy. The initial evaluation must be directed toward establishing an exact etiologic diagnosis in order to select appropriate therapy and make an accurate prognosis. For example, the patient with recurrent corneal erosion in one eye should also be carefully examined for epithelial basement membrane (map-dot-fingerprint) dystrophy in the asymptomatic eye as evidenced by intraepithelial microcysts or subepithelial geographic and fingerprint lines. As treatment for extensive devitalization and disadhesion of the epithelium and associated cellular debris, simple localized debridement to provide a smooth basement membrane or Bowman's layer substrate for healthy epithelium to resurface and readhere should be performed. This is best accomplished by gentle scrubbing with a cellulose sponge (Weck-cel) and removal of the epithelial fragments with jeweler's forceps (Fig. 6-5). Sharp instruments (such as scalpel blades) and chemical cauterizers (such as iodine) are never appropriate.

Medical therapy. Adjunctive medical therapy for routine recurrent erosion should include continuous pressure patching during the 24- to 72-hour interval of epithelial wound healing followed by continuation of lubricants, especially ointments applied at bedtime, for approximately 8 weeks until the newly restored epithelium has been able to completely reconstruct the basement membrane complexes. Nonpreserved petrolatum ointments, such as Refresh PM, Duolube, Hypotears, and Aquatears, are preferred and appear to be as effective as hypertonic preparations, which can be irritating. If conventional lid closure and lubrication therapy are not successful, a therapeutic soft contact lens remains an excellent approach because it is compatible with vision, comfort, and cosmesis during the 2 months required for epithelial readhesion. For topical antibiotic prophylaxis, current preferences include sulfacetamide or an aminoglycoside plus frequent instillation of unpreserved saline or other lubricant. In eyes that still have residual inflammation following a recent erosive episode, tolerance of a bandage soft contact lens may be increased by the use of an antibiotic ointment for both lubrication and infection prophylaxis, and cycloplegia (such as atropine 1%), especially during the first few days of wear when the "tight lens syndrome" is most likely to develop. With extreme caution, topical steroids

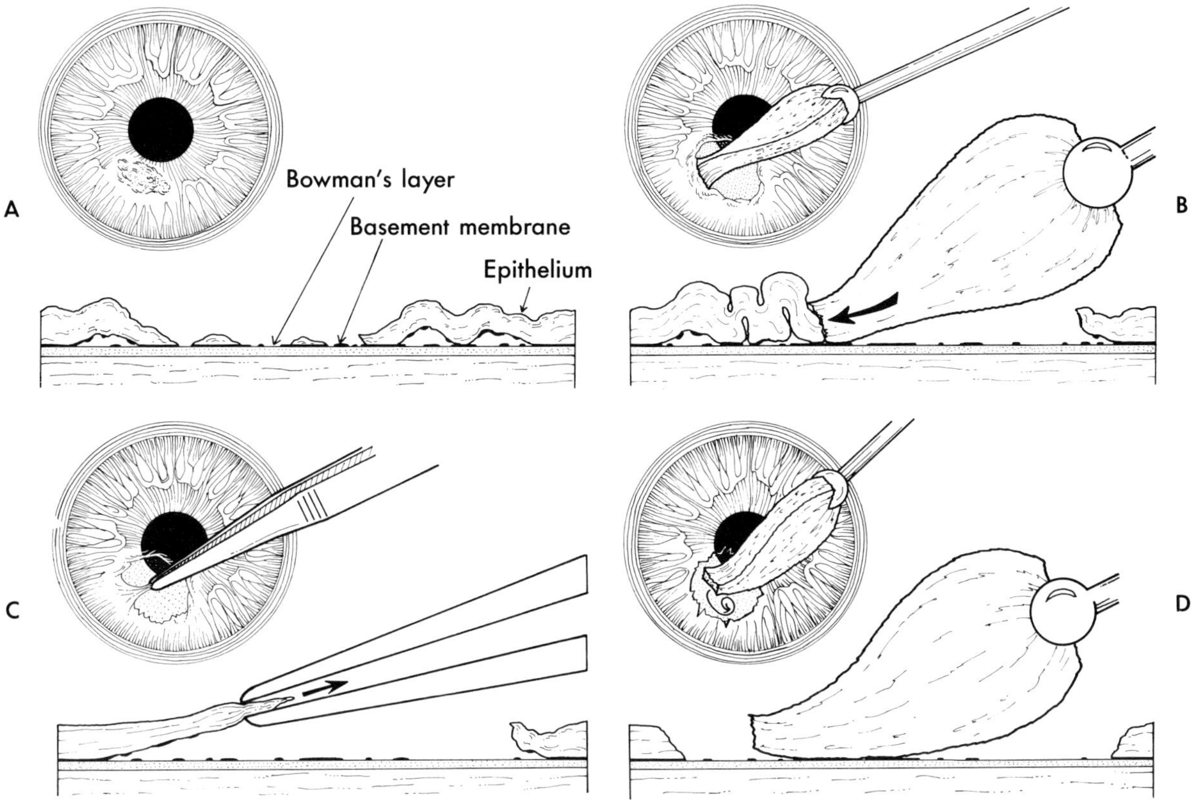

Fig. 6-6. Technique of epithelial debridement involves removal of devitalized epithelium and debris (**A**) with dry cellulose sponges (**B** and **D**) and jeweler's forceps (**C**), thereby facilitating subsequent epithelial recovery and adhesion.

(such as dexamethasone ointment) may be used when inflammation causes significant discomfort and retards epithelial wound healing. Close follow-up is mandatory for those patients with concomitant ocular surface disorders who use multiple topical medications, especially steroids, and are thus at increased risk of microbial superinfection. In the presence of a therapeutic soft contact lens, the progress of epithelial wound healing can be monitored by applying topical anesthesia and fluorescein, sliding the lens aside with a cotton-tipped applicator, observing the staining pattern at the slit lamp, and then repositioning the contact lens on the cornea (Fig. 6-7). This simple maneuver obviates the time and manipulation required to remove and replace the contact lens, and the fluorescein will be rapidly diluted from the lens without permanent staining.

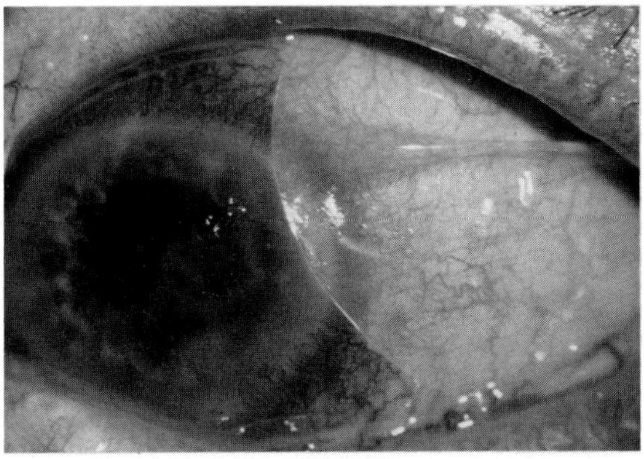

Fig. 6-7. To assess corneal epithelial recovery in the presence of a bandage soft contact lens, topical anesthesia and fluorescein are instilled, and the lens is slid aside and then repositioned.

Surgical therapy. For the most recalcitrant erosive cases, surgical therapy may be indicated. Particularly in situations where there is excessive aberrant epithelial basement membrane and subepithelial collagenous pannus (most commonly in map-dot-fingerprint dystrophy but also in numerous other superficial dystrophic or degenerative disoders), the extremely simple and noninvasive procedure of superficial epithe-

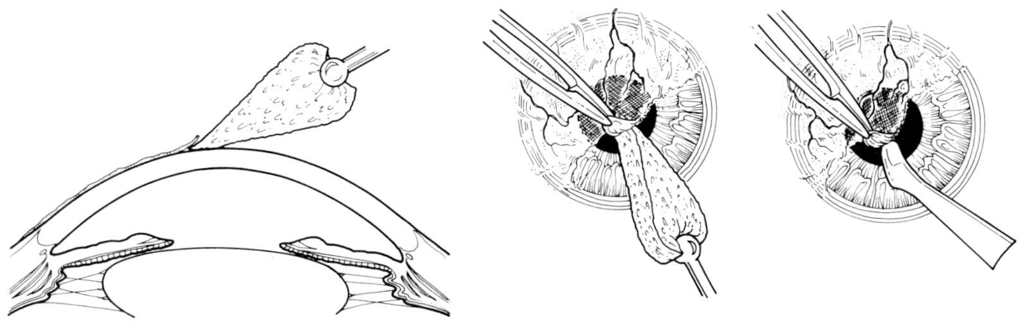

Fig. 6-8. Technique of superficial keratectomy. A dry cellulose sponge is used to identify a cleavage plane beneath fibrocellular tissue. The pannus is then stripped using a dry sponge and tissue forceps. A scarifier may be used for firmly adherent tissue by scraping without sharp incision or dissection to avoid stromal damage.

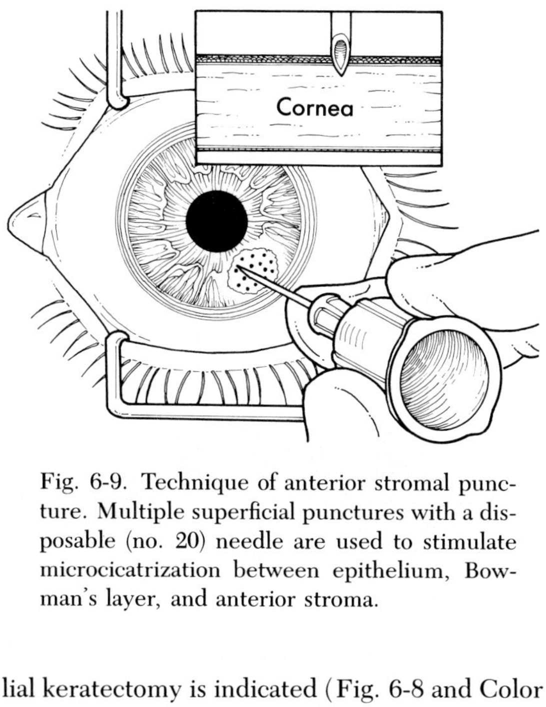

Fig. 6-9. Technique of anterior stromal puncture. Multiple superficial punctures with a disposable (no. 20) needle are used to stimulate microcicatrization between epithelium, Bowman's layer, and anterior stroma.

lial keratectomy is indicated (Fig. 6-8 and Color Plate 6-1, *G* to *J*).[5] The procedure is performed using the operating microscope and topical anesthesia. The area appropriate for debridement is identified with fluorescein staining or slit-lamp biomicroscopy or both. The epithelium and any loosely adherent subepithelial debris is debrided by gentle scraping with a disposable scarifier blade (Grieshaber 681.01 or Beaver 59). The corneal surface is then kept dry to visualize any topographic irregularities that may represent focal accumulations of aberrant basement membrane or pannus. With the leading edge of a dry cellulose sponge, cleavage planes can be identified between the anterior abnormal accumulations and the underlying Bowman's layer or stroma. Jeweler's forceps may then be used to strip these cellophane-like membranes from the surface. Further polishing of the peeled surface is accomplished with additional cellulose sponges or careful scraping. Sharp dissection (as in lamellar keratectomy or diamond burr polishing) is never used. Furthermore, although reports have suggested that debridement be carried broadly over the entire corneal surface,[6] we perform only focal debridement in areas of definite biomicroscopic abnormality and avoid damage to the limbal epithelium. Postoperatively, pressure patching with topical antibiotic followed by copious lubrication, and in some cases soft contact lens application, has produced excellent visual and symptomatic results.

Occasionally, when conventional medical therapy and superficial epithelial keratectomy fail, the anterior stromal puncture technique of McLean, MacRae, and Rich[7] may be used (Fig. 6-9; Color Plate 6-1, *K* and *L*). In this technique, 15 to 25 micropunctures are made into the anterior stroma in the area of erosion using a no. 20 hypodermic needle to encourage epithelial adhesion by inciting focal microcicatrization to "spot weld" epithelium to stroma. Although easily and safely performed at the slit lamp, this procedure is perhaps best reserved for posttraumatic or postinfection areas of focal erosion that do not involve the visual axis. In erosions involving the visual axis (where even nebular stromal haze might compromise vision) and conditions of more diffuse basement membrane complex abnormality (such as map-dot-fingerprint dystrophy), epithelial debridement, superficial keratectomy, or both are preferred.

The use of surface cautery or diathermy is not indicated in the management of recurrent erosion or persistent epithelial defect in any eye with visual potential but may be useful in providing relief of painful bullous keratopathy in eyes that are not tolerant of bandage soft contact lens therapy and are not candidates for penetrating keratoplasty. Using the operating microscope and topical anesthesia, approximately 100 focal burns are made with a disposable thermal cautery or diathermy instrument over the entire corneal surface, followed by cellulose sponge debridement of the devitalized epithelium. Pressure patching with topical antibiotic is continued for 1 to 2 weeks until the epithelium has recovered.

The excimer laser may also have potential application for ocular surface disorders because it can be directed to photoablate fibrocellular pannus and band keratopathy, leaving a smooth, anterior stromal surface suitable for optical clarity and epithelial stability. The long-term success of such procedures depends on the extent to which anterior stromal scarring can be avoided or pharmacologically suppressed. At present, however, conventional techniques of superficial epithelial keratectomy remain both simple and effective for such purposes.

Persistent Epithelial Defect and Noninfected Stromal Ulceration

Diagnosis and primary therapy, medical therapy, and surgical therapy are also mainstays of the approach to persistent epithelial defects and noninfected stromal ulceration (see box).[8] A nonhealing epithelial defect with elevated margins that have undergone mitotic and migratory arrest is particularly ominous because of its predisposition to sterile ulceration or microbial superinfection. (Color Plate 6-1, *D* to *F*). Conversely, because stromal ulceration seldom progresses in the presence of an intact epithelium, closure of an epithelial defect should be encouraged by every possible medical and surgical means.

THERAPY OF PERSISTENT EPITHELIAL DEFECT AND NONINFECTED STROMAL ULCERATION

Diagnosis and primary therapy

- Determine etiology—Examine lids, tears, sensation—examine for systemic (e.g., collagen-vascular) and dermatologic (e.g., rosacea) disease
- Debride devitalized tissue
- Culture as indicated
- Initiate appropriate antimicrobial/antiinflammatory therapy (avoid preservatives and toxic antibiotics and antivirals)
- Close lid (pressure patch, taping, botulism toxin)

Medical therapy

- Lubricants, hypertonics, visco substances (avoid preservatives)
- Fibronectin (investigational)
- Epidermal growth factor (investigational)
- Retinoids (investigational)
- Ascorbate/citrate (investigational)
- Medroxyprogesterone
- Tetracycline
- Immunosuppression (e.g., cyclophosphamide, azathioprine)
- Therapeutic soft contact lens
- Collagen shield
- Tissue adhesive (for sterile ulceration)
- Glued-on contact lens (for total persistent epithelial defect and high ulceration risk)

Surgical therapy

- Punctum occlusion (collagen inserts, punctum plugs, cauterization)
- Tarsorrhaphy
- Conjunctival resection
- Limbal or conjunctival autograft
- Tenon-plasty
- Mucous membrane graft (oral or nasal)
- Keratoepithelioplasty
- Conjunctival flap (partial or total)
- Lamellar keratoplasty (± limbal tissue)
- Penetrating keratoplasty
- Keratoprosthesis

Diagnosis and primary therapy. Given the management complexities of these conditions, it is particularly important to determine their precise causes. Although it is compelling to focus on the corneal problem, it is equally important to examine the eyelids, tears, and corneal sensation. For example, clinically unsuspected keratoconjunctivitis sicca is probably the most prevalent cause of persistent epithelial defects following anterior segment surgery and nonsurgical trauma. Moreover, dermatologic conditions (most commonly rosacea) and systemic disorders (especially collagen-vascular disease) should be sought because the former are frequent concomitants of ocular surface disorders and the latter may be life- as well as sight-threatening.

Once cause has been established, it is important to initiate appropriate antimicrobial and antiinflammatory therapy and to discontinue unneeded lubricants, antibiotics, or antivirals that may have inadvertently resulted in a chronic medicamentosa reaction.

Medical therapy. Particularly in the dry eye patient, avoidance of preservatives, especially where medicamentosa toxicity is suspected, may be curative. Newer lubricant preparations, including viscoelastics such as dilute hyaluronate and hydroxymethyl cellulose (Celluvisc), are of potential interest although awaiting clinical verification. Other biologic agents to promote epithelial wound healing and adhesion, specifically fibronectin[9,10] and epidermal growth factor,[11,12] also remain investigational (see box on p. 73).

In severe chemical and possibly thermal burn (see Chapter 7), the ocular anterior segment is rendered scorbutic and thereby unable to secrete collagen for proper wound healing. Although direct beneficial effects on epithelial recovery are uncertain, topical and systemic ascorbate (10% sodium ascorbate drops every 2 hours and ascorbic acid 8 g by mouth daily) appear useful in reducing sterile stromal ulceration.[13] In these situations, citrate (10% sodium citrate in tears without EDTA every hour plus sodium citrate 2 g by mouth every 6 hours) may be important to inhibit metalloprotease enzymes (including collagenase) of acute inflammatory cells and injured keratocytes, thereby decreasing their ability to ulcerate the corneal stroma. Because human experience with citrate is extremely limited, its clinical efficacy is as yet uncertain.

Vitamin A analogs have been applied topically for the treatment of various dry eye disorders, especially those of major severity that result in keratinization of the ocular surface epithelium such as advanced keratoconjunctivitis sicca, Stevens-Johnson syndrome, ocular cicatricial pemphigoid, and radiation keratitis. In a series of selected patients with these severe disorders, Tseng et al[14] observed major improvement in ocular surface characteristics, including reversal of keratinization and closure of persistent epithelial defects, while using topical Tretinoin (all-*trans*-retinoic acid) 0.01% once or twice daily. However, subsequent trials attempting to extend these initial observations to mild dry eye cases failed to demonstrate efficacy. Thus, it is likely that clinical use of topical retinoids will be appropriate only in situations of severe ocular surface keratinization.

Surgical therapy. For patients with significant and chronic dry eye disorders, which can both produce and promote the persistence of a corneal epithelial defect, punctum occlusion is extremely beneficial. Collagen inserts and silicone plugs (Eagle Vision) have recently gained popularity because of their respectively temporary and reversible characteristics. However, temporary surface cauterization or deeper permanent cauterization using the hyfrecater continues to be technically simple, rapid, economical, and complication-free. Punctum occlusion by laser seems to offer no technical advantage.

The recently introduced collagen shield (Bausch & Lomb; Chiron)—collagen in the configuration of a bandage soft contact lens—is said to improve patient comfort and promote corneal epithelial wound healing despite its dissolution within 24 to 72 hours in currently available designs.[15] This advantage is still somewhat uncertain because no laboratory investigation has established a biologic effect of the collagen gel alone upon wound healing and no extensive prospective clinical study has proven its superiority over conventional patching or hydrogel contact lenses. However, an important additional benefit of the device is as a sustained-release drug delivery system; the collagen gel concentrates topical medications and releases the medication continuously to the ocular surface. This application is especially useful in the management of bacterial keratitis.[16]

Transplantation of autologous bulbar conjunctiva has become an effective means of restoring ocular surface epithelial integrity in patients with unilateral chemical or thermal burns.[17] Recent laboratory evidence that limbal epithelium is the "stem cell" from which corneal epithelium is derived prompted us to devise the technique of limbal autograft transplantation (Fig. 6-10).[18] This procedure can be performed early (about 2 months after injury) for corneal and conjunctival epithelial defects that persist despite aggressive medical management. It is done to facilitate reepithelialization, promote stability of the ocular surface epithelium, minimize risk of sterile or microbial ulceration, and suppress chronic inflammation and neovascularization. Limbal transplantation can also be used for later-stage rehabilitation in cases where regenerating epithelium has retained conjunctival

A-C

D-F

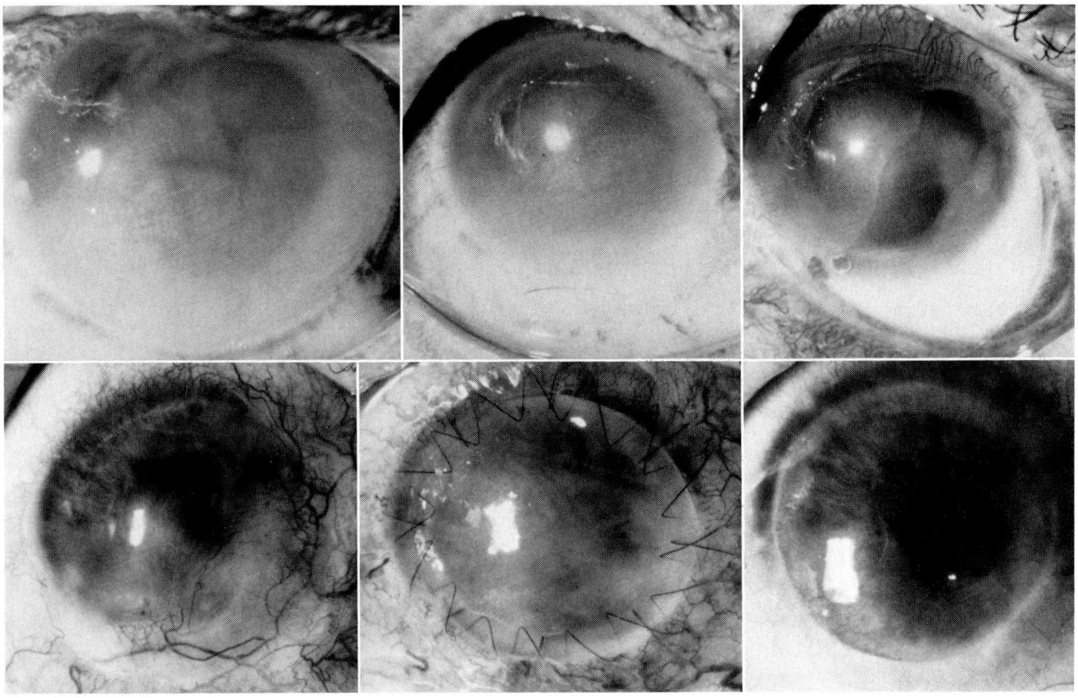

Fig. 6-10. Limbal autograft transplantation for chemical burn. **A,** Severe acute chemical burn with total destruction of ocular surface epithelium. **B,** An extensive persistent epithelial defect with limbal and scleral ischemia develops. **C,** A nonhealing defect of corneal and conjunctival epithelium with necrosis of totally ischemic sclera ensues. **D,** Within days after limbal autograft and conjunctival advancement, the epithelial defects have healed completely. **E,** Deep lamellar keratoplasty is then performed. **F,** One year following lamellar-keratoplasty visual acuity is 20/60 with intact epithelial surface, clear stroma and regression of neovascularization.

characteristics, thereby limiting vision and making penetrating keratoplasty hazardous. In some cases this approach with removal of superficial fibrovascular pannus will not only rehabilitate the ocular surface but also improve media clarity and hence visual acuity. In cases requiring subsequent lamellar or penetrating keratoplasty, the prognosis for graft success is improved by prior limbal grafting.

In cases of bilateral severe chemical injury, healthy conjunctival or limbal epithelium may not be available for autograft transplantation. In this situation, surgical advancement of posterior Tenon's tissue provides vascular support for areas of ischemic sclera and limbus, thereby encouraging conjunctival reepithelialization. Autografts of buccal mucous membrane have long been in use for conjunctival replacement, but goblet cell-containing nasal mucosa may be more suitable. Thoft[19] has advocated the use of allogenic keratoepithelioplasty, as performed by denuding the recipient cornea of epithelium and pannus followed by suturing donor lenticules of epithelium and superficial stroma from a fresh donor cornea. We have modified this approach by using large-diameter (11- to 12-mm) lamellar allografts, which also facilitate the transfer of viable limbal tissue. Unfortunately, the success of such allograft procedures is often limited by epithelial rejection and a tendency for abnormal, conjunctivally derived epithelium to eventually repopulate the ocular surface.

Infected Ulceration

Infectious microbial keratitis seldom occurs in the absence of predisposing factors, and ocular trauma is a frequent precipitating cause. In recent years, the stress of contact lens wear, particularly with extended overnight use, has become a particularly prevalent cause of microbial keratitis. Detailed consideration of differential diagnosis and management is well beyond the scope of this discussion power. However, basic principles in the approach to bacterial, *Acan-*

thamoeba, and fungal keratitis will be outlined here.

The clinical presentation of microbial keratitis is usually accompanied by pain, inflammation, photophobia, decreased vision, and discharge. Objective findings include conjunctival injection, single or multiple inflammatory infiltrates of the corneal stroma, usually with overlying epithelial defects and potentially with necrosis of stroma leading to descemetocoele formation and perforation (Fig. 6-5, *E*). Anterior chamber inflammatory reaction is evidenced by keratic precipitates, anterior chamber flare and cell, hypopyon, and posterior synechiae. Most commonly, especially where traumatic causes are involved, infectious keratitis is bacterial, although in special circumstances fungal keratitis (following vegetable matter trauma, especially in tropical climates) or *Acanthamoeba* keratitis (usually in a soft contact lens wearer using saline rinsing solution prepared from salt tablets) may develop.

Any stromal infiltrate with overlying epithelial defect should be considered a potential microbial keratitis, and the work-up should proceed in standard fashion, including complete history to search for predisposing factors and slit-lamp microscopy with careful documentation of ulceration size and depth. Smears and cultures of not only the corneal lesion and conjunctiva, but also all concurrent contact lenses, solutions, and topical medications must be taken. The last is especially important given the high prevalence of contamination of typical medications (about 30%). Cultures are performed routinely on blood agar (for bacteria), thioglycollate (for anaerobic bacteria), chocolate agar (for *Neisseria* species), Sabouraud's medium (for fungus), Lowenstein-Jensen medium (for mycobacteria), and nonnutrient agar with *E. coli* (for *Acanthamoeba*). Smears of the ulcer base are routinely taken for Gram and Giemsa stain. The GMS-silver and Calcofluor White stains are appropriate for fungus and *Acanthamoeba*. Corneal biopsies may be indicated, especially in partially treated cases that have proven recalcitrant to therapy and hence where an unusual organism is suspected.

Treatment is directed toward broad coverage of the organism suspected on the basis of history, clinical findings, and microscopic examination of corneal smears. Subsequent modifications are dictated by response to therapy and microbial culture results.

In general, a corneal epithelial abrasion or geographic defect with no significant focal stromal infiltrate and no anterior chamber reaction is appropriately managed with broad-spectrum topical antibiotic ointment (such as polymyxin-bacitracin four times a day), except in the situation of contact lens use, where the increased probability of gram-negative keratitis mandates addition of an aminoglycoside antibiotic (such as tobramycin or gentamicin ointment 4 times a day). Cycloplegia (e.g., atropine 1% daily) is optional. Patching may be appropriate to improve epithelial healing and increase patient comfort; however, in the presence of any stromal infiltrate and in all patients with contact lens–related abrasions (Fig. 6-11), the infected eye should *not* be patched. Although such patients can be managed on an outpatient basis, 24-hour follow-up is mandatory for all cases with stromal infiltrates and all contact lens-related cases.

With more substantial stromal infiltrate and anterior chamber reaction or purulent discharge, intensive antibiotic therapy with fortified cefazolin and tobramycin or gentamicin is used hourly, so that the patient is compelled to alternate these medications every half hour around the clock. In such circumstances, depending on the severity of the ulceration, patient compliance, and other social and medical factors, either outpatient management or hospital treatment may be appropriate. Given the extreme efficacy of fortified topical antibiotics alone, subconjunctival antibiotics (such as cefazolin 100 mg and gentamicin 20 mg) are almost never used except in situations of extreme severity, or when fortified antibiotics cannot be initiated immediately, or when there is difficulty with compliance (e.g., for pediatric patients).

When fungal keratitis is suspected in a clinical setting of trauma (especially with vegetable matter foreign bodies, a prolonged course of indolent ulceration unresponsive to multiple antibiotic therapies and complicated by steroid use, and slit-lamp findings of gray stromal infiltrate with feathery edges and satellite lesion), then appropriate cultures, smears, and possibly corneal biopsies must be taken for pathologic and microbiologic study. Treatment includes combinations of Natamycin 5% (every 1 to 2 hours), amphotericin B 0.15% (every hour), and/or ketoconazole (200 to 400 mg by mouth daily). Topical steroids should be discontinued or withheld and the response to therapy monitored fre-

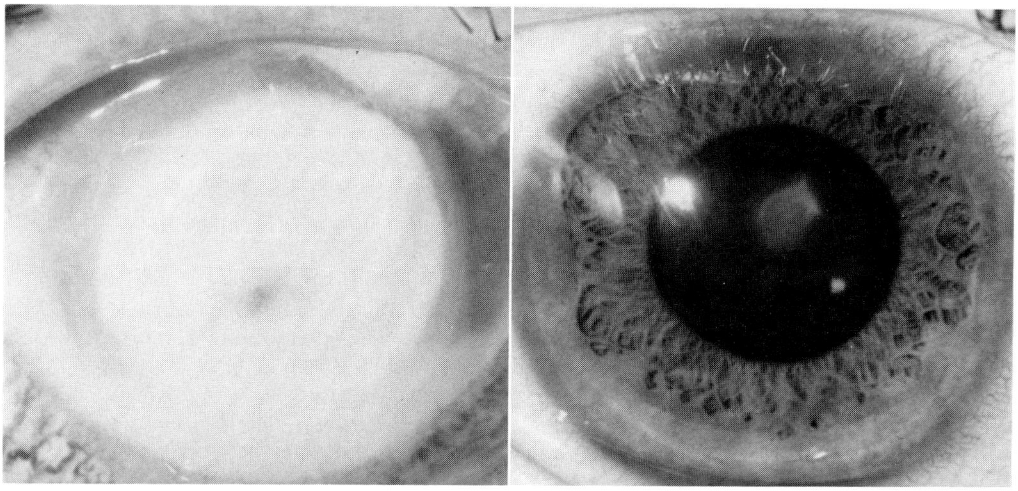

Fig. 6-11. *Pseudomonas* keratitis related to soft contact lens wear. **A,** Intense stromal infiltration and liquefaction. **B,** Small superficial ulcer is also *pseudomonas* culture positive.

quently, with the expectation that the clinical course will be prolonged.

Acanthamoeba keratitis is especially prevalent in patients who wear soft contact lenses, use nonsterile saline solution from salt tablets, and swim while wearing the lenses. Disproportionately severe and prolonged ocular pain, photophobia unresponsive to antibiotics or antivirals, and possibly some symptomatic improvement from topical steroids are typically accompanied by clinical findings of a stromal ring infiltrate or subepithelial infiltrates in a radial perineural pattern. Treatment is prolonged and complex. It involves combinations of Brolene (propamidine isethionate 0.1% every hour), clotrimazole 1% (every 2 hours), neomycin (every hour), and ketoconazole (400 mg by mouth daily). A topical steroid may be necessary to control inflammation and pain but should otherwise be avoided. The course of recovery is extremely prolonged, often requiring months of continuous topical therapy, close monitoring, and slow tapering of the medical regimen. Corneal transplantation is hazardous but sometimes successful. (Note that Brolene, available over the counter in Europe, can be obtained only with FDA approval in the United States.)

Ultraviolet Radiation and Electrical Injury

Ultraviolet radiation injury to the cornea usually occurs after accidental exposure to a welder's arc or sunlamp without protective eye wear. Pain, foreign body sensation, and photophobia usually develop 6 to 12 hours after exposure. Biomicroscopy reveals superficial punctate keratopathy in an interpalpebral distribution. Other etiologies to be differentiated include toxic epithelial keratopathy following chemical or drug exposure, nocturnal lagophthalmos, and exposure keratitis from other mechanical or neurologic causes. Treatment involves topical cycloplegia and antibiotic ointment with pressure patching, and possibly systemic analgesics. Antibiotic ointment is continued for several days until irritative symptoms abate, vision improves, and superficial punctate keratitis resolves.

Chronic ultraviolet light exposure, as found in fishermen or agricultural workers, may be associated with the development of pterygia. Long-term exposure to infrared light, classically the occupational hazard of glassblowers, may result in cataracts. Similarly, electrical injury, as caused by lightning or electrocution, may cause cataracts months to years later.[20] In the absence of appropriate corneal shielding, x-radiation to the orbit can result in cataracts as well as radiation keratitis.

References

1. Slingsby JG and Forstot SL: Effect of blunt trauma on the corneal endothelium, Arch Ophthalmol 99:1041-1043, 1981.
2. Topping TM et al: Traumatic wound dehiscence following penetrating keratoplasty, Br J Ophthalmol 66:174-178, 1982.
3. Karr DJ, Grutzmacher RD, and Reeh MJ: Radial keratotomy complicated by sterile keratitis and corneal perforation: histopathologic case report and review of complications, Ophthalmology 92:1244-1248, 1985.

4. Kenyon KR: Recurrent corneal erosion: pathogenesis and therapy, Int Ophthalmol Clin 19(2):169-195, 1979.
5. Wood TO et al: Treatment of Reis-Bücklers' corneal dystrophy by removal of subepithelial fibrous tissue, Am J Ophthalmol 85:360-362, 1978.
6. Buxton JN and Fox ML: Superficial epithelial keratectomy in the treatment of epithelial basement membrane dystrophy: a preliminary report, Arch Ophthalmol 101:392-395, 1983.
7. McLean EN, MacRae SM, and Rich LF: Recurrent erosion: treatment by anterior stromal puncture, Ophthalmology 93:784-788, 1986.
8. Wagoner MD and Kenyon KR: Noninfected corneal ulceration. Focal points: clinical modules of ophthalmology, vol III, no. 7, San Francisco, 1985, American Academy of Ophthalmology.
9. Fujikawa LS et al: Fibronectin in healing rabbit corneal wounds, Lab Invest 45:120-129, 1981.
10. Nishida T et al: Fibronectin: a new therapy for corneal trophic ulcer, Arch Ophthalmol 101:1046-1048, 1983.
11. Schultz GS, Davis JB, and Eiferman RA: Growth factors and corneal epithelium, Cornea 7:96-101, 1988.
12. Singh G and Foster CS: Epidermal growth factor in alkali-burned corneal epithelial wound healing, Am J Ophthalmol 103:802-807, 1987.
13. Pfister RR and Paterson CA: Ascorbic acid in the treatment of alkali burns of the eye, Ophthalmology 87:1050-1057, 1980.
14. Tseng SCG et al: Topical retinoid treatment for various dry-eye disorders, Ophthalmology 92:717-727, 1985.
15. Ruffini JJ, Aquavella JV, and LoCascio JA: Effect of collagen shields on corneal epithelialization following penetrating keratoplasty, Ophthalmic Surg 20:21-25, 1989.
16. Sawusch MR et al: Use of collagen corneal shields in the treatment of bacterial keratitis, Am J Ophthalmol 106:279-281, 1988.
17. Thoft RA: Conjunctival transplantation, Arch Ophthalmol 95:1425-1427, 1977.
18. Kenyon KR and Tseng SCG: Limbal autograft transplantation for ocular surface disorders, Ophthalmology 96:709-723, 1989.
19. Thoft RA: Keratoepithelioplasty, Am J Ophthalmol 97:1-6, 1984.
20. Johnson EV, Kline LB, and Skalka HW: Electrical cataracts: a case report and review of the literature, Ophthalmic Surg 18:283-285, 1987.

CHAPTER 7

Chemical injuries

MICHAEL D. WAGONER
KENNETH R. KENYON

- Alkali burns
  - Etiology
  - Pathophysiology
    - Effect of pH
    - Epithelium
    - Stroma
    - Endothelium
    - Anterior chamber and lens
  - Clinical course and evaluation
    - Immediate phase
    - Acute phase (0 to 7 days)
    - Early reparative phase (7 to 21 days)
    - Late reparative phase (21 days to several months)
  - Medical therapy
    - Tear substitutes
    - Bandage soft contact lens
    - Antibiotics
    - Antiglaucoma medications
    - Cycloplegics
    - Corticosteroids
    - Medroxyprogesterone
    - Ascorbate
    - Citrate
    - Retinoic acid
    - Fibronectin
    - Epidermal growth factor (EGF)
    - Superoxide scavengers
    - Collagenase inhibitors
    - Abandoned therapy
  - Surgical therapy
    - Paracentesis
    - Punctal occlusion
    - Tarsorrhaphy
    - Tissue adhesive
    - Ocular surface replacement
    - Mucous membrane grafts
    - Keratoepithelioplasty
    - Keratoplasty
    - Keratoprosthesis
- Acid burns
  - Etiology
  - Pathophysiology
  - Clinical course and therapy
- Specific therapy for chemical injury
  - Immediate phase
  - Acute phase (0 to 7 days)
  - Early reparative phase (7 to 21 days)
  - Late reparative phase (21 days to several months)
- References

Chemical injuries are potentially devastating ocular surface injuries that may result in permanent unilateral or bilateral visual impairment. Because alkalies readily penetrate the eye, they may damage the ocular surface, corneal stroma, and endothelium, as well as other anterior segment structures such as the iris, lens, and ciliary body. Alkali injuries are usually more severe than acid injuries, the latter tending to remain confined to the ocular surface and producing more superficial damage. Extensive laboratory and clinical studies of the basic reparative and ulcerative processes of the chemically injured eye have contributed to our understanding of the ocular response to such injury and of other important biological phenomena such as mechanisms of epithelial wound healing and stromal ulceration and repair. This knowledge has led to the development and application of new ocular medical regimens and surgical procedures for managing severely injured eyes.

ALKALI BURNS

Etiology

The most common chemicals causing alkali burns are ammonia (NH_3), lye (NaOH), potassium hydroxide (KOH, caustic potash), magnesium hydroxide [$Mg(OH)_2$], and lime [$Ca(OH)_2$].[1] Ammonia is found in fertilizers, refrigerants, and cleaning agents (7% solution). Because ammonia dissolves in water to form NH_4OH, fumes from ammonia-containing compounds can be toxic to the eye. When ammonia is in direct contact with the eye, its lipid solubility results in extremely rapid penetration. Lye, commonly found in drain cleaners, penetrates almost as rapidly as ammonia. Magnesium hydroxide is found in sparklers and flares and may add to the thermal injury produced by fireworks.[2] Lime, present in plaster, mortar, cement, and whitewash, is the most common cause of alkali injuries in the construction workplace. Because it exists as particulate matter, lime can be retained in the eye (especially in the upper fornix) and provide a continuous reservoir of alkali. Fortunately, it penetrates poorly into the corneal stroma.

Pathophysiology

Because of their tendency to penetrate the eye easily, alkali compounds may produce injury to the entire anterior segment. Postinjury sequelae related to inflammation and repair processes may increase the severity of the original injury.

Effect of pH

The presence of the hydroxyl (OH) ion in alkali injury elevates the pH. With high pH, there is saponification of fatty components of the cell membrane resulting in cell disruption and death.[1] Depending on the depth of penetration, cell membrane destruction and death occur in conjunctival and corneal epithelium, stromal keratocytes, stromal nerve endings, endothelium, lens epithelium, and the epithelium and vascular endothelium of the iris and ciliary body. The pH of the aqueous rises almost immediately after ammonia injury and within 3 to 5 minutes after sodium hydroxide injury.[3] With or without external irrigation, the aqueous pH levels return to normal in 30 minutes to 3 hours.[3]

Epithelium

Because of the instantaneous cell death associated with a high pH, all corneal and conjunctival epithelium sloughs following contact with alkali. The size of the epithelial defect is a good indicator of the overall extent of alkali exposure. Normal intact corneal epithelium provides an effective barrier against microbial pathogens. It is also capable of producing both a cytokine, which inhibits collagenase production by corneal fibroblasts,[4-7] and superoxide dismutase,[8] a free radical scavenger. A persistent epithelial defect deprives the corneal stroma of all three of these protective mechanisms and can contribute to both microbial and sterile ulceration of the stroma. In addition, injured or migrating corneal epithelium may produce cytokines that stimulate collagenase production by keratocytes.[4-7]

Repair of the injured ocular surface is a two-stage process involving primary reepithelialization (early) and differentiation (late). Reepithelialization occurs with centripetal movement of the surviving corneal and/or conjunctival epithelium into the region of cell loss.[9] The rate of reepithelialization is influenced by the source of the migrating epithelium. If any corneal epithelium remains or if limbal epithelium (palisades of Vogt) is present, reepithelialization occurs much more rapidly than if nonlimbal conjunctival epithelium must be the sole source of epithelium. Reepithelialization is even more delayed if alkali-induced cell death has resulted in conjunctival necrosis involving more than half the limbus. Epithelial migration is often initially poor because of inflammation, and the limited migration seen in this period often stops about 72 hours after injury, correlating with loss of motility of the advancing epithelium at the leading edge of the cell layer.[10] In addition, the regenerating epithelium cannot utilize the existing but often damaged basement membrane. Accumulations of polymorphonuclear neutrophils (PMNs) at the leading edge of the migrating epithelium can also retard epithelial migration.[11] Topical medications containing benzalkonium chloride decrease cell migration as a result of damage to cell membranes, loss of adherence, decreased membrane activity, and actual retraction of the epithelial sheet.[10,12] Contrary to popular belief, epithelial migration does not seem to be directly decreased by corticosteroids.[13] The degradation of fibronectin on the basement membrane after alkali injury may result in poor adherence of the advancing epithelium.[14]

Factors that would be expected to improve reepithelialization are those that improve the tear layer or lubricate the ocular surface (tear substitutes); minimize trauma to the regenerating epithelium (pressure patch, bandage lens, tarsorrhaphy); reduce inflammation (corticosteroids and progestational steroids); promote epithelial mitosis (epidermal growth factor); or facilitate adhesion (fibronectin).

Following restoration of an intact epithelial layer, the epithelium continues to undergo morphologic transdifferentiation with assumption of either the normal, clear, stable characteristics of corneal epithelium or the poor clarity, vascularization, and superficial pannus formation characteristic of epithelium derived conjunctivally. Reepithelialization accomplished with corneal or limbal epithelium resembles normal corneal epithelium morphologically and biochemically.[9,15,16] If complete reepithelialization occurs from nonlimbal conjunctival epithelium, but the injury is not severe, the conjunctival epithelium will ultimately transdifferentiate into normal corneal epithelium in both its morphological and physiological function.[15,16] In severe injuries, however, the resurfacing epithelium retains its conjunctival characteristics with resultant corneal vascularization, pannus formation, and loss of clarity.[15] Despite copious tearing, abnormalities of goblet cells may result in tear film instability with chronic ocular surface abnormalities. Corneal epithelial transdifferentiation during this late phase can be favorably influenced by factors that control inflammation (corticosteroids, progestational steroids) and promote corneal epithelial transdifferentiation (retinoic acid).

Following reepithelialization, there is slow regeneration of basement membrane complexes and hence a tendency for epithelial erosion[17] to recur and secondary epithelial defects to persist.

Stroma

The severity of stromal injury is related to the depth of penetration, which in turn is related to the alkali's cation.[1] Cation binding to collagen and glycosaminoglycans results in hydration, thickening, and shortening of collagen fibrils.[18] The trabecular meshwork is distorted and produces an early increase in intraocular pressure. Stromal hydration results in loss of corneal clarity. Damage to stromal nerve endings may cause relative or absolute corneal anesthesia. Keratocytes may be completely obliterated from areas of significant alkali penetration.

Within 12 to 24 hours after injury, infiltration of the peripheral cornea with PMNs is seen. This inflammatory reaction peaks at approximately 72 hours and will subside if reepithelialization occurs. If the injury is severe, the PMN reaction remains constant for 14 to 21 days, at which time a second progressive increase in PMN and mononuclear leukocyte infiltration occurs.[19] Increased levels of PMN collagenase,[20] aldolase,[21] β-N-acetylglucoamidase,[22] lysosomal phosphatase,[23] glycosidase,[23] and other lysosomal enzymes[22] are found in the stroma correlating with the inflammatory response. Mononuclear leukocytes release interleukin-1, which can stimulate fibroblast collagenase.[24] Progressive leukocyte infiltration occurs if the epithelial defect is persistent or antiinflammatory medications are not used. Factors that inhibit leukocyte infiltration include reepithelialization, cyanoacrylate adhesive or glued-on hard contact lens,[25] citrate,[26] and corticosteroids or progestational steroids.[27,28]

Keratocyte repopulation of the injured stroma begins early in the repair process. In cases of incomplete destruction of the entire keratocyte population, proliferation probably occurs from adjacent regions. In severe injuries the site of the new keratocytes has not been established. Keratocyte repopulation is a necessary event because these pluripotential cells possess the unique ability to remodel damaged stroma, being able to secrete collagenase,[4-7,29] collagen, and extracellular matrix mucopolysaccharides. When the delicate regulation of this remodeling process becomes disordered, excessive collagenolysis or "sterile ulceration" may occur if net collagen breakdown exceeds collagen synthesis. The pathogenetic mechanisms of this process are depicted schematically in Fig. 7-1.

Mammalian collagenase,[30] not normally present in the cornea,[31] has been identified in ulcerating corneas[31] as soon as 9 hours after injury but not in significant amounts until 14 to 21 days later.[32] Although damaged corneal epithelium was originally thought to produce collagenase,[33] the epithelium is now felt not to be a source of collagenase.[31] Both keratocytes[4,7,29] and PMNs[20] produce collagenase in the ulcerating cornea, although the relative contribution of collagenases from these two sources to stromal degradation is not well defined. Keratocyte collagenase production may be induced by stimulatory

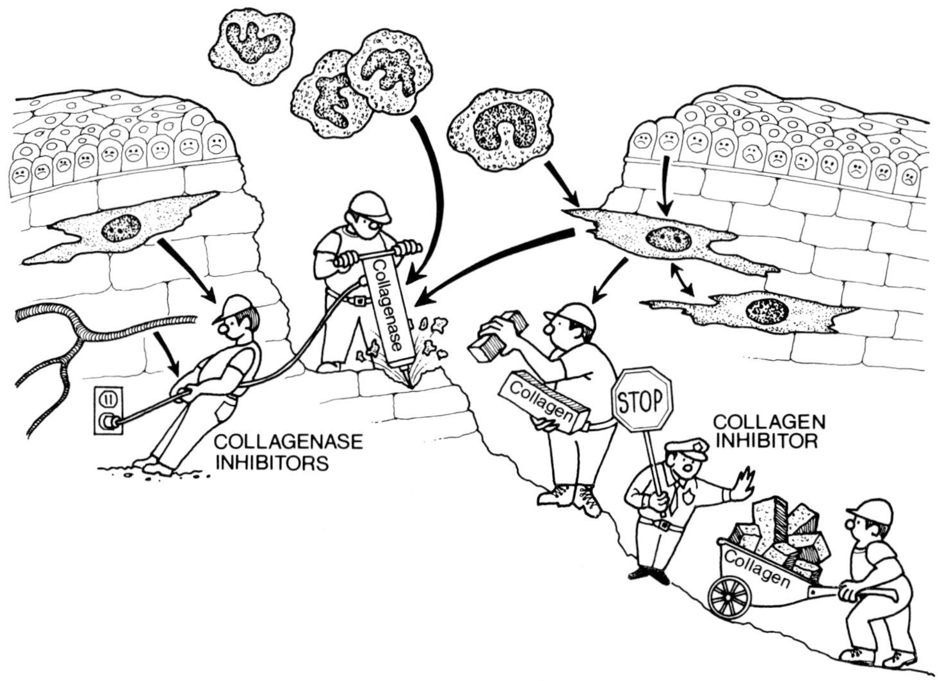

Fig. 7-1. Schematic depiction of the mechanism of corneal ulceration and repair following alkali injury. Although an epithelial defect persists, collagenase debridement of the stromal matrix occurs concurrently with new collagen synthesis. The net result of these two repair mechanisms determines whether successful repair or dissolution of the corneal stroma occurs.

cytokines from injured or migrating epithelium,[4-6] interleukin-1,[24] or stimulatory autocrine factors from proliferating fibroblasts.[7] The efficacy of collagenase in degrading the cornea is increased by factors that promote activation of the latent form[34] of the enzyme (e.g., plasmin[35]) and inhibited by those that inactivate the enzyme (e.g., serum α-2-macroglobulins[36]).

Several mechanisms can delay keratocyte proliferation and synthesis of new collagen. Because ascorbate is essential to collagen synthesis, the scorbutic state of the anterior chamber may result in depletion of intracellular levels of ascorbate and impair collagen synthesis. Topically and systemically administered ascorbate has been shown experimentally to reverse this phenomenon.[37] Steroids may impair keratocyte collagen synthesis; corticosteroids have a far greater inhibitory effect than do progestational steroids.[38,39]

Collagenolysis invariably ceases upon complete reepithelialization, possibly because of the discontinued secretion of cytokines that stimulate keratocyte collagenase, the resumed synthesis of cytokines that inhibit keratocyte collagenase, and the exclusion of inflammatory cells and their mediators from the corneal stroma. Collagenolysis is also arrested following application of tissue adhesives,[40] presumably on the basis of exclusion of inflammatory cells and their mediators. Neovascularization of the corneal stroma, whether induced by persistent inflammation or iatrogenically by tissue adhesives, arrests further collagenolysis, probably because of the diffusion of serum antiproteases into the corneal stroma.[36]

Endothelium

Alkali that fully penetrates the stroma can damage the corneal endothelium severely.[41] Transient or even permanent corneal edema may follow. Proliferation of Descemet's membrane and even retrocorneal membranes may occur in the most severe cases.

Anterior Chamber and Lens

Intraocular penetration of alkali results in a decrease in aqueous glucose and ascorbate,[37] both of which interfere with normal keratocyte metabolism. Injury to the iris and ciliary body produces intraocular inflammation, decreased aqueous production, and secondary decrease in aqueous outflow through the trabecular meshwork. This usually causes increased intraocular pressure, although hypotony may occur in especially severe injuries. Damage to the lens capsule and epithelium may result in early or delayed cataract formation.

Clinical Course and Evaluation

McCulley[1] has divided the clinical course of chemical injuries into four phases: immediate, acute (minutes to 1 week), early reparative (1 to 3 weeks), and late reparative (more than 3 weeks). Although severe injuries may completely heal early in the course and without long-term sequelae, they typically progress through each of these phases, with various clinical characteristics.

Immediate Phase

All the clinical findings present immediately after a chemical injury are related to the area of involvement, depth of penetration, and relative toxicity of the substance. A detailed examination must wait until copious irrigation is complete, but the initial findings provide important information regarding the ultimate prognosis. A proper examination should test for visual acuity, intraocular pressure, presence of particulate matter (particularly following plaster injury), extent of corneal and conjunctival epithelial cell loss, presence and extent of conjunctival ischemic necrosis, corneal clarity, anterior chamber inflammation, and lenticular clarity.

The Hughes classification[42] is the most widely used of the several classification schemes that relate early findings to long-term prognosis. It divides injuries into four groups (Color Plate 7-1 and Fig. 7-2).

Grade I: Good prognosis
Corneal epithelial damage
No ischemia

Grade II: Good prognosis
Cornea hazy but iris details seen
Ischemia of less than one third of limbus

Grade III: Guarded prognosis
Total loss of corneal epithelium
Stromal haze blurring iris details
Ischemia of one third to one half of limbus

Grade IV: Poor prognosis
Cornea opaque, obscuring view of iris or pupil
Ischemia of more than one half of limbus

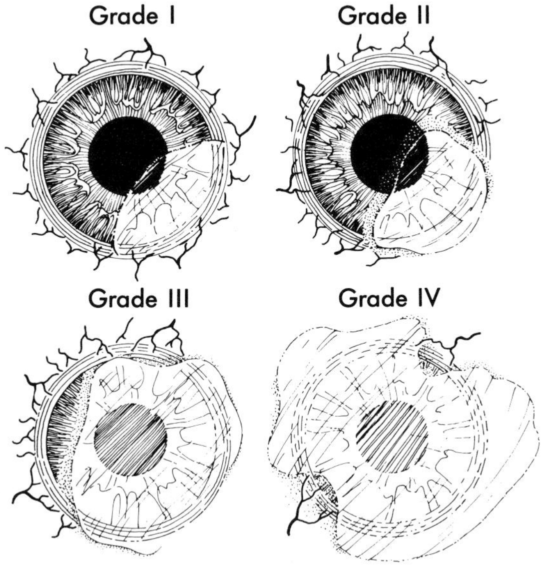

Fig. 7-2. Hughes classification of ocular alkali burns:
Grade I—Corneal epithelial damage, no limbal ischemia.
Grade II—Cornea hazy, iris details seen. Ischemia less than one third of limbus.
Grade III—Total loss of corneal epithelium. Stromal haze blurring iris details. Ischemia of one third to one half of limbus.
Grade IV—Cornea opaque, obscuring view of iris or pupil. Ischemia of more than one half of limbus.

Acute Phase (0 to 7 Days)

The acute phase after injury is approximately the first week.[1] The slow initiation of reepithelialization and keratocyte proliferation and migration occurs concurrently with progressive ocular surface and intraocular inflammation. Failure to attempt to control this progressive inflammatory response is a significant clinical error because uncontrolled inflammation may lead to complete epithelial arrest and increase the occurrence and severity of late cicatricial changes. Intraocular pressure may rise as intraocular inflammation increases.[43] With the use of prophylactic antibiotics, microbial superinfection is seldom seen. Collagenolysis rarely, if ever, occurs in this period.

Early Reparative Phase (7 to 21 Days)

During this phase, corneal and conjunctival epithelium and keratocytes continue to proliferate in an effort to restore structurally and functionally normal ocular surface and stroma. In less severe cases, reepithelialization may be completed at this time; it is associated with well-regulated corneal stroma repair, clearing of the opacification, and elimination of the risk of sterile ulceration. The degree of reepithelialization should be monitored carefully and any areas of stromal thinning identified. This is particularly critical because of the rapidity with which stromal ulceration may now occur and progress to perforation.

Late Reparative Phase (21 Days to Several Months)

Injured eyes entering this phase can be classified into two groups. In the first group, reepithelialization has been completed or is nearly complete. In general, only those injured eyes with some residual corneal or limbal epithelium will reepithelialize without incident within this time period. As a result of corneal anesthesia, persistent goblet cell and mucin abnormalities, and slow regeneration of new basement membrane and epithelial adhesions, a persistent epitheliopathy may occur that can produce prolonged suboptimal vision. In more severe cases a fibrovascular pannus may overgrow the cornea.

In the second group, conjunctival reepithelialization is required for all resurfacing, and corneal reepithelialization has proceeded poorly or not at all. The lack of epithelial migration at this stage portends a high likelihood of sterile stromal ulceration. Even if perforation can be avoided or treated successfully with tissue adhesives, the ocular surface will often heal with severe corneal vascularization, conjunctival and corneal scarring, goblet cell and mucin deficiency, and recurrent or persistent epithelial erosions. Progressive symblepharon formation may produce lid abnormalities and trichiasis and further worsen the ocular surface difficulties. Permanent loss of corneal sensation may result in neurotrophic keratitis. Intraocular abnormalities including retrocorneal membranes, peripheral anterior synechiae, cataract, glaucoma, hypotony, and phthisis bulbi may progressively occur.

Medical Therapy

Tear Substitutes

Although most chemical injuries occur in young healthy individuals with the ability to produce copious tearing, the use of tear substitutes and lubricating ointments may provide a coating for the ocular surface that minimizes the trauma of eyelid movement and indirectly facilitates reepithelialization. To avoid additional complications for an already damaged epithelium, only nonpreserved preparations should be used. Following reepithelialization, frequent tear substitutes and bedtime ointments may ameliorate persistent superficial punctate epitheliopathy and reduce the risk of recurrent erosion.

Bandage Soft Contact Lens

Bandage lenses promote epithelial migration, basement membrane regeneration, and epithelial-stromal adhesion by protecting the ocular surface from the "windshield-wiper" effect of the lids. Unfortunately these lenses are usually poorly tolerated in the acutely inflamed eye, and the increased risk of such complications as "tight-lens syndrome" and microbial superinfection may make the use of pressure patching, lid taping, or tarsorrhaphy the preferred initial therapy. A bandage soft contact lens is better tolerated if introduced several days after injury. It may also be used even more effectively following tarsorrhaphy. Prophylactic administration of topical antibiotics is mandatory. Concomitant topical cycloplegics and steroids may reduce the likelihood of sterile hypopyon. Long-lasting collagen shields may eventually prove to be a useful alternative to bandage soft contact lenses.

Antibiotics

Prophylactic antibiotics should be used in all chemical injury cases until reepithelialization is complete, especially if a contact lens or topical corticosteroids are used. The antibiotic selected should have broad-spectrum coverage and be nontoxic to the regenerating corneal epithelium. We prefer the use of a combination antibiotic ointment such as bacitracin/polymyxin (Polysporin). Prophylactic antiviral or antifungal medications are not advocated because of the low incidence of secondary infection with herpes simplex or fungi and the relative high epithelial toxicity of these compounds.

Antiglaucoma Medications

Because the principal mechanism of glaucoma in the alkali-burned cornea is obstruction of trabecular outflow, the most effective means of lowering intraocular pressure is decreasing aqueous production with carbonic anhydrase inhibitors or topical beta blockers or both. Agents that promote improved trabecular meshwork outflow are minimally effective. The control of intraocular inflammation may secondarily improve aqueous outflow and lower intraocular pressure.

Cycloplegics

Cycloplegic agents promote comfort, reduce photophobia, and prevent posterior synechiae.

Corticosteroids

Although corticosteroids have traditionally been the mainstay of therapy for the reduction of tissue injury related to acute or chronic inflammatory conditions, there has been an unfounded reluctance on the part of many clinicians to use antiinflammatory agents in the severely inflamed, acutely chemically injured cornea. Perhaps this is related to injudicious use of corticosteroids after corneal ulceration has begun, and the inaccurate extrapolation that corticosteroids themselves "melt the cornea" or potentiate collagenase. Further, there is a widely held but fallacious belief that the use of topical corticosteroids worsens the delay in reepithelialization. In fact, corticosteroids have no direct effect on the rate of epithelial migration.[13]

The beneficial effect of decreasing ocular tissue destruction by reducing inflammation with corticosteroids is well documented in a variety of ocular disorders. Intensive use of corticosteroids after chemical injury may indirectly facilitate reepithelialization by reducing the inhibitory effect of ocular surface inflammation, reduce the incidence of subsequent corneal ulceration by limiting the stromal inflammatory response, and limit the severity of late sequelae. This effect is related to stabilization of cytoplasmic and lysosomal membranes of PMNs with resultant decreased release of inflammatory mediators and chemotaxis of additional leukocytes.

The use of topical corticosteroids is not without potential adverse effects, including potential of secondary microbial keratitis and diminution of stromal wound healing,[44,45] although their effect on tensile wound strength is equivocal.[39,66] Approximately 14 days after alkali injury, stromal repair processes become important, as both collagen and collagenase synthesis begin.[32] The continued use of topical corticosteroids in this period may limit repair processes and permit collagenolytic debridement of the stroma to result in corneal dissolution because of the imbalance between repair and debridement rates. This occurs despite the anticollagenolytic effect of corticosteroids.[39] For this reason, the intensive use of topical corticosteroids should be continued beyond 10 to 14 days only with extreme caution and close follow-up, unless reepithelialization is complete.

Medroxyprogesterone

Medroxyprogesterone (Provera 1%), a progestational steroid with weaker antiinflammatory properties than corticosteroids, has been shown experimentally to inhibit collagenase and reduce ulceration after alkali injury.[38,46] Contradictory reports exist regarding its direct effect in reducing corneal ulceration after alkali burns,[47] and no controlled clinical studies have been reported that assess its antiulcerogenic properties. Its principal benefit lies not in its anticollagenolytic properties, but in its minimal suppression of corneal wound repair.[39] Because of this, it may be substituted for topical corticosteroids after 10 to 14 days when suppression of inflammation is needed but interference with corneal stroma repair is undesirable, as in the situation of actual or impending stromal ulceration.

Ascorbate

Ascorbate is a cofactor in the hydroxylation of proline and lysine in collagen synthesis. Because this is the rate-limiting step of collagen formation, keratocyte depletion of ascorbate, secondary to decreased aqueous levels of ascorbate, could hinder new collagen synthesis.[37] Both topical and systemic ascorbate have been shown to reduce the incidence of ulceration after alkali burns in experimental animal models.[37,48] After severe burns, topical administration of ascorbate appears to be superior to systemic therapy in preventing ulceration.[48] Once ulceration begins, ascorbate seems to be ineffective[26] in arresting further ulceration.

Citrate

Citrate is a natural food ingredient with physical properties similar to ascorbate. Its calcium-chelating effect decreases the membrane and intracellular Ca^{2+} levels of PMN, with resultant impaired chemotaxis, phagocytosis, and release of lysosomal enzymes.[49] Topical 10% citrate decreases early-phase and late-phase PMN infiltration by 63% and 92%, respectively.[19] Citrate has been shown to be effective in decreasing corneal ulceration and perforation after alkali burns in experimental animal models,[26] but this has not been confirmed in controlled human studies.

Retinoic Acid

Major interest has been generated concerning the application of topical vitamin A analogs for treating ocular surface disorders associated with abnormal keratinization and goblet cell abnormalities. This approach appears to have some promise for severe keratinizing disorders such as erythema multiforme.[50] After reepithelialization of severe chemical injuries, retinoic acid could play a role in promoting goblet cell recovery and corneal epithelial differentiation during the late reparative period, but this has not been formally studied in either experimental animals or humans.

Fibronectin

Fibronectin is a multimeric glycoprotein present in the extracellular matrix that is responsible for cell-matrix adhesion.[14] It facilitates cell spreading by the promotion of cell-cell and cell-matrix adhesions, although it has no direct effect on cell mitosis or migration. After corneal injury, fibronectin is produced by epithelial cells[51] and keratocytes[52] within 8 hours and is distributed on the bare basement membrane ahead of and under the advancing epithelium where it persists until wound closure is complete.[51] After alkali burns, plasminogen produced by basal epithelial cells may degrade fibrin and fibronectin at the basement membrane and interfere with hemidesmosome adhesion.[14] Theoretically, exogenous fibronectin should facilitate reepithelialization by improving epithelial adhesion. Despite considerable contradictory data in the literature, several experimental studies have demonstrated a beneficial effect of fibronectin in promoting reepithelialization after alkali injury.[53,54] Fibronectin is currently not available for clinical use.

Epidermal Growth Factor (EGF)

Epidermal growth factor (EGF), a polypeptide originally isolated from the mouse submaxillary gland, has been shown to enhance the rate of healing and induce hyperplasia in the healing corneal epithelium,[13,55] although it does not promote adherence of the migrating epithelium to damaged basement membrane.[55] In experimental alkali burns, EGF enhances epithelial wound healing, although recurrent erosions occur when it is discontinued.[55] EGF is currently not available for clinical use.

Superoxide Scavengers

In experimental models, the superoxide scavengers superoxide dismutase, ascorbic acid, and dimethyl sulfoxide have been shown to decrease corneal ulceration and corneal opacification after alkali burns.[56] These compounds are not available for clinical use.

Collagenase Inhibitors

The collagenase inhibitors 0.2 M sodium EDTA, 0.2 M calcium EDTA, 0.2 M cysteine, penicillamine, and 10% or 20% acetylcysteine have not been effective clinically in the treatment of chemical injury. Only acetylcysteine (Mucomyst) is clinically available, but is no longer used in the treatment of chemical burns.

Abandoned Therapy

Other medical therapies that have fallen into disuse because of a lack of proven efficacy include the subconjunctival injection of serum or heparin, and topical vasodilators.

Surgical Therapy

Paracentesis

Although the use of paracentesis and anterior chamber irrigation may help restore a normal aqueous pH, it has not been shown to improve the overall prognosis of chemical injury.[3]

Punctal Occlusion

Excessive reflex tearing is normally present after alkali injury. The need for improved lubrication of the ocular surface becomes apparent only many months later when a chronic persistent epitheliopathy occurs as a result of goblet cell-mucin abnormalities. In these cases, temporary punctal occlusion with either collagen plugs or canalicular sutures may augment the effect of tear substitutes. In patients with preexisting keratoconjunctivitis sicca, temporary or permanent punctal occlusion may be necessary to facilitate reepithelialization.

Tarsorrhaphy

The importance of reestablishing an epithelial cover within 2 to 3 weeks after injury to prevent the serious complications of bacterial superinfection and sterile ulceration should lead to increasingly aggressive intervention when epithelial recovery is delayed. A temporary lateral tarsorrhaphy can be performed easily with minimal morbidity, may dramatically facilitate reepithelialization, and can be reversed when the situation stabilizes. Tarsorrhaphy also facilitates the use and retention of a bandage soft contact lens.

Tissue Adhesive

Tissue adhesives, particularly isobutyl cyanoacrylate (Histoacryl), remain the best tool for treating impending or actual perforations related to sterile ulceration of the corneal stroma.[25,40,57] Other polymers, such as Krazy-Glue, have similar tectonic properties but may be inflammatogenic or toxic and should not be used. Experimental and clinical experience shows that application of adhesives prevents further ulceration and supports the stroma during neovascularization and repair. In almost all cases of persistent epithelial defect with progressive ulceration, tissue adhesives should be used before perforation occurs. In cases of small perforations (<1 mm), successful closure of the defect with tissue adhesive may eliminate the need for tectonic keratoplasty. Using the slit lamp, cyanoacrylate glue can be easily and quickly placed on the area of ulceration or perforation, after which a durable bandage soft contact lens (e.g., Bausch & Lomb T-series) is usually applied to provide comfort and reduce the chances of the glue dislodging (see Chapter 13). The adhesive can be left in place until it loosens spontaneously as a result of reepithelialization, or it can be easily removed with jeweler's forceps after 6 to 8 weeks once the inflammation has subsided and neovascularization of the area has eliminated the risk of recurrent ulceration.[56] Prophylactic antibiotics are usually administered while the contact lens is in place.

Ocular Surface Replacement

Autograft transplantation of ocular surface epithelium (conjunctival or limbal transplantation) has become an effective means of restoring surface integrity in patients with unilateral chemical injury. The success of the procedure depends upon the availability of healthy epithelium, which migrates over the ocular surface of the injured eye and assumes the biochemical and morphological features of normal corneal epithelium.[15] As initially described by Thoft,[58] bulbar conjunctival tissue was transplanted to the injured eye following a superficial keratectomy. This procedure was usually performed more than 6 months after the injury and following resolution of ocular inflammation with the intention of improving the status of the ocular surface to permit subsequent penetrating keratoplasty.

Recent evidence, however, suggests that limbal epithelium is the "stem cell" from which corneal epithelium is derived. Accordingly, Kenyon and Tseng[59] have developed the technique of transplanting limbal tissue (Fig. 7-3). This procedure can be performed early (<3 months) in cases with persistent epithelial defects to facilitate reepithelialization, minimize the risk of ulceration and its attendant complications, and prepare for future visually rehabilitative procedures. Limbal transplantation can also be used for late rehabilitation in cases where reepithelialization has occurred with retention of conjunctival characteristics, thereby limiting useful vision and making penetrating keratoplasty hazardous. In some cases, removal of superficial pannus combined with limbal autograft will not only rehabilitate the ocular surface but also restore media clarity and improve visual acuity. In cases where subsequent lamellar or penetrating keratoplasty is required, the prognosis for graft clarity is improved by prior limbal grafting (Color Plate 7-2).

Mucous Membrane Grafts

Mucous membrane grafts have largely been abandoned in favor of conjunctival or limbal autograft transplantation. They may be necessary, however, in cases of severe bilateral burn, where no healthy ocular surface tissue is available for transplantation.

Keratoepithelioplasty

In cases of bilateral, severe chemical injury, Thoft[60] has advocated the use of allogenic corneal donor epithelium in an effort to repopulate the ocular surface with epithelium that has corneal morphology and biochemical characteristics. The procedure is performed by denuding the recipient epithelium and pannus and suturing to the corneal limbus several donor lenticules consisting of a thin crescent of stroma with intact epithelium from a fresh whole donor cornea. Postoperatively, topical steroids are required to prevent immune system rejection of the donor epithelium. Success is limited by epithelial rejection and a tendency of the abnormal con-

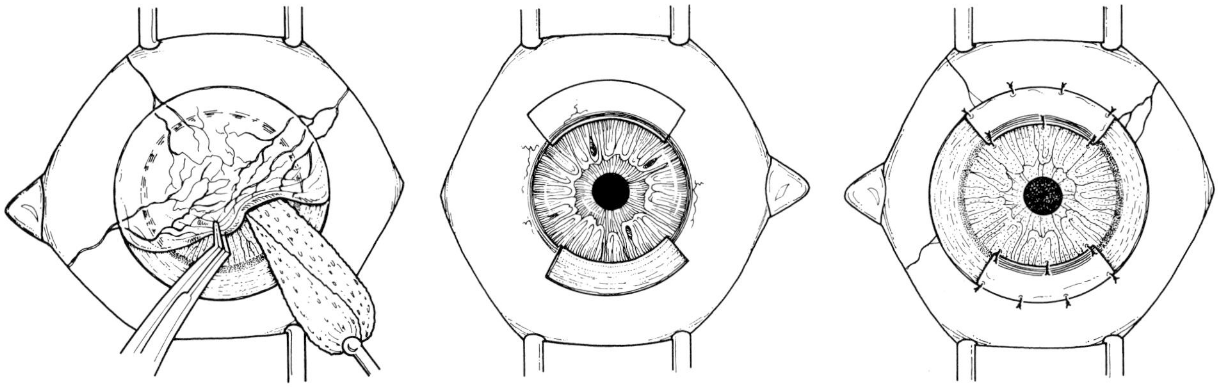

Fig. 7-3. Technique of limbal autograft transplantation. *Left,* Following conjunctival peritomy ≈2 mm posterior to limbus, corneal pannus is stripped using predominantly blunt dissection. *Middle,* Preparation of donor grafts usually involves two limbal tissue segments, each ≈2 × 10 mm in size. *Right,* Limbal grafts are transferred to corresponding location in recipient eye and sutured to bare sclera and peripheral cornea.

junctivalized epithelium to subsequently repopulate the injured ocular surface.[60]

Keratoplasty

Lamellar or penetrating keratoplasty may be used for tectonic stabilization of the globe or visual rehabilitation. Because keratoplasty procedures in an acutely inflamed eye with an unstable ocular surface are almost invariably associated with rejection and graft failure, early keratoplasty should be reserved for globe-threatening perforations that are too large to be managed successfully by application of cyanoacrylate glue. Aggressive management of persistent epithelial defects with limbal transplantation, and the use of tissue adhesive for areas with rapid thinning before perforation, will make this procedure unnecessary in all but the most severe chemical injuries. Because the graft will almost invariably be rejected and opacify, it should be no larger than necessary to reestablish the integrity of the globe. Especially if the area of perforation is peripheral, extension of the grafted tissue into the visual axis is to be avoided. A penetrating graft is usually preferred, because the area of perforation is often surrounded by a zone of corneal thinning and necrosis that precludes the successful preparation of a lamellar bed. Because the patch graft is placed in a site of active ulceration, the major postoperative complications include persistent epithelial defect, ulceration of the donor graft, "cheese-wiring" of the sutures through the surgical wound with dehiscence, and rapid loss of graft clarity. To minimize these complications, additional interrupted 10-0 nylon sutures are used, a tarsorrhaphy is placed, and tissue adhesive is applied if progressive thinning occurs.

Penetrating keratoplasty for visual rehabilitation can be definitively performed only after all corneal repair processes and inflammation have been inactive for some time, preferably more than 1 year. The most unfavorable prognostic indicator is an unstable ocular surface with conjunctival characteristics. In such cases, bulbar or limbal autograft transplantation should precede penetrating keratoplasty by at least 6 months. If no tissue is available for conjunctival transplantation, a 6-month to 1-year trial of all-*trans*-retinoic acid 0.01% daily may improve ocular surface stability. Despite these measures, all too often an initially clear graft will ultimately fail.

Factors that may adversely affect success with penetrating keratoplasty include abnormalities of the lids and lashes; tear deficiency; conjunctival scarring; corneal epithelial defects and stromal neovascularization; previous failed grafts; persistent intraocular abnormalities such as glaucoma, hypotony, anterior segment fibrosis, and retrocorneal membrane formation; and difficulties with postoperative follow-up and compliance. Postoperative complications include significantly increased risks of graft rejection and failure, vascularization, glaucoma, hypotony, and phthisis bulbi, compared with penetrating keratoplasty for other indications.

Keratoprosthesis

Keratoprosthesis has enjoyed cyclical popularity in attempts to rehabilitate the badly scarred, alkali-injured eye where there is no hope for primary or repeat penetrating keratoplasty.[61] Early visual results may be good, but the prosthesis invariably fails because of retroprosthetic membranes, glaucoma, retinal detachment, scleral ulceration, dehiscence, and extrusion. In general, the poorest results have been obtained with the "nut-and-bolt," or collar-button, prosthesis. Better results, at least in the short term, have been achieved with the "through-and-through" keratoprosthesis placed through the closed upper lid.

ACID BURNS

Etiology

The acids that are the most clinically important sources of chemical eye injuries are sulfuric acid (H_2SO_4), sulfurous acid (H_2SO_3), hydrofluoric acid (HF), hydrochloric acid (HCl), nitrous acid (HNO_3), and acetic acid (CH_3COOH).[1]

Sulfuric acid is the one most commonly encountered. It is a common industrial acid and a component of automobile battery acid. Battery explosions, which can be caused by improper use of battery cables or use of a match to read directions on the battery, run the combined danger of acid injury to the globe and injury from high-velocity particulate matter, with attendant risk of ocular perforation. Sulfuric acid reacts with water in the precorneal tear film producing heat and charring of the corneal and conjunctival epithelium.

Sulfurous acid is formed from sulfur dioxide and water. It is commonly used as a fruit and vegetable preservative, in bleach, and as a refrigerant. When an injury occurs from a refrigerant, the severity is related to the penetration of the acid, not the freezing.[62] Because the acid is combined with oil, prolonged contact with the globe occurs. The acid penetrates corneal stroma with subsequent denaturation of corneal proteins and enzymes and damage to corneal nerves.

Hydrofluoric acid is a weak inorganic acid that produces skin burns and severe ocular injury, mainly because of the toxicity of the fluoride ion.[63] It is used in refining uranium, tantalum, and beryllium and in alkylating high-octane gasoline. The fluoride ion penetrates easily into the corneal stroma, where it produces rapid destruction of cell membranes.[63]

Hydrochloric acid, despite its reputation from movie thrillers, produces severe ocular injury relatively infrequently. Because of its poor penetration and its tendency to produce heavy reflex tearing, severe injuries occur only when there is prolonged contact. Nitrous acid behaves similarly. It has the unique feature of producing a yellow epithelial opacity.[1] Acetic acid requires a high concentration ($>10\%$) and prolonged contact to produce severe injury. Fortunately, it is used commercially in more dilute concentrations of 4% to 10%.

Pathophysiology

As with alkali injuries, the severity of injury after exposure to acidic compounds is related to the area of exposure and the penetration. The coagulation of proteins in the corneal epithelium and superficial stroma caused by acids tends to function as a barrier to further penetration and limit and localize the injury.[64] Because of the poor corneal penetration, acid injuries tend to be less severe than alkali injuries and result in fewer corneal stromal and intraocular complications. The ocular surface complications, however, including vascularization and scarring of the cornea, can be just as severe. Sulfuric acid tends to char the ocular surface from the release of heat following its reaction with water in the preocular tear film.

Hydrofluoric acid readily penetrates the corneal stroma.[63] The precipitation of the extracellular glycosaminoglycans leads to corneal opacification.[62-64] Collagen fibrils are shortened with secondary distortion of the trabecular meshwork and consequent rise in intraocular pressure.[43] Depending on the amount of intraocular penetration, the entire spectrum of intraocular changes, including endothelial damage, anterior segment inflammation, and cataract formation, may occur.

Clinical Course and Therapy

As in alkali injuries, acid injuries progress through the immediate, acute, and early and late reparative phases. The principal difference is the relative infrequency of sterile ulceration and perforation of the corneal stroma after acid injuries, although this may be seen following hydrofluoric acid burns or if there is a prolonged epithelial defect. The evaluation of the extent of

THERAPY FOR CHEMICAL EYE INJURY

I. Initiate primary therapy
  A. Irrigate
  B. Remove particulate matter
  C. Debride devitalized tissue
  D. Initiate antimicrobial therapy
  E. Initiate antiinflammatory therapy
II. Promote epithelial wound healing, using one or more of the following:
  A. Tear substitutes and lubricants
  B. Punctal occlusion in severely dry eyes
  C. Lid closure (taping, pressure patch, tarsorrhaphy)
  D. Therapeutic soft contact lens
  E. Fibronectin (investigational)
  F. Epidermal growth factor (investigational)
  G. Ocular surface (conjunctival or limbal) transplantation
  K. Keratoepithelioplasty
III. Limit ulceration and support repair by:
  A. Minimizing corticosteroid use after 10 days, unless reepithelialization is complete
  B. Use of one or more of the following:
    1. Progestational steroids (Provera 1%)
    2. Ascorbate
    3. Citrate
    4. Tissue adhesive (isobutyl cyanoacrylate) and soft contact lens
    5. Conjunctival flap
    6. Keratoplasty: patch graft, lamellar keratoplasty, penetrating keratoplasty
IV. Avoid complications by use of one or more of the following:
  A. Antiglaucoma medications (inhibitors of aqueous production)
  B. Cycloplegics
  C. Lysis of conjunctival adhesions (glass rods)
  D. Long-term antiinflammatory therapy
  E. Retinoic acid
  F. Ocular surface transplantation prior to penetrating keratoplasty

injury and classification based on degree of epithelial cell loss and evidence of limbal ischemia are the same in acid burns as in alkali injury. Late consequences of severe injury or inadequate therapy are usually related to conjunctival scarring, corneal scarring, and corneal vascularization.

We use the same treatment strategies (see the box above) for acid injuries as for alkali injuries with only minor variations. Because of the lack of penetration and effect on aqueous ascorbate levels, topical and systemic ascorbate is not needed after acid injuries. Although a similar level of medical aggressiveness is used to promote reepithelialization, the lower risk of sterile ulceration, except with prolonged epithelial defects, makes it less critical to perform early ocular surface transplantation. Typically, this can be delayed until the epithelial defect has been present for 2 months. Following reepithelialization, we apply the same method of prolonged corticosteroid use and recurrent erosion prophylaxis. As with alkali injuries, consideration of keratoplasty for visual rehabilitation is recommended only after the ocular surface has been stabilized for approximately 1 year by limbal transplantation.

SPECIFIC THERAPY FOR CHEMICAL INJURY

The goals at each stage after chemical injury are to maximize the benefits of medical and surgical therapy by tailoring them to the predominant pathophysiologic mechanisms. After initiating primary therapy, the management of each stage should specifically address the issues of promoting epithelial wound healing, limiting ulceration while supporting repair, and avoiding complications. The basic therapeutic "menu" for each of these objectives is shown in the box. Obviously, all of these modalities are not used in each case, and we recommend increasingly aggressive techniques in each category only as the clinical situation warrants. The case presented in Color Plate 7-2, for example, demonstrates the combination of early medical therapy, intervention with limbal autograft transplantation for a persistent epithelial defect before the development of sterile ulceration, and a subsequent lamellar keratoplasty for visual rehabilitation.

Immediate Phase

The most important immediate therapy for any chemical injury is copious irrigation. Since the extent of chemical contact is probably the most important prognostic indicator, the rapidity with which the ocular surface is neutralized determines the subsequent clinical course. Unfortunately, initial irrigation attempts, usually performed by the patient or co-workers, are usually wholly inadequate, thereby prolonging chemical contact time and penetration. Nonetheless, immediate and copious irrigation should be initiated (or resumed) and continued for at least 30 minutes, using any nontoxic irrigating solution.

It is impossible to overirrigate the chemically injured eye. Some clinicians prefer an irrigating contact lens. The pH should be rechecked at the end of the irrigation, and, if still abnormal, irrigation should continue until neutrality is achieved. There is no need to use acidic or basic irrigation solutions.[63,65]

Any particulate matter present should be completely removed. In the case of plaster injuries, the eyelids should be everted to examine for the presence of retained particles. All particles should be removed under topical anesthesia with fine forceps or by scraping with a disposable scalpel (e.g., Bard-Parker No. 15 blade).

Acute Phase (0 to 7 Days)

In cases of severe chemical injury, hospitalization is required. In milder cases, outpatient therapy is acceptable, but follow-up must be at intervals frequent enough to allow therapy to be modified to match the evolving course.

A typical set of admission orders for a patient with a chemical injury might read:

1. Dexamethasone 0.1% (or equivalent) topically QIh
2. 10% sodium ascorbate topically QIh
3. Sodium ascorbate 2 g po QID
4. 10% sodium citrate topically QID
5. Polysporin ointment topically QID
6. Homatropine 2% (or equivalent) topically TID
7. Timolol 0.5% (or equivalent) topically BID
8. Acetazolamide 500 mg po BID
9. Pressure patch or tape lids between applications of topical medications

The mainstay of therapy during this period is the use of topical corticosteroids and prophylactic antibiotics. These should be continued throughout this phase whether or not reepithelialization is complete. Ascorbate and citrate should be continued unless reepithelialization is complete, in which case they can be discontinued. Glaucoma medications and cycloplegics are adjusted as indicated. Conjunctival adhesions are lysed with glass rods as they occur.

Early Reparative Phase (7 to 21 Days)

During this stage the same basic principles are applicable. Complete reepithelialization is of paramount importance. If reepithelialization appears to be headed for completion, the regimen described above is maintained. Upon completion of reepithelialization, ascorbate and citrate can be discontinued and topical antibiotics tapered. Topical corticosteroids may be tapered as the resolution of inflammation dictates.

If reepithelialization is delayed and appears to be potentially persistent, increasingly aggressive measures should be employed. Unpreserved lubricating ointments should be used frequently. A temporary lateral tarsorrhaphy may be utilized in conjunction with a bandage soft contact lens. If available, topical fibronectin and epidermal growth factor may be tried. Repair mechanisms can be supported by continuation of topical and systemic ascorbate and citrate. Topical corticosteroids may be continued at appropriately reduced doses if no stromal thinning or ulceration has occurred, but in the presence of any stromal loss, corticosteroids should be discontinued and medroxyprogesterone (Provera 1%) initiated at least every 2 hours to control inflammation.

Late Reparative Phase (21 Days to Several Months)

In cases where reepithelialization is progressing but is not quite complete, it is advisable to continue with the therapy outlined above. The corneal stroma should be monitored carefully for any evidence of thinning in areas of incomplete epithelialization. If reepithelialization is then completed without incident, topical corticosteroids are continued to suppress inflammation and vascular pannus formation. Unpreserved tear ointments are used at bedtime to minimize the risk of recurrent erosion; topical lubrication is used as needed for any persistent epitheliopathy. A trial of retinoic acid 0.01% may be initiated to promote goblet cell recovery and support appropriate corneal epithelial differentiation.

In cases with little or no reepithelialization, the risk of sterile ulceration is very high. If progressive thinning with impending or actual perforation occurs, it may be necessary to use tissue adhesives. Despite their effectiveness in arresting further ulceration, tissue adhesives virtually insure corneal vascularization and limit the possibility of later penetrating keratoplasty. Because the ocular surface will ultimately be in need of rehabilitation anyway, the increasingly aggressive approach of recommending surgical intervention at this stage has been adopted. This is performed before corneal thinning if possible, both to enhance corneal reepithelialization and to avoid stromal breakdown. If available, limbal autograft transplantation from the contralateral eye is performed at this time. In bilateral injuries, where conjunctival tissue is not available for transplantation, keratoepithelioplasty or large-diameter (>11 mm) lamellar keratoplasty with viable epithelium may be required. Following such surgery, there may still be a considerable delay before reepithelialization is complete. Continued careful monitoring for evidence of stromal breakdown is mandatory, and the use of tissue adhesives is still indicated for any impending perforation. Pending completion of reepithelialization, topical medroxyprogesterone, ascorbate, citrate, antibiotics, cycloplegics, and tear substitutes should be continued. After reepithelialization, topical corticosteroids are reinstituted, prophylactic antibiotics tapered, and citrate and ascorbate discontinued.

Despite optimal management, a scarred and vascularized cornea is a not uncommon end result. If success has been achieved in minimizing intraocular complications, limiting deep stromal vascularization, and providing a source of appropriately differentiated ocular surface epithelium, then keratoplasty (lamellar or penetrating) may be attempted after approximately 1 year.

References

1. McCulley JP: Chemical injuries. In Smolin G and Thoft RA, editors: The cornea: scientific foundations and clinical practice, ed 2, Boston, 1987, Little, Brown, 527-542.
2. Harris LH, Cohn K, and Galin MA: Alkali injury from fireworks, Ann Ophthalmol 3:849-851, 1971.
3. Paterson CA, Pfister RR, and Levinson RA: Aqueous humor pH changes after experimental alkali burns, Am J Ophthalmol 79:414-419, 1975.
4. Johnson-Muller B and Gross J: Regulation of corneal collagenase production: epithelial-stromal cell interactions, Proc Natl Acad Sci USA 75:4417-4421, 1978.
5. Johnson-Wint B: Regulation of stromal cell collagenase production in adult rabbit cornea: in vitro stimulation and inhibition by epithelial cell products, Proc Natl Acad Sci USA 77:5531-5535, 1980.
6. Johnson-Wint B and Gross J: Regulation of connective tissue collagenase production: stimulation from adult and fetal epidermal cells, J Cell Biol 98:90-96, 1984.
7. Johnson-Wint B: Autocrine regulation of collagenase production by passaged corneal stromal cells in vitro, Invest Ophthalmol Vis Sci 28(suppl):230, 1987.
8. Wright P: The chemically injured eye, Trans Ophthalmol Soc UK 102:85-87, 1982.
9. Shapiro MS, Friend J, and Thoft RA: Corneal reepithelialization from the conjunctiva, Invest Ophthalmol Vis Sci 21:135-142, 1981.
10. Pfister RR: The alkali-burned cornea. I. Epithelial and stromal repair, Exp Eye Res 23:519-535, 1976.
11. Wagoner MD et al: Polymorphonuclear neutrophils delay corneal epithelial wound healing in vitro, Invest Ophthalmol Vis Sci 25:1217-1222, 1984.
12. Pfister RR and Burstein N: The effects of ophthalmic drugs, vehicles, and preservatives on corneal epithelium: a scanning electronmicroscopic study, Invest Ophthalmol Vis Sci 15:246-259, 1976.
13. Ho PC and Elliott JH: Kinetics of corneal epithelial regeneration. II. Epidermal growth factor and topical corticosteroids, Invest Ophthalmol Vis Sci 14:630-633, 1975.
14. Berman MB et al: Ulceration is correlated with degradation of fibrin and fibronectin at the corneal surface, Invest Ophthalmol Vis Sci 24:1358-1366, 1983.
15. Thoft RA and Friend J: Biochemical transformation of regenerating ocular surface epithelium, Invest Ophthalmol Vis Sci 16:14-20, 1977.
16. Kinoshita S and Manabe S: Chemical burns. In Brightbill FS, editor: Corneal surgery, St Louis, 1986, The CV Mosby Co, 370-379.
17. Hirst LW et al: Corneal epithelial regeneration and adhesion following acid burns in the rhesus monkey, Invest Ophthalmol Vis Sci 23:764-773, 1982.
18. Chung JH and Fagerholm P: Stromal reaction and repair after corneal alkali wound in the rabbit: a quantitative microradiographic study, Exp Eye Res 45:227-237, 1987.
19. Paterson CA, Williams RN, and Parker AV: Characteristics of polymorphonuclear leukocyte infiltration into the alkali-burned eye and influence of sodium citrate, Exp Eye Res 39:701-708, 1984.
20. Lazarus GS et al: Human granulocyte collagenase, Science 159:1483-1485, 1968.
21. Chayakul V and Reim M: The enzymatic activities in the alkali-burned rabbit cornea, Graefes Arch Clin Exp Ophthalmol 218:145-148, 1982.
22. Cejkova J et al: Alkali burns of the rabbit cornea. I. A histochemical study of β-glucuronidase, β-galactosidase, and N-acetyl-β-d-glucosaminidase, Histochemistry 45:65-69, 1975.
23. Pahlitzsch T and Sinha P: The alkali burned cornea: electron microscopical, enzyme histochemical, and biochemical observations, Graefes Arch Clin Exp Ophthalmol 223:278-286, 1985.

24. Wagoner MD and Johnson-Wint B: Intact stromal explants in vitro behave like monolayers of primary stromal fibroblasts in their collagenase response to epithelial cytokines and interleukin-1, Invest Ophthalmol Vis Sci 28(suppl):222, 1987.
25. Kenyon KR et al: Prevention of stromal ulceration in the alkali-burned rabbit cornea by glued-on contact lens: evidence for the role of polymorphonuclear leukocytes in collagen degradation, Invest Ophthalmol Vis Sci 18:570-587, 1979.
26. Pfister RR, Nicolaro ML, and Paterson CA: Sodium citrate reduces the incidence of corneal ulcerations and perforations in extreme alkali-burned eyes—acetylcysteine and ascorbate have no favorable effect, Invest Ophthalmol Vis Sci 21:486-490, 1981.
27. Srinivasan BD and Kulkarni PS: Polymorphonuclear leukocyte response: inhibition following corneal epithelial denudation by steroidal and nonsteroidal anti-inflammatory agents, Arch Ophthalmol 99:1085-1089, 1981.
28. Donshik PC et al: Effect of topical corticosteroids on ulceration in alkali-burned corneas, Arch Ophthalmol 96:2117-2120, 1978.
29. Newsome DA and Gross J: Regulation of corneal collagenase production: stimulation of serially passaged stromal cells by blood mononuclear cells, Cell 16:895-900, 1979.
30. Eisen AZ, Jeffrey JJ, and Gross J: Human skin collagenase: isolation and mechanism of attack on the collagen molecule, Biochim Biophys Acta 151:637-645, 1968.
31. Gordon JM, Bauer EA, and Eisen AZ: Collagenase in the human cornea: immunologic localization, Arch Ophthalmol 98:341-345, 1980.
32. Berman MB et al: Characterization of collagenolytic activity in the ulcerating cornea, Exp Eye Res 11:255-257, 1971.
33. Pfister RR et al: Collagenase activity of intact corneal epithelium in peripheral corneal alkali burns, Arch Ophthalmol 86:308-313, 1971.
34. Berman MB, Leary R, and Gage J: Latent collagenase in the ulcerating rabbit cornea, Exp Eye Res 25:435-445, 1977.
35. Berman M, Leary R, and Gage J: Evidence for a role of the plasminogen activator-plasmin system in corneal ulceration, Invest Ophthalmol Vis Sci 19:1204-1221, 1980.
36. Berman MB et al: Corneal ulceration and the serum antiproteases. I. α-1-antitrypsin, Invest Ophthalmol Vis Sci 12:759-770, 1973.
37. Pfister RR and Paterson CA: Ascorbic acid in the treatment of alkali burns of the eye, Ophthalmology 87:1050-1057, 1980.
38. Gross J et al: Inhibition of tumor growth, vascularization, and collagenolysis in the rabbit cornea by medroxyprogesterone, Proc Natl Acad Sci USA 78:1176-1180, 1981.
39. Philips K et al: Effects of prednisolone and medroxyprogesterone on corneal wound healing, ulceration, and neovascularization, Arch Ophthalmol 101:640-643, 1983.
40. Fogle JA, Kenyon KR, and Foster CS: Tissue adhesive arrests stromal melting in the human cornea, Am J Ophthalmol 89:795-802, 1980.
41. Matsuda H and Smelser GK: Endothelial cells in alkali-burned corneas, Arch Ophthalmol 89:402-409, 1973.
42. Hughes WF: Alkali burns of the cornea. II. Clinical and pathologic course, Arch Ophthalmol 36:189-214, 1946.
43. Chiang TS, Moorman LR, and Thomas RP: Ocular hypertensive response following acid and alkali burns in rabbits, Invest Ophthalmol Vis Sci 10:270-273, 1971.
44. Gasset AR et al: Quantitative corticosteroid effect on corneal wound healing, Arch Ophthalmol 81:589-591, 1969.
45. Francois J and Feher J: Studies with the polarization microscope of the fibroblastic activity of the regenerating rabbit's cornea under the influence of corticosteroids, Exp Eye Res 15:471-483, 1973.
46. Newsome DA and Gross J: Prevention by medroxyprogesterone of perforation in the alkali-burned rabbit cornea: inhibition of collagenolytic activity, Invest Ophthalmol Vis Sci 16:21-31, 1977.
47. Lass JH et al: Medroxyprogesterone on corneal ulceration: its effects after alkali burns on rabbits, Arch Ophthalmol 99:673-676, 1981.
48. Pfister RR et al: The efficacy of ascorbate treatment after severe experimental alkali burns depends upon the route of administration, Invest Ophthalmol Vis Sci 19:1526-1529, 1980.
49. Pfister RR: Polymorphonuclear leukocyte inhibition by citrate, other heavy metal chelators, and trifluorperazine, Invest Ophthalmol Vis Sci 25:955-970, 1984.
50. Soong K et al: Topical retinoid therapy for squamous metaplasia of various ocular surface disorders, Ophthalmology 95:1442-1446, 1988.
51. Fujikawa LS et al: Fibronectin in healing rabbit corneal wounds, Lab Invest 45:120-129, 1981.
52. Colvin RB et al: Fibronectin therapy of persistent corneal epithelial defects, Invest Ophthalmol Vis Sci 26(suppl):92, 1985.
53. Spigelman AV, Vernot AJ, and Deutsch TA: Fibronectin in alkali burns of rabbit cornea, Cornea 4:169-173, 1985.
54. Tenn PF et al: Fibronectin in alkali-burned rabbit cornea: enhancement of epithelial wound healing, Invest Ophthalmol Vis Sci 26(suppl):92, 1985.
55. Singh GA and Foster CS: Epidermal growth factor in alkali-burned corneal epithelial wound healing, Am J Ophthalmol 103:802-807, 1987.

56. Nirankari VS et al: Superoxide radical scavenging agents in treatment of alkali burns, Arch Ophthalmol 99:886-887, 1981.
57. Wagoner MD and Kenyon KR: Noninfected corneal ulceration. In Focal points: clinical modules of ophthalmology, vol III, no 7, San Francisco, 1985, American Academy of Ophthalmology.
58. Thoft RA: Conjunctival transplantation, Arch Ophthalmol 95:1425-1427, 1977.
59. Kenyon KR and Tseng SCG: Limbal autograft transplantation for ocular surface disorders, Ophthalmology 96:709-723, 1989.
60. Thoft RA: Keratoepithelioplasty, Am J Ophthalmol 97:1-6, 1984.
61. Rao GN, Blatt HL, and Aquavella JV: Results of keratoprosthesis, Am J Ophthalmol 88:190-196, 1979.
62. Grant WM: Ocular injury due to sulfur dioxide. II. Experimental study and comparison with ocular effects of freezing, Arch Ophthalmol 38:762-774, 1947.
63. McCulley JP et al: Ocular hydrofluoric acid burns. In Henkind P, editor: Acta: XXIV International Congress of Ophthalmology, San Francisco, 1982, vol 2, Philadelphia, 1983, JB Lippincott, 1058-1062.
64. Friedenwald JS, Hughes WF, and Herrmann H: Acid burns of the eye, Arch Ophthalmol 35:98-108, 1946.
65. McCulley JP, Pettit M, and Lauber S: Treatment of experimental ocular hydrofluoric acid burns, Invest Ophthalmol Vis Sci 19(suppl):228, 1980.
66. Hersh PS et al: Topical nonsteroidal agents and corneal wound healing, Arch Ophthalmol 108:577-583, 1990.

CHAPTER 8

Iris trauma

ROGER F. STEINERT

Penetrating injury
- Presenting signs
- Initial management

Blunt trauma
- Presenting signs
- Initial management

Laser and surgical repair
- Assessment
- Laser treatment
- Surgical reconstruction

References

Penetrating wounds of the cornea commonly result in iris injury, either as a result of direct laceration or as a consequence of iris prolapse through the wound. Blunt, non-penetrating trauma to the anterior segment may also injure the iris.[1-3] The most common patterns of iris injury after severe blunt trauma are sphincter tears and dialysis of the iris root.[4] Iridoschisis and iris atrophy can also occur. Because of the vascularity of the iris and ciliary body, such injuries are often accompanied by hyphema (see Chapter 9).

This chapter will describe the presenting symptoms, acute management, and reconstruction of the injured iris. A large, nonreactive, or distorted pupil is cosmetically undesirable and may cause glare and photophobia that disturb the patient for the remainder of his or her life. A secluded pupil will block vision. The initial goal in management of iris trauma is to preserve as much iris tissue and normal architecture as possible. Options for subsequent secondary repair may be limited by unnecessary iris injury or loss at the time of initial repair (see Chapter 16).

PENETRATING INJURY

Presenting Signs

A sharp object that penetrates the cornea and traverses an anterior chamber that is rapidly shallowing because of aqueous release will commonly lacerate both the iris and the anterior lens capsule. The patient, therefore, commonly suffers a corneal or corneoscleral laceration, flat anterior chamber, rapidly hydrating and opacifying crystalline lens, iris incarceration in the wound, and/or external iris prolapse. Smaller wounds, particularly when located toward the periphery where the anterior chamber is shallower, typically result in iris incarceration or prolapse plugging the wound and, consequently, a shallow but not flat anterior chamber. Lens injury may be avoided entirely or appear later as a progressive cortical and subcapsular opacity.

Initial Management

As described in Chapter 13, an incarcerated but nonprolapsing iris should rarely be sacrificed. During acute repair of the corneal laceration, the initial sutures should avoid the incarcerated

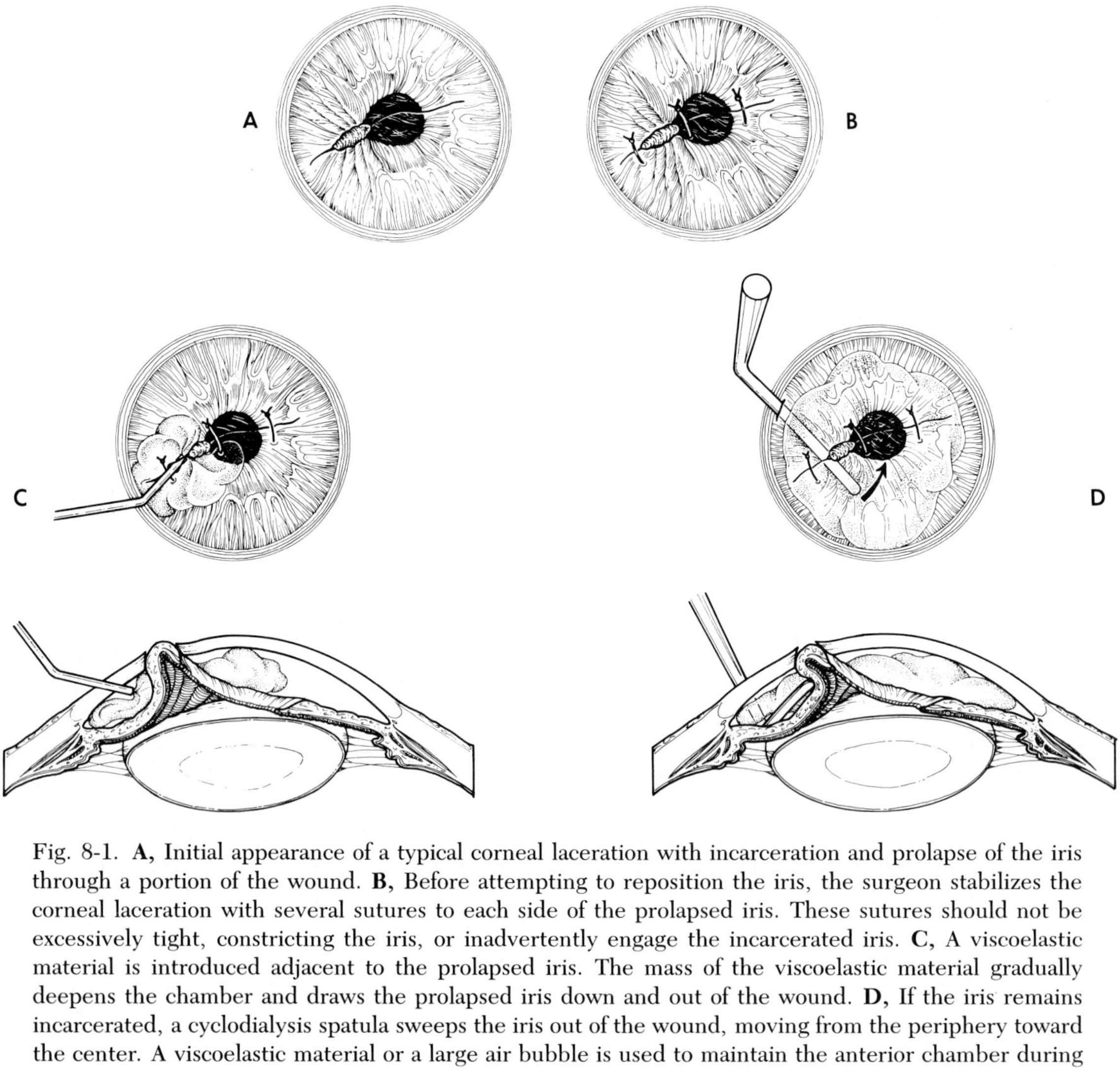

Fig. 8-1. **A,** Initial appearance of a typical corneal laceration with incarceration and prolapse of the iris through a portion of the wound. **B,** Before attempting to reposition the iris, the surgeon stabilizes the corneal laceration with several sutures to each side of the prolapsed iris. These sutures should not be excessively tight, constricting the iris, or inadvertently engage the incarcerated iris. **C,** A viscoelastic material is introduced adjacent to the prolapsed iris. The mass of the viscoelastic material gradually deepens the chamber and draws the prolapsed iris down and out of the wound. **D,** If the iris remains incarcerated, a cyclodialysis spatula sweeps the iris out of the wound, moving from the periphery toward the center. A viscoelastic material or a large air bubble is used to maintain the anterior chamber during this maneuver.

iris if such areas exist (Fig. 8-1, *A* and *B*). An exquisitely fine, sharp needle is required for the initial sutures so that the wound does not separate when the suture is passed. Separation of the wound will lead to further iris incarceration or frank prolapse. A 4-mil needle is preferred (e.g., Alcon AU15, Ethicon TG 160-4) with 10-0 nylon suture material. The initial stabilizing sutures often may prove to be temporary, shallow, too long, or too short; they can be replaced later in the repair if necessary. The initial objective is simply to stabilize the wound to allow iris reposition.

Once the wound is stabilized, the most atraumatic method of repositioning the incarcerated iris is with viscoelastic material injected either directly through the wound or obliquely to deepen the chamber and draw the iris away from the cornea (Fig. 8-1, *C*). A high-viscosity agent has less tendency to be regurgitated from the wound (e.g., chondroitin sulfate and hyaluronic acid 30 mg/ml [Viscoat]). If a viscoelastic agent is not available, an air bubble injected from the periphery can be helpful.

If the iris remains incarcerated despite these measures, and reinspection of the wound confirms that no sutures have inadvertently impaled the iris, a fine cyclodialysis spatula passed through a peripheral paracentesis wound is gently swept across the anterior chamber to free the incarcerated tissue (Fig. 8-1, *D*).

Frankly prolapsed, exposed iris must be evaluated thoughtfully before deciding to either reposition or excise it. Prolonged prolapse leads to ischemia and subsequent necrosis. The exposed iris can become colonized with microorganisms. Under these circumstances, repositing the exposed iris will lead to prolonged inflammation and potential endophthalmitis. Most trauma surgeons would reposition a prolapsed iris that has been exposed only several hours and excise a severely macerated iris or one that has been prolapsed longer than 24 hours. If a decision is made to reposition the prolapsed iris, a cellulose surgical sponge and balanced salt irrigation should be used to gently remove any accumulated mucus and debris, and the cellulose sponge sent for culture.

Surgical repair of iris damage is usually best deferred to a secondary operation. The acute corneal injury itself and accompanying inflammation and hemorrhage reduce visualization. The principal reason for surgical iris repair is to improve visual function, and this cannot be assessed accurately until the eye heals from the initial injury and primary repair. The type of repair, if any, is often determined as much by the healing of the iris as by the original injury. Frequently other secondary surgery is indicated, such as penetrating keratoplasty, and repair of the iris is readily accomplished at that time. Finally, a zealous attempt at primary repair of an injured iris may interfere with critical aspects of diagnosis and treatment postoperatively, such as visualization of the peripheral retina or cataract extraction.

BLUNT TRAUMA

Presenting Signs

Mild iris injury results in transient iritis. Pigment may be liberated and deposited on the corneal endothelium, trabecular meshwork, or lens.[1]

Iris stromal tears from nonpenetrating anterior segment injury appear either centrally as sphincter damage or peripherally at the iris root as iridodialysis or, as a split in the iris stroma, as iridoschisis.

Sphincter muscle injury may be minimal, resulting in mild anisocoria with retained pupil reactivity. In more severe cases a profound mydriasis results that is unresponsive to light or miotic agents. Local sphincter tears can cause a nearly imperceptible teardrop deformation of the pupil or a more pronounced sector deformity. Pigment epithelium may migrate from the pupil over the injured anterior iris stroma.

Stretching at the iris root frequently results in hyphema. The residual anatomic deformity can be a hyperpigmented angle with synechia formation, angle recession, dialysis of the iris root, or, rarely, creation of a cyclodialysis cleft.[1-3]

Initial Management

Conservative supportive treatment continues until the eye has completely recovered from the initial injury. Mild contusion may result in an iritis without other damage. Cycloplegia alone is often adequate treatment; in more intense iritis, topical steroids improve comfort and speed clearing of the reaction.

Management of hyphema is discussed in detail in Chapter 9. Avoidance of prolonged elevated intraocular pressure reduces the chance of ischemic injury to the sphincter muscle, as well as optic nerve injury, and corneal bloodstaining. Aggressive use of topical and systemic antiinflammatory medications reduces formation of anterior and posterior synechiae. Pharmacologic mydriasis and cycloplegia, when indicated, should be performed with short-acting agents in pulses. This may reduce the likelihood of irreversible dilation.

LASER AND SURGICAL REPAIR

Assessment

Conservative measures frequently are adequate and appropriate to manage the long-term sequelae of iris injury. The ophthalmologist should not treat the patient's cosmetic concerns as unimportant but rather address them with appropriate compassion and empathy. Although cosmetic concerns are secondary to the preservation of vision, iris deformities can be quite pronounced, especially in individuals with light-colored irides, which contrast strongly with the black pupil. Tinted contact lenses, with either a general tint or an artificial pupil, frequently correct the appearance adequately.

Complaints about glare and photophobia first require an evaluation of the source. Corneal scars may result in severe glare, and an irregular epithelium will cause photophobia. If the pupil responds to topical miotics, administration of pilocarpine or carbachol can be both diagnostic and therapeutic. Similarly, if the pupil is nonreactive, a heavily tinted contact lens with an artificial pupil can be diagnostic and, if tolerated, therapeutic. Sunglasses relieve photophobia and glare from sunlight but cannot help patients troubled by headlight glare at night.

Simulation of glare and multiplopia should be attempted with point light sources and other targets in the office. If the patient can appreciate a recreation of real-world symptoms, the edge of an occluder can be advanced across the pupil, as close as possible to the cornea, to determine the anatomic source of the symptoms.

If the pupil is eccentric or secluded, dilation should be attempted. If this is successful, long-acting agents may be adequate treatment.

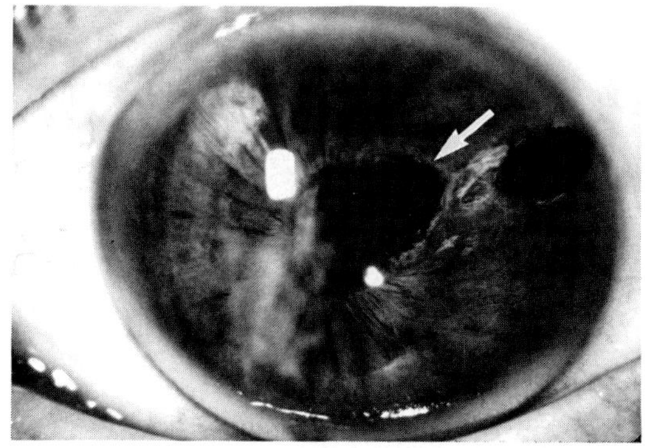

Fig. 8-2. An Nd-YAG laser sphincterotomy expanded the pupil away from the scarred area and into normal cornea *(arrow)*. Visual acuity improved, and a penetrating keratoplasty was avoided. (Reprinted with permission from Steinert RF and Puliafito CA: The Nd-YAG laser in ophthalmology: principles and clinical applications of photodisruption, Philadelphia, 1985, WB Saunders.)

Laser Treatment

Laser therapy can perform sphincterotomy and lysis of strands, bands, and adhesions. Sphincterotomy can result in marked improvement in some patients with eccentric or secluded pupils. This approach is particularly useful in patients unresponsive to or intolerant of topical dilating drops. Sphincterotomy can also be helpful in improving visual acuity if the visual axis can be shifted away from a scar toward a clear, optically regular portion of the cornea.

In aphakic or pseudophakic patients, the Nd-YAG laser can rupture the iris stroma and achieve an adequate sphincterotomy (Fig. 8-2). Typically, pulses are 6 mJ. Because bleeding occurs principally from the sphincter, treatment should begin where the opening should end and then work back toward the sphincter (Fig. 8-3). In this manner, bleeding is avoided until near the end of the procedure and can usually be easily controlled with 1 minute of pressure on the globe.

Phakic patients undergoing sphincterotomy should be treated with the argon laser. Linear photocoagulation can achieve a sphincterotomy without the risk of lens capsule rupture that is present with Nd-YAG photodisruption. Typical argon laser settings are a 50μ spot, power of 1000 to 1500 W, and duration of 0.1 second. A converging contact lens such as an Abraham lens with a central lens button should be employed to improve beam concentration and reduce the chance of inadvertent photocoagulation injury to the retina. The beam must never be directed toward the macula.

Laser treatment is also effective in the lysis of strands, bands, and adhesions. Lens capsule remnants, vitreous strands, or fibrin may become incarcerated in or adhere to the wound and lead to optically significant pupillary distortion. If pigment precipitates form on such a strand, the argon photocoagulator can rupture the strand thermally. In most cases, however, the Nd-YAG photodisruptor is the preferred instrument.

Lens capsule remnants are usually delicate and readily rupture with pulses of 2 to 3 mJ. Vitreous strands typically rupture more readily when higher energies of at least 5 mJ are used. Rupturing fibrinous adhesions requires a wide range of energy levels, depending upon the density of the bands. The configuration of the strand, pupil, and wound determines whether the laser beam should be aimed directly, with the aid of a central or peripheral button Abraham lens, or whether it should be aimed obliquely, using a gonioscopy lens.

Generally, strands, bands, and membranes

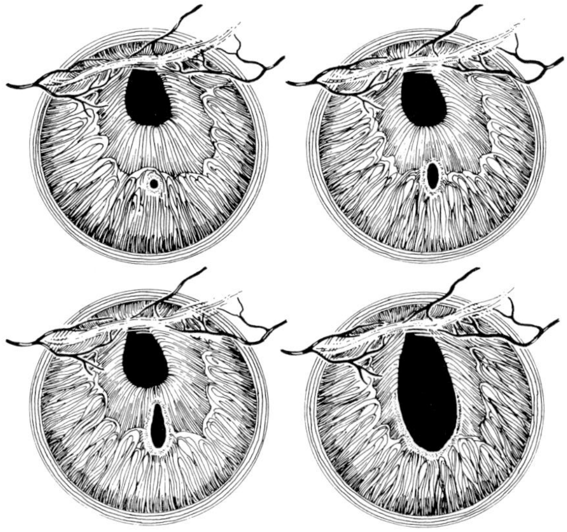

Fig. 8-3. Technique for Nd-YAG laser sphincterotomy. **A,** Treatment is begun in the peripheral iris stroma. **B, C,** Progressive cutting is made toward the iris sphincter. **D,** The sphincter is cut last so that bleeding is minimized for as long as possible to increase the chance of completing the treatment in one session.

are best treated as soon as they cause clinically significant iris distortion. Prolonged presence of a strand causes permanent pupillary distortion, synechiae, and increased density of the strand or band. Surgical intervention with scissors or a vitrector is required only in unusual cases of extensive adhesions.

Surgical Reconstruction

Repair of sphincter lacerations and tears in a closed chamber is based on the concepts first described by McCannel.[5] If repair is performed in the course of a penetrating keratoplasty, the open-sky suturing is straightforward.

Suture material of 10-0 polypropylene (Prolene) should be used because it is less subject to hydrolysis and biodegradation. Use of a noncutting vascular needle will avoid the tendency of cutting needles to lacerate the delicate iris stroma. An excellent short needle for open-sky suturing is the Ethicon BV 100-4 series. For McCannel techniques, a longer needle such as the Ethicon CIF-4 is needed.

Figs. 8-4 and 8-5 illustrate the McCannel suture technique for repairing an inferior sphincter laceration in a closed chamber. One must use caution in stretching the iris to close a coloboma. Excessive tension may distort the globe because of the internal "trampoline" of the iris or may cause an iridodialysis and hemorrhage. Repair of a sphincter tear will usually be in an aphakic eye. In the rare case of a repair in an eye with an intact and clear crystalline lens, great care must be taken to avoid injury to the lens capsule and secondary cataract. Placement of viscoelastic between the posterior iris and lens may help to protect the lens in these cases.

A traumatic iridodialysis should be repaired when it is large enough to cause multiplopia or glare.[4,5] Color Plate 8-1 and Fig. 8-6 illustrate the suspension of the peripheral iris stroma to the sclera. Creating a scleral flap is mandatory to permanently cover the external portion of the suture. The suture exits through the sclera about 1 mm posterior to the limbus, where Tenon's capsule and the conjunctiva are thin. If the suture is not cut short and well buried, it may eventually erode through the conjunctiva. It can then serve as a conduit of access for microorganisms, leading to endophthalmitis, or be removed unwittingly by an ophthalmologist unaware of the suture's function.[6]

Additional surgical techniques in anterior segment reconstruction involving the iris are described in Chapter 16.

A

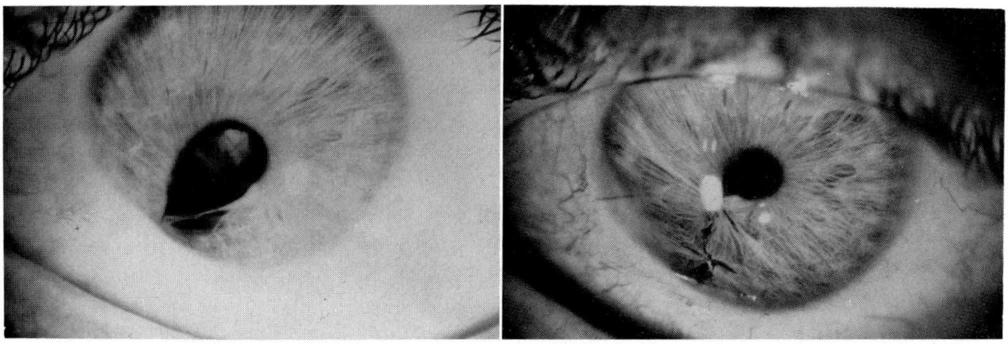

B

Fig. 8-4. **A,** A cataract can be seen through a trauma-induced sector iris defect. **B,** After extracapsular cataract extraction and implantation of a posterior chamber intraocular lens, the iris defect has been closed with two interrupted 10-0 polypropylene sutures using the McCannel suture technique.

A

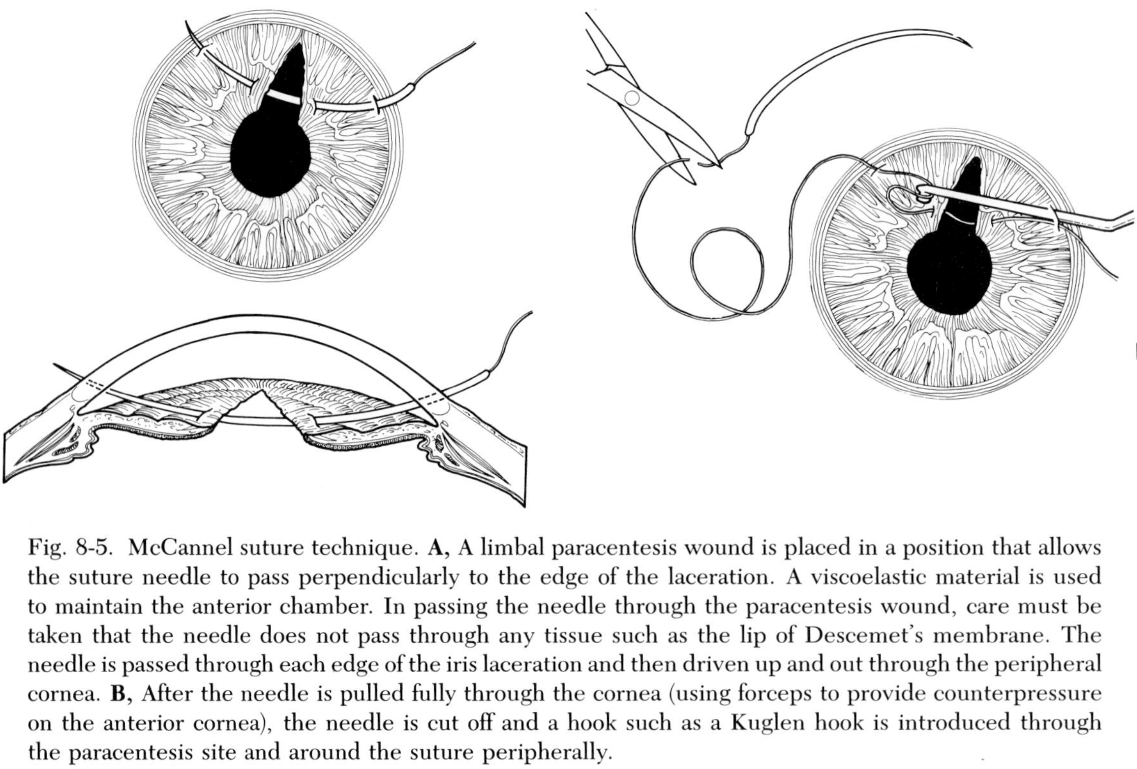

B

Fig. 8-5. McCannel suture technique. **A,** A limbal paracentesis wound is placed in a position that allows the suture needle to pass perpendicularly to the edge of the laceration. A viscoelastic material is used to maintain the anterior chamber. In passing the needle through the paracentesis wound, care must be taken that the needle does not pass through any tissue such as the lip of Descemet's membrane. The needle is passed through each edge of the iris laceration and then driven up and out through the peripheral cornea. **B,** After the needle is pulled fully through the cornea (using forceps to provide counterpressure on the anterior cornea), the needle is cut off and a hook such as a Kuglen hook is introduced through the paracentesis site and around the suture peripherally.

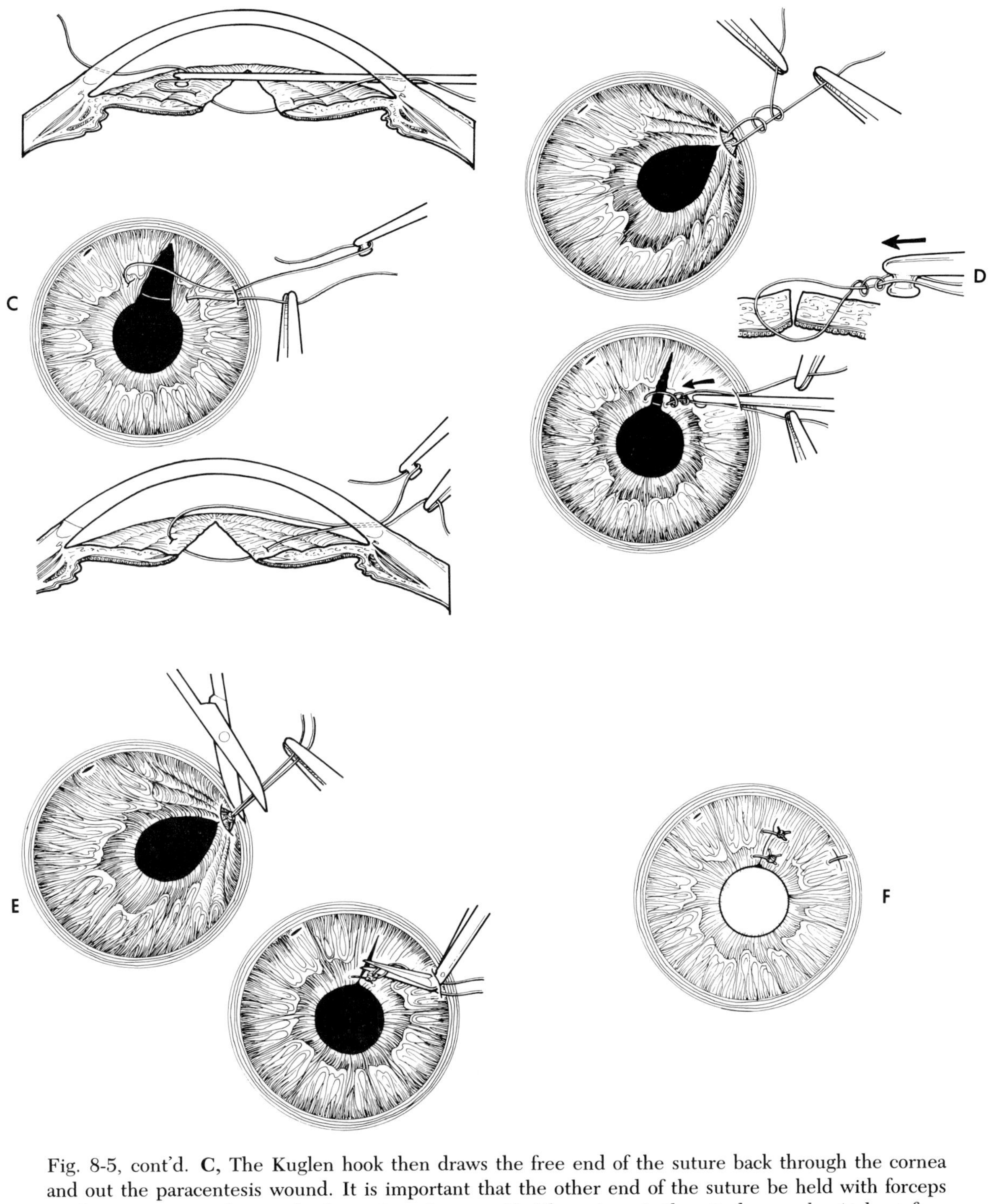

Fig. 8-5, cont'd. **C,** The Kuglen hook then draws the free end of the suture back through the cornea and out the paracentesis wound. It is important that the other end of the suture be held with forceps so that it is not inadvertently drawn into the eye. **D,** The suture is then tied securely. At least four square knots are recommended for 10-0 polypropylene sutures. A flaccid iris may allow the knot to be tied in a normal fashion by pulling the iris up to the wound. If the iris will not allow this, the knot is tied within the anterior chamber. The assistant holds one suture end under minimal tension, preventing laxity of the suture but not displacing the iris. The surgeon holds the other suture end under similar tension with tying forceps in the nondominant hand and uses a Kuglen hook to advance the looped suture down to the knot. **E,** After the knot is tight and secure, the ends are cut short, either by drawing the knot up to the wound if possible or by a Gills-Vannas scissors introduced through the paracentesis wound. **F,** In the case of large repairs, two or more sutures may be needed to close the iris adequately. A single 10-0 nylon suture is usually sufficient to close the paracentesis wound.

A

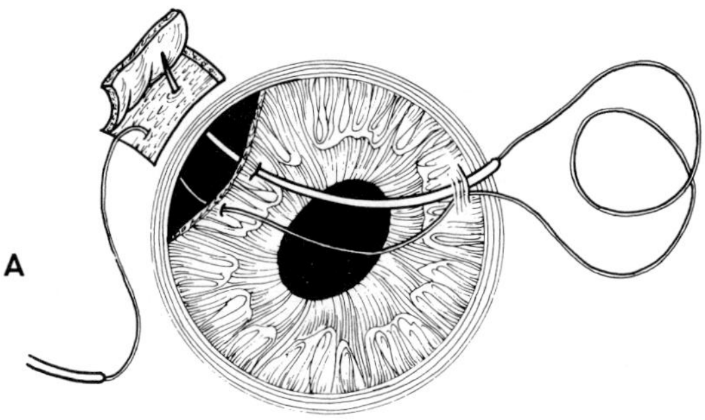

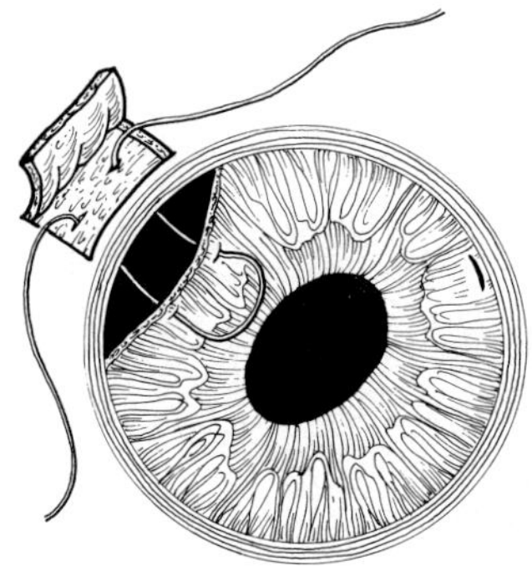

B

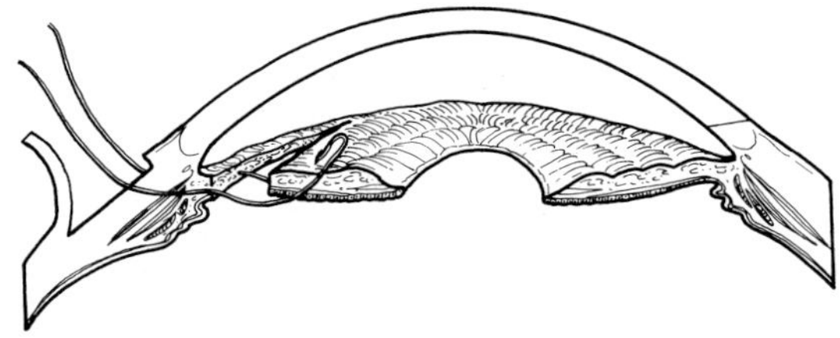

C

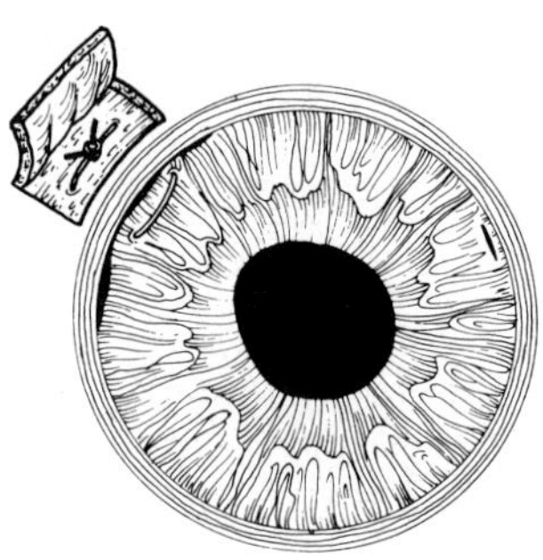

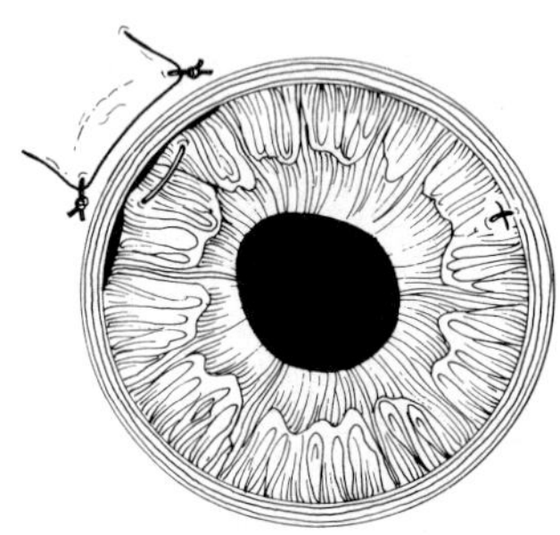

D

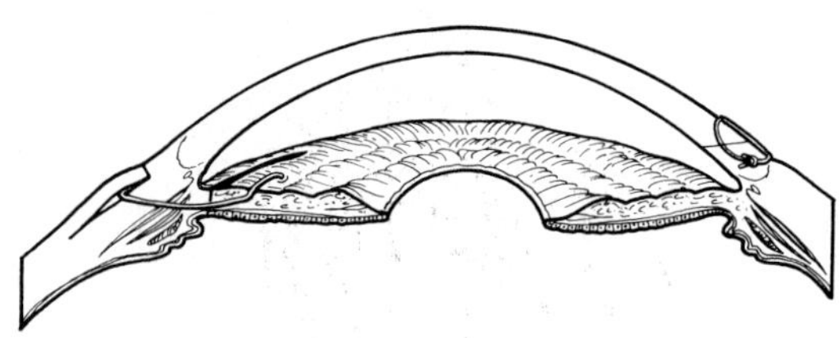

Fig. 8-6. **A, B,** An iridodialysis is repaired with one or more mattress sutures of double-armed 10-0 polypropylene sutures tied externally under a scleral flap. Both arms of the polypropylene suture are introduced through a paracentesis opening on the opposite side of the anterior chamber. The dialyzed edge of iris is engaged by each needle in turn, and the needle is passed through the sclera into the bed of the scleral flap. **C,** The mattress suture is tied in the bed of the scleral flap. The paracentesis wound is closed with a single 10-0 nylon suture. **D,** The scleral flap is then closed over the polypropylene mattress suture with corner sutures of 8-0 Vicryl or other absorbable suture material. The conjunctiva is then closed over the scleral flap.

References

1. Britten MJA: Follow-up of 54 cases of ocular contusion with hyphaema, with special reference to the appearance and function of the filtration angle, Br J Ophthalmol 49:120-127, 1965.
2. Weidenthal DT: Experimental ocular contusion, Arch Ophthalmol 71:77-81, 1964.
3. Wolff SM and Zimmerman LE: Chronic secondary glaucoma: associated with retrodisplacement of iris root and deepening of the anterior chamber angle secondary to contusion, Am J Ophthalmol 54:547-563, 1962.
4. Paton D and Craig J: Management of iridodialysis, Ophthalmic Surg 4(1):38-39, 1973.
5. McCannel MA: A retrievable suture idea for anterior uveal problems, Ophthalmic Surg 7(2):98-103, 1976.
6. Epstein E: Suture problems, J Cataract Refract Surg 15:116, 1989.

CHAPTER 9

Traumatic hyphema

BRADFORD J. SHINGLETON
PETER S. HERSH

Causes and demographics
Classification
Pathophysiology
- Mechanism of injury
- Associated ocular findings
- Clot formation and dissolution

Evaluation of traumatic hyphema
- History
- Physical examination
- Laboratory tests

Treatment of traumatic hyphema
- Inpatient versus outpatient treatment
- Supportive treatment
- Medical treatment
  - Salicylates
  - Cycloplegics and miotics
  - Steroids
  - Antifibrinolytic agents
  - Fibrinolytic agents
  - Medical treatment summary

Surgical intervention for traumatic hyphema
- Indications for surgical intervention
  - Intraocular pressure criteria
  - Corneal bloodstaining
  - Prolonged clot duration
- Techniques of surgical intervention
  - Paracentesis and anterior chamber washout
  - Clot expression and limbal delivery
  - Automated hyphemectomy
  - Peripheral iridectomy and trabeculectomy
  - Other techniques

Complications of hyphema
- Rebleeding
- Glaucoma
- Corneal bloodstaining

Special considerations
- Sickle cell disease
- Children with traumatic hyphema

Clinical outcomes and prognosis
References

Hyphema is a common manifestation of blunt trauma to the globe. Although blood clears from the anterior chamber without problem in most cases, a significant number of short- and long-term complications may develop. Because such complications can threaten vision, hyphema patients must be followed carefully. Based on the constellation of signs and symptoms, hyphema patients may be referred to various ophthalmic subspecialists. All ophthalmologists, therefore, must develop a systematic approach to evaluating and treating this problem.

CAUSES AND DEMOGRAPHICS

Hyphema patients are preponderantly male (in a striking 3:1 ratio), and 70% are under 20 years of age.[1] External causes are multiple and include, among others, fists, rocks, sticks, and BBs.[1-7] Schein et al.[8] confirmed these hazardous projectiles as frequent causes of ocular injuries in children and noted that sports may account for up to 60% of traumatic hyphemas. North American studies in children and adults estimate the incidence of hyphema at 17 to 20 per 100,000 per year.[9,10]

CLASSIFICATION

Microscopic hyphema is a term used for circulating red blood cells in the anterior chamber without gross collection of blood. The importance of microscopic hyphema, as it relates to treatment and prognosis, remains unclear because of the lack of systematic evaluation and confusion with traumatic iritis. Two studies, however, cite a rebleed rate of approximately 7% in children with microscopic hyphema, so this population must be monitored closely.[9,10]

Grading schemes for traumatic hyphema are based on the amount of blood in the anterior chamber (Table 9-1): initially after injury 50% to 60% of the patients fall into the Grade I category, 20% to 30% into Grade II, and approximately 15% into Grade III.[1,2,9] Five percent to 10% of the patients have "eight-ball," or total, hyphemas; if rebleeding patients are included, this percentage may be as high as 15%.[11]

PATHOPHYSIOLOGY

Mechanism of Injury

Blunt ocular trauma causes stretching of limbal tissues, equatorial scleral expansion, posterior displacement of the lens/iris diaphragm, and acute elevation of intraocular pressure (IOP), with consequent tearing of tissues near the anterior chamber angle (Fig. 9-1).[12] Most hyphemas result from tears in the anterior face of the ciliary body with disruption of the major arterial circle and its branches, recurrent choroidal arteries or ciliary body veins.[12] Approximately 15% of hyphemas arise from ruptured iris vessels, cyclodialysis, or iridodialysis.

Blood in the anterior chamber less commonly arises from rubeosis iridis, vitreous hemorrhage, occult perforating injury, neoplasm (retinoblastoma, malignant melanoma, metastatic tumor, juvenile xanthogranuloma), or intraocular lenses. Spontaneous iris bleeding rarely occurs in the setting of abnormal clotting factors.

Table 9-1. Grading scheme for traumatic hyphema

Grade	Size of hyphema (fraction of anterior chamber filled with blood)
Microscopic	No layered blood; circulating red blood cells only
I	< ⅓
II	⅓–½
III	½–near total
IV	Total ("eight-ball")

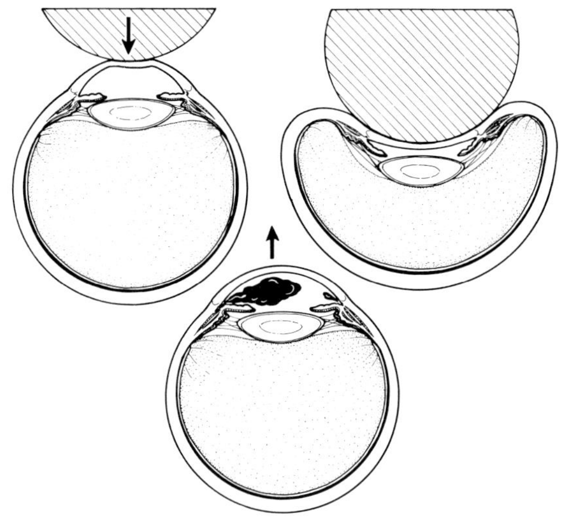

Fig. 9-1. Compressive force to the globe results in vascular disruption and bleeding into the anterior chamber.

Associated Ocular Findings (Fig. 9-2)

Angle recession, a separation between the longitudinal and circular muscle fibers of the ciliary muscle,[13] is the most important associated anterior segment finding in traumatic hyphema. The amount of angle recession does not necessarily correlate with the size of the hyphema or degree of acute IOP elevation. The incidence of angle recession is variably reported as 30% to 85%.[2,9,10] More extensive recession is associated with a higher incidence of late-onset glaucoma, and it is estimated that approximately 6% to 10% of hyphema patients will develop angle recession glaucoma[12] (see Chapter 10 for treatment). A cyclodialysis cleft with separation of the scleral spur from its ciliary body attachments occurs less commonly and may cause postinjury hypotony.

Traumatic iritis invariably accompanies hyphema. Furthermore, pigment liberation may result in endothelial pigment dusting and increased trabecular meshwork pigmentation. Iris atrophy occurs less commonly,[4] and a Vossius ring, signifying compression of the pupillary margin on the anterior lens capsule, may develop.

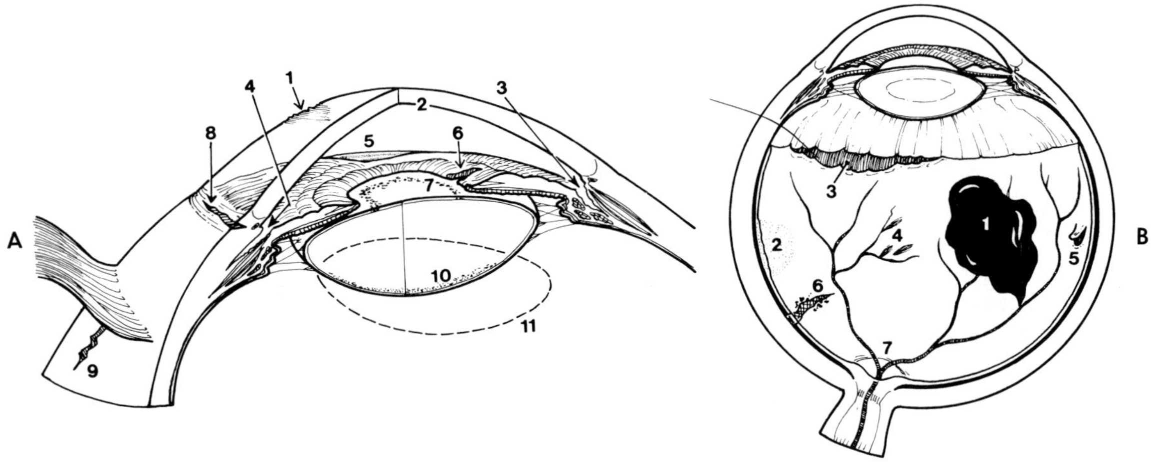

Fig. 9-2. Associated ocular injuries in eyes with traumatic hyphema. **A,** *1,* Corneal abrasion; *2,* corneal endothelial injury with or without bloodstaining; *3,* angle recession; *4,* cyclodialysis; *5,* iridodialysis; *6,* iris sphincter tears; *7,* Vossius ring; *8,* corneoscleral rupture; *9,* scleral rupture; *10,* cataract; *11,* lens subluxation. **B,** *1,* Vitreous hemorrhage; *2,* retinal edema; *3,* retinal dialysis; *4,* retinal hemorrhages; *5,* horseshoe tear; *6,* choroidal rupture; *7,* optic nerve injury.

Traumatic mydriasis occurs in about 10% of cases secondary to sphincter muscle paresis and tears.[4,9] In contrast, miosis may be associated with severe traumatic iritis. Iridodialysis occurs in less than 10% of cases. Treatment of symptomatic iris damage is discussed in Chapter 8.

Corneal abrasions are common after blunt trauma, and the possibility of an occult globe rupture must always be kept in mind when evaluating cases of traumatic hyphema. Corneoscleral rupture most commonly occurs near the limbus parallel to the equator or just behind the rectus muscle insertions perpendicular to the limbus. Rupture may be heralded by chemosis, subconjunctival hemorrhage, alteration in anterior chamber depth, hypotony, and scleral show on indirect ophthalmoscopy. The corneal endothelium may also be damaged by blunt injury, which may lead to early and late corneal edema and, especially if IOP is increased, to blood-staining. Cataract formation may develop in 5% to 15% of cases secondary to blunt trauma.[4,9] Subluxation is less frequent (see Chapter 11).

Posterior segment injuries are a common cause of reduced vision following clearing of traumatic hyphemas. Significant vitreous hemorrhage, retinal edema, holes, hemorrhages, and choroidal rupture may occur in as many as 33% of cases (see Chapters 17 and 18).[4,9] Optic atrophy may develop as a direct result of trauma to the optic nerve (see Chapter 34) or following marked IOP elevation. Such associated injuries are the predominant cause of irretrievable visual loss in patients with traumatic hyphema.

Clot Formation and Dissolution

Bleeding of the injured vessel in traumatic hyphema stops as a result of IOP tamponade, vascular spasm, and formation of a fibrin/platelet clot.

Histopathology studies show that blood in the anterior chamber clots to form a fibrin/platelet coagulum.[14,15] There is an outer pseudocapsular membrane with firm attachments to surrounding structures. Total hyphema may be molded into a bilobed configuration with contiguous blood in both the anterior and posterior chambers. Maximum clot integrity is achieved about 4 to 7 days after injury. However, the clot demonstrates no fibroblastic activity or neovascularization characteristic of clots in other parts of the body.

The anterior chamber is fibrinolytically active.[16] Plasminogen (profibrinolysin) is converted to plasmin (fibrinolysin) by activators. Plasmin, in turn, breaks down fibrin, leading to clot dissolution.

Free blood cells and fibrin degradation products in the anterior chamber clear by normal trabecular outflow pathways.[2,17] Absorption by iris vasculature may play a minor role.

EVALUATION OF TRAUMATIC HYPHEMA

History

Patients with hyphema usually have complaints of reduced vision and pain. Somnolence is relatively common in children. Careful questioning is indicated to assess the type of trauma involved and to focus the subsequent clinical examination. Both blunt and lacerating traumas may cause hyphema but commonly have different associated ocular problems. Particular attention should be paid to any history of bleeding disorders; pregnancy; sickle cell, kidney, and liver disease; and recent anticoagulant therapy, including aspirin.

Physical Examination

A complete eye examination is required of every patient with hyphema. Blunt rupture of the globe is the most important associated clinical finding to be ruled out, and all patients should be considered ruptured globe suspects until proven otherwise.

To facilitate later comparison, the hyphema should be described in detail. Size of the hyphema may be described in terms of height (mm), percentage of anterior chamber filled with blood, or clock-hour extent. Clotted hemorrhage should be distinguished from unclotted blood. Free, circulating red blood cells should be quantified as much as possible (1+ to 4+). Early examination may permit identification of an anterior chamber bleeding site. Rebleeding is not always easy to identify, but it is suggested by the presence of bright red blood layered over darker clotted blood and increased hyphema size.

Vision, hyphema status, and IOP are documented at every follow-up examination. Critical, high-magnification slit-lamp evaluation is required to detect corneal bloodstaining. Gonioscopy may be performed acutely to search for an active bleeding vessel and is required to detect angle recession at the 1-month postinjury examination. Dilated funduscopy is recommended at the time of presentation, but scleral depression is generally reserved for the 1-month follow-up visit to avoid precipitating a rebleed.

Laboratory Tests

Laboratory tests of importance include a "sickle prep" and hemoglobin electrophoresis for black patients. A history of bleeding disorder may lead to performance of liver function tests, protime, partial thromboplastin time, platelet counts, and bleeding time assessment. Baseline BUN and creatinine levels should be obtained if aminocaproic acid is to be used.

TREATMENT OF TRAUMATIC HYPHEMA

Management of traumatic hyphema has tended to be institutionally ritualistic, but although data remain inexact, current information is now available to allow formation of a reasonable approach to the care of this difficult problem.

Inpatient versus Outpatient Treatment

Noncontrolled studies[9,18,19] do not show significant differences in rebleeding rates and clinical outcomes in patients treated at home or in a hospital. Advantages of hospitalization include ease of follow-up examination, confirmation of medical compliance, and possible earlier detection of complications. Cost is the overriding disadvantage. Outpatient care has the advantage of being the usual preference of family and patient.

Supportive Treatment

In 1967 Darr and Passmore[20] suggested that bed rest with bilateral patching may decrease rebleeding in hyphema patients. Rakusin[6] found a more rapid rate of hyphema resorption with bed rest but no decrease in the rate of rebleeding. Since then most authors[2,9,21] have noted no significant difference in results between moderate activity and strict bed rest. Bilateral versus unilateral patching did not produce differences in clinical results,[22] and patching may increase patient anxiety, especially in children. Reading restrictions do not appear to be necessary.

Sedation is rarely required when mild activity is permitted. Metal shield protection to minimize further injury to the globe is accepted by most ophthalmologists as a reasonable preventive measure. Head elevation to approximately 30° while at rest enhances dependent settling of blood and may permit earlier posterior segment clinical examination.

Medical Treatment

Miotics and cycloplegics, antifibrinolytics and fibrinolytics, estrogens and corticosteroids, and numerous other pharmacologic adjuncts have all been suggested for the medical treatment of hyphema.[4] Few have proven to be efficacious, and interest has waned in many of these treatments.

Salicylates

Aspirin[23-25] may increase bleeding after hyphema. This view is shared by most ophthalmologists. However, Marcus et al.[26] found no significant increase in bleeding if aspirin (500 mg by mouth 3 times a day) was used after hyphema, and Palmer et al.[27] found no difference in rebleeding in patients taking aminocaproic acid with or without aspirin. The antiplatelet effect of aspirin and subsequent prolongation of bleeding time remain a concern and suggest that aspirin should be avoided, if possible. A similar caveat holds for the use of nonsteroidal anti-inflammatory agents.

Cycloplegics and Miotics

Gilbert and Jensen[28] found that topical atropine 1% had no beneficial effect on rebleeding, blood resorption, or vision. Cycloplegia, however, may enhance patient comfort in the setting of traumatic iritis, and the associated mydriatic effect often facilitates fundus examination. Miotics are generally avoided because of their tendency to increase intraocular inflammation in the acute setting.

Steroids

Topical steroids are commonly used in the setting of hyphema to help minimize discomfort related to traumatic iritis. Efficacy in improving clinical outcome remains to be proven.[6] Systemic steroids are more controversial. There is theoretical evidence supporting their use to enhance clot stabilization. Retrospective, noncontrolled reviews by Yasuna[29] and Rynne and Romano[30] supported the use of oral prednisone to reduce rebleeding. A prospective study of 43 adults, by Spoor, Hammer, and Belloso[31] found no statistically significant difference in blood resorption and rebleeding when prednisone 40 mg per day was used. No studies are definitive, and further prospective work is required. Given their lack of proven efficacy in reducing rebleeding and their potential adverse consequences, even for short treatment courses in healthy patients,[32] systemic steroids are best reserved for special situations.

Antifibrinolytic Agents

Antifibrinolytic agents such as aminocaproic acid and tranexamic acid have been proposed for use in traumatic hyphema to reduce rebleeding.[33] The rationale for their use is based on the fact that the anterior chamber is a fibrinolytically active system and on the hypothesis that a reduced rate of hyphema clot lysis may allow the injured bleeding vessel more time to heal (Fig. 9-3).[34]

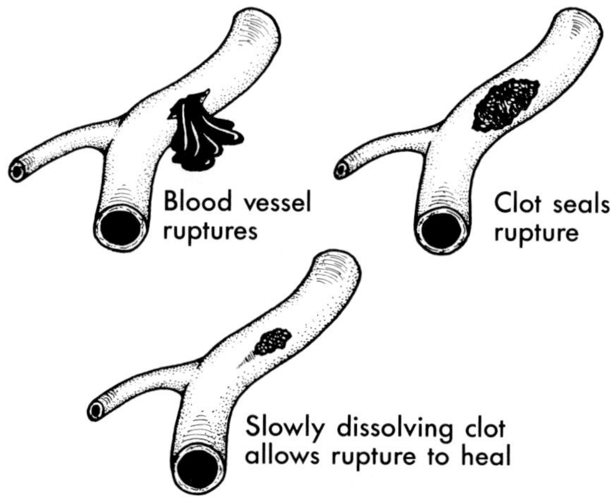

Fig. 9-3. Antifibrinolytic agent theoretically stabilizes clot and thus enhances healing of the injured blood vessel.

Structure and mechanism of action of aminocaproic acid. Aminocaproic acid (Amicar) is a monoaminocarboxylic acid similar to lysine. It is the most commonly used antifibrinolytic agent for traumatic hyphema in the United States. It is a competitive inhibitor of the activating substance that converts plasminogen into the proteolytic enzyme plasmin. It also has a secondary inhibitory effect on plasmin itself. Plasmin lyses fibrin into smaller polypeptides and accelerates clot breakdown. Therefore, its inhibition will theoretically stabilize the clot-vessel wall interface, decreasing the potential for rebleeding.

Administration, dosage, and contraindications. Aminocaproic acid is administered orally and is cleared by the kidneys. The current recommended dosage is 50 mg/kg orally every 4 hours, up to 30 g/day, for a total of 5 days. Use is contraindicated in cases of active intravascular clotting disorders, pregnancy, and cardiac, hepatic, and renal disease.

Efficacy. The use of aminocaproic acid to reduce rebleeding in traumatic hyphema in the United States was first studied by Crouch and Frenkel.[35] With a dosage of 100 mg/kg by mouth every 4 hours for 5 days, they found a rebleeding rate of 1 in 32 for the treated group and 9 in 27 for the placebo group. Other authors[36-39] have confirmed a reduced rate of rebleeding in white and black hyphema patients treated with antifibrinolytic agents.

Side effects. Complications commonly encountered include nausea, vomiting, and postural hypotension. Less common are tinnitus, lethargy, skin rash, myopathy, and hematuria. Symptoms may be severe enough to require discontinuation of the medication.[37]

Stopping aminocaproic acid before completion of a full 5-day course may be associated with a greater tendency to rebleed.[36] Palmer et al.[27] minimized side effects and maintained efficacy in reducing rebleeding by using aminocaproic acid at one half the Crouch and Frenkel[35] dosage.

Dieste et al.[40] showed that rapid clot dissolution may occasionally occur in large hyphemas (greater than 30%) 1 to 2 days after cessation of aminocaproic acid with resultant marked elevation in IOP. The rise is transient but may reach such levels that surgical intervention is required (Color Plate 9-1).

Topical antifibrinolytics. Allingham et al.[41] demonstrated that aqueous humor levels comparable to those achieved by systemic administration of aminocaproic acid can be achieved with topical agents in the rabbit model; topical aminocaproic acid in carboxypolymethylene gel reduced rebleeding in experimentally induced rabbit hyphemas.[42] Human studies are planned.

Summary of antifibrinolytic use. The clinical efficacy of antifibrinolytic agents in reducing rebleeding in traumatic hyphema has been demonstrated.[27,35-39] The rate of rebleeding in traumatic hyphema is less well established, however, with the rates varying from 3.5% to 38%.[19,35] In populations with lower rebleeding rates, some authors feel that cost issues and potential complications and side effects of aminocaproic acid do not justify its use on a routine basis, especially with outpatients.[9,19] All of these issues must be considered in determining the optimum treatment protocol for a given hyphema patient.

Fibrinolytic Agents

Tissue plasminogen activator (TPA) is receiving attention as it relates to hyphema and vitreous hemorrhage.[43] It may have theoretical applications for large clots of prolonged duration where angle closure and corneal bloodstaining are of concern.

ROUTINE ADMISSION ORDERS FOR TRAUMATIC HYPHEMA

Supportive

1. Routine vital signs.
2. Moderate activity; may sit in chair and walk in hall.
3. Elevate head of bed 30°.
4. Metal shield.
5. CBC, PT, PTT, platelet count; BUN, creatinine, electrolytes.
6. Sickle prep, hemoglobin electrophoresis (black patients).

Medications

1. Oral acetaminophen as needed.
2. No aspirin-containing compounds.
3. Laxative of choice.
4. Sleeping pill as needed.
5. Atropine 1% 1 drop twice daily.
6. Prednisolone acetate 1% 1 drop 4 times daily.
7. Oral aminocaproic acid 50 mg/kg every 4 hours up to 30 g/day, for a total of 5 days.

Medical Treatment Summary

We favor hospital admission for hyphema patients (see the box above). Patients receive metal shield protection and are permitted moderate activity. The head of the bed is elevated 30°. Aspirin-containing products are avoided. Topical medications include atropine 1% twice a day and topical steroids 4 times a day. Aminocaproic acid is used at a dosage of 50 mg/kg orally every 4 hours up to a total of 30 g/day for 5 days. If aminocaproic acid is tolerated well, there are no signs of rebleeding or other complicating problems, and there is adequate support at home, selected patients may be discharged after 2 days. Daily follow-up is recommended for the first 5 days of therapy. Patients with large clots are seen 2 days after cessation of aminocaproic acid for evaluation of exaggerated clot lysis and consequent IOP elevation.

SURGICAL INTERVENTION FOR TRAUMATIC HYPHEMA

Despite medical therapy, about 5% of hyphema patients require surgical intervention.[1,11,12]

Indications for Surgical Intervention[11,44]

Intraocular Pressure Criteria

Traditional IOP criteria for surgery are > 50 mm Hg for 5 days or > 35 mm Hg for 7 days to avoid optic nerve damage. Earlier intervention is indicated in patients with sickle cell disease or preexisting glaucomatous optic atrophy.

Corneal Bloodstaining

Surgical intervention to remove blood from the anterior chamber and reduce IOP is indicated at the earliest sign of corneal bloodstaining. Moreover, patients with total or near-total hyphemas and IOP > 25 mm Hg for 5 days should undergo surgery to prevent bloodstaining. Earlier intervention is indicated in patients with compromised endothelial function.

Prolonged Clot Duration

Patients with large clots that persist longer than 10 days, which may lead to peripheral anterior synechiae formation, are candidates for surgery. Moreover, total hyphemas that are not resolving by day 5 should be evacuated.

Techniques of Surgical Intervention

Paracentesis and Anterior Chamber Washout

This represents the simplest and safest surgical procedure for traumatic hyphema and is our initial surgical procedure of choice. It is effective in evacuating anterior chamber red blood cells and lowering IOP.[45] If rebleeding or elevated IOP recurs, the procedure can easily be repeated. The technique of anterior chamber washout is illustrated in Fig. 9-4. Simple evacuation of suspended anterior chamber cells and debris is all that is desired; removal of the entire clot is not required. Advantages of the technique include its ease of performance, repeatability, sparing of conjunctiva for future filtration sur-

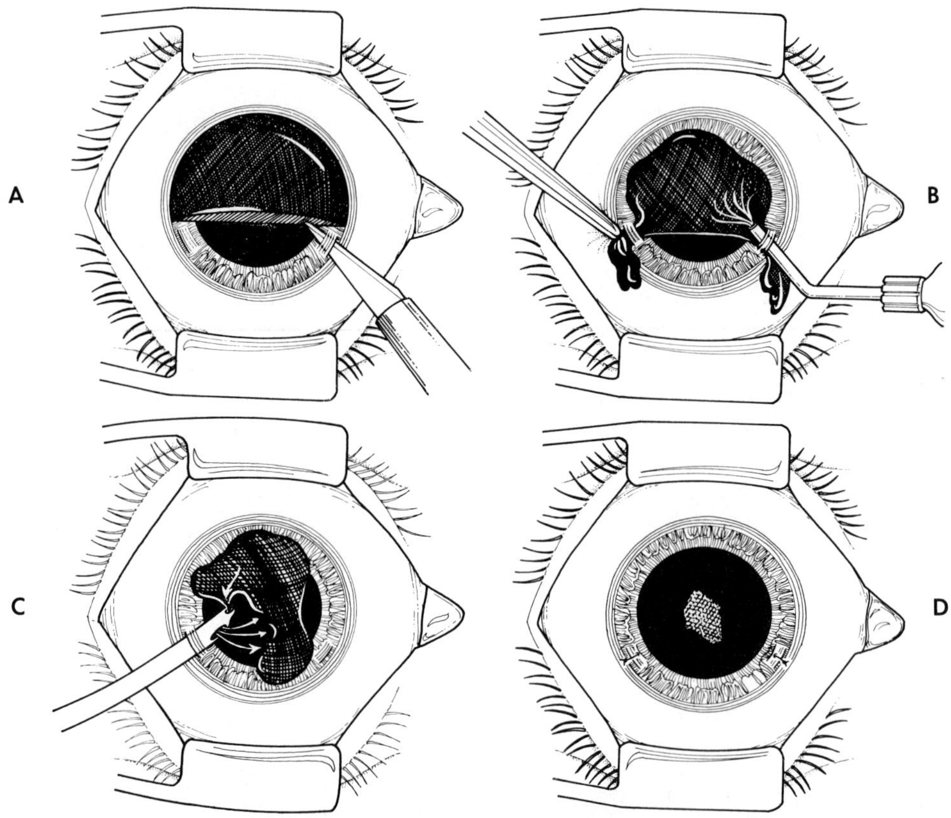

Fig. 9-4. Technique of anterior chamber washout (surgeon's view). **A,** Two clear corneal paracentesis incisions 2 mm in size with internal opening equal to external opening. Incisions enlarged as necessary to accommodate irrigation and aspiration instruments. **B,** Simultaneous balanced salt solution irrigation with 30-gauge blunt irrigator via one paracentesis and depression of posterior lip of second paracentesis incision. **C,** Conversion to irrigation and aspiration unit after enlargement of one paracentesis incision. This is performed if simple irrigation is inadequate to remove enough blood. **D,** Residual clot remains after evacuation of suspended red blood cells and debris. Paracentesis incisions closed with buried 10-0 nylon sutures.

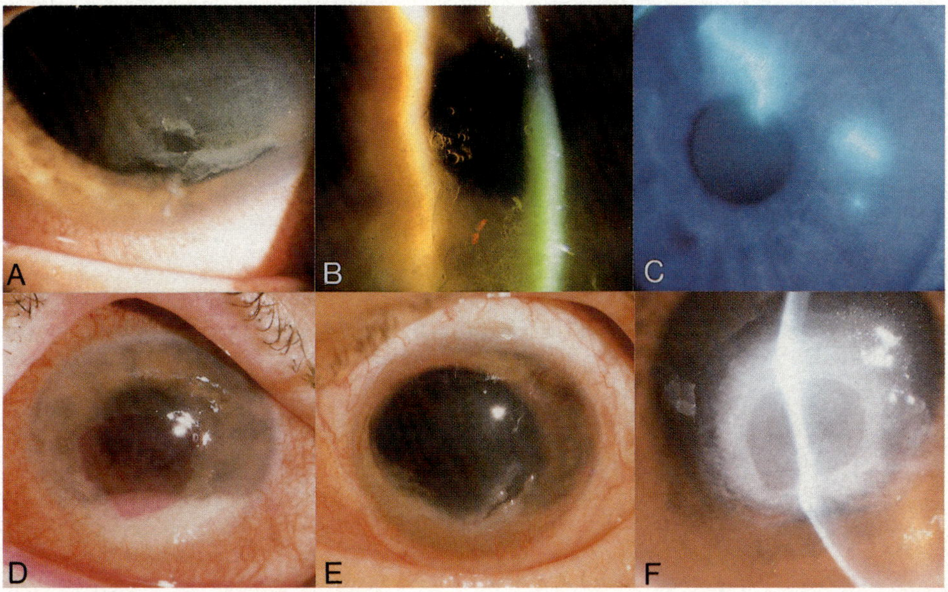

Color Plate 6-1. *Top: Recurrent epithelial erosion*. **A,** Posttraumatic erosion shows extensive area of devitalized, nonadherent epithelium. **B,** Map-dot-fingerprint with intraepithelial pseudocysts. **C,** Rupture of confluent pseudocysts results in pseudodendrite pattern of fluorescein staining. *Persistent epithelial defect*. **D,** In a patient with herpes zoster neurotrophic keratitis and sterile hypopyon, a geographic persistent epithelial defect stains with rose bengal. **E,** Incomplete healing of the corneal epithelium in a diabetic patient several weeks after vitrectomy. **F,** In combined neurotrophic and neuroparalytic keratitis, persistence of the epithelial defect is complicated by noninfected stromal ulceration.

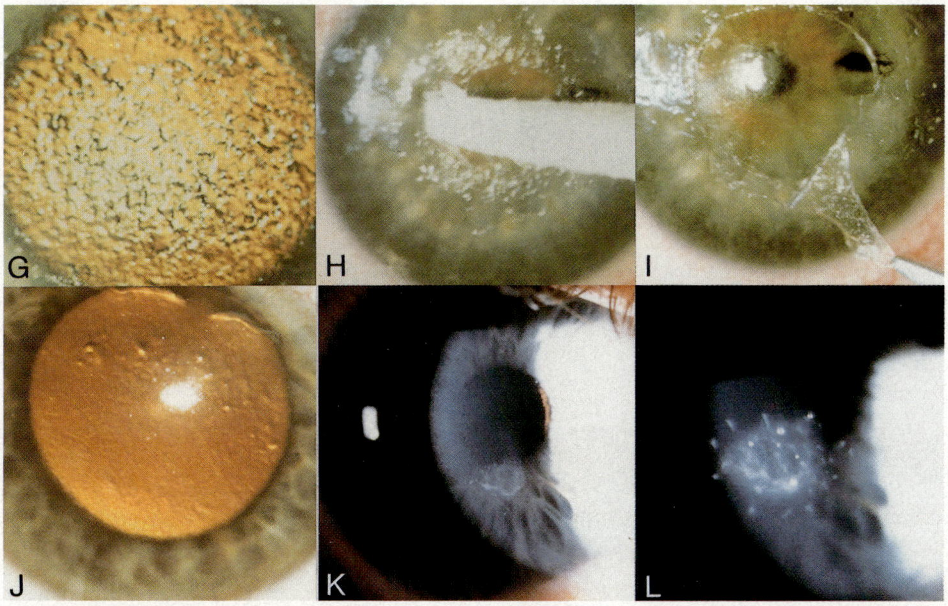

Bottom: Technique of superficial epithelial keratectomy. **G,** In a patient with Reis-Bückler dystrophy, reticular subepithelial pannus is extensive. **H,** Dry cellulose sponges to expose and develop dissection planes between fibrocellular pannus and stroma. **I,** Cellophane-like membranes are stripped with jeweler's forceps. **J,** At conclusion of procedures, optically smooth and clear surface is restored.
Anterior stromal puncture. **K,** A focal zone of devitalized epithelium outside the visual axis is appropriate for treatment. **L,** Following treatment, multiple puncture sites are visible. (Clinical photos **K** and **L** reproduced with permission of Dr. S. MacRae.)

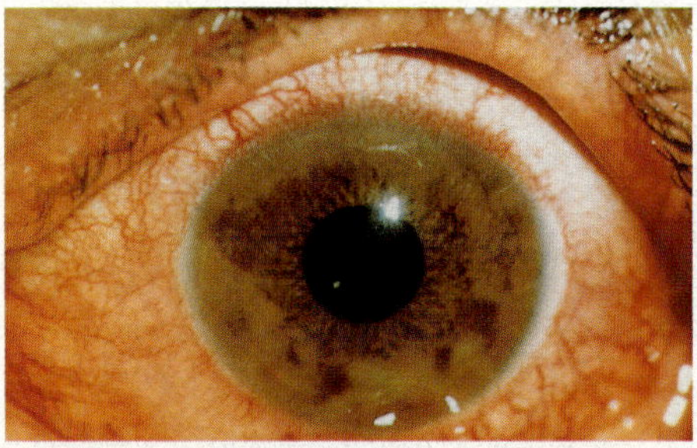

A, Grade I—Corneal epithelial defect without stromal haze or limbal ischemia.

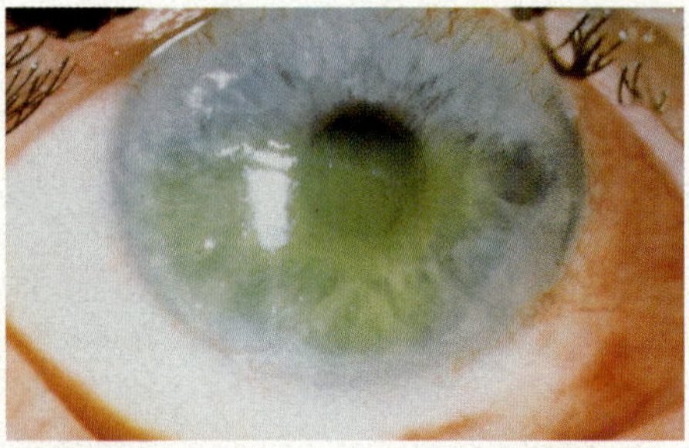

B, Grade II—Corneal epithelial defect and mild stromal haze with sectoral limbal ischemia.

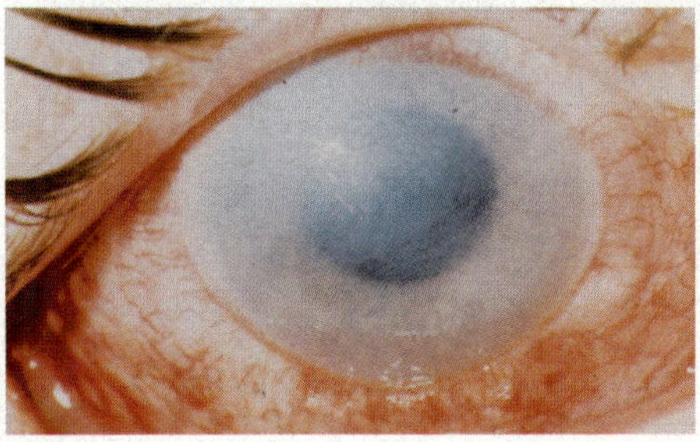

C, Grade III—Total corneal epithelial defect and stromal haze with sectoral limbal ischemia.

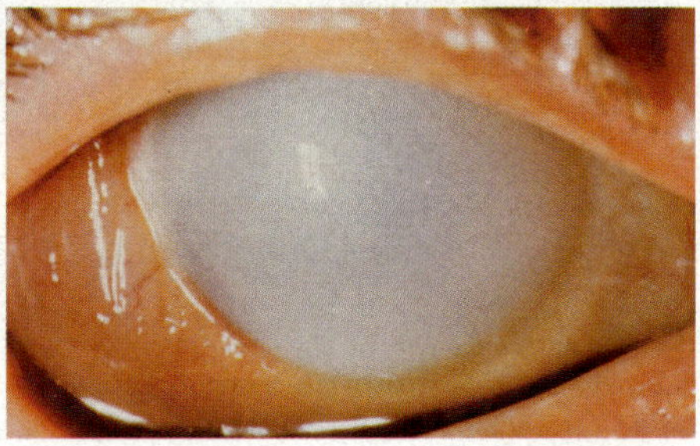

D, Grade IV—Total ocular surface epithelial loss, stromal opacity, and extensive limbal ischemia.

Color Plate 7-1. Alkali injury, Hughes classification.

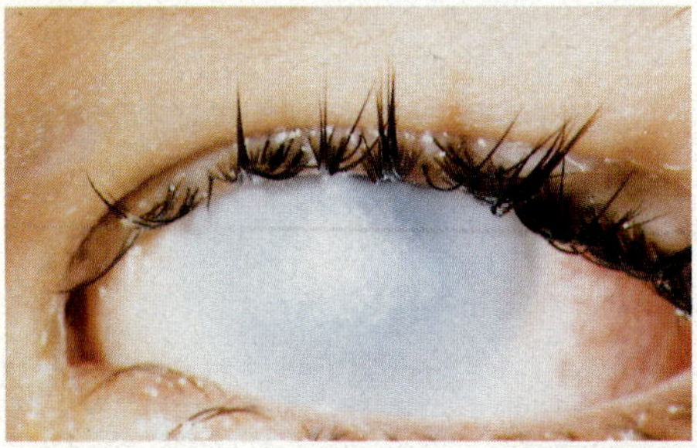

A, This 5-year-old boy sustained severe alkali injury to the left eye with total ocular surface epithelial loss and extensive limbal and scleral ischemia.

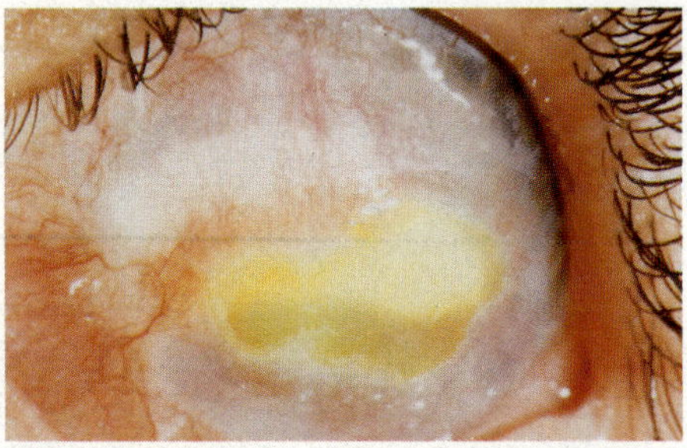

B, Despite maximal medical therapy, including corticosteroids and ascorbate, an extensive corneal epithelial defect persisted. Limbal autograft transplantation was performed at 4 weeks postinjury with slow resolution of the epithelial defect.

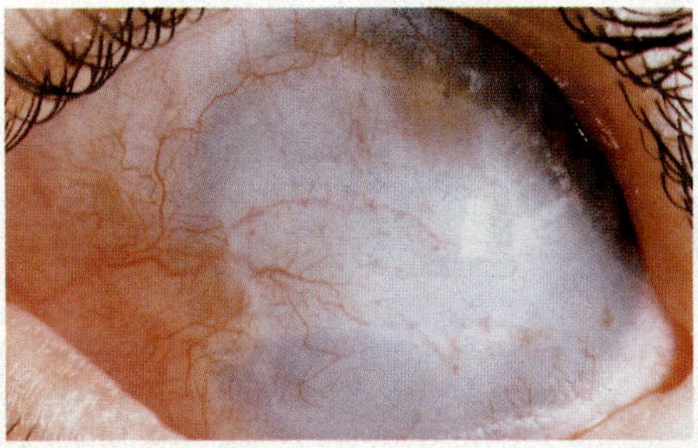

C, The ocular surface epithelium is intact and stable 6 months after injury, and stromal neovascularization and edema have subsided albeit with dense scarring.

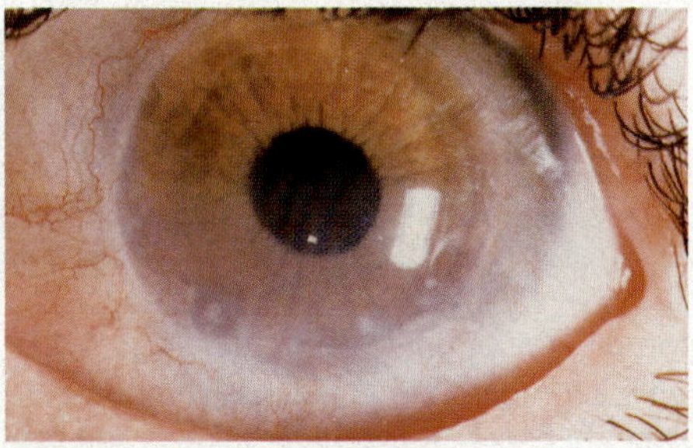

D, A deep lamellar keratoplasty was performed 1 year after injury. Visual acuity is 20/60 2 years later, and the cornea remains stable, uninflamed, and avascular without topical medications or lubricants.

Color Plate 7-2. Severe alkali injury managed by limbal autograft transplantation and lamellar keratoplasty.

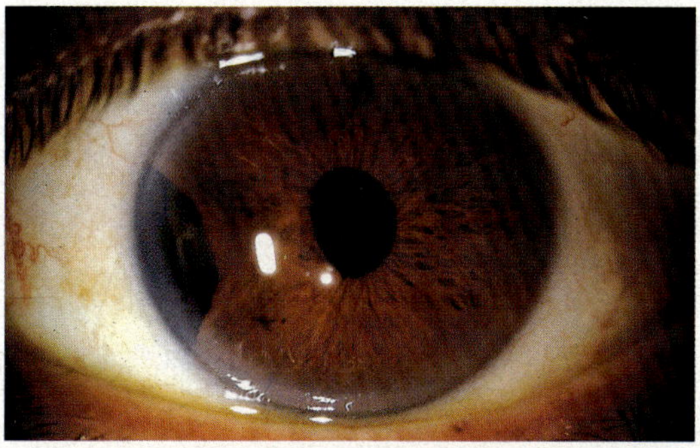

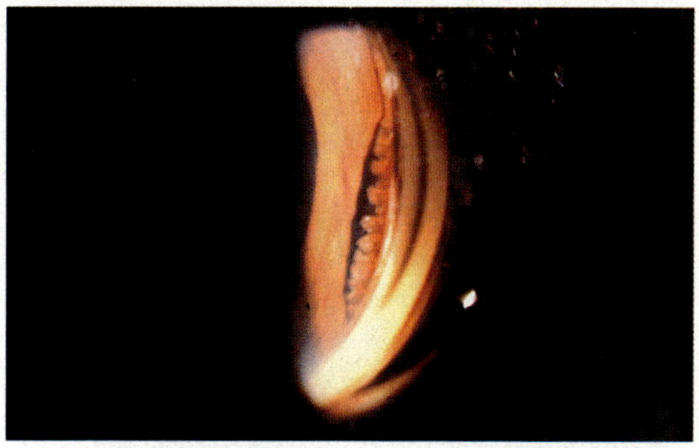

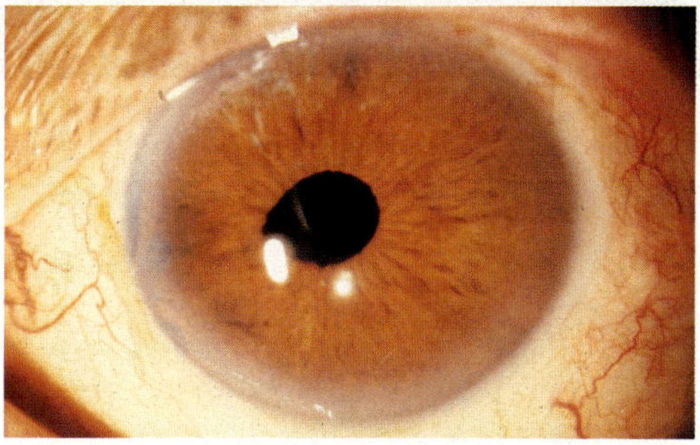

Color Plate 8-1. **A,** A patient with multiplopia due to a traumatic iridodialysis. **B,** Gonioscopy reveals the ciliary processes visible through the iridodialysis. **C,** A double-armed 10-0 polypropylene mattress suture from the peripheral iris to the sclera just anterior to the ciliary body repaired the defect.

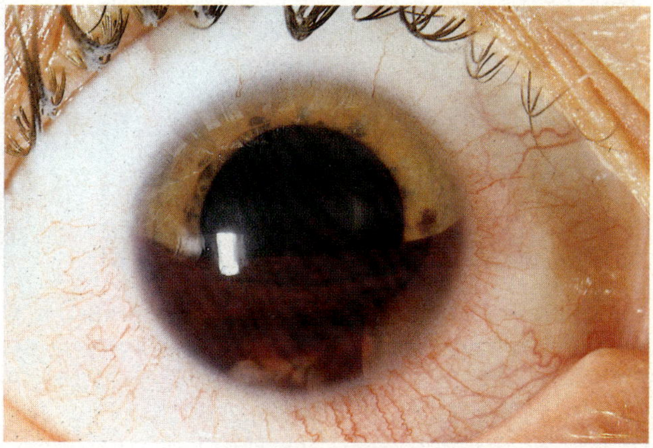

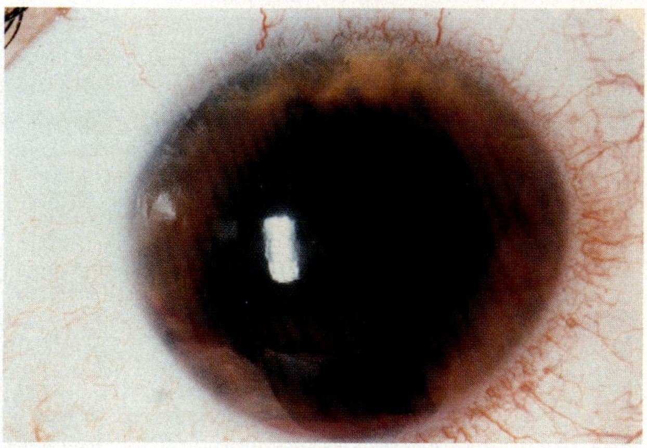

Color Plate 9-1. **A,** 5 days following traumatic hyphema on aminocaproic acid treatment. Blood is layered and anterior chamber is otherwise clear. Applanation tension = 16 mm Hg. **B,** 24 hours after discontinuation of aminocaproic acid. Note obscuration of iris details by free-floating red blood cells without evidence of rebleed. Applanation tension = 46 mm Hg. (Published with permission from the American Journal of Ophthalmology, vol 106, pp 383-390, 1988. Copyright by The Ophthalmic Publishing Company.)

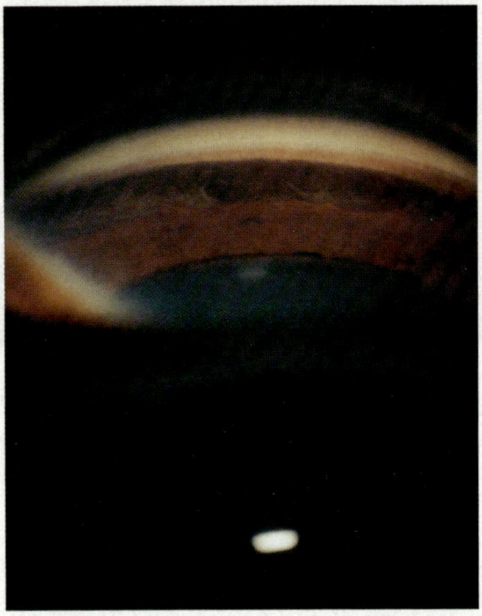

Color Plate 10-1. Massive total angle recession, gonioscopic view.

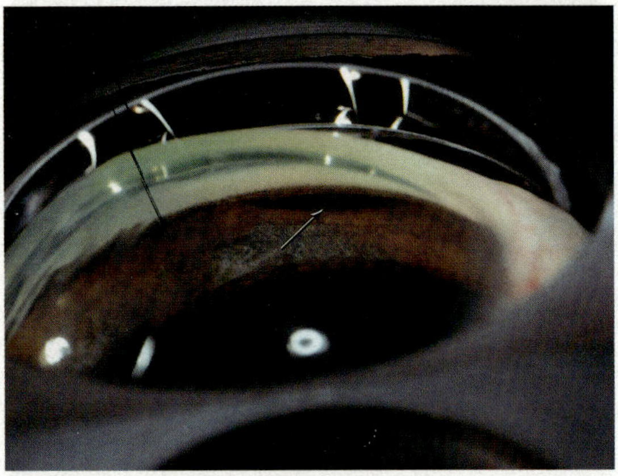

Color Plate 10-2. Traumatic cyclodialysis cleft *(arrow)*, gonioscopic view.

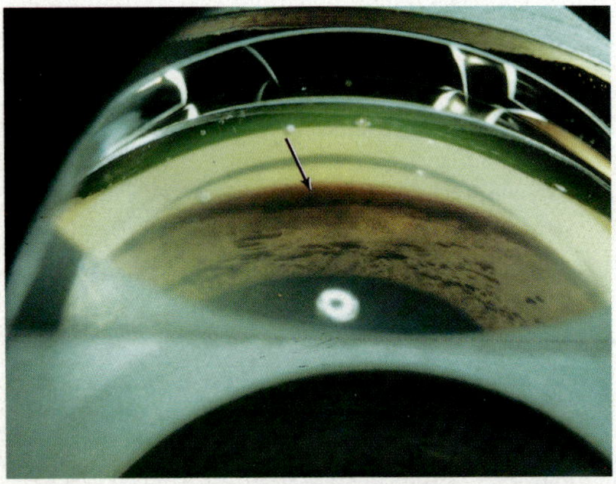

Color Plate 10-3. Hemorrhage of the trabecular meshwork *(arrow)* following blunt injury, gonioscopic view.

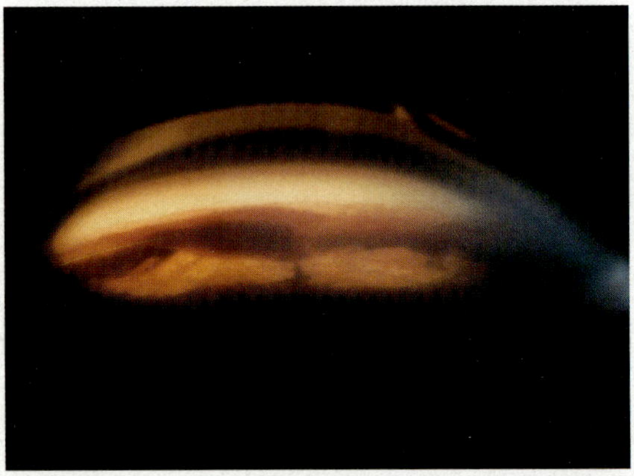

Color Plate 10-4. Hemorrhagic clot protruding from torn trabecular meshwork a few days following blunt injury, gonioscopic view.

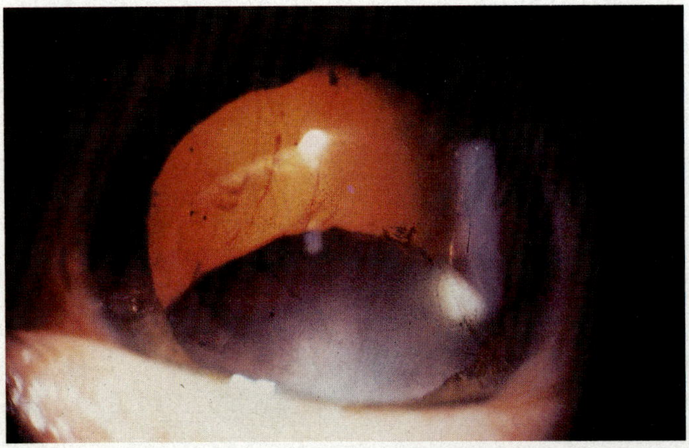

Color Plate 11-1. Subluxed cataractous lens following blunt trauma. The lens was removed using a pars plana lensectomy technique.

gery if required, ability to convert intraoperatively to automated hyphemectomy or bimanual irrigation and aspiration with use of the same ports, and ability to lower IOP postoperatively via the corneal paracentesis incisions at slit-lamp examination.

Techniques involving injection of air[46] and washout with fibrinolytic agents[47-49] do not appear to be more efficacious than simple irrigation with balanced salt solution.

Clot Expression and Limbal Delivery

Hyphema clots reach maximal consolidation and retraction by days 4 to 7[14,15] and are most amenable to expression at that time.[50] If large clot removal is required, clot expression and limbal delivery may be helpful and may be combined with peripheral iridectomy and anterior chamber washout (Fig. 9-5). Disadvantages include the large limbal incision required, the violation of limbal conjunctiva if future filtration surgery is required, and the possibility of delivering attached uveal tissue, lens material, and vitreous coincident with expression of the clot. Hill[51] described the use of cryoapplication to facilitate clot delivery through a large limbal wound.

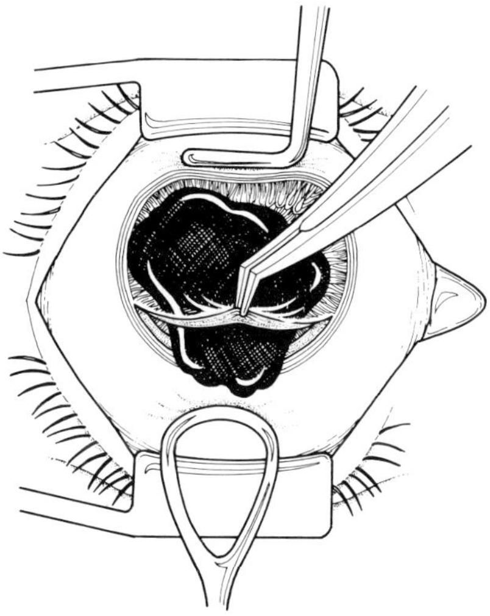

Fig. 9-5. Expression of clot via limbal incision.

Automated Hyphemectomy

Automated cutting/aspiration instruments may be used in evacuating an anterior chamber hemorrhage (Fig. 9-6, *A*).[52] They may be used primarily or after intraoperative conversion from a simple anterior chamber washout procedure. Conversion to bimanual cutting, aspiration, and irrigation instrumentation may be indicated after anterior chamber washout in special situations. Intraoperative bleeding occasionally develops during anterior chamber washout, and conversion to a bimanual irrigation and aspiration system provides expanded opportunities for controlling bleeding. Bleeding may be simultaneously irrigated and aspirated until it spontaneously ceases. The bottle height of the infusion fluid can be elevated to raise IOP and thus tamponade bleeding. Intraocular bimanual diathermy, as described by Michels and Rice,[53] may be applied directly to bleeding vessels in aphakic or pseudophakic eyes (Fig. 9-6, *B*). If

A

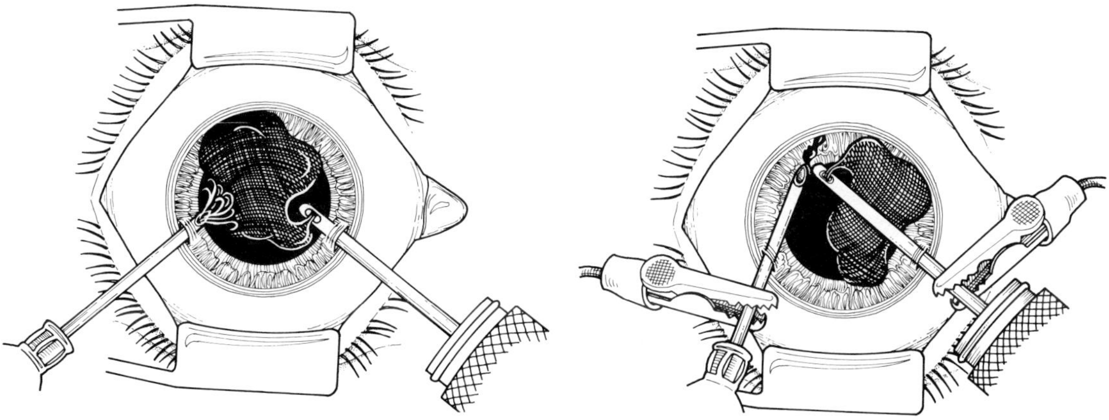

B

Fig. 9-6. **A,** Conversion to bimanual cutting, aspiration, and irrigation instrumentation to facilitate hyphema removal. Balanced salt solution irrigation is provided by butterfly intravenous needle infusion. Standard vitrectomy instruments are used for cutting and aspiration. **B,** Intraocular cautery may be performed by attaching bipolar alligator clips to the metal infusion and cutting/aspiration instruments and touching the bleeding vessel between the instrument tips.

anterior segment reconstruction is required, automated cutting and aspiration instruments permit removal of blood and excision of iris, lens, and vitreous material in a single procedure. As with simple anterior chamber washout, clear corneal incisions preserve virgin conjunctiva in case later filtration surgery is required.

Peripheral Iridectomy and Trabeculectomy

Pupillary block glaucoma may develop with hyphemas, particularly large ones, that extend into the posterior chamber. Simple anterior chamber irrigation is usually adequate to restore normal anterior segment dynamics, but occasionally a peripheral iridectomy is required. This is indicated at the time of washout by inability to restore a normal anterior segment configuration and IOP. If this is the case, a peripheral iridectomy can be performed directly through an enlarged washout entry site. Parrish and Bernardino[54] recommend peripheral iridectomy in cases of hyphema, and Weiss, Parrish, and Anderson[55] advocate trabeculectomy with peripheral iridectomy, with the expectation that long-term filtration success will be low but short-term pressure control will be improved.

Other Techniques

Gilbert and Smith[56] described the use of cyclodiathermy to stop recurrent rebleeding in traumatic hyphemas. Kelman and Brooks[57] reported a case of ultrasonic emulsification and aspiration of a traumatic hyphema.

COMPLICATIONS OF HYPHEMA

Rebleeding

Rebleeding occurs in 3.5% to 38% of patients with traumatic hyphema.* This occurs most frequently during days 2 to 5 following injury and may be caused by clot lysis and retraction. Such retraction may open a vessel that was incompletely healed. Rebleeding is associated with a poorer pronosis because of the significant percentage of eyes that develop a total hyphema (30% to 40%) or increased IOP (up to 50%) or both. Edwards and Layden[1] noted a complication rate of 58% in rebleeding eyes and 22% in eyes that did not rebleed. In one study, 7 of 25 rebleed patients required surgery compared with only 1 of 131 nonrebleed patients.[58]

Most studies cite a higher rebleed rate with larger hyphemas,[1,2,9,10] but this is not supported by all studies.[27,31] Aspirin ingestion is most consistently cited as a factor leading to more frequent rebleeding,[24,25] but even this risk factor has been questioned.[26] Younger age[2] may be associated with increased rebleeding. Race may also be a factor as higher rebleeding rates have been cited in studies with a large percentage of black or Hispanic patients[2,27,35,36] than in those with a predominantly white population.[9,10,19]

Treatment of rebleeding depends on the presence of associated IOP elevation, bloodstaining, and peripheral anterior synechiae formation.

Glaucoma

IOP may rise in the early and late stages following hyphema. An acute rise in IOP to > 25 mm Hg occurs in 25% with 10% to 15% of these patients reaching levels > 35 mm Hg.[2] This acute IOP rise is due to trabecular meshwork obstruction by red blood cells, platelets, and fibrin and to direct concussive damage to the outflow channels. Steroid-induced IOP elevation must also be kept in mind. Most hyphema patients are young and healthy and can withstand moderate IOP elevations without nerve damage and do not require antiglaucoma treatment. As a general guideline, we favor initiating medical treatment for IOP > 40 mm Hg in the acute setting and for persistent elevation of IOP > 30 mm Hg for 2 weeks or more. Aqueous suppressants, both topical beta blockers and oral carbonic anhydrase inhibitors, are the mainstays of therapy (e.g., topical timolol meleate 0.5% twice a day or oral acetazolamide 250 mg 4 times a day). Oral and intravenous hyperosmotic agents are used as necessary for spikes in IOP (e.g., oral isosorbide 2 ml/kg, or intravenous mannitol 20% solution 2 ml/kg over 30 minutes). Miotics and epinephrine derivatives are to be avoided. Criteria for surgical intervention after failed medical management are cited earlier in this chapter. It is important to emphasize that IOP treatment must be tailored to the patient. Much more aggressive and selective medical management, along with earlier surgical intervention, may be indicated for certain patients, such as those with sickle cell disease, previous glaucomatous optic nerve damage, or large clots with corneal endothelial dysfunction.

Larger hyphemas may be associated with

*References 1-3, 9-12, 19, 24, 27, 35, 36, 38, 39, 58.

higher IOP.[6] Pupillary block most commonly occurs in eyes with larger hyphemas. Rebleeds are frequently complicated by significant IOP elevation and represent the most common setting for surgical intervention.

Late glaucoma, developing weeks to years after hyphemas, may be due to posterior synechiae formation with iris bombé, peripheral anterior synechiae, ghost cell glaucoma, and angle recession. These entities are discussed in detail in Chapter 10.

Corneal Bloodstaining

Corneal bloodstaining occurs in up to 5% of hyphema patients.[2,11,12] It is associated with larger hyphemas, rebleeding, prolonged clot duration, elevated IOP, and compromised corneal endothelial cell function. Pathologic studies of bloodstaining demonstrate erythrocyte breakdown products and hemosiderin in the keratocytes. Early clinical signs are difficult to detect but include yellow granular changes in the posterior corneal stroma and reduced definition of the posterior stromal fibrillar structure on high-powered slit-lamp examination.[59,60] If bloodstaining is detected, paracentesis and anterior chamber washout are indicated.

Generally, corneal bloodstaining resolves over several months to several years without the need for penetrating keratoplasty. Clearing begins peripherally and posteriorly. Early penetrating keratoplasty may be considered in the amblyopic age group or with other select patients.

SPECIAL CONSIDERATIONS

Sickle Cell Disease

Sickle cell disease presents particular problems for the ophthalmologist in the management of traumatic hyphema. The anterior chamber environment does not tolerate sickled red blood cells well. Sickle cells are elongated and relatively rigid, characteristics that reduce their egress through normal trabecular outflow pathways. Even relatively small hyphemas, therefore, may clog the trabecular meshwork, leading to marked elevation of intraocular pressure. This, consequently, may cause hypoperfusion of the anterior segment, leading to even more anterior chamber hypoxia, acidosis, and hypercarbia, all factors that encourage further sickling. Therefore, a self-propagating cycle develops with increased sickling and resultant increase in IOP.

Sickle cell patients, moreover, are predisposed to optic nerve damage and central retinal artery occlusion with only a marginal increase in the IOP, presumably a consequence of vascular sludging by sickled cells leading to ischemia and vaso-occlusion.[17] Intraocular pressure as low as the mid-20s may lead to these grave consequences. Therefore, the IOP must be monitored closely and treated aggressively in sickle cell patients.

The prevalence of sickle cell trait is approximately 10% in the black population. In the stagnant environment of the anterior chamber after hyphema, not only homozygotic (SS) red blood cells, but also heterozygote (SA, SC) carriers are predisposed to sickling. Therefore, even carriers of the trait, without clinical manifestations of the systemic disease, are at risk for IOP elevation and its consequences. Hence, all black patients should have an immediate screen for sickle cell disease (sickle prep) and a specimen sent for hemoglobin electrophoresis when a hyphema is diagnosed.

The goal of treatment is to keep the IOP low without exacerbating the hypoxia or acidosis which will cause further sickling. Topical beta-adrenergic antagonists are the mainstay of therapy. Topical epinephrine derivatives may be used, but vasoconstriction may increase hypoxia and vascular sludging. Miotics may increase inflammation. Carbonic anhydrase inhibitors lead to hemoconcentration, systemic acidosis, and elevated ascorbic acid (a reducing agent), all of which may increase sickling. Methazolamide is theoretically preferable to acetazolamide in such patients because of a lesser tendency toward acidosis. Hyperosmotic agents also lead to hemoconcentration, and their use should be minimized. Treatment is a balance between acceptable IOP control and factors that exacerbate sickling. We strive for a consistent IOP < 25 mm Hg and consider anterior chamber washout if chronic use of carbonic anhydrase inhibitors or hyperosmotic agents is required for control.

Surgery may be indicated if, despite medical therapy, the IOP exceeds 25 mm Hg for more than 24 hours. Control during the first 24 hours after injury may be an important prognostic sign.[61] If the IOP remains at an acceptable level during these initial 24 hours, the prognosis is improved.

Aminocaproic acid has not been extensively studied directly in sickle cell patients. There is no absolute contraindication to its use. However, since it may cause the clot to remain in the anterior chamber for a longer time, it may theoretically be a disadvantage in the sickle cell patient. Hyperbaric oxygen delivered transcorneally has received experimental attention and may reduce sickling.[62]

Children with Traumatic Hyphema

The incidence of traumatic hyphema in children is probably not very different from that in the general population.[9,10] The prognosis in children younger than 6 years may be poorer, however.[2] Rebleeding occurred in 7.6% of children in a Canadian white population, and 1% of the total hyphemas developed bloodstaining.[10] Amblyopia was uncommon. The use of oral antifibrinolytic agents in children has undergone the same debate as in adults. Uusitalo, Ranta-Kemppainen, and Tarkkanen[63] found that tranexamic acid reduced rebleeding in children. In a small series, Kraft et al.[64] showed no reduction in rebleeding with or without aminocaproic acid. Intuition suggests that antifibrinolytic agents would act similarly in adults and children. It appears reasonable that these drugs may be used in children who do not have specific contraindications.

CLINICAL OUTCOMES AND PROGNOSIS

Three quarters of all hyphema eyes end up with vision better than 20/50.* Larger hyphemas are most often associated with a poorer prognosis,[2,11] and rebleeds are consistently associated with elevated IOP, bloodstaining, more frequent surgery, and poorer long-term vision. Poorer overall results are documented in surgically treated patients than in medically treated patients, but this may be related in large part to more severe associated injuries. Persistent visual reduction is most commonly due to cataract, posterior pole injury, or optic atrophy.[2,11,58]

References

1. Edwards WC and Layden WF: Traumatic hyphema, Am J Ophthalmol 75:110-116, 1973.
2. Read J and Goldberg MF: Comparison of medical treatment for traumatic hyphema, Trans Acad Ophthalmol Otolaryngol 78:799-815, 1974.

*References 1, 2, 6, 11, 12, 58.

3. Cassel GH, Jeffers JB, and Jaeger EA: Wills Eye Hospital traumatic hyphema study, Ophthalmic Surg 16:441-443, 1984.
4. Thygeson P and Beard C: Observations on traumatic hyphema, Am J Ophthalmol 35:977-985, 1952.
5. Pilger IS: Medical treatment of traumatic hyphema, Surv Ophthalmol 20:28-34, 1975.
6. Rakusin W: Traumatic hyphema, Am J Ophthalmol 74:284-292, 1972.
7. Collet BI: Traumatic hyphema: a review, Ann Ophthalmol 14:52-56, 1982.
8. Schein OD et al: The spectrum and burden of ocular injury, Ophthalmology 95:300-305, 1988.
9. Kennedy RH and Brubaker RF: Traumatic hyphema in a defined population, Am J Ophthalmol 106:123-130, 1988.
10. Agapitos PJ, Noel LP, and Clarke WN: Traumatic hyphema in children, Ophthalmology 94:1238-1241, 1987.
11. Read J: Traumatic hyphema: surgical vs medical management, Ann Ophthalmol 7:659-670, 1975.
12. Wilson FM: Traumatic hyphema: pathogenesis and management, Ophthalmology 87:910-919, 1980.
13. Wolfe SM and Zimmerman LE: Chronic secondary glaucoma associated with retrodisplacement of iris root and deepening of the anterior chamber angle secondary to contusion, Am J Ophthalmol 54:547-563, 1962.
14. Caprioli J and Sears ML: The histopathology of black ball hyphema: a report of two cases, Ophthalmic Surg 15:491-495, 1985.
15. Wolter JR, Henderson JW, and Talley TW: Histopathology of a black ball clot around four days after total hyphema, J Pediatr Ophthalmol Strabismus 8:15-17, 1971.
16. Pandolfi M, Nilsson IM, and Martinsson G: Coagulation and fibrinolytic components in primary and plasmoid aqueous humor of rabbit, Acta Ophthalmol 42:820-825, 1964.
17. Goldberg MF: Sickled erythrocytes, hyphema and secondary glaucoma, Ophthalmic Surg 10:17-31, 1979.
18. Clever VG: Home care of hyphemas, Ann Ophthalmol 14:25-27, 1982.
19. Wittenman GJ et al: The incidence of rebleeding in traumatic hyphema, Ann Ophthalmol 17:525-529, 1985.
20. Darr JL and Passmore JW: Management of traumatic hyphema, Am J Ophthalmol 63:134-136, 1967.
21. Wright KW, Sunal PM, and Urrea P: Bed rest versus activity ad lib in the treatment of small hyphemas, Ann Ophthalmol 20:143-145, 1988.
22. Edwards WC and Layden WF: Monocular versus bilateral patching in traumatic hyphema, Am J Ophthalmol 76:359-362, 1973.

23. Crawford JS: The effect of aspirin on rebleeding in traumatic hyphema, Trans Am Ophthalmol Soc 73:357-362, 1975.
24. Gorn RA: The detrimental effect of aspirin on hyphema rebleed, Ann Ophthalmol 11:351-355, 1979.
25. Ganley JP et al: Aspirin and recurrent hyphema after blunt ocular trauma, Am J Ophthalmol 96:797-801, 1983.
26. Marcus M et al: Aspirin and secondary bleeding after traumatic hyphema, Ann Ophthalmol 20:157-158, 1988.
27. Palmer DJ et al: A comparision of two dose regimens of epsilon aminocaproic acid in the prevention and management of secondary traumatic hyphemas, Ophthalmology 93:102-108, 1986.
28. Gilbert HD and Jensen AD: Atropine in the treatment of traumatic hyphema, Ann Ophthalmol 5:1297-1300, 1973.
29. Yasuna E: Management of traumatic hyphema, Arch Ophthalmol 91:190-191, 1974.
30. Rynne MV and Romano PE: Systemic corticosteroids in the treatment of traumatic hyphema, J Pediatr Ophthalmol Strabismus 17:141-143, 1980.
31. Spoor TC, Hammer M, and Belloso H: Traumatic hyphema: failure of steroids to alter its course: a double-blind prospective study, Arch Ophthalmol 98:116-119, 1980.
32. Fujikawa LS, Meisler DM, and Nozik RA: Hyperosmolar hyperglycemic nonketotic coma: a complication of short-term systemic corticosteroid use, Ophthalmology 90:1239-1242, 1983.
33. Goldberg MF: Antifibrinolytic agents in the management of traumatic hyphema, Arch Ophthalmol 101:1029-1030, 1983.
34. Lowey D et al: Systemic aminocaproic acid reduces fibrinolysis in aqueous humor, Arch Ophthalmol 105:272-276, 1987.
35. Crouch ER and Frenkel M: Aminocaproic acid in the treatment of traumatic hyphema, Am J Ophthalmol 81:355-360, 1976.
36. McGetrick JJ et al: Aminocaproic acid decreases secondary hemorrhage after traumatic hyphema, Arch Ophthalmol 101:1031-1033, 1983.
37. Kutner B et al: Aminocaproic acid reduces the risk of secondary hemorrhage in patients with traumatic hyphema, Arch Ophthalmol 105:206-208, 1987.
38. Varnek L et al: The effect of tranexamic acid on secondary hemorrhage after traumatic hyphema, Acta Ophthalmol 58:787-792, 1980.
39. Vangsted P and Nielsen PJ: Tranexamic acid and traumatic hyphema, Acta Ophthalmol 61:447-453, 1983.
40. Dieste MC et al: Intraocular pressure increase associated with epsilon-aminocaproic acid therapy for traumatic hyphema, Am J Ophthalmol 106:383-390, 1988.
41. Allingham RR et al: Topically applied aminocaproic acid concentrates in the aqueous humor of the rabbit in therapeutic levels, Arch Ophthalmol 105:1421-1423, 1987.
42. Allingham RR et al: Topical aminocaproic acid significantly reduces the incidence of secondary hemorrhage in traumatic hyphema in the rabbit model, Arch Ophthalmol 106:1436-1438, 1988.
43. Lambrou FH, Snyder RW, and Williams GA: Use of tissue plasminogen activator in experimental hyphema, Arch Ophthalmol 105:995-997, 1987.
44. Deutsch TA and Feller DB: Paton and Goldberg's management of ocular injuries, ed 2, Philadelphia, 1985, WB Saunders.
45. Belcher CD, Brown SVL, and Simmons RJ: Anterior chamber washout for traumatic hyphema, Ophthalmic Surg 16:475-479, 1985.
46. Wilson JM et al: Air injection in the treatment of traumatic hyphema, Am J Ophthalmol 37:409-411, 1954.
47. Jukofsky SL: A new technique in the treatment of hyphema, Am J Ophthalmol 34:1692-1696, 1951.
48. Scheie HG, Ashley BJ, and Burns DT: Treatment of total hyphema with fibrinolysin, Arch Ophthalmol 69:147-153, 1963.
49. Liebman SD, Pollen A, and Podos SM: Treatment of experimental total hyphema with intraocular fibrinolytic agents, Arch Ophthalmol 68:72-78, 1962.
50. Sears ML: Surgical management of black ball hyphema, Trans Am Acad Ophthalmol Otolaryngol 74:820-827, 1970.
51. Hill K: Cryoextraction of total hyphema, Arch Ophthalmol 80:368-370, 1968.
52. McCuen BW and Fung WE: The role of vitrectomy instrumentation in the treatment of severe traumatic hyphema, Am J Ophthalmol 88:930-934, 1979.
53. Michels RG and Rice TA: Bimanual bipolar diathermy for treatment of bleeding from the anterior chamber angle, Am J Ophthalmol 84:873-874, 1977.
54. Parrish RK and Bernardino V: Iridectomy in the surgical management of eight ball hyphema, Arch Ophthalmol 100:435-437, 1982.
55. Weiss JS, Parrish RK, and Anderson DR: Surgical therapy of traumatic hyphema, Ophthalmic Surg 14:343-345, 1983.
56. Gilbert HD and Smith RE: Traumatic hyphema: treatment of secondary hemorrhage with cyclodiathermy, Ophthalmic Surg 7(3):31-35, 1975.
57. Kelman CD and Brooks DL: Ultrasonic emulsification and aspiration of traumatic hyphema: preliminary report, Am J Ophthalmol 71:1289-1291, 1971.
58. Thomas MA, Parrish RK, and Feuer WJ: Rebleeding after traumatic hyphema, Arch Ophthalmol 104:206-210, 1986.

59. McDonell PJ et al: Blood staining of the cornea: light microscopic and ultrastructural features, Ophthalmology 92:1668-1674, 1985.
60. Slingsby JG and Forstot SL: Effect of blunt trauma on the corneal endothelium, Arch Ophthalmol 99:1041-1043, 1981.
61. Deutsch TA, Weinreb RN, and Goldberg MF: Indications for surgical management of hyphema in patients with sickle cell trait, Arch Ophthalmol 102:566-569, 1984.
62. Jampol LM et al: Hyperbaric oxygen and transcorneal delivery of oxygen to the rabbit and monkey anterior segment, Arch Ophthalmol 106:825-829, 1988.
63. Uusitalo RJ, Ranta-Kemppainen L, and Tarkkanen A: Management of traumatic hyphema in children, Arch Ophthalmol 106:1207-1209, 1988.
64. Kraft SP et al: Traumatic hyphema in children, Ophthalmology 94:1232-1237, 1987.

CHAPTER 10

Traumatic glaucoma

DAVID G. CAMPBELL

The seven anterior rings of tissue
Anterior injury associated with tissue disruption
Response to tearing of tissues: inflammation and hemorrhage
Glaucomas associated with blunt injury to the angle
  Acute glaucoma without hemorrhage
  Chronic glaucoma with angle recession
  Examination
  Histopathologic changes
  Fibrous ingrowth following nonpenetrating injury
Treatment of blunt injury and IOP elevation
Ghost cell glaucoma
References

Injuries to the anterior segment following blunt injury arise from the momentary anatomic deformation that occurs during impact (Fig. 10-1). As the cornea and anterior sclera are suddenly displaced posteriorly, there is compensatory expansion at the equator of the eye.[1] Inside the eye, seven rings, or circles, of tissue anterior to the equator are suddenly required to expand because the internal fluids of the eye cannot compress. This forceful expansion may cause tissue separation, resulting in a characteristic splitting or tearing of the tissues. Such damage may lead to both acute and long-term glaucoma in the injured eye.

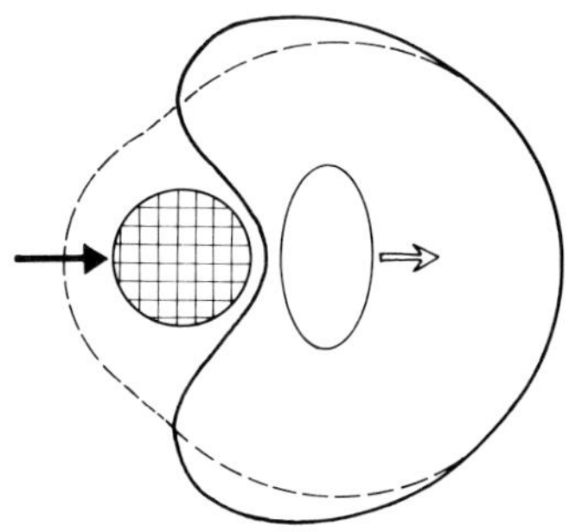

Fig. 10-1. Eye at moment of blunt impact showing equatorial expansion.

THE SEVEN ANTERIOR RINGS OF TISSUE

The seven rings of tissue that expand and characteristically tear (and the resultant changes) (Fig. 10-2) are, in order:

1. Sphincter pupillae (rupture with radial tears)
2. Peripheral edge of the iris—that is, the iris base (iridodialysis)
3. Anterior ciliary body (angle recession)
4. Attachment of the ciliary body to the scleral spur (cyclodialysis cleft)
5. Trabecular meshwork (splits and separations in this tissue)
6. Zonules (subluxation and dislocation of the lens)
7. Attachment of the retina to the ora serrata (retinal dialysis and detachment)

In all except the first tissue ring, the damage

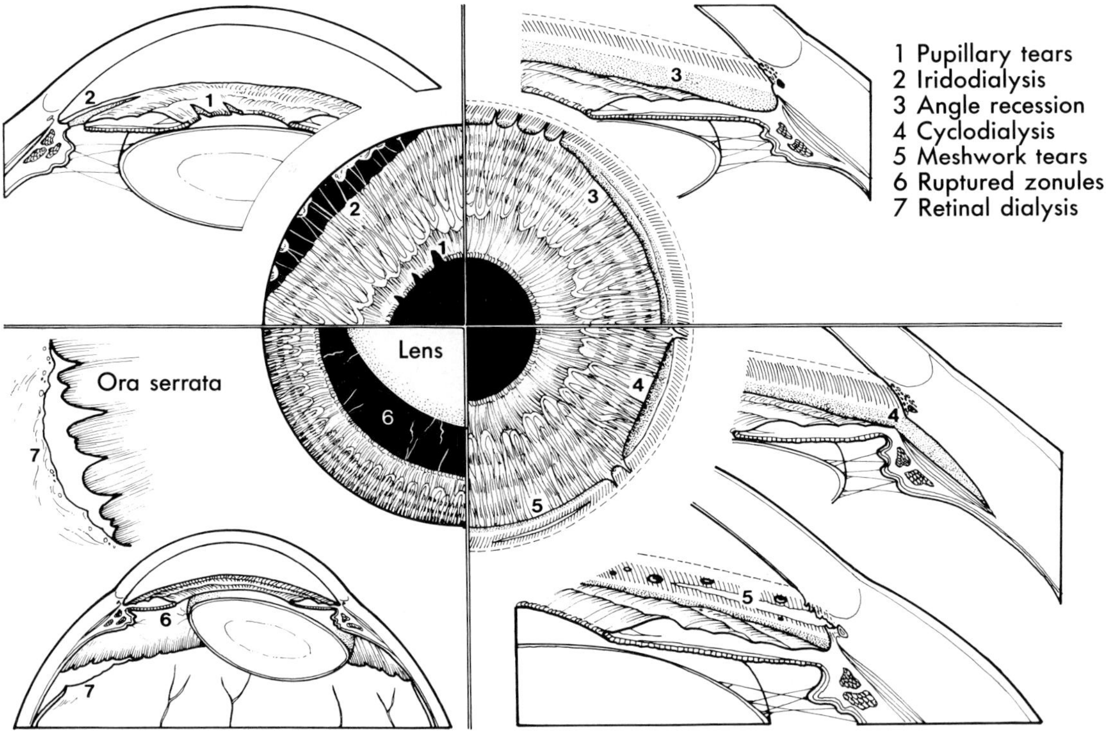

Fig. 10-2. The seven typical anterior tears that occur following blunt trauma to the eye.

and tearing are typically circumferential because the rings are bounded on each side. In the sphincter pupillae, the tears are radial, perhaps because the sphincter is unbounded internally. Following blunt injury, these seven rings of tissue should be systematically examined, the examiner should look at each individually for signs of damage.

ANTERIOR INJURY ASSOCIATED WITH TISSUE DISRUPTION

Damage to each of the seven sites produces typical and predictable injuries.

1. The tearing of the pupillary margin, typically fine radial tears (Fig. 10-3), may cause mild distortion of the pupil, failure of the pupil to respond normally to light either temporarily or permanently, and permanent traumatic mydriasis. The mydriasis has been variably attributed to direct sphincter, ciliary body ganglion, and nerve damage.
2. The typical tear of the peripheral iris attachment, or iris base, is an iridodialysis, representing traumatic separation between the iris and ciliary body (Fig. 10-4). Because the iris thins substantially at its insertion, it is a likely area for separation. These tears, often not larger than a third of the circumference, can disfigure the iris and pupil. The latter is displaced slightly away from the tear. The first two

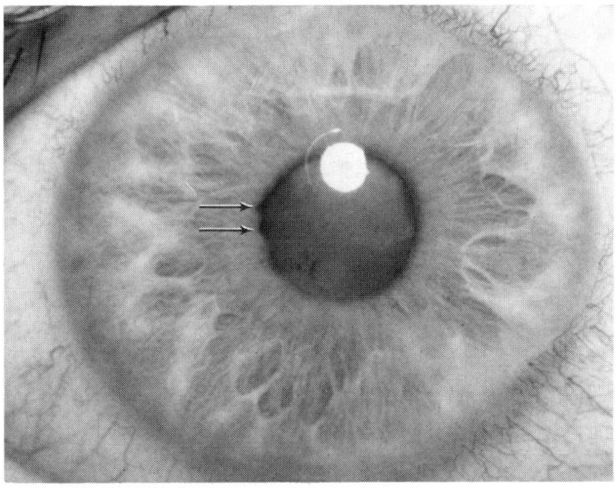

Fig. 10-3. Radial, notchlike tears *(arrows)* at 9 o'clock following blunt injury.

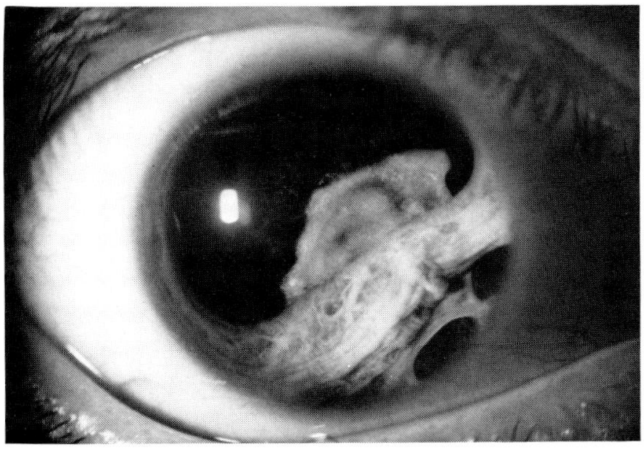

Fig. 10-4. Massive iridodialysis at 5 o'clock following blunt injury.

rings can be seen easily at slit-lamp examination.

3. A tear of the ciliary body itself results in angle recession.[2] The typical tear occurs into the face of the ciliary body between the scleral spur and the region of iris insertion (i.e., into the ciliary body band). This tear, which often occurs between the circular and longitudinal muscles of the ciliary body,[3,4] causes the band to enlarge as the iris root is displaced posteriorly (Color Plate 10-1). This tearing, the most common anterior finding in blunt trauma, is the hallmark of that trauma.

   Angle recession can be suspected at slit-lamp examination by comparing the peripheral depth at the limbus of the anterior chamber in the injured eye with that of the uninjured eye. A large difference usually indicates that recession will be found.

   The diagnosis of angle recession is made by careful gonioscopic examination. The normal ciliary body band is generally even in width throughout its circumference, and the two eyes are usually symmetric. The band usually is not wider than the trabecular meshwork itself. Unevenness in the width of the ciliary body band or a band greater than one trabecular meshwork in width usually constitutes recession. To be certain, however, one must carefully compare the normal eye with the damaged eye. A useful technique is to examine the uninvolved eye first to establish the normal appearance, and then to examine and carefully draw the damaged eye. Bilateral simultaneous Koeppe gonioscopy[5] with two lenses is an excellent way to detect these differences, particularly if they are subtle.

4. A separation of the ciliary body attachment to the scleral spur, much rarer than a ciliary body tear, results in a cyclodialysis cleft (Color Plate 10-2). The muscle is entirely torn from the spur, exposing the internal scleral wall, allowing passage of aqueous from the anterior chamber into the suprachoroidal space, and permitting direct access to the uveoscleral outflow pathway. This can result in temporary or permanent hypotony. Cyclodialysis clefts, which should be suspected and searched for if the intraocular pressure is below episcleral venous pressure (9 to 10 mm Hg), are usually small, rarely greater than one quarter of the circumference of the angle. Like angle recession, cyclodialysis clefts are discovered and diagnosed by careful gonioscopic examination.

5. The surface and substance of the trabecular meshwork itself may tear. This tearing is very important in the etiology of both early and late glaucoma and results in some of the more subtle gonioscopic findings associated with angle damage.[6] The uveoscleral meshwork, which extends from the surface of the iris to Schwalbe's line and constitutes the surface of the trabecular meshwork, can be torn and separated from the deeper tissue. This can result in three gonioscopic findings: torn iris processes, an abnormally prominent or white appearance to the scleral spur (Fig. 10-5), and circumferential tears in the surface of the trabecular meshwork. If the tear is deeper and extends through the corneoscleral meshwork and into Schlemm's canal, the white, glistening back wall of the canal may be apparent. These fine circumferential tears are somewhat easier to see immediately after injury; they are less obvious after healing. In these cases, there may be a temporary initial increase in outflow facility. However, healing by fibrosis in the meshwork may later contribute to glaucoma. These subtle findings are dis-

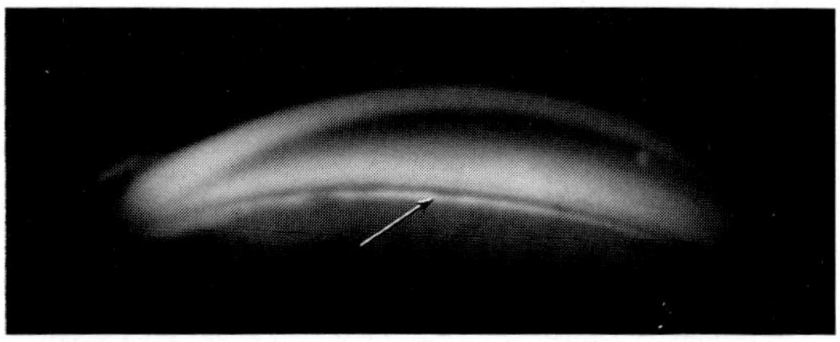

Fig. 10-5. Abnormally white scleral spur *(arrow)* following mild recession, gonioscopic view.

covered by careful gonioscopic inspection (see Chapter 12).

6. Zonular injury can result in symmetric loosening, subluxation, or lens dislocation. With maximal iris dilation, the separation of the zonules from the lens can frequently be seen. The damaged lens can cause post-traumatic glaucoma by a variety of mechanisms (see Chapter 11).
7. Tears in the attachment of the retina to the ora serrata[7,8] are discussed in Chapter 18.

RESPONSE TO TEARING OF TISSUES: INFLAMMATION AND HEMORRHAGE

The two major pathologic responses that occur immediately following these tearing injuries, especially tearing into the ciliary body, are inflammation and hemorrhage. Inflammation causes light sensitivity, ocular tenderness, and white blood cell infiltration into the aqueous. These cells can temporarily obstruct the trabecular meshwork leading to immediate pressure elevation. The accumulation of blood in the anterior chamber is called a hyphema. The blood may be minimal and visible only as circulating RBCs within the aqueous, or it may consist of a layer of cells of various heights in the anterior chamber or a clot emanating from some portion of the angle (see Chapter 9).

Immediate gonioscopy of traumatized patients reveals that the most common cause of hemorrhage is the rupture of fine vessels deep within the angle, specifically vessels within the ciliary body (Fig. 10-6). A second source of bleeding may be tears deep in the trabecular meshwork itself, which can cause bleeding into the meshwork (Fig. 10-6 and Color Plate 10-3) or through the meshwork and into the anterior chamber (Color Plate 10-4). This bleeding presumably originates from vessels surrounding the trabecular meshwork, because the mesh itself has characteristically few or no vessels within it. Any clots attached to a deeply torn angle directly indicate the source of bleeding. Later, after the hemorrhage has resolved, dark ovoid deposits may persist on the meshwork or the ciliary body band as a hallmark of the prior hemorrhage.

GLAUCOMAS ASSOCIATED WITH BLUNT INJURY TO THE ANGLE

Glaucoma can occur either early or late following blunt injury and with or without angle recession. The great majority of these glaucomas are associated with recession, with or without hyphema.

The glaucomas associated with blunt injury can be classified as follows: acute glaucoma with hemorrhage, acute glaucoma without hemorrhage, chronic glaucoma with recession (angle recession glaucoma), and chronic glaucoma without recession. Glaucoma associated with acute hemorrhage and hyphema is discussed in Chapter 9.

Acute Glaucoma without Hemorrhage

Immediately following blunt injury, the intraocular pressure may often be slightly depressed.[9,10] This may be due to decreased aqueous production by the traumatized and inflamed ciliary body or to increased outflow either through the conventional pathway (via splits in the trabecular meshwork) or the uveoscleral pathway.[11]

Occasionally, however, the pressure may be immediately elevated in association with the presence of inflammatory cells in the anterior chamber, which transiently obstruct the intertrabecular spaces. In addition, this elevation is usually associated with severe angle recession, although it is rare to have recession without hemorrhage. The increased resistance to outflow, in association with significant recession, is presumed to be due to associated trabecular meshwork disruption. In clinical and laboratory studies, Herschler and Cobo[12,13] showed that when the angle was recessed, there was frequent concomitant meshwork damage. If the damage is severe, the glaucoma may be permanent.

Acute, severe, and often permanent glaucoma will rarely ensue without persistent in-

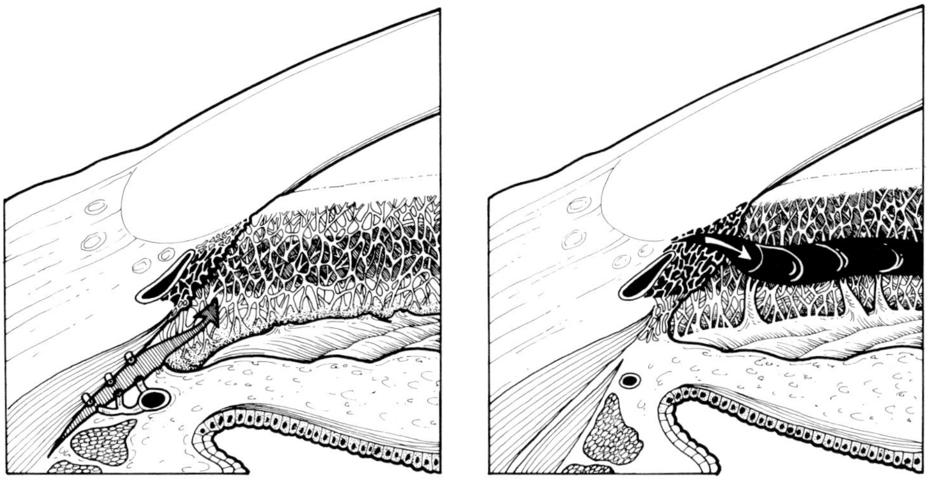

Fig. 10-6. The two sources of anterior bleeding following blunt injury. **A,** Bleeding from torn ciliary body vessels is most common. **B,** Bleeding from torn trabecular meshwork is less common. Rarely, hemorrhage into the meshwork in its entirety occurs.

flammation and without visible angle recession.[14] The etiology is unknown.

Chronic Glaucoma with Angle Recession

Almost all patients who develop a hyphema following blunt injury have some degree of either recession or direct trabecular meshwork damage.[15,16] Rarely, a recession can occur without significant bleeding.

If the hyphema clears without complication and the pressure normalizes, the patient should be examined gonioscopically approximately 6 weeks following the initial injury. If more than 180° of the angle is recessed, there is up to a 10% chance of subsequent development of chronic glaucoma.[17-20]

Examination

Gonioscopy immediately following injury can be revealing but should be done only with the utmost care to avoid hemorrhage. The procedure should be performed only (1) with a lens or technique that assiduously avoids central corneal indentation and peripheral angle widening, which might precipitate hemorrhage; (2) on a comfortable and cooperative patient; (3) by an expert gonioscopist; and (4) for therapeutic or research purposes. Unless the source of the bleeding is covered, gonioscopy usually reveals it.

Approximately 6 weeks following the injury, the bluntly traumatized but now recovered eye should undergo a thorough evaluation, recognizing that initial examination at the time of injury has usually excluded gonioscopy and peripheral retinal examination. All seven rings of tissue should be thoroughly and systematically examined and the angle carefully evaluated gonioscopically. The pupils should be dilated to look for subtle signs of lens trauma and zonular disruption, and the periphery of the retina should undergo indirect ophthalmoscopic examination with scleral depression to examine the ora serrata.

In regard to gonioscopy, the normal eye should be examined first to establish a baseline. For examining the injured eye, the clear view of a mirrored, vaulting gonioscopic lens is helpful. The entire circumference should be examined twice, first for signs of recession, including widening of the ciliary body band and circumferential torn edges of tissue on the ciliary body band that can appear gray in color. During the second sweep, the spur and the trabecular meshwork should be carefully inspected, and all findings should be recorded on a gonioscopic chart.

Glaucoma that develops years later is believed to be due to direct trabecular meshwork damage at the time of injury with subsequent scarring.[21] It is possible that the normal age-related decrease in outflow facility may tip a compensated but damaged eye into decompensation and abnormal elevation of pressure. Some patients who develop angle recession glaucoma

A B

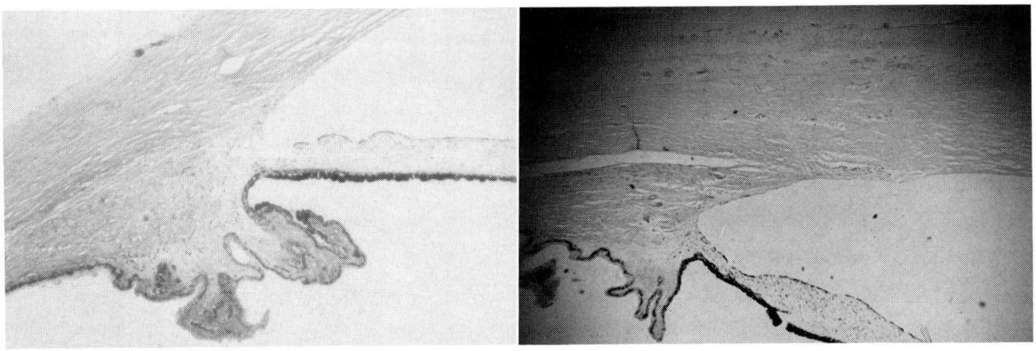

Fig. 10-7. Histology of **A,** normal and **B,** massively recessed angles. Note widened ciliary body band and retrodisplacement of the iris root.

may be borderline open-angle glaucoma patients[3,22,23] who have a preexisting reduced outflow facility unrelated to trauma.

Because of the risk of the development of late angle recession glaucoma, all patients who have had a hyphema or an angle recession should have intraocular pressures checked annually for life.

Histopathologic Changes

In both clinical observations and animal experiments, Herschler and Cobo[12,13] found an association between direct damage to the trabecular meshwork and traumatic angle recession and glaucoma. Wolff and Zimmerman[24] observed sclerosis and fibrosis of the trabecular meshwork and a greatly widened ciliary body band in these chronically damaged eyes (Fig. 10-7).

Occasionally a cuticular membrane (i.e., an extension of Descemet's membrane) has been found covering the trabecular meshwork.[25,26] This membrane, unlike the membrane seen in essential iris atrophy, rarely if ever grows beyond the angle. It apparently grows over a damaged and perhaps nonfunctioning trabecular meshwork and may not be a primary factor in the development of glaucoma, although its exact role is unknown.

Peripheral anterior synechiae can occur following recession injury but do not appear to play an important role in the etiology of glaucoma. Occasionally a recessed angle filled with blood and fibrin will partially close, but this occurs rarely and does not constitute a progressive process involving significant portions of the undamaged angle.

Fibrous Ingrowth Following Nonpenetrating Injury

Rarely, both clinically and pathologically, a limited fibrous ingrowth can develop from a severely damaged angle. Fibroblasts, apparently using the hyphema as a scaffold, can grow into the angle, sometimes in shelflike fashion (Figs. 10-8 and 10-9). This growth is limited and seems to do no further harm to a region of the angle already badly damaged by the initial trauma.

TREATMENT OF BLUNT INJURY AND IOP ELEVATION

Following blunt trauma, unless contraindicated, vigorous use of topical steroids is advised. If glaucoma has developed acutely and appears to be due to inflammation or acute angle recession and damage, topical steroids should reduce inflammation and cellular infiltration of the meshwork. Also, because direct trabecular damage with scarring and fibrosis probably play a major role in the development of late or angle recession glaucoma, topical steroids should be used 4 to 6 times per day for approximately 6 weeks to avoid or minimize this scarring.

If the pressure is elevated, drugs that reduce aqueous production should be used—topical beta-adrenergic antagonists and oral carbonic anhydrase inhibitors. These medications can be supplemented with topical sympathomimetic agents. Following the resolution of severe inflammation, topical parasympathomimetic agents can also be given.

For chronic glaucoma, standard glaucoma medications should be used. If they fail, laser trabeculoplasty can be considered but should be

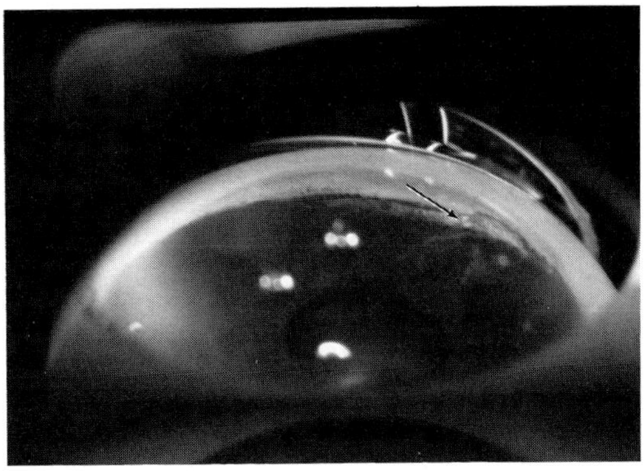

Fig. 10-8. Fibrous ingrowth *(arrow)* from the angle following blunt injury, gonioscopic view.

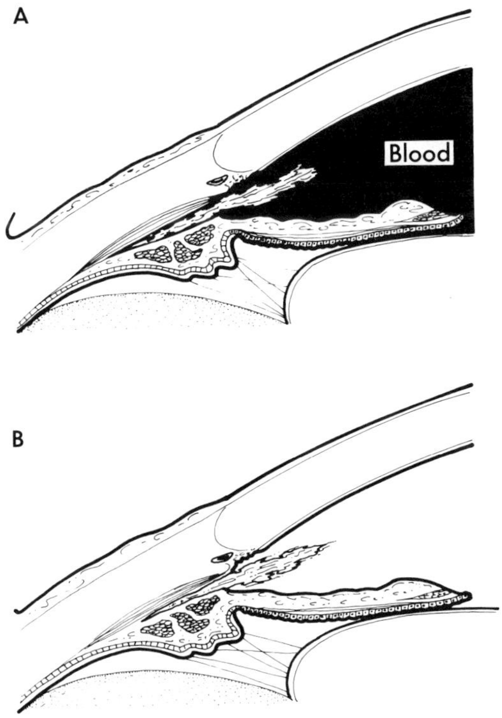

Fig. 10-9. **A** and **B**, Fibrous ingrowth following nonpenetrating injury to the eye with hyphema.

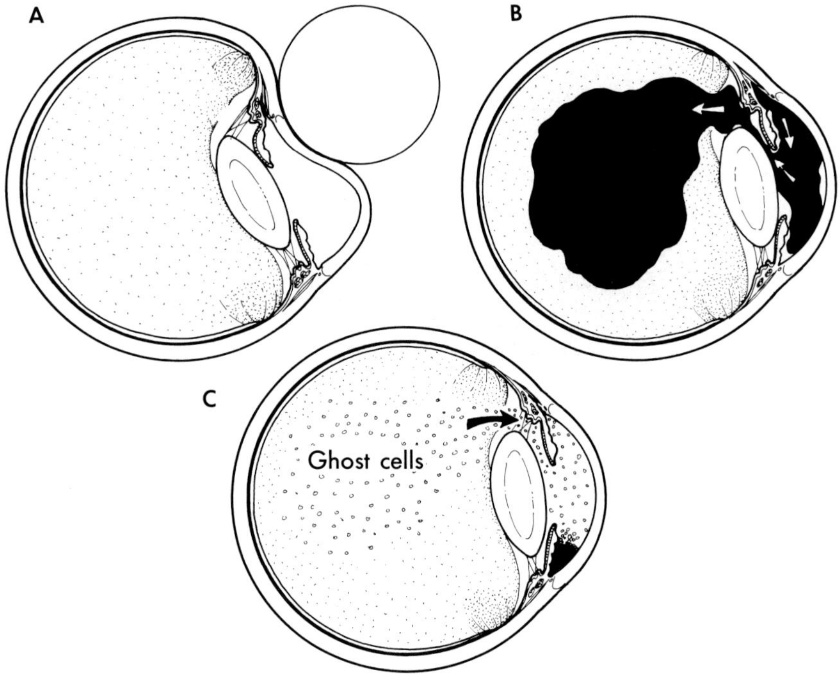

Fig. 10-10. Illustration of mechanism of ghost cell glaucoma following trauma. **A,** Blunt injury with globe deformation. **B,** Vitreous hemorrhage accompanies initial injury. **C,** Degenerated red blood cells, ghost cells, migrate from the vitreous into the anterior chamber weeks after the original injury.

approached cautiously because the success rate is low. If laser trabeculoplasty is attempted, only one third of the meshwork should be treated initially, followed by another third, and the final third if the first treatments are successful. Filtration surgery may be necessary.

The argon laser can be used to stop angle bleeding following injury or minor rebleeding if the bleeding points can be clearly seen on gonioscopy.

GHOST CELL GLAUCOMA

Ghost cell glaucoma[27,28] can occur following blunt injury to the eye. If the injury causes a disruption in the anterior hyaloid face and is associated with significant collection of blood in the vitreous in addition to a hyphema, the stage can be set for a second elevation of intraocular pressure, usually at a time when the anterior chamber hemorrhage has almost resolved (Fig. 10-10). In 1 to 3 weeks after the injury, the fresh blood cells in the vitreous convert to less pliable, khaki-colored, ghost cells and slowly begin a leak into the anterior chamber, where they can be recognized on slit-lamp examination by their color. They can then cause a severe, usually secondary, pressure elevation at this time secondary to blockage of the trabecular outflow channels. The treatment for this condition is medication, lavage of the anterior chamber, and, if necessary, vitrectomy.

References

1. Delori F, Pomerantzeff O, and Cox MS: Deformation of the globe under high-speed impact: its relation to contusion injuries, Invest Ophthalmol 8:290-301, 1969.
2. Alper MG: Contusion angle deformity and glaucoma: gonioscopic observations and clinical course, Arch Ophthalmol 69:455-467, 1963.
3. Mooney D: Angle recession and secondary glaucoma, Br J Ophthalmol 57:608-614, 1973.
4. Pettit TH and Keates EU: Traumatic cleavage of the chamber angle, Arch Ophthalmol 69:438-444, 1963.
5. Epstein DL, editor: Chandler and Grant's glaucoma, ed 3, Philadelphia, 1986, Lea & Febiger.
6. Béchetoille A: Aspects gonioscopiques des lesions traumatiques de l'angle, Clin Ophthalmol 3:17-23, 1971.

7. Cox MS, Schepens CL, and Freeman HM: Retinal detachment due to ocular contusion, Arch Ophthalmol 76:678-685, 1966.
8. Weidenthal DT and Schepens CL: Peripheral fundus changes associated with ocular contusion, Am J Ophthalmol 62:465-477, 1966.
9. Hoskins HD and Kass MA: Diagnosis and therapy of the glaucomas, St Louis, 1989, The CV Mosby Co.
10. Shields MB: Textbook of glaucoma, ed 2, Baltimore, 1987, Williams & Wilkins.
11. Bleiman BS and Schwartz AL: Paradoxical intraocular pressure response to pilocarpine: a proposed mechanism and treatment, Arch Ophthalmol 97:1305-1306, 1979.
12. Herschler J and Cobo M: Trauma and elevated intraocular pressure. In Ritch R, Shields MB, and Krupin T, editors: The glaucomas, St Louis, 1989, The CV Mosby Co.
13. Herschler J: Trabecular damage due to blunt anterior segment injury and its relationship to traumatic glaucoma, Trans Am Acad Ophthalmol Otolaryngol 83:239-243, 1977.
14. Richardson K: Acute glaucoma after trauma. In Freeman HM, editor: Ocular trauma, New York, 1979, Appleton-Century-Crofts.
15. Howard GM, Hutchinson BT, and Frederick AR Jr: Hyphema resulting from blunt trauma: gonioscopic, tonographic, and ophthalmoscopic observations following resolution of the hemorrhage, Trans Am Acad Ophthalmol Otolaryngol 69:294-306, 1965.
16. Tonjum AM: Gonioscopy in traumatic hyphema, Acta Ophthalmol 44:650-664, 1966.
17. Blanton FM: Anterior chamber angle recession and secondary glaucoma: a study of the aftereffects of traumatic hyphemas, Arch Ophthalmol 72:39-43, 1964.
18. Kaufman JH and Tolpin DW: Glaucoma after traumatic angle recession: a ten-year prospective study, Am J Ophthalmol 78:648-654, 1974.
19. Thiel H-J, Aden G, and Pulhorn G: Changes in the chamber angle following ocular contusions, Klin Monatsbl Augenheilkd 177:165, 1988.
20. Tonjum AM: Intraocular pressure and facility of outflow late after ocular contusion, Acta Ophthalmol 46:886-908, 1968.
21. D'Ombrain A: Traumatic monocular chronic glaucoma, Trans Ophthalmol Soc Aust 5:116-121, 1945.
22. Armaly ME: Steroids and glaucoma. In Transactions of the New Orleans Academy of Ophthalmology: symposium on glaucoma, St Louis, 1967, The CV Mosby Co.
23. Tesluk GC and Spaeth GL: The occurrence of primary open-angle glaucoma in the fellow eye of patients with unilateral angle-cleavage glaucoma, Ophthalmology 92:904-912, 1985.
24. Wolff SM and Zimmerman LE: Chronic secondary glaucoma: associated with retrodisplacement of iris root and deepening of the anterior chamber angle secondary to contusion, Am J Ophthalmol 54:547-562, 1962.
25. Iwamoto T, Witmer R, and Landolt E: Light and electron microscopy in absolute glaucoma with pigment dispersion phenomena and contusion angle deformity, Am J Ophthalmol 72:420-434, 1971.
26. Lauring L: Anterior chamber glass membranes, Am J Ophthalmol 68:308-312, 1969.
27. Campbell DG and Essigman EM: Hemolytic ghost cell glaucoma: further studies, Arch Ophthalmol 97:2141-2146, 1979.
28. Campbell DG, Simmons RJ, and Grant WM: Ghost cells as a cause of glaucoma, Am J Ophthalmol 81:441-450, 1976.

CHAPTER 11

Lens injuries

JOHN A. IRVINE
RONALD E. SMITH

Pathophysiology
Evaluation
Approaches to management
Contusion cataracts
Dislocation or subluxation of lenses
Surgical treatment and considerations
Anterior surgical approach
Cataract with intact posterior capsule, no displacement, and no vitreous in anterior chamber
Lens dislocation into the anterior chamber
Posterior surgical approach
Intraocular lenses
References

Lens injury is a major complication of blunt ocular trauma. Contusion cataracts may occur as either early or late sequelae of the injury. Moreover, blunt, nonperforating ocular trauma can partially or totally dislocate the lens. The management of such lenticular trauma depends upon numerous factors, including visual acuity, intraocular pressure, intraocular inflammation, associated anterior segment trauma, and ability to visualize posterior segment damage.

Contusion cataracts are not invariably progressive; some remain stable and do not require surgery. Similarly, many dislocated or subluxated clear lenses do not immediately threaten vision; hence surgery, if deemed necessary, can be performed electively. Other contusion cataracts require urgent intervention to prevent further ocular complications. In general, decreased visual acuity, lens-induced glaucoma or inflammation, or poor visualization of an injured posterior segment are indications for surgical intervention.

PATHOPHYSIOLOGY

The pathogenesis of lens changes following blunt ocular trauma has been suggested by Wolter[1] and by Weidenthal and Schepens.[2] These authors have described "coup" and "contrecoup" injuries, along with equatorial expansion of the globe due to trauma, as the pathophysiologic mechanisms responsible for ocular damage. "Coup" refers to direct damage resulting in abrasion or laceration; "contrecoup" denotes injury occurring along a plane of trajectory, causing damage at a distal site as a result of shock waves. Contusion cataract formation, for instance, may result from contrecoup damage following a blow to the orbital area. Shock waves pass through the eye, possibly rupturing the anterior or posterior lens capsule with subsequent lens opacification.

The equatorial expansion theory suggests that blunt trauma applied to the globe in an anterior or posterior direction causes shortening of that meridian, with concomitant equatorial stretching. The equatorial expansion may cause a rupture in the lens capsule at its equator, resulting in lens opacification. Zonular disruption during a sudden increase in the equatorial meridian causes incomplete and asymmetric lens support, with resultant dislocation or subluxation.

EVALUATION

In the absence of perforating ocular trauma or symptomatic trauma-induced inflammation or bleeding, the patient with a contusion cataract or dislocated lens frequently does not seek immediate medical care. Initial visual problems, which may not occur for several days, weeks, or months after the trauma, may consist of fluctuating vision (subluxated lens) or decreased vision (progressive cataract formation or dislocated lens). Depending on the degree of subluxation, there may also be monocular diplopia, glare, functional aphakia, or marked astigmatism.

The past history of the patient who has sustained ocular trauma is important to reveal preexisting conditions such as glaucoma, previous eye surgery, or a predisposition to retinal pathology, as in diabetes mellitus.

Especially important for the evaluation is the assessment of vision, presence or absence of hyphema, type and extent of lens opacity (cortical, nuclear, or capsular; total or focal), ocular inflammation, lens swelling, lens capsule integrity (anterior and posterior), and presence or absence of iridodonesis and phacodonesis (Figs. 11-1 and 11-2). Lens dislocation can be subtle and may be apparent only on dilated retroillumination (Fig. 11-3). Iridodonesis or phacodonesis are variably present. Comparison of the anterior chamber depth in both eyes may reveal a deeper chamber in the eye with the dislocated or subluxated lens; the angle may be shallower in an eye with an intumescent cataract or anteriorly displaced lens.

Posterior capsule status is of major importance when planning the surgical approach to a traumatic cataract without dislocation or subluxation. If opacification precludes viewing the posterior capsule, water immersion ultrasonography may be helpful[3] (Fig. 11-4) (see Chapter 2).

If marked intraocular inflammation is present, the patient may seek medical care soon after blunt ocular trauma. If the inflammation is lens induced, prompt intervention—medical, surgical, or both—is necessary.

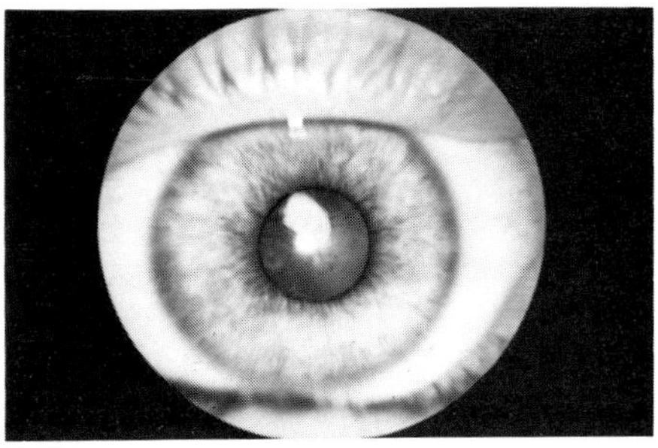

Fig. 11-1. Focal anterior cortical traumatic cataract.

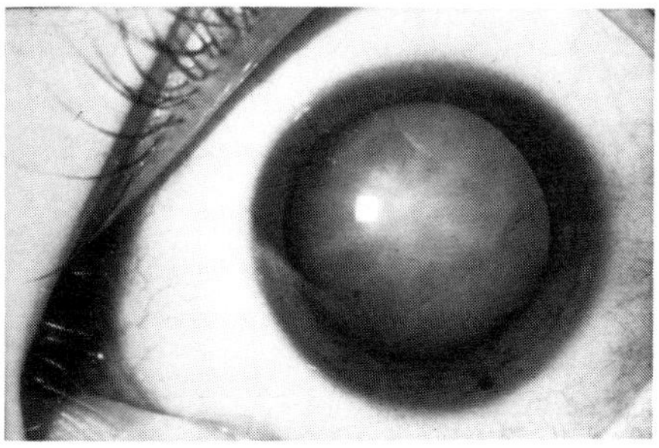

Fig. 11-2. Diffuse traumatic cataract with pigment on the anterior lens capsule.

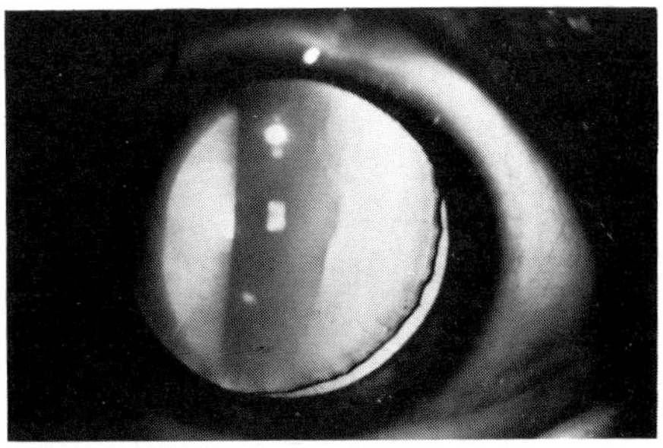

Fig. 11-3. Retroillumination through a dilated pupil demonstrating lens subluxation.

Lens-induced intraocular inflammation may occur secondary to release of lens proteins following traumatic rupture of the lens capsule. Phacoanaphylactic (or phacoantigenic) uveitis, first described by Verhoeff and characterized by the presence of polymorphonuclear leukocytes, eosinophils, and giant cells surrounding lens ma-

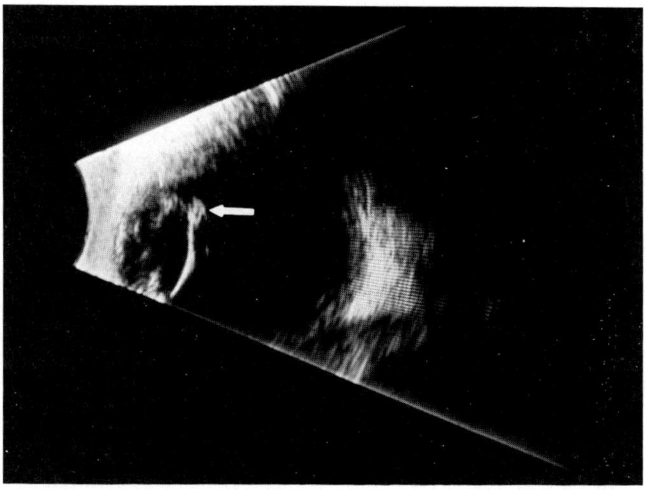

Fig. 11-4. B-scan ultrasonogram demonstrating traumatic posterior capsular disruption.

terial, is thought to be an immunopathologic reaction to lens proteins.

Phacolytic glaucoma may result from phagocytosis of lens proteins by macrophages in patients with mature cataracts. The macrophages and high-density lens proteins occlude the trabecular meshwork, causing an acute rise in intraocular pressure (IOP).[4] An attempt should be made to treat inflammation and elevated IOP with corticosteroids and antiglaucoma medications, respectively. However, prompt cataract extraction is usually required to eliminate inflammation and restore normal IOP.

Glaucoma can also result from inflammation-induced alterations in the anterior segment anatomy, such as peripheral anterior synechiae or seclusion of the pupil by posterior synechiae, which can lead to relative pupillary block. Lens swelling can also cause relative pupillary block to aqueous outflow and thus may be a cause of secondary (phacomorphic) glaucoma (see Chapter 10).

APPROACHES TO MANAGEMENT

Historically, various techniques have been advocated for extracting traumatic cataracts[5] and dislocated lenses.[6] The most common have been aspiration, loop extraction of the lens, erysophake extraction, extraction with a loop plus needle, a double-needle operation (in which the lens is trapped and supported by passing two needles through the pars plana posterior to the lens), a Calhoun-Hagler double needle (a double-pronged needle introduced behind the lens to trap it), and cryoextraction. The large number and diversity of the techniques reflect the great variability of trauma cases and the fact that no one surgical technique proved universally satisfactory.

The development of vitrectomy, phacoemulsification instrumentation, and sophisticated irrigation and aspiration systems has added a safer dimension to the surgical treatment of these lens injuries.[7-9] An understanding of the principles of these endosurgical techniques is critical to the management of ocular trauma, including complicated traumatic cataracts.

Contusion Cataracts

Contusion cataract refers to any lens opacification attributable to blunt, nonperforating trauma. The distribution of the opacities may be focal, sectoral, or total, and they may be stationary or progressive (see Chapter 12). Good visual acuity is possible despite focal opacification of the lens. In the absence of decreased visual acuity, glaucoma, or lens-induced uveitis, observation is the preferred management.

If the lens capsule is intact, contusion cataracts may not develop until several months after injury. If the lens capsule is ruptured, thereby allowing hydration of the cortical material, such cataracts can develop rapidly. In the latter situation, marked inflammation is often present, and secondary glaucoma due to angle damage or relative pupillary block is not uncommon.

The medical treatment of a traumatic cataract

is directed against focal, off-axis opacities or inflammation. Small focal opacities that are paraaxial may decrease visual acuity because of glare and diplopia. Miotics may help to maintain a small but clear visual axis and decrease the debilitating optical effects of the opacity.

Intraocular inflammation, secondary to the blunt trauma itself or to lens-induced uveitis, can result in trabecular meshwork congestion, peripheral anterior synechiae with subsequent angle closure, and posterior synechiae formation with subsequent pupillary block. Intensive treatment with topical corticosteroids is indicated in these situations to control inflammation, and systemic and periocular corticosteroids may be added if necessary. Topical betablockers, mydriatics, and systemic carbonic anhydrase inhibitors may be necessary to control IOP.

Capsular rupture will influence the timing and technique of cataract removal. A pars plana surgical approach is favored in cases of posterior capsular rupture to minimize the risk of nucleus dislocation into the vitreous during surgical removal. Removal of the vitreous/lens admixture also prevents subsequent traction retinal detachment.[10] Other factors influencing the timing of and necessity for surgical intervention include preexisting ocular abnormalities such as chronic open-angle glaucoma or diabetic retinopathy, both of which require ongoing observation of the optic disc and retina. If the lens has entered the anterior chamber or blocks the pupil causing glaucoma, emergency removal of the lens is required. Thus, the indications for surgical removal of a traumatic cataract are the same as for any cataract, but with some additional indications unique to the traumatized eye: (1) vision decreased to a level unacceptable to the patient; (2) the need to access, treat, or follow retinal or optic nerve pathology; (3) capsule rupture with lens swelling; (4) lens-induced inflammation; (5) secondary glaucoma caused by the cataract; and (6) other trauma-related ocular pathology requiring surgical treatment.

Dislocation or Subluxation of Lenses

Rapid equatorial expansion of the globe secondary to sudden anterior/posterior compression during blunt trauma can cause zonular disruption, which may result in partial or complete dislocation of the lens. If zonular rupture is incomplete, the lens will be drawn to the side opposite the rupture. A minimally dislocated

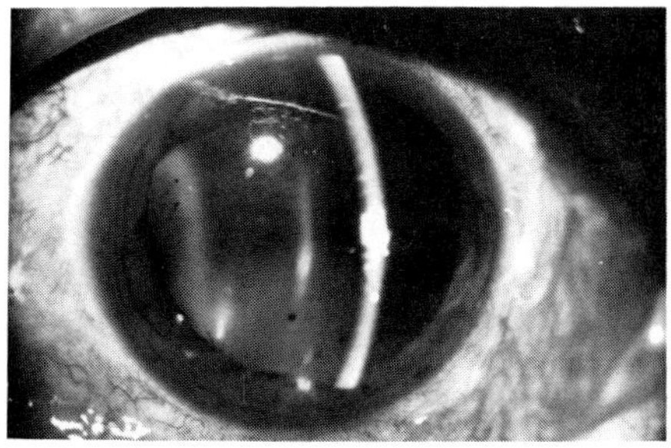

Fig. 11-5. Examination of an eye in the immediate postinjury period reveals inferior lens subluxation.

lens may cause induced myopia or astigmatism as it is decentered. If the lens dislocation is more extreme and its edge is in the visual axis, monocular diplopia may develop. Complete lens dislocation follows total zonular dehiscence.

Evaluation of an eye with a dislocated lens may reveal iridodonesis, phacodonesis, or a deeper anterior chamber than in the fellow eye (judged by slit-lamp examination or gonioscopy). Displacement of the lens will be apparent if its edge is within the visual axis (Fig. 11-5 and Color Plate 11-1). Zonular disruption may be detected gonioscopically through a dilated pupil. Vitreous herniation between broken zonules, with bulging into the anterior chamber, confirms the diagnosis of zonular rupture and lens displacement (Figs. 11-6 and 11-7). Frank angle recession or an apparent widening of the ciliary body band may also be evident. If the lens is completely dislocated posteriorly, funduscopic examination will reveal the lens within the vitreous cavity. Alternatively, a dislocated lens may block the pupillary aperture, predisposing to relative pupillary block, or the lens may be dislocated forward into the anterior chamber, resulting in lens-endothelial cell contact and corneal damage (Fig. 11-8).

Medical therapy for a traumatically dislocated lens includes the use of dilating or constricting drugs to minimize astigmatism resulting from off-centering of the lens or effects of the lens edge within the visual axis. In minimally dislocated lenses, miotic therapy may help to decrease the astigmatism and monocular diplopia if the lens edge is encroaching on the visual axis of a large pupil. By relaxing zonules, miotics may also lead to forward displacement of a subluxated lens. However, anterior chamber shal-

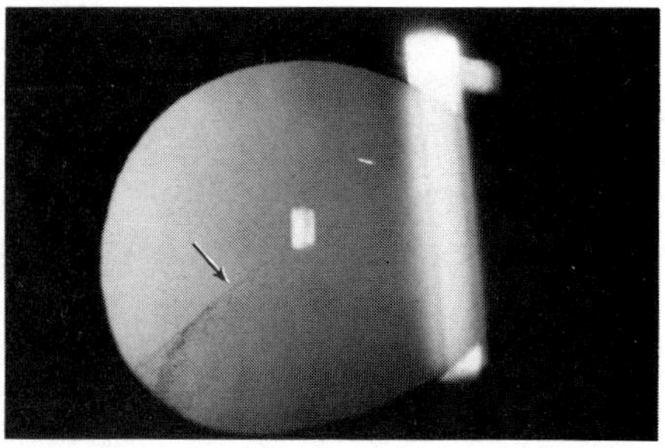

Fig. 11-6. Vitreous herniation *(arrow)* into the anterior chamber demonstrated by retrolumination confirms zonular disruption.

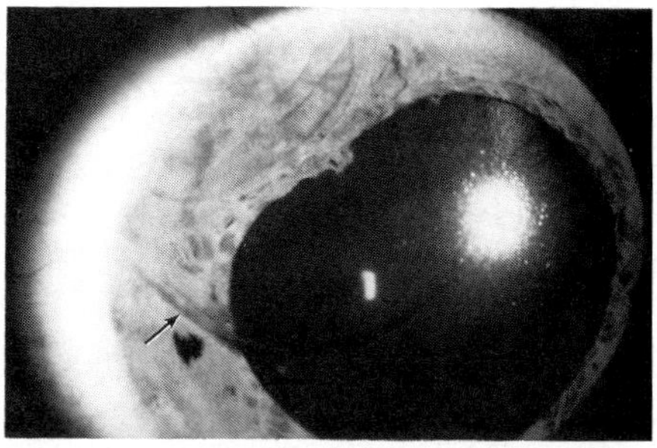

Fig. 11-7. Pupillary eccentricity and a vitreous strand *(arrow)* present temporally in an eye confirm zonular disruption and lens subluxation following injury.

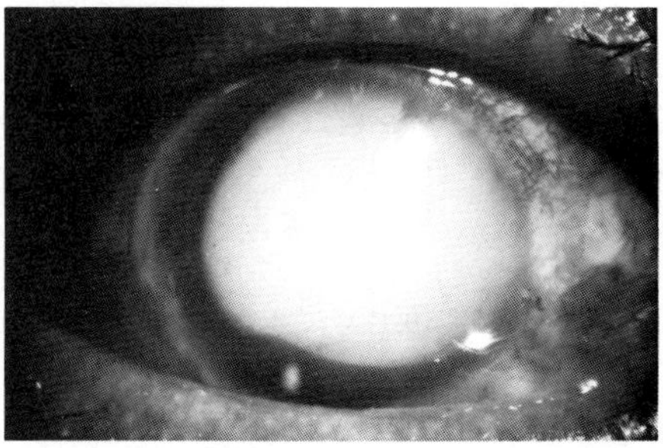

Fig. 11-8. Opaque traumatic cataract with dislocation into the anterior chamber.

lowing may occur and must be looked for if miotics are used. Mydriatics, conversely, may allow some patients to view around a subluxated, cataractous lens using aphakic correction.

The presence of a dislocated or subluxated lens is not necessarily an indication for surgical removal. Emergency surgical intervention is required only when there is an immediate threat to the health of the eye, as with relative pupillary block or dislocation into the anterior chamber. Induced myopia, astigmatism, or extreme monocular diplopia that cannot be corrected with glasses or miotic therapy are relative indications for elective lens extraction.

SURGICAL TREATMENT AND CONSIDERATIONS

If surgical removal of a traumatic cataract or dislocated lens is deemed necessary, the likelihood of vitreous loss must be considered in planning the surgical approach.[9] Cases may be classified as (1) nondislocated cataract with intact capsule and intact zonular-capsular ligament, (2) cataract with ruptured posterior capsule, (3) subluxated lens with or without cataract, or (4) dislocated lens with or without cataract. To facilitate lens removal and minimize complications, the surgeon must decide between an anterior (limbal) and posterior (pars plana) approach.

An anterior (limbal) approach is preferred to remove a traumatic cataract in the presence of an intact posterior capsule, or if the lens has been dislocated completely into the anterior chamber. Conversely, if the posterior capsule is ruptured, or the lens is dislocated posteriorly, or if there is traumatic rupture of the zonules with vitreous herniation through the pupillary space, a pars plana approach using vitrectomy techniques may be preferred. An anterior approach may be attempted to extract a minimally subluxated lens, as long as it is kept in mind that an anterior vitrectomy, conversion to a pars plana approach, or both may prove to be necessary during the procedure. If the lens is dislocated into the vitreous cavity out of the visual axis, is not causing inflammation or glaucoma, and is not obstructing vision, surgery may be avoided.

Anterior Surgical Approach

Cataract with Intact Posterior Capsule, No Displacement, and No Vitreous in Anterior Chamber

An anterior or limbal approach is preferred for a traumatic cataract in an eye with an intact posterior capsule and in the absence of zonular disruption or lens displacement. Because most eye injuries occur in young patients with soft lenses, many traumatic cataracts can be removed by an aspiration technique and do not require nucleus expression or phacoemulsification. In an older

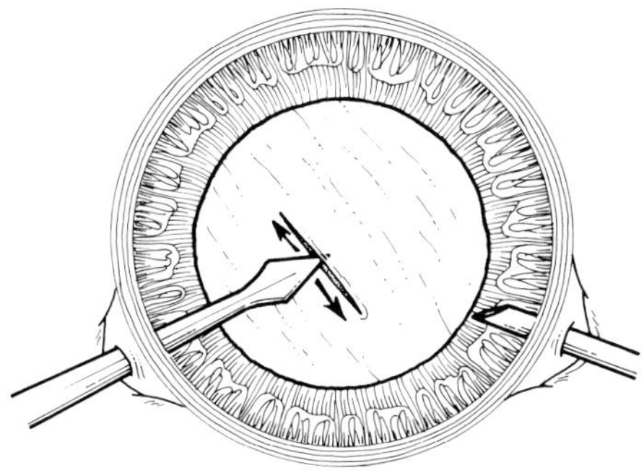

Fig. 11-9. After a hand-held infusion line is introduced into the anterior chamber, a second incision is made 135° away with a disposable blade, which can then be used to open the anterior capsule.

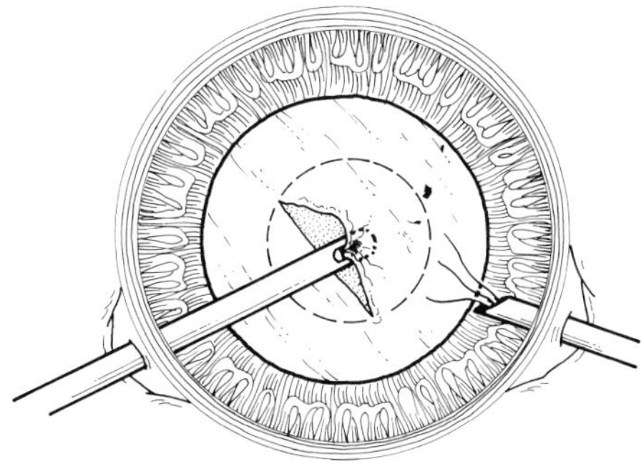

Fig. 11-10. The cutting and aspiration handpiece is introduced into the anterior chamber through the limbal incision. The cutting handpiece allows for easy enlargement of the capsulotomy.

patient, standard phacoemulsification or extracapsular techniques may be preferred, depending upon the surgeon's experience. It must be remembered that occult zonular incompetence may become apparent during surgery, necessitating intraoperative modification of the planned procedure.

In young patients the entire lens can be aspirated with automated irrigation-aspiration instrumentation using a bimanual technique. The entry sites of the two instruments are made approximately 135° apart to facilitate manipulation of the globe while the instruments are in the eye (Fig. 11-9). Two small conjunctival incisions are made. It is important to achieve adequate hemostasis so that blood does not enter the anterior chamber. The nasal incision is created first by advancing a sharp knife (e.g., MVR blade) through the limbus parallel to the iris. A handheld cannula is then inserted into the anterior chamber through this nasal incision, taking care not to strip Descemet's membrane or injure the iris. Instrumentation for this infusion line can vary from an infusion cannula to a bent 23-gauge butterfly needle. If the anterior chamber is formed and the intraocular pressure is normal, a second incision is made approximately 135° from the nasal incision to enhance maneuverability within the eye. This incision is made of appropriate size to allow insertion of the automated cutting-aspiration instrument. The 20G MVR blade may be used to perform a capsulotomy in addition to providing an adequate but relatively watertight opening for the instrument (Fig. 11-9). Alternatively, a cystotome may be used to perform the capsulotomy in standard extracapsular fashion. The cutting-aspiration handpiece is introduced into the anterior chamber with the cutting tip open. A maximum suction of 150 mm Hg is usually sufficient for lens aspiration in young patients; older individuals may require up to 400 mm Hg. Cutting rate may be varied depending on the density of the lens material. The anterior chamber is irrigated to remove blood and fibrin obscuring the view. The cutting-aspiration instrument is then used to remove as much of the capsule as necessary (Fig. 11-10); the cortical material, which may be fluffy secondary to hydration, can also be aspirated. If vitreous is present in the anterior chamber, the cutting and aspiration capability of the vitrectomy instrument allows for greater flexibility in its management.

In patients with more advanced nuclear sclerosis and no evidence of dislocation, the wound can be enlarged and the nucleus expressed with standard extracapsular cataract extraction techniques. An irrigating vectus may be helpful in nucleus removal to avoid undue external pressure on the globe.

Following removal of the sclerotic nucleus, cortical material can be engaged and aspirated by capturing lens material in the port for aspiration from the eye as in standard techniques of extracapsular cataract extraction.

Because of the many unanticipated variables that may occur in trauma cases (such as clinically undetected vitreous prolapse), aspiration with a manual irrigation and aspiration unit may allow a more controlled approach. Curved cannulas

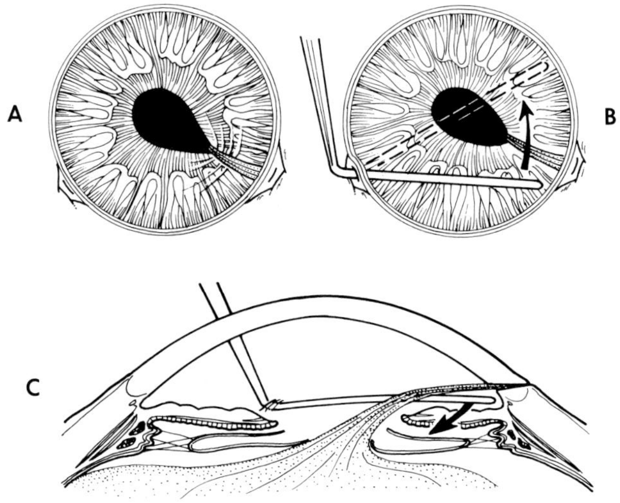

Fig. 11-11. **A,** After introduction of an intracameral miotic, constriction of the pupil reveals peaking secondary to vitreous to the wound. **B, C,** The vitreous may be removed from the angle by passing a sweep or spatula from the opposite port. This may be done under fluid, air, or viscoelastic material.

may allow easier access to certain areas beneath the iris, with less risk of inflicting further damage to a possibly traumatized capsule-zonular ligament. There is also less chance of uncontrolled vitreous aspiration, which can exert subsequent traction on the retina.

Following removal of cortical material, care should be taken to ensure that no vitreous is present in the anterior chamber. A cholinergic agonist is injected into the anterior chamber to induce miosis. If there is peaking of the pupil, the vitrectomy instrument can then be used to perform an anterior vitrectomy. If necessary, air or a small amount of a viscoelastic substance can be injected through the wound to push the iris back from the limbal incisions and the internal wound can be swept with a cyclodialysis spatula (Fig. 11-11). On completion of the vitrectomy the instruments are removed and the wounds closed with 10-0 nylon sutures; the conjunctiva is closed as needed. Subconjunctival corticosteroids and antibiotics are recommended.

Lens Dislocation into the Anterior Chamber

If the lens is dislocated anteriorly, miotic drops are instilled to trap the lens in the anterior chamber while the patient is being prepared for immediate surgery (Fig. 11-12). This is especially important if retrobulbar anesthesia is administered since the pupil may dilate, allowing the lens to migrate posteriorly. A soft lens, as in young patients, can be surgically aspirated but there is a risk of losing lens material into the vitreous cavity as the aspiration proceeds. If aspiration is not considered safe, a limbal incision is made through which the lens can be extracted with either an irrigating vectus or a cryoprobe (Fig. 11-13). The lens often can be delivered through the incision by external pressure, without introducing instrumentation into the eye (Fig. 11-14). An anterior vitrectomy will be necessary if vitreous is present. This can be performed through the limbal incision or by the pars plana approach. The limbal incision is then closed with interrupted 10-0 nylon sutures.

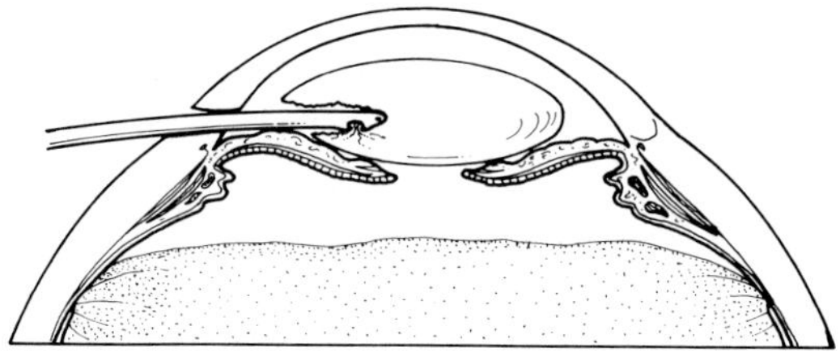

Fig. 11-12. Pharmacologically induced miosis may trap a dislocated lens in the anterior chamber where aspiration or anterior segment delivery can be performed. This may prevent posterior dislocation of the lens.

Posterior Surgical Approach

A posterior or pars plana approach for removing a traumatic cataract may be preferred when the

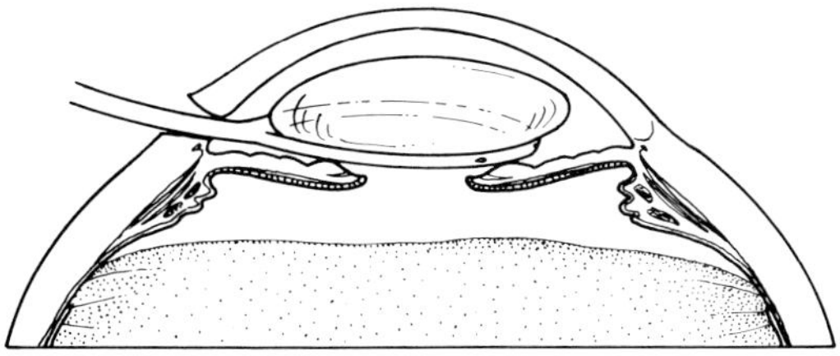

Fig. 11-13. An irrigating vectus may be inserted under the anteriorly displaced traumatic cataract to facilitate removal.

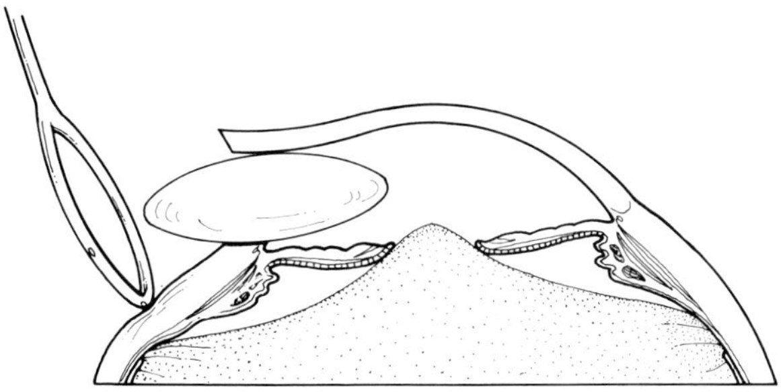

Fig. 11-14. External scleral pressure alone may deliver a traumatically dislocated lens from the anterior chamber. A broad corneoscleral section is required.

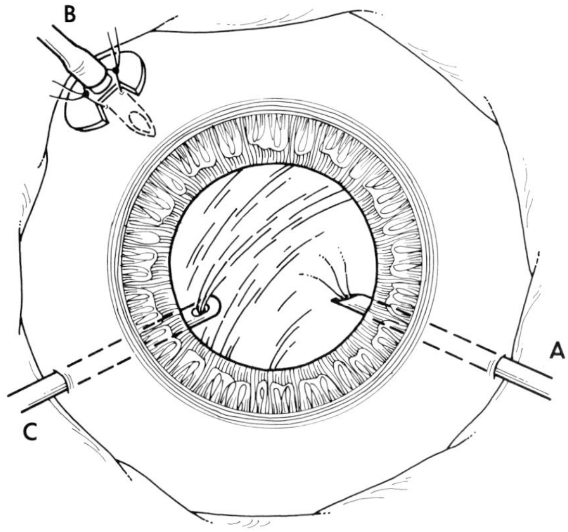

Fig. 11-15. Sclerotomies are made 3 mm posterior to the limbus. *A*, The superonasal incision may be used temporarily for a hand-held infusion until *B*, the infusion cannula is sewn into place inferotemporally. *C*, The cutting tip is introduced via the superotemporal sclerotomy. Site A may then be used for a second instrument to permit bimanual manipulation of the posterior segment.

posterior capsule is ruptured or when there is lens dislocation or subluxation with vitreous prolapse into the anterior chamber. During surgery, care should be taken to maintain the intraocular pressure within the normal range by manipulating the height of the infusion line. If the pressure is low, sterile balanced salt solution can be injected through the pars plana before making the incision, using a 30-gauge needle inserted 3 mm posterior to the limbus, in the area to be used for a sclerotomy. Hyperosmotics, such as mannitol (50 ml of 25% solution), may be given by intravenous push just before the start of surgery if the intraocular pressure is high. To minimize the risk of choroidal hemorrhage, pressure control several hours before surgery is recommended.

A bimanual approach is preferred, with the infusion line inserted nasally and the cutting and suctioning instrumentation inserted temporally via the pars plana. After a peritomy is made, sclerotomies are performed approximately 135° apart with an MVR blade 3 mm posterior to the limbus. A separate 4-mm infusion cannula is sutured into place through an inferotemporal sclerotomy with 5-0 vicryl suture to facilitate bimanual extraction techniques (Fig. 11-15).

Infusion should be turned on only when the surgeon can visualize the infusion cannula port; infusion should not be started until it is verified that the tip of the cannula is through the uveal tract, to prevent inadvertent suprachoroidal infusion. If lens opacification prevents visualization of the tip, a hand-held, bent 20-gauge infusion needle is placed through the sclerotomy and into the center of the pupil. This infusion needle is then brought forward into the lens until it is possible to see that the tip of the needle has penetrated the uveal tract and is indeed in the vitreous cavity. The eye is then infused through this hand-held needle (Fig. 11-15). With suction and cutting modes, the opacified lens material can be removed from the eye until the anterior segment is sufficiently clear to permit accurate determination of the location of the pars plana infusion cannula. Gravity infusion can then be introduced through the pars plana cannula, obviating the need for the hand-held infusion line. The infusion is controlled by adjusting the bottle height to maintain the anterior chamber while using the vitrectomy instrument. With a full-function probe, the second sclerotomy may be used to accommodate an endoilluminator or, if necessary, another instrument to aid in manipulating lens material.

The goal of this procedure is to remove the entire lens and as much vitreous as is safely possible. The cutting port should be open wide with a cutting rate of approximately 300 to 450 per minute; suction of up to 300 mm Hg may be required. Because vitreous is present around the lens, it is important that a combination of cutting and suction, rather than aspiration alone, be used to remove the lens material. Ideally, any visible vitreous should be removed first.

A traumatically dislocated lens and a posterior rupture carry the risk of movement of lens material into the vitreous cavity. Care should be taken to avoid this complication, but the surgeon must be prepared to deal with it using standard pars plana vitrectomy techniques. Most traumatic cataracts can be removed using such techniques.

Although pars plana vitrectomy is usually adequate for young patients, those over 40 years of age may require ultrasonic fragmentation or removal of the entire nucleus through an enlarged limbal incision. Lens remnants may fall posteriorly with this technique. If possible, the nucleus should be removed first, since the surrounding cortex helps to stabilize it in position. After removal of the nucleus, removal of the cortex and capsule is facilitated with a suction cutter and intraocular forceps, respectively. Following removal of the entire lens through a pars plana sclerotomy, a generous vitrectomy and iridectomy are performed to prevent the development of a vitreous wick to the wound and aphakic pupillary block. At the conclusion of the procedure, the sclerotomies are sutured with 4-0 Dexon, and the conjunctiva is closed.

Intraocular Lenses

Intraocular lens implantation at the time of surgery for a traumatic cataract raises important questions. First, the use of anterior chamber lenses should probably be avoided since there is a high probability of preexisting contusion damage to the angle, and the patients are usually young. Placement of a posterior chamber intraocular lens in the capsular bag may result in postoperative lens decentration if there is undetected zonular incompetence. Therefore, sulcus fixation may be the safest technique for lens fixation. Contact lens rehabilitation should be seriously considered when the extent of angle and sulcus damage is unknown. In the event of contact lens intolerance, a secondary posterior chamber lens may be implanted even in the absence of capsular support using a suture fixation technique.[9] However, there is as yet no significant reported experience using intraocular lenses (IOLs) in traumatized eyes.

Traditionally, many surgeons have not advocated IOL implantation in children because of the uncertainty of the natural history over many years. However, the minimum age for lens implantation has continued to decrease as experience has increased and improved lens design and materials have been developed. Hemo and Ben Ezra[11] described a series of 37 children (age 2 to 10 years) who, because of behavior or economic problems, could not be treated with contact lenses and underwent IOL insertion following removal of traumatic cataracts.

No major complications were encountered if posterior capsulotomy and anterior vitrectomy were performed before IOL insertion. Although the natural history of early IOL insertion in these patients is yet to be determined, selected pediatric patients who cannot be treated with contact lenses may benefit from early IOL insertion following cataract removal to minimize the degree of amblyopia that may develop if left otherwise untreated. More time and experience are needed to determine the overall efficacy of this mode of visual rehabilitation in pediatric patients. In selected cases of pediatric lens injury and aphakia, epikeratophakia[12] may be a reasonable alternative to intraocular lens implantation.

References

1. Wolter JR: Coup-contrecoup mechanism of ocular injuries, Am J Ophthalmol 56:785-796, 1963.
2. Weidenthal DT and Schepens CL: Peripheral fundus changes associated with ocular contusion, Am J Ophthalmol 62:465-477, 1966.
3. Jarrett WH: Dislocation of the lens: a study of 166 hospitalized cases, Arch Ophthalmol 78:289-296, 1967.
4. Epstein DL, Jedziniak JA, and Grant WM: Obstruction of aqueous outflow by lens particles and heavy-molecular weight soluble lens proteins, Invest Ophthalmol Vis Sci 17:272-277, 1978.

5. Ryan SJ and Von Noorden GK: Further observations on the aspiration technique in cataract surgery, Am J Ophthalmol 71:626-630, 1971.
6. Calhoun FP Jr and Hagler WS: Experience with the José Barraquer method of extracting a dislocated lens, Am J Ophthalmol 50:701-715, 1960.
7. Sellyei LF Jr and Barraquer J: Surgery of the ectopic lens, Ann Ophthalmol 5:1127-1133, 1973.
8. Shock JP and Appleton B: Continuous irrigation for removal of congenital and traumatic cataracts, Ann Ophthalmol 5:361-368, 1973.
9. Stern WH, Diddie KR, and Smith RE: Vitrectomy techniques for the anterior segment surgeon: a practical approach, New York, 1983, Grune & Stratton.
10. Cleary PE and Ryan SJ: Method of production and natural history of experimental posterior penetrating eye injury in the rhesus monkey, Am J Ophthalmol 88:212-220, 1979.
11. Hemo Y and Ben Ezra D: Traumatic cataracts in young children: correction of aphakia by intraocular lens implantation, Ophthalmic Pedriatr Genet 8:203-207, 1987.
12. Morgan KS et al: The nationwide study of epikeratophakia for aphakia in children, Am J Ophthalmol 103:366-374, 1987.

CHAPTER 12

Pathophysiology of anterior segment wound healing

J. DOUGLAS CAMERON

Pathophysiology of corneal wound healing
- Early events
- Epithelial healing
- Endothelial healing
- Stromal healing
- Anomalies of corneal wound healing
- Medical management

Pathophysiology of scleral and limbal healing
- Scleral healing
- Limbal healing

Iris and angle changes after trauma

Lens changes after trauma

References

Healing of injured tissues is a complex process involving coagulation (to achieve hemostasis), inflammation (to remove necrotic debris), proliferation of fibrovascular tissue and surface cells (to reestablish anatomic integrity), and tissue remodeling (to reestablish tissue function).

The basic functional component of both the cornea and the sclera is collagen.[1] Collagen is one of the components of the extracellular matrix that must be produced and maintained by living cells. The goal of ideal healing in corneal and scleral tissues is restoration of the collagenous components to their original composition and structure—a goal, particularly in corneal tissue, that is never fully accomplished.

The cornea and sclera provide architectural support (a function of collagenous tissues throughout the body) for the internal components of the eye and for the extraocular muscles. In addition, the collagen of the cornea is highly modified to transmit light. The different functions of the cornea and sclera are reflected in the composition and arrangement of the collagen and the type of adjacent tissue that produces and maintains the collagen. It is not surprising that the wound-healing process of these two tissues is distinct in several clinically important areas.

The corneal collagen fibers resemble embryonic connective tissue—thin fibers embedded in a mucopolysaccharide matrix—and retain those characteristics throughout life. Corneal stromal collagen is aggregated into broad, tapelike bands of uniform thickness but variable breadth that run parallel to each other and to the surface. These bands, or lamellae, extend throughout the length of the cornea. The most superficial layers are oriented vertically; the middle layers are directed toward the insertions of the rectus muscles; and the deeper peripheral layers are circular.[2-4] Bowman's layer is a modified superficial layer of the stroma that ends abruptly at the limbus. The specialized nature of the avascular cornea requires specialized support. The stroma is protected and maintained externally by nonkeratinized squamous epithelial cells with a high reactive potential and internally by endothelial-like cells with a limited reactive potential.

Scleral collagen fibers are thicker than corneal collagen fibers and lack a mucoid sheath. The collagenous fibers of the sclera interlace, and generally are parallel to the surface of the sclera. The arrangement of collagen fibers is oriented by prevailing tissue tension in the region of the limbus, optic canal, and insertions of the rectus muscles. The collagen and extracellular matrix of the sclera are supported by fibrovascular tissue of the extrascleral tissue externally and of the choroid internally. A sparse population of fibroblasts is located within the sclera.

Given the complexity of the contents and arrangement of the cornea and sclera, regeneration of the native tissue is not possible. However, there are many avenues of intervention for the ophthalmic surgeon in guiding the wound healing process toward successful repair of injured tissue and restoration of function.

PATHOPHYSIOLOGY OF CORNEAL WOUND HEALING

Rigorous requirements must be met if function is to be restored to the cornea following trauma: the tissue must remain avascular, the corneal stroma must be precisely realigned, the anterior and posterior contours of the cellular layers of the cornea must be reproduced, stromal deturgescence must be reestablished, and the tensile strength of the stroma must be restored. Detailed examination of the cellular events involved in a linear, perforating, noncontaminated laceration of the central cornea reveals how the wound healing process attempts to meet these requirements (Fig. 12-1).[5,6]

Early Events

Cell death begins the wound healing process. The delicate and loosely adherent corneal epithelium is damaged for a variable distance from the anterior aspect of the wound; the long, wispy cellular processes of the stromal keratocytes are transected; and endothelial cells are destroyed or dislodged for a variable distance from the posterior aspect of the wound.[5] Damaged cells are swept away by the action of the tears and lids externally and by the aqueous convection currents internally. Hemostasis per se does not occur because no blood vessels are directly involved. There is, however, a type of aqueostasis to prevent excessive loss of aqueous by formation of a fibrin clot of secondary aqueous and swelling of exposed corneal stroma.[5]

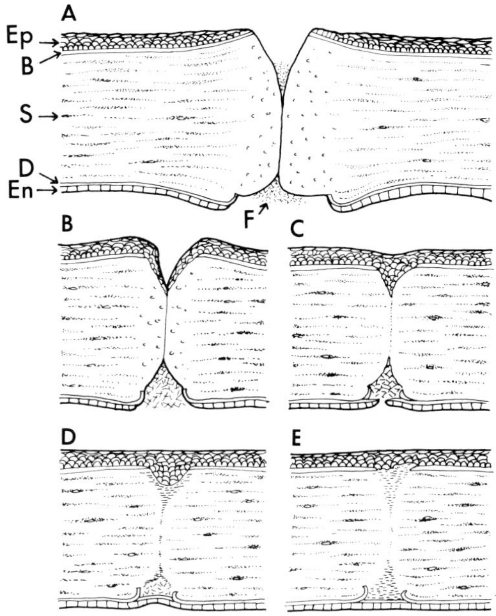

Fig. 12-1. Central corneal wound healing. **A,** A linear laceration of the cornea may seal spontaneously because of swelling of exposed corneal stroma (*S*) if the wound edges are well-apposed and by formation of a fibrin clot (*F*) from secondary aqueous. **B,** Rapid migration of the epithelium (*E*) serves to protect the underlying stroma from infection, drying, or additional swelling. **C,** The surface contour will be reestablished by the epithelium despite a defect in the underlying stroma, which allows for return of the refractive properties at the air/fluid interface of the cornea. **D,** Healing of the stroma generally proceeds from the center of the stroma outward. **E,** The breach in Bowman's membrane (*B*) is not reestablished, and a new (thinner) Descemet's membrane (*D*) is formed posteriorly. The tensile strength of the cornea in the wound area is less than that of the surrounding tissue. The scar tissue does not become transparent.

Surgical approximation of the corneal stroma, depending upon the extent of the wound, sets the stage for the cellular events of the wound healing process. Both Bowman's layer and Descemet's membrane have elastic qualities that cause the membranes to retract from the wound edge. The edges of Bowman's layer can often be surgically reapposed; however, the free ends of Descemet's membrane will remain retracted into the corneal stroma even with perfect stromal realignment.

Epithelial Healing

Undamaged epithelial cells aggregate, and after a refractory period they reform a continuous leading edge of cells.[7,8] The tissue migrates toward the wound guided by topographic features of the epithelium itself, by chemical messages in solution (chemotaxis), and by chemical messages incorporated in the matrix over which the cells travel (haptotaxis).[9] The epithelium extends downward over exposed Bowman's layer and corneal stroma until it meets a physical obstruction such as intact or well-apposed corneal stroma, a fibrin clot, or perhaps healthy endothelial cells (contact inhibition of migration).[10] Upon completion of migration, the epithelium increases in thickness by mitotic division to fill any available space in the wound and to reestablish the corneal epithelial external contour.[11,12]

Endothelial Healing

Endothelial cells follow a pattern of recovery and migration similar to that of epithelial cells although over a much longer period of time.[12-15] Endothelial cells migrate as a monolayer following the posterior contour of the wound. Once migration is complete, a limited amount of mitosis may occur depending on the age of the tissue. As the endothelium recovers, corneal deturgescence will occur. When the wound is stabilized, the endothelial cells will produce a new Descemet's membrane contiguous with the original one. In cases of severe endothelial cell injury, the cells are capable of metaplasia, or transformation to a different type of mature cell, and take on cytologic characteristics of fibroblasts. The fibrous tissue produced by these cells under these conditions is opaque.

Stromal Healing

Keratocytes have the longest refractory period following injury. Very little distinct cellular activity can be seen until the surface cells have stabilized. After several days, keratocytes will repopulate the wound area and begin producing new collagen. Repair collagen lacks the mucoid sheath of the native collagen fibers. Initially the collagen is deposited with a random orientation. Later, during maturation of the wound, the fibers reorient according to prevailing tissue tensions, but the strictly layered lamellar pattern is not reestablished. The repair tissue does not transmit light.[16-18]

Anomalies of Corneal Wound Healing

Full-thickness lacerations of the central cornea rarely occur in isolation from other potentially complicating factors, such as hemorrhage, tissue incarceration, tissue loss, and bacterial contamination. Any of these factors may substantially alter the wound healing process. Less extensive injuries such as corneal abrasion or penetrating injury of the cornea follow the same healing process, but it is truncated at the epithelial stage for abrasions and at the stromal stage for penetrating injuries.

Uncontrolled cellular growth as an aberration of the corneal wound healing process may cause far-ranging damage to the eye. If epithelial migration is not controlled, the epithelial cells may grow on any available surface of the anterior chamber.[19] Epithelial cells covering the trabecular meshwork may cause intractable glaucoma. Similarly, endothelial cells may proliferate over the trabecular meshwork or onto the surface of the iris in cases of iris incarceration.[20] Fibrous tissue may extend from the wound[21] or be formed by metaplastic endothelial cells, creating an opaque retrocorneal fibrous plaque (posterior collagenous layer).[22]

Medical Management

Medical management of corneal wounds has been limited to antibacterials, to prevent infection, and steroids, to prevent undue inflammation and scarring. New treatment modalities are being sought to control various aspects of wound healing directly. It is now possible, through recombinant DNA technology, to produce growth-regulating proteins that are normally present in trace amounts in tissue. These substances, which have been named by the tissue of origin rather than by type of regulating activity, include epidermal growth factor (EGF), fibroblast growth factor (FGF), platelet-derived growth factor (PDGF), and many others.[23-29] Along with inhibiting factors,[30,31] they have the potential to control the cellular events of corneal healing. In addition, matrix proteins—proteins that make up the membranes and other supportive structures of tissues—applied as purified peptides may be able to selectively influence aspects of cell migration and adhesion.[9] The role of zinc and other trace metals and of certain vitamins[32] is also being investigated.

PATHOPHYSIOLOGY OF SCLERAL AND LIMBAL HEALING

Scleral Healing

The wound-healing requirements of the sclera are less rigorous. The scleral fibroblasts appear to play only a minor role in scleral wound healing. The repair tissues originate from the fibrovascular components of the episclera and the uveal tract. Fibrovascular tissue from both areas will participate in healing of full-thickness injuries of the sclera. The resulting collagen is similar to the native collagen of the sclera. With maturation of the wound, the orientation of the healed fibers will come to resemble that of the original sclera more closely than is seen in corneal tissue.

Limbal Healing

Limbal wound healing combines features of corneal and scleral wound healing. The exact nature of the wound-healing process in cataract surgery depends to a large degree on the placement of the wound. More anteriorly placed limbal wounds, not involving the substantia propria of the conjunctiva, will heal in a manner similar to more centrally placed corneal wounds. If the vascular structures of the episclera are crossed, however, wound healing is accomplished, at least in part, by direct participation of blood vessels. The surface of a limbal wound is quickly covered by corneal and conjunctival epithelial cells.[33-35] Endothelial cells in the posterior portion of the wound eventually resurface the tissue exposed to aqueous. Blood vessels from the episclera migrate through the extent of the wound along with accompanying fibrous repair tissue. Repair collagen is initially oriented perpendicular to the surface of the limbus. With maturation of the wound, collagen fibers extend across the wound, thereby increasing the tensile strength of the limbus.[36,37]

IRIS AND ANGLE CHANGES AFTER TRAUMA

Several anatomic features make the anterior uveal tract particularly vulnerable to trauma (Fig. 12-2, *A*). The sphincter muscle of the iris is supported only by delicate fibrous tissue of the iris stroma. Sudden dilation of the pupil may cause radial tears in the muscle fibers, resulting in notching of the pupillary contour. These tears rarely have functional significance.

Similarly, the iris base is attached by only a small number of collagenous fibers attached to the medial face of the ciliary body. Traction on the iris leaf may cause dialysis of the iris at this point. The major vessels that supply the iris and traverse the iris base may rupture, causing anterior chamber hemorrhage. Even when surgically reapproximated, these tissues rarely proliferate or heal.

The face of the ciliary body is exposed to variations in the hydrostatic forces of the anterior chamber. Sudden increases of intraocular pressure may cause a dissection of tissue along a plane of relative weakness between the longitudinal and oblique muscle fiber bundles (Fig. 12-2, *B*).[38] The unsupported internal muscles of the ciliary body are then displaced posteriorly, causing a contusion angle deformity. This injury may be associated with two clinically significant problems. First, the major arterial circle of the ciliary body and its rich surrounding vasculature may rupture, causing arterial hemorrhage into the anterior chamber. Second, the adjacent trabecular meshwork may be injured subclinically by the same traumatic episode, causing clinically detectable angle recession. Angle recession may then serve as a clinical marker for possible substantial damage to the filtering apparatus of the eye. Immediate or delayed intractable open- or closed-angle glaucoma may result.

The entire anterior uveal tract is anchored by the insertion of the longitudinal muscles of the ciliary body to the scleral spur. Tissue rupture (traumatic cyclodialysis) at this site allows free access of the anterior chamber fluid to the suprachoroidal space (Fig. 12-2, *C*). Increased filtration of fluid combined with dysfunction of aqueous production leads to hypotony. These tissues may abruptly reappose at a later time, reversing the hypotony and possibly causing increased intraocular pressure.

Any inflammatory process in the anterior chamber may cause peripheral anterior synechiae formation, obstructing the anterior chamber angle. The synechiae may result from mechanical displacement of tissue, adhesive factors of secondary aqueous, fibrosis of the angle struc-

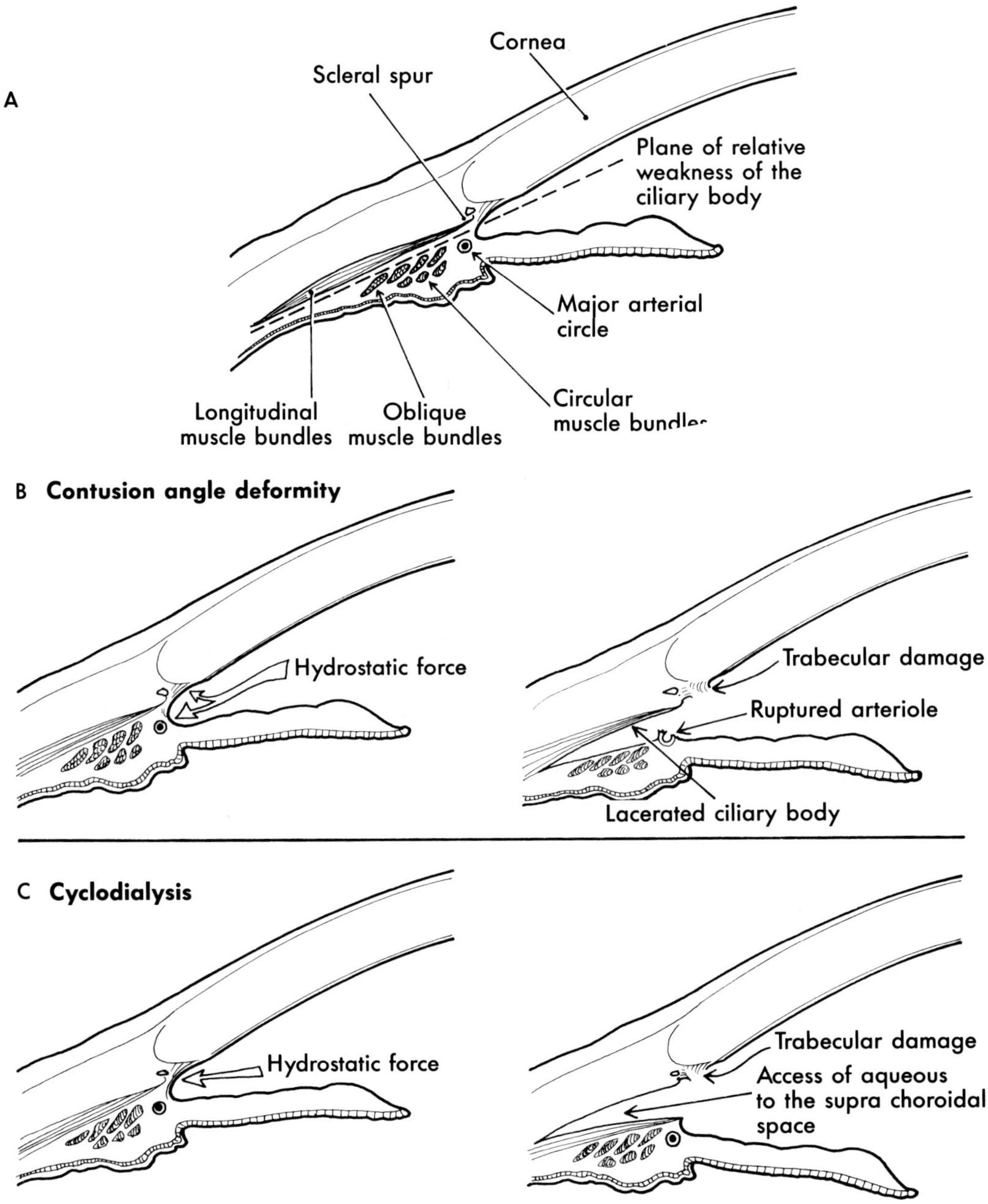

Fig. 12-2. Anterior chamber angle tissue damage from closed eye trauma. **A,** Anterior chamber angle tissue is vulnerable at the attachment of the ciliary body to the scleral spur, along the plane between the longitudinal and oblique fibers of the ciliary body, and at the trabecular meshwork. Deforming the eye by external pressure will cause an increase in anterior chamber hydrostatic pressure, which tends to be directed toward the structures of the anterior chamber angle. **B,** Contusion angle deformity results from rupture along the plane between the longitudinal and oblique muscles of the ciliary body. The potential functional damage to the eye is due to the rupture of either the rich vascular system of the ciliary body, leading to hyphema in the immediate posttrauma period, or the trabecular meshwork, leading to secondary angle glaucoma in the late posttrauma period. The angle recession is a clinical marker of the risk for hyphema or glaucoma. **C,** Cyclodialysis results from rupture of the ciliary body attachment at the scleral spur. The aqueous has unrestricted access to the suprachoroidal space, leading to altered fluid dynamics, which in turn may result in either decreased or increased intraocular pressure.

tures, or fibrovascular proliferation associated with ocular ischemia. Established synechiae are rarely reversible. Even surgical separation of the iris from the posterior cornea may not be beneficial because of associated microscopic damage and fibrosis of the trabecular meshwork.

LENS CHANGES AFTER TRAUMA

The crystalline lens is surrounded by a single layer of ectodermally derived surface epithelium that has become highly differentiated and is metabolically and immunologically isolated. These cells therefore have a limited reactive capability and are highly vulnerable.

Any physical or metabolic change in microenvironment may cause the lens epithelial cell to undergo fibrous metaplasia (i.e., transformation into a cell with characteristics of a fibroblast).[39] If the integrity of the lens capsule is maintained during injury, as in cases of anterior chamber inflammation or acute rises in intraocular pressure, an opaque fibrous plaque will form in the area of injury. Small rents in the lens capsule, as caused, for example, by trauma during paracentesis, may be healed by this process. However, with extensive exposure of the lens epithelial cells to the hostile environment of an inflamed aqueous, the epithelial cells are easily overwhelmed, causing the cells to swell, become opaque, and die, thus forming a cataract. Individual cells or small groups of cells may be protected by becoming enveloped in residual fragments of lens capsule. These cells may recover and proliferate, resulting in the formation of Elschnig's pearls.

References

1. Lindberg KA and Pinnell SR: Collagen and its disorders. In Garner A and Klintworth GK, editors: Pathobiology of ocular disease: a dynamic approach, New York, 1982, Marcel Dekker.
2. Fine BS and Yanoff M: Ocular histology: a text and atlas, New York, 1972, Harper & Row.
3. Duke-Elder S: System of ophthalmology, vol II, The anatomy of the visual system, St Louis, 1961, The CV Mosby Co.
4. Hogan MJ, Alvarado JA, and Weddell JE: Histology of the human eye, Philadelphia, 1971, WB Saunders.
5. Matsuda H and Smelser GK: Electron microscopy of corneal wound healing, Exp Eye Res 16:427-442, 1973.
6. Spencer W, editor: Ophthalmic pathology: an atlas and textbook, vol I, Philadelphia, 1985, WB Saunders.
7. Khodadoust AA et al: Adhesion of regenerating corneal epithelium: the role of the basement membrane, Am J Ophthalmol 65:339-348, 1968.
8. Buck PC: Cell migration in repair of mouse corneal epithelium, Invest Ophthalmol Vis Sci 18:767-784, 1979.
9. Cameron JD et al: Effects of matrix proteins on rabbit corneal epithelial cell adhesion and migration, Curr Eye Res 7:293-301, 1988.
10. Cameron JD, Flaxman BA, and Yanoff M: In vitro studies of corneal wound healing: epithelial-endothelial interactions, Invest Ophthalmol Vis Sci 13:575-579, 1974.
11. Danjo S, Friend J, and Thoft RA: Conjunctival epithelium in healing of corneal epithelial wounds, Invest Ophthalmol Vis Sci 28:1445-1449, 1987.
12. Kinoshita S et al: Limbal epithelium in ocular surface wound healing, Invest Ophthalmol Vis Sci 23:73-80, 1982.
13. Olsen EG and Davanger M: The healing of human corneal endothelium: an in vitro study, Acta Ophthalmol 62:885-892, 1984.
14. Matsuda H et al: Cellular migration and morphology in corneal endothelial wound repair, Invest Ophthalmol Vis Sci 26:443-449, 1985.
15. Tuft SJ, Williams KA, and Coster DJ: Endothelial repair in the rat cornea, Invest Ophthalmol Vis Sci 27:1199-1204, 1986.
16. Cintron C, Schneider H, and Kublin C: Corneal scar formation, Exp Eye Res 17:251-259, 1973.
17. Cintron C and Kublin CL: Regeneration of corneal tissue, Dev Biol 61:346-357, 1977.
18. Davison PF and Galbavy EJ: Connective tissue remodeling in corneal and scleral wounds, Invest Ophthalmol Vis Sci 27:1478-1484, 1986.
19. Weiner MJ et al: Epithelial downgrowth: a 30-year clinicopathological review, Br J Ophthalmol 73:6-11, 1989.
20. Colosi NJ and Yanoff M: Reactive corneal endothelialization, Am J Ophthalmol 83:219-224, 1977.
21. Bloomfield SE, Jakobiec FA, and Iwamoto T: Fibrous ingrowth with retrocorneal membrane, Ophthalmology 88:459-465, 1981.
22. Waring GO III: Posterior collagenous layer of the cornea: ultrastructural classification of abnormal collagenous tissue posterior to Descemet's membrane in 30 cases, Arch Ophthalmol 100:1022-1034, 1982.
23. Fujikawa LS et al: Fibronectin in healing rabbit corneal wounds, Lab Invest 45:120-129, 1981.
24. Nishida T et al: Fibronectin enhancement of corneal epithelial wound healing of rabbits in vivo, Arch Ophthalmol 102:455-456, 1984.

25. Brightwell JR et al: Biosynthetic human EGF accelerates healing of neodecadron-treated primate corneas, Invest Ophthalmol Vis Sci 26:105-110, 1985.
26. Singh G and Foster CS: Epidermal growth factor in alkali-burned corneal epithelial wound healing, Am J Ophthalmol 103:802-807, 1987.
27. Mathers WD and Jester JV: Full thickness corneal wound strength enhancement by epidermal growth factor, Invest Ophthalmol Vis Sci 29(ARVO suppl):312, 1988.
28. Woost PG et al: Enhancement of corneal endothelial cell mitosis in corneal storage media using EGF and other defined agents, Invest Ophthalmol Vis Sci 29(ARVO suppl):112, 1988.
29. Hersh PS: Effects of platelet-derived growth factor on cultured keratocytes and its uptake by the cornea, Invest Ophthalmol Vis Sci 29(ARVO suppl):313, 1988.
30. Del Vecchio PJ et al: Inhibition of human scleral fibroblast proliferation with heparin, Invest Ophthalmol Vis Sci 29:1272-1276, 1988.
31. McGuigan LJ et al: D-penicillamine and β-aminopropionitrile effects on experimental filtering surgery, Invest Ophthalmol Vis Sci 28:1625-1629, 1987.
32. Kastl PR et al: Topical vitamin A ointment increases healing of cataract incisions, Ann Ophthalmol 19:175-177, 1987.
33. Desjardins DC et al: Wound healing after filtering surgery in owl monkeys, Arch Ophthalmol 104:1835-1839, 1986.
34. Geggel HS, Friend J, and Thoft RA: Conjunctival epithelial wound healing, Invest Ophthalmol Vis Sci 25:860-863, 1984.
35. Jampel HD et al: Cellular proliferation after experimental glaucoma filtration surgery, Arch Ophthalmol 106:89-94, 1988.
36. Flaxel JT and Swan KC: Limbal wound healing after cataract extraction, Arch Ophthalmol 81:653-659, 1969.
37. Flaxel JT: Histology of cataract extractions, Arch Ophthalmol 83:436-444, 1970.
38. Wolff SM and Zimmerman LE: Chronic secondary glaucoma: associated with retrodisplacement of iris root and deepening of the anterior chamber angle secondary to contusion, Am J Ophthalmol 54:547-563, 1962.
39. Font RA and Brownstein S: A light and electron microscopic study of anterior subcapsular cataracts, Am J Ophthalmol 78:972-984, 1974.

CHAPTER 13

Management of corneoscleral lacerations

PETER S. HERSH
BRADFORD J. SHINGLETON
KENNETH R. KENYON

Preoperative management
Injury hierarchy and repair techniques
- Nonperforating corneal lacerations
- Simple full-thickness corneal lacerations
  - Bandage soft contact lens
  - Tissue adhesive
  - Corneal sutures
- Stellate corneal lacerations
- Corneal laceration with iris incarceration
- Corneal laceration with lens involvement
- Corneal laceration with vitreous involvement
- Simple corneoscleral lacerations
- Corneoscleral lacerations with uveal and vitreous prolapse
- Posterior scleral lacerations
- Corneoscleral lacerations with tissue loss
  - Lamellar inlay grafting
  - Full-thickness patch grafting
  - Penetrating keratoplasty
- Irreparable Penetrating Injury

Postoperative management
References

The primary objective of surgery for penetrating corneoscleral injuries is complete, watertight closure of the globe with restoration of structural integrity. Secondary goals include removal of disrupted lens and vitreous, avoidance of uveal and vitreous incarceration in the wound, removal of intraocular foreign bodies, and restoration of normal anatomic relationships with minimal tissue distortion. When one considers the appropriate surgical management of these diverse injuries, it is useful to follow a hierarchical protocol starting with the most simple laceration and progressing to more complex injuries and repair techniques. Such a systematic approach allows for stepwise planning and control at each step during surgical repair. Following this management protocol will bring the eye into a progressively simpler injury configuration, with each new stage calling for a relatively standard surgical approach.

PREOPERATIVE MANAGEMENT

A complete eye examination is performed preoperatively to ascertain the extent of damage and rule out an intraocular foreign body or infection. Radiologic testing and appropriate microbial cultures are obtained. (See Chapters 1 to 3 for a detailed discussion of the preoperative management of the lacerated globe.)

In general, broad-spectrum intravenous antibiotics are administered for prophylaxis of infection. For "routine" cases, one commonly used regimen includes cefazolin (1 g every 6 hours) and gentamicin (80 mg every 8 hours adjusted for body weight and renal status) for 3 to 5 days. In some cases, vancomycin may be preferred to the cephalosporin. Topical antibiotics typically are avoided preoperatively in an open globe to prevent inadvertent intraocular administration and lid squeezing with additional damage to intraocular contents. Antibiotic therapy is modified as dictated by culture results, and any sign of new infection is cultured promptly. Prevention and treatment of posttraumatic endophthalmitis are discussed in Chapter 23.

INJURY HIERARCHY AND REPAIR TECHNIQUES

Nonperforating Corneal Lacerations

All suspected nonperforating corneal lacerations must be examined carefully to rule out occult perforation of Descemet's membrane. Seidel's test with 2% fluorescein should be performed to check for microscopic leaks (Color Plate 13-1). Provocation with gentle finger pressure against the upper lid during testing might reveal an otherwise self-sealing wound. Because many small perforating injuries will self-seal as a result of stromal swelling when raw stroma is exposed to tears and aqueous fluid after breakdown of the epithelial and endothelial barriers, Descemet's membrane should be examined closely with the slit beam in search of breaks. This distinction is of utmost importance because the finding of an intraocular entry site, no matter how small, drastically changes management strategy. All perforating injuries are at risk for endophthalmitis and require patient hospitalization for antibiotic therapy, whereas a partial-thickness injury often may be treated on an outpatient basis.

The treatment goals in a nonperforating corneal laceration include the prevention of infection and optimization of reepithelialization and stromal healing (see Chapter 6). Also important are efforts to minimize scarring and postoperative surface irregularity that may cause poor epithelial adhesion and irregular astigmatism (see Chapter 14 for a detailed discussion of topographic considerations in wound repair).

If the edges of the wound are not overriding and there is no significant wound gape, pressure patching with an antibiotic ointment may be sufficient to promote epithelialization and subsequent stromal repair. If the wound is somewhat unstable (for example, deep nonperforating injury), a bandage soft contact lens may be used to support the wound by its splinting effect and to enhance reepithelialization by shielding the cornea from lid movement (Fig. 13-1).

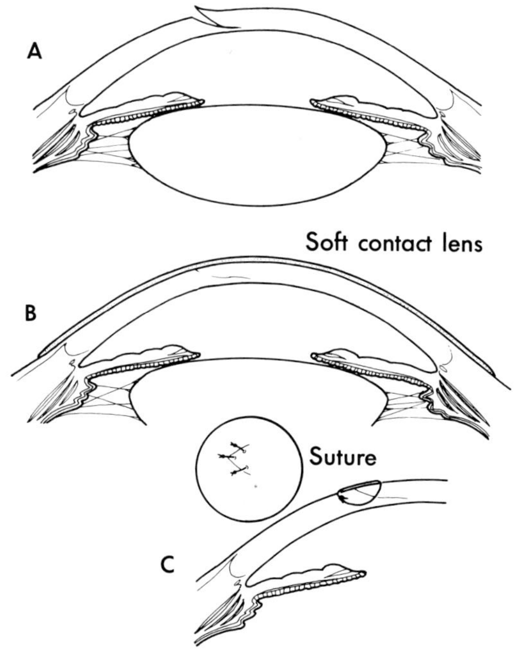

Fig. 13-1. **A,** Partial-thickness, bevelled corneal laceration. **B,** Wound is splinted and protected by bandage soft contact lens. **C,** Wound secured with sutures. Note orientation of sutures toward apex of the triangular avulsion to improve tissue apposition.

A number of bandage soft contact lenses are available. In trauma cases, thicker, stiffer, larger lenses are generally preferred because of their greater stability and ability to splint the cornea. The durable Bausch & Lomb Plano T lens is often useful in the trauma setting. Other thicker, high–water content lenses such as Permalens (Cooper) and Sauflon (Visiontech) may be better tolerated by some corneas. For cases with persistent epithelial defects, these high–water content lenses or a thin lens such as the CSI or Bausch & Lomb O-series may be preferred. In any case, the lens must be fitted properly to ensure adequate oxygenation and patient comfort. To improve wound stabilization, excessive lens movement should be avoided.

While the bandage lens is in place, antibiotic prophylaxis is recommended. An aminoglycoside drop given 2 to 4 times daily is well tolerated and gives broad coverage. A cycloplegic should be used to prevent ciliary spasm and reduce discomfort. The lens should remain in place until the stromal wound has become relatively stabilized (3 to 6 weeks) and epithelialization is complete. In cases where epithelialization is problematic, the lens should be kept in place for about 2 months to allow formation of epithelial-basement membrane adhesion complexes, thus minimizing subsequent recurrent erosion.

Occasionally a flap of tissue will be avulsed from the cornea, remaining attached at its base. Although a bandage soft contact lens may stabilize the tissue in its proper position, in some cases sutures may be necessary to ensure good reapproximation (Fig. 13-1). Sutures also may be advisable in some long, partial-thickness wounds and in those with significant wound override or gape. The principles of corneal suturing discussed later in the chapter also apply in these cases.

Simple Full-Thickness Corneal Lacerations

For this discussion, a simple corneal laceration is defined as one that does not violate the limbus and has neither iris, lens, or vitreous incarceration nor traumatic lens damage. A number of treatment modalities are available.

Bandage Soft Contact Lens

For small, self-sealing corneal perforations, a bandage lens may be sufficient to protect and support the wound as it heals. Bandage lenses are often useful for nondisplaced, bevelled, or edematous lacerations less than 3 mm in length, particularly if self-sealing (Fig. 13-2). The selection of lens type is similar to that described for partial-thickness lacerations.

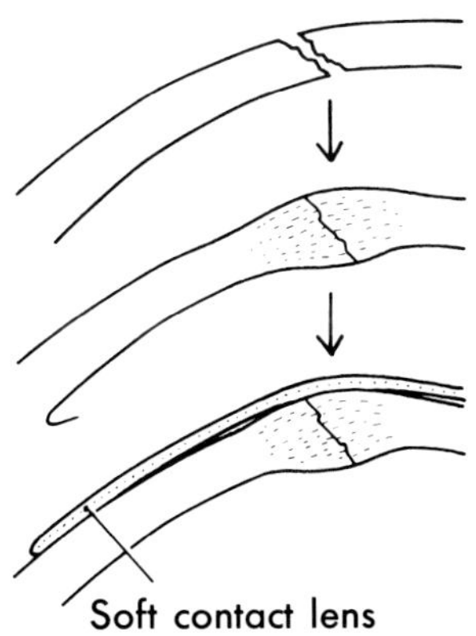

Fig. 13-2. Corneal stroma swells and self-seals laceration. Bandage soft contact lens supports and protects wound.

If, after lens application, the anterior chamber reforms and remains stable, further intervention is often unnecessary. However, if the chamber does not reform in 24 hours, if aqueous leakage persists, if there is progressive shallowing of the anterior chamber, or if iris or lens incarceration supervenes, further surgical intervention is warranted. In cases where follow-up is uncertain or in children who may accidentally traumatize the wound, treatment exclusively with a bandage soft contact lens should be undertaken only with extreme caution.

In cases that respond satisfactorily, the lens should be kept in place until the wound has stabilized, usually 3 to 6 weeks. A protective metal shield should be worn at all times. Topical antibiotic prophylaxis and cycloplegia are recommended with the lens in place.

Tissue Adhesive

Cyanoacrylate tissue adhesive is useful either alone or as adjunctive treatment for puncture wounds with small amounts of central tissue loss, stellate wounds with poor central apposition, selected small (< 2 mm) lacerations that do not self-seal, and those that would require excessive suture placement in the visual axis (Color Plate 13-2).

Application of the adhesive is best performed with the patient lying down under the operating microscope. In cooperative patients, the adhesive may be applied at the slit-lamp. Topical anesthesia is used and a lid speculum placed. Using jeweler's forceps, dry cellulose sponges, or the back edge of a scarifier type of blade, the epithelium is removed carefully for 1 to 2 mm around the perforation site to allow for adhesion. The site of application is then dried meticulously with cellulose sponges. If the perforation persistently leaks and wets the site, cellulose sponges may be used to carefully drain some aqueous immediately before applying the tissue adhesive.

A capillary microapplicator or fine-gauge disposable needle may be used to apply a very thin film of adhesive over the site (Fig. 13-3). Alternatively, adhesive may be applied using a sterile 2- to 4-mm polyethylene or silicone disc affixed to the end of an applicator stick with sterile ophthalmic ointment, with the tissue adhesive placed in mortarboard fashion (Fig. 13-4).[1] The disc may be left in place or removed with care.

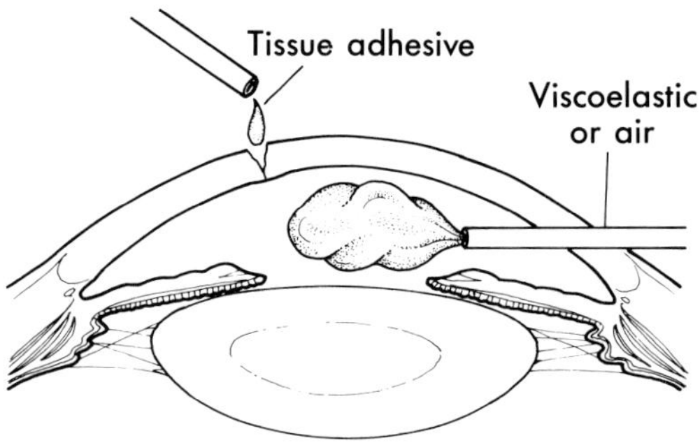

Fig. 13-3. Application of tissue adhesive using a capillary microapplicator or fine-gauge needle. The anterior chamber is maintained with viscoelastic or air.

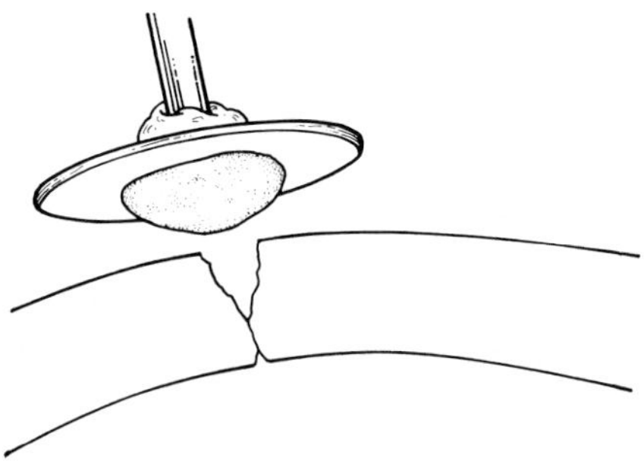

Fig. 13-4. Tissue adhesive applied with a polyethylene or silicone disc affixed to the end of an applicator stick.

In an eye with a shallow anterior chamber, a viscoelastic or air may be irrigated through the wound or a separate paracentesis incision to deepen the chamber and prevent iris incarceration during adhesive placement. After application, the lid speculum is kept in place for 3 to 5 minutes to allow for polymerization of the adhesive.

The efficacy of the application may be ascertained by performing a Seidel test with 2% fluorescein or awaiting spontaneous reformation of the anterior chamber (usually within 30 minutes). A bandage soft contact lens should be applied over the dried tissue adhesive; the Bausch & Lomb Plano T lens is preferable because of its durability.

The tissue adhesive is often dislodged with time as the wound surface reepithelializes. Alternatively, it may be gently removed with forceps in 6 to 8 weeks if the glued area has vascularized (peripheral wound) or in 12 to 16 weeks after adequate stromal scar formation (central wound). Despite its efficacy, cyanoacrylate is not currently approved for clinical use by the U.S. Food and Drug Administration.

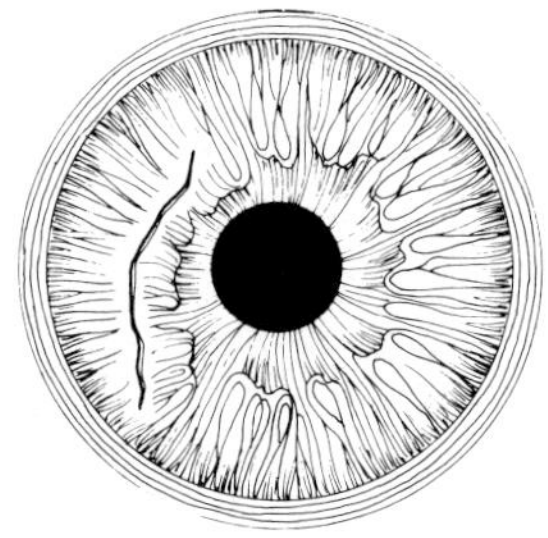

Fig. 13-5. Simple corneal laceration.

Corneal Sutures

Most corneal lacerations require suture placement (Fig. 13-5). Prompt, secure wound closure is especially important in children, who are at greater risk of inadvertently rubbing the eye with consequent reopening of a tissue adhesive– or contact lens–supported wound. Large lacerations (> 2 to 3 mm), displaced wounds, wounds with loss of corneal tissue, and lacerations with accompanying iris or lens incarceration are not amenable to treatment with a bandage soft contact lens or tissue adhesive. Patients with such conditions must be brought to the operating room for surgical repair and suture placement.

Presurgical preparation and appropriate anesthesia for the patient with an open globe are discussed in detail in Chapters 3 and 4. Surgery is performed under general anesthesia unless medically contraindicated or in selected cases of small or self-sealing wounds. Rarely, with extremely cooperative patients, topical anesthesia may suffice.

The eye is prepared and draped, and a lid speculum is placed using caution to avoid applying pressure to the globe. If a speculum cannot be used without undue pressure to the eye, lid retraction sutures of 4-0 silk may be used. In simple corneal lacerations, stay sutures may be unnecessary. If stabilization or manipulation of the globe is necessary, stay sutures of 6-0 silk may be placed at the limbus 90° to the wound, again taking care not to press on the eye. It may also be possible to place rectus bridle sutures after the wound is stabilized with sutures. Bridle

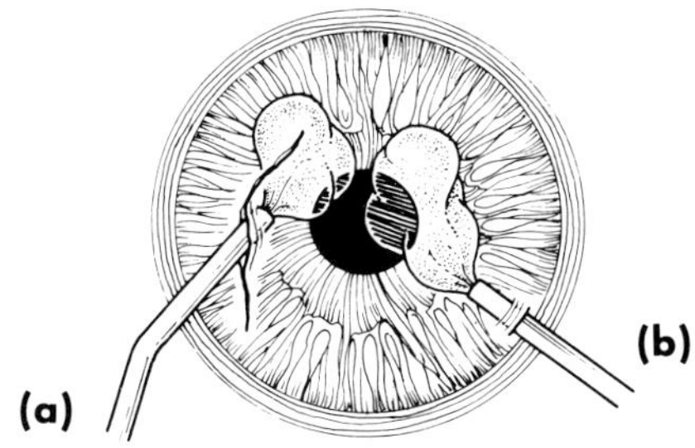

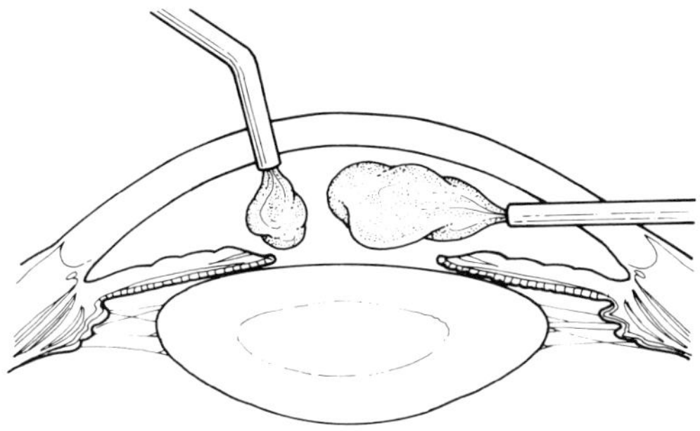

Fig. 13-6. Anterior chamber is maintained with viscoelastic or air irrigated through *a*, the wound itself or *b*, limbal paracentesis site.

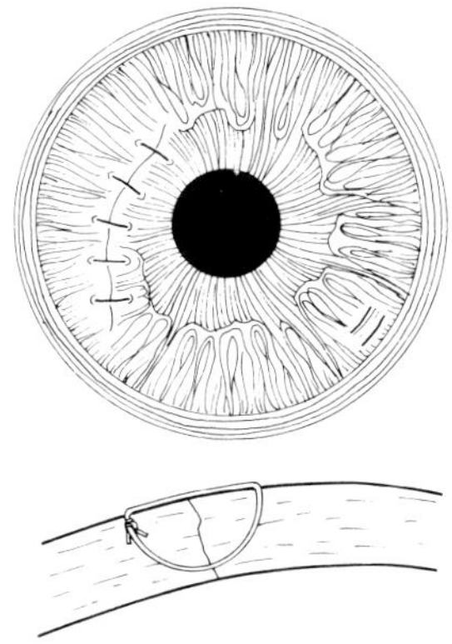

Fig. 13-7. Simple corneal laceration closed with interrupted sutures. Note symmetric and deep suture placement. Paracentesis site at 10 o'clock (surgeon's view) has been used for intraocular manipulation.

sutures placed initially in the open globe may apply untoward pressure and cause chamber flattening and tissue incarceration.

A relatively watertight wound with a formed anterior chamber may be sutured directly. If the anterior chamber will remain formed during suturing, the eye need not be entered with instruments. If the wound is less stable, however, a viscoelastic should be irrigated into the anterior chamber either directly through the wound or through a separate limbal stab incision to maintain the chamber and protect the lens, iris, and corneal endothelium (Fig. 13-6). Air may also be used for chamber reformation.

In many cases a limbal stab incision is preferable, because it is often less traumatic than repeatedly disrupting the wound edges with instruments and may provide better access.[2] Importantly, this site also may be used to sweep the wound and reposition the iris if tissue incarceration supervenes. The limbal incision may be made with a 15° sharp microsurgical knife and should be placed approximately 90° from the wound, where it can be used to best advantage. In an eye with a flat chamber, care should be taken to avoid damage to the iris or lens.

Regardless of whether initial reformation of the anterior chamber is necessary, the ultimate goal of corneal suturing is definitive placement of corneal sutures to make the wound watertight, minimize scarring, and reconstruct the native nonastigmatic corneal contour. If initial placement of deep, definitive sutures would cause loss of the anterior chamber, it is useful to place temporary sutures first. Although such temporary sutures may be shallow and less than optimally positioned, they may be placed without wound distortion and chamber collapse, subsequently allowing more accurate placement of the final definitive sutures. The number of temporary sutures should be minimized, however, to avoid trauma to the wound margins and surrounding stroma.

Monofilament 10-0 nylon suture material on a fine spatula-design microsurgical needle is used for corneal suturing (Color Plate 13-3). Some surgeons prefer the even finer 11-0 nylon suture for work near the visual axis. A number of strategies for corneal suturing are available. The simplest involves progressively halving the wound with simple interrupted sutures. These definitive corneal sutures should be approximately 1.5 mm long, approximately 90% deep in the stroma, and of equal depth on both sides of the wound (Fig. 13-7). Shallow sutures will cause internal wound gape; sutures that are asymmetric or of unequal depth will result in wound override. Conversely, full-thickness bites should be avoided, because the suture may then act as a conduit for microbial invasion from the ocular surface. In shelved lacerations, sutures should be placed equidistant with respect to the internal aspect of the wound and tied without undue tension to optimize tissue apposition (see Chapter 14). Wounds with macerated or edematous margins may require longer sutures for security.

Suture bites through the visual axis should be avoided. If sutures must be placed near the visual axis, a number of techniques can be used to minimize scarring. First, the suture bite proximal to the central cornea may be made shorter, avoiding the visual axis. Second, the visual axis may be straddled by sutures placed at each side of, but not directly through, the axis itself. Finally, a no-touch technique, in which forceps are used to secure the globe away from the cornea rather than at the wound margin, may be used (Fig. 13-8). The tip of the suture needle is placed perpendicular to the corneal surface, and the needle is rotated through the wound following its curvature. If this is done properly, the corneal tissue is not distorted, the anterior chamber remains formed, the wound margin is not disrupted with forceps, and suture placement is effected as atraumatically as possible.

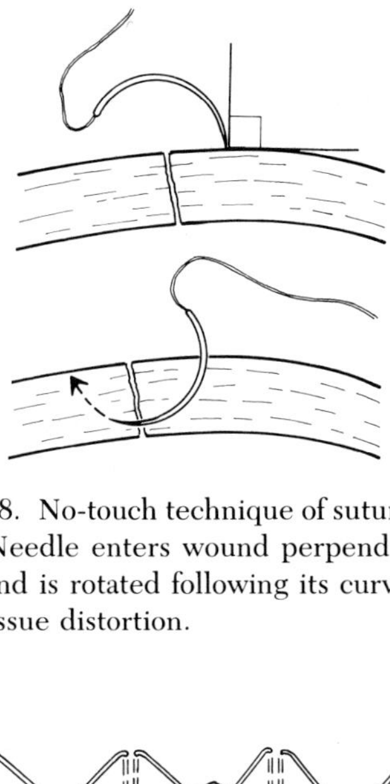

Fig. 13-8. No-touch technique of suture placement. Needle enters wound perpendicular to tissue and is rotated following its curvature to avoid tissue distortion.

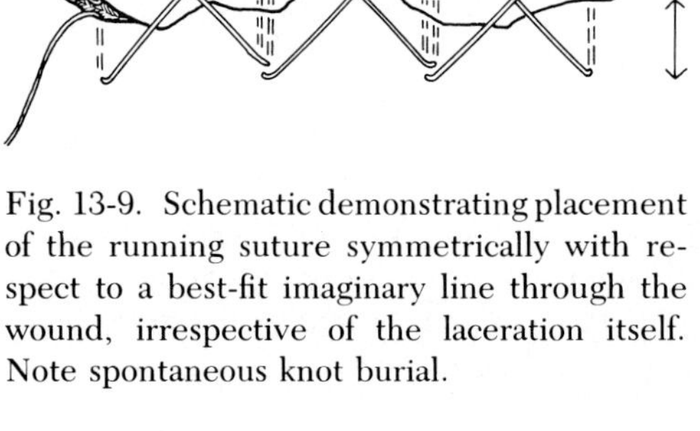

Fig. 13-9. Schematic demonstrating placement of the running suture symmetrically with respect to a best-fit imaginary line through the wound, irrespective of the laceration itself. Note spontaneous knot burial.

With increased understanding of corneal topography and the micromechanical effects of incisions and suturing on corneal contour, a number of different suture techniques and patterns have been suggested.[3] In some cases of straight lacerations, a running shoestring closure may minimize astigmatism and facilitate subsequent suture removal (Color Plate 13-4). A running suture, however, will tend to linearize and thus distort an irregular or curvilinear wound. If a running suture is used, therefore, the bites should be placed perpendicular and equidistant to a best-fit imaginary line through the wound, irrespective of the laceration itself (Fig. 13-9). In contradistinction, when using an interrupted suture technique for curvilinear or irregular lacerations, all sutures should be placed perpendicular to the wound to avoid transverse shifting of the wound margins.

Complicated lacerations require planning to achieve optimal wound approximation with minimal distortion. Perpendicular rather than beveled areas of the wound are sutured first, and an irregular wound is divided into relatively straight segments before proceeding with usual suture techniques. Moreover, strategic placement of long, deep sutures at the wound's periphery combined with shorter, shallower appositional sutures toward the visual axis may resurrect the normal corneal contour.[4] Such techniques and their theoretical mechanical underpinnings are discussed in detail in Chapter 14.

A locked 2-1-1 knot or a 1-1-1 slipknot may facilitate subsequent suture removal compared with a standard 3-1-1 surgeon's knot, which may be relatively large. To minimize scarring, all knots should be trimmed short and superficially buried on the side away from the visual axis. The ends of the buried knot should be directed away from the surface to facilitate subsequent removal (Fig. 13-10).

After repair, the anterior chamber may be deepened through either the paracentesis or the wound itself. The wound should be checked for leaks by using gentle pressure with a dry cellulose sponge. Fluorescein 2% may also be used to verify watertightness. Usually, the paracentesis is self-sealing and may be left unsutured. If leaking, it may be closed with one 10-0 nylon suture.

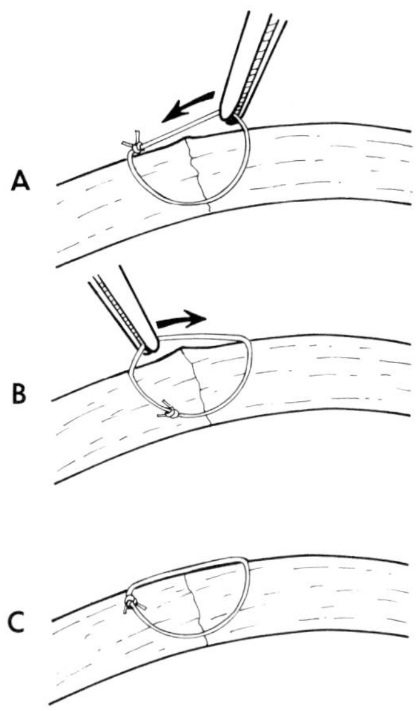

Fig. 13-10. Technique of burying suture knot. **A,** The knot is trimmed short and rotated beneath the surface with smooth forceps. **B,** The orientation of the knot is reversed, directing the cut ends away from the surface to facilitate subsequent suture removal. **C,** The knot is buried superficially on the side of the wound away from the visual axis.

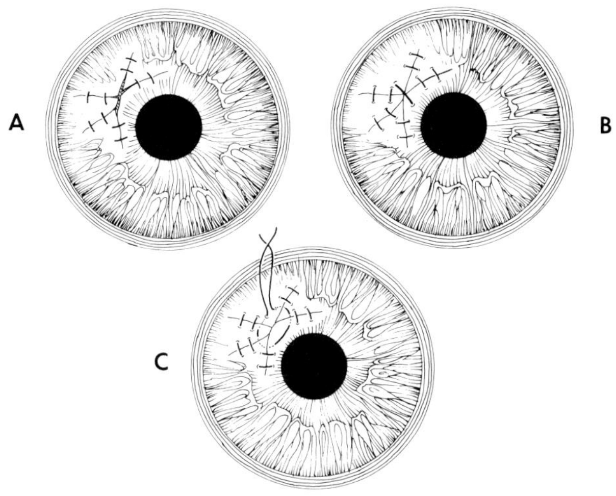

Fig. 13-11. **A,** Multiple simple interrupted sutures may not adequately close stellate laceration. **B,** Bridge suture used to close center of laceration. **C,** Pursestring suture technique.

Stellate Corneal Lacerations

Achieving watertight closure of stellate lacerations and partial tissue avulsions presents a challenge. Techniques useful for a stellate laceration include multiple interrupted sutures, bridging sutures, and pursestring sutures (see Chapter 14) (Fig. 13-11). Occasionally, the center of a stellate laceration is difficult to appose and persistently leaks, requiring bandage lens application, tissue adhesive or patch grafting.

Some avulsive injuries result in a pedicle flap of tissue. This should be properly repositioned and sutured with minimal tissue distortion. Sutures should be angled toward the apex of such a wound to pull the avulsed tissue back into place (Fig. 13-1).

Corneal Laceration with Iris Incarceration

Often after an extensive corneal laceration, the anterior chamber will shallow with consequent iris incarceration or actual prolapse from the wound. If prolapsed, the tissue must be critically evaluated with regard to the advisability of tissue repositioning versus excision. Obviously devitalized tissue should be excised, as should extremely macerated, feathery, or depigmented iris. Certainly, any foreign body that is present within the tissue should be removed. Especially if laceration repair is delayed more than 24 hours, the tissue should be inspected for signs of surface epithelialization, and if present, the affected iris should be excised to avoid seeding the anterior chamber with epithelial cells that may subsequently proliferate. Finally, tissue that has been prolapsed for over 24 hours generally should be removed to minimize infectious risks. Healthy-appearing tissue occasionally may be repositioned with caution even after this time period.

If excision is necessary, the tissue is grasped with fine forceps but not pulled from the wound (Fig. 13-12). It is cut flush with the cornea using Vannas scissors. This technique conserves tissue and prevents further iris damage. In all cases, the surgeon should attempt to preserve as much tissue as possible to maintain a normal iris diaphragm and conserve tissue for subsequent reconstructive efforts.

During surgery, attention is directed toward both properly repositing incarcerated tissues and definitively closing the corneal wound. A flat or shallow anterior chamber should first be deepened with either a viscoelastic or air. Occasionally this may be done directly through the wound but, more frequently, preliminary placement of a paracentesis site, as previously described, affords easier access and better control.

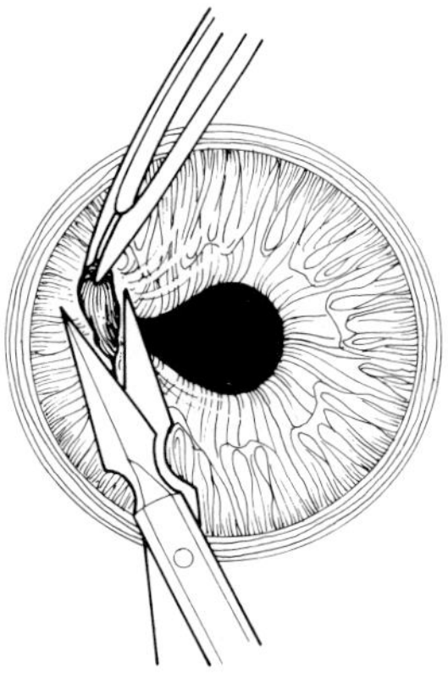

Fig. 13-12. Excision of prolapsed iris. Tissue is grasped without tension and cut flush with wound.

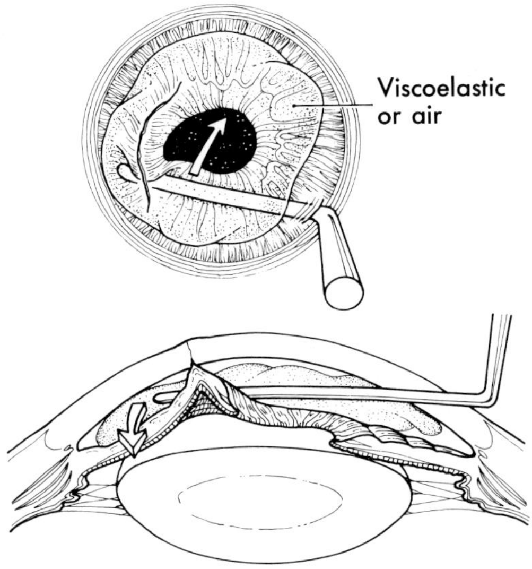

Fig. 13-13. Technique of iris repositioning. Anterior chamber is maintained with viscoelastic or air. Vitreous sweep, placed through paracentesis site, is used to remove incarcerated tissue from the wound.

Occasionally, the wound architecture does not allow for chamber reformation. In such cases, preliminary, temporary corneal sutures may be placed to stabilize the wound for chamber deepening.

In some instances of minimal incarceration, iris repositioning may be achieved pharmacologically. Intraocular acetylcholine or carbachol is irrigated into the anterior chamber, the consequent pupillary constriction pulling the iris atraumatically from the wound. If the iris is incarcerated in the central cornea, mydriasis with intraocular epinephrine 1:10,000 may have a similar effect.

More often than not, however, the incarcerated tissue must be mechanically reposited. Simply deepening the chamber may pull incarcerated tissues from the wound. Viscoelastic irrigated through the wound or paracentesis site and directed toward the incarcerated iris may be effective in mobilizing the tissue.[5] The mainstay of iris repositioning, however, remains direct sweeping with a spatula (e.g., cyclodialysis spatula or vitreous sweep) or irrigating cannula. After chamber deepening, the spatula is placed through the paracentesis site, advanced behind the incarcerated tissue, and carefully swept through the tissue, dragging it from the wound (Fig. 13-13). Care is taken to avoid causing iatrogenic iridodialysis or damage to the corneal endothelium and lens.

If excessive bleeding from the iris or anterior chamber angle is encountered, a number of interventions are valuable. First, irrigation of viscoelastic around the bleeding site can keep the blood localized, preserving the surgeon's view while preventing leakage of blood into the vitreous in an aphakic eye. In a globe already watertight, increasing the intraocular pressure with infusion may tamponade the bleeding site. Bleeding may also be controlled pharmacologically. Epinephrine 1:10,000 may be irrigated into the anterior chamber, causing vessel constriction. The use of intraocular thrombin (100 units/ml) has been advocated for hemostasis in vitrectomy surgery and would probably be useful in the anterior chamber as well.[6] However, there have been conflicting reports regarding adverse effects on the corneal endothelium.[7,8] Finally, where a bleeding site is visible, it may be directly cauterized. A fine-gauge, underwater bipolar cautery (Mentor) is especially useful in this situation. Alternatively, bimanual, bipolar diathermy may be used. In this technique, alligator clips are placed on the ends of each lead of the cautery wire. These are clipped to two intraocular instruments (e.g., irrigating cannula, spatula, vitrector tip), which then act as the two poles of the cautery (Fig. 13-14).[9]

After adequate iris repositing, the corneal laceration is sutured as previously described and the wound is carefully inspected for any remaining tissue incarceration. If necessary, sweeping is again performed through the para-

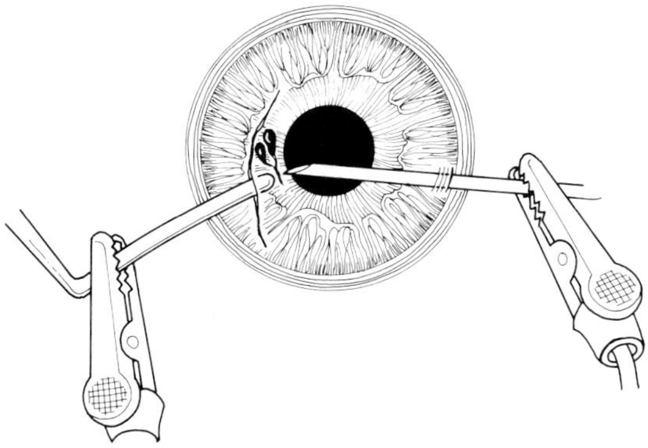

Fig. 13-14. Technique of bipolar, bimanual diathermy. Alligator clips from cautery leads are placed on intraocular instruments, which are used to cauterize the bleeding site.

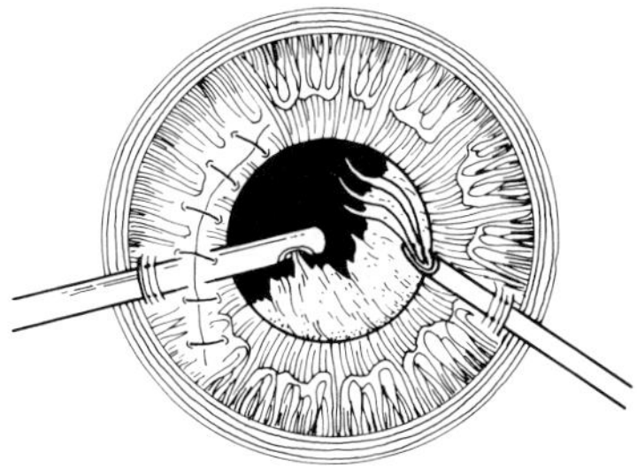

Fig. 13-15. Bimanual lensectomy performed through limbal entry site using microvitrectomy instrumentation.

centesis. An air bubble may be placed in cases in which iris strands tend to migrate anteriorly into the wound. The anterior chamber is fully restored through the paracentesis site and, finally, the wound is tested for leakage.

Corneal Laceration with Lens Involvement

Eyes with large corneal lacerations and concomitant iris involvement often have lens disruption as well. Small penetrating injuries, especially those caused by small projectiles or puncture wounds, also may cause significant lens damage.

The decision about lens removal depends on critical preoperative and intraoperative assessment. The removal of a cataractous lens is rarely an emergency procedure. Of course, if assessment is correct and surgical visualization adequate, it is better to complete all operative interventions at a single surgical session.[10] However, a number of situations would make lens extraction inadvisable in the setting of an acute injury. For instance, a fibrinous anterior chamber reaction and pupillary membrane may occasionally masquerade as a flocculent cataract.[11] Moreover, poor visualization through an edematous cornea makes immediate lens intervention inadvisable. Waiting even just a few days often will allow the cornea to clear, the fibrin to resorb, and inflammation to abate, optimizing subsequent lens removal. When in doubt, the lens should be left undisturbed and, if necessary, removed in a second procedure.

A number of factors support primary removal of the lens. A lens with disrupted capsule and flocculent cortical material liberated into the anterior chamber is best removed to prevent ongoing phacogenic postoperative inflammation (Color Plate 13-5). An admixture of lens remnants and violated vitreous also should be addressed in the primary procedure if possible. A clearly cataractous lens may be removed in the initial surgery. Importantly, however, a stable lens with an intact capsule and without liberated cortical material can be treated in a secondary procedure. In any case, lens intervention should be undertaken only under controlled circumstances with the appropriate equipment and good visualization.

Before attention is turned to the lens in the lacerated globe, all tissues are reposited and the cornea sutured as described. The nature of the injury will dictate the lens removal technique appropriate in a particular setting. If the lens capsule is intact, standard cataract extraction techniques may be used. Because much eye trauma occurs in a young population, the lens may often be removed through a small incision using manual or automated aspiration techniques. Extracapsular cataract extraction and phacoemulsification also may be used if the posterior capsule has not been violated (Color Plate 13-6). After repair of the laceration, the necessary section is made and surgery done in standard fashion. However, the surgeon always should be aware of the possibility of poor zonular integrity in the posttrauma patient and plan nucleus delivery techniques accordingly.

In cases with capsular rupture, significant vitreous involvement, or lens dislocation, lensectomy techniques using microvitrectomy instrumentation are advisable (Fig. 13-15). Surgery may be done from either the limbus or pars plana depending on the surgeon's preference. Usually the lens-vitreous admixture can be removed using aspiration and cutting alone. Sonication may be necessary with hard nuclei. At the conclusion of surgery, all lens remnants should have been removed and all vitreous cleared from the anterior chamber.

The propriety of intraocular lens placement at initial trauma surgery is as yet controversial, especially given the youth of the patient population. In patients of appropriate age, a posterior chamber intraocular lens would be suitable if the posterior capsule were intact. If a vitrectomy is necessary in older adults, an anterior chamber lens could be used if all cortical remnants and anterior segment vitreous strands have been removed. Posterior chamber lenses may also be placed in the absence of capsular support, suspended by iris or transcleral sutures.[12,13] This requires adequate anterior vitrectomy. The advisability of such a procedure in the acute setting of ocular trauma remains to be seen.

Chapter 11 further describes the management of traumatic lens injuries.

Corneal Laceration with Vitreous Involvement

Violation of the vitreous face frequently accompanies corneal laceration with lens involvement (Color Plate 13-7). The primary goal in the acute surgical setting is to relieve any vitreous incarceration in traumatic or surgical wounds. This helps prevent the associated complications of chronic inflammation, cystoid macular edema, vitreous fibrosis and retinal detachment, and infection mediated by a vitreous wick exposed to the environment. It is important to remove disrupted vitreous from the anterior chamber to minimize subsequent corneal endothelial damage.

Automated microvitrectomy instrumentation is preferred. Bimanual techniques are particularly useful to optimize control. Surgery may be performed through limbal, pars plana, or combined limbal irrigation/pars plana cutting sites, depending on the surgeon's preference and the surgical situation. An irrigation sleeve also may be used, allowing vitrectomy through a single limbal site or the wound itself.

Definitive attention usually is given to the vitreous after iris repositing and wound closure. Before closing, however, vitreous should be removed as best as possible from the wound. If visualization allows, the vitrectomy probe may be placed directly through the wound or through the paracentesis site. Often, however, the chamber is flat, and placing the vitrector through the wound would cause further disruption. In such cases, the wound may be freed of vitreous using dry cellulose sponges to attach, immobilize, and gently withdraw gel without placing it under traction. The vitreous is then cut flush with the wound using sharp, spring-action scissors (Fig. 13-16).

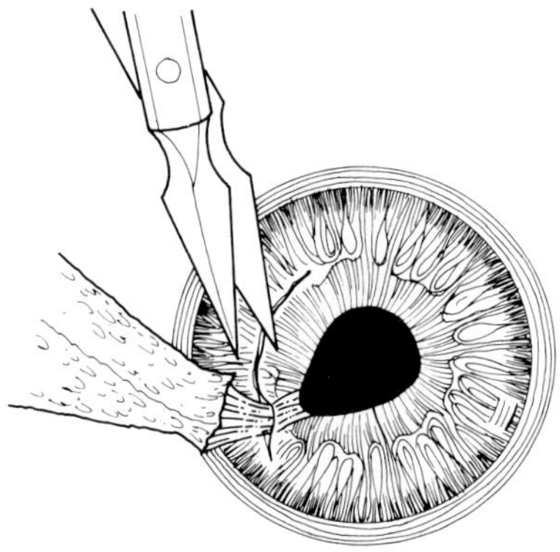

Fig. 13-16. Dry cellulose sponges gently withdraw vitreous strands, which are cut flush with the wound. Traction on the vitreous should be minimized.

After wound closure, limbal entry sites are prepared and vitrectomy performed to the extent necessary. Vitreous strands to the wound are lysed, cortical remnants removed, and anterior vitrectomy performed if necessary. High cutting rates (approximately 400 cps) and low suction (approximately 100 mm Hg) should be used. Lower cutting and higher suction will be required to remove lens remnants and intraocular membranes.

The wound may be swept with a vitreous sweep via the paracentesis site to dislodge any remaining incarcerated vitreous, observing the pupil for movement or peaking, which indicate overriding vitreous strands (Fig. 13-17). Acetylcholine solution is irrigated into the anterior chamber to constrict the pupil, making areas of peaking more apparent. Moreover, an air bubble may be placed to better visualize and tamponade remaining vitreous. A fiberoptic light pipe may also aid identification of further vitreous strands. Additional vitrectomy is performed if needed. After vitrectomy, the pupil should be round without peaking, the wound free of incarceration, and the vitreous behind the iris.

Simple Corneoscleral Lacerations

Lacerations extending beyond the limbus and into the sclera should be explored to delineate their full extent. Fixation sutures of 6-0 silk may

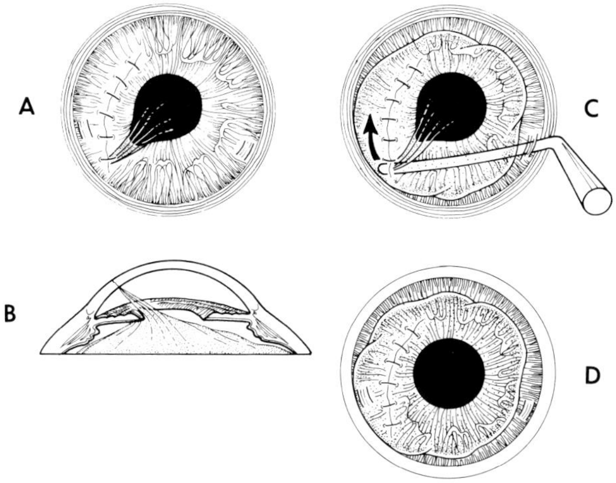

Fig. 13-17. **A,B,** Vitreous strand incarcerated in sutured laceration causing peaked pupil. **C,** Vitreous sweep, placed through paracentesis site, is used to remove incarcerated vitreous from the wound. Anterior chamber is maintained with an air bubble, facilitating visualization of vitreous strands. **D,** After vitrectomy, the pupil is round and the wound free of vitreous incarceration.

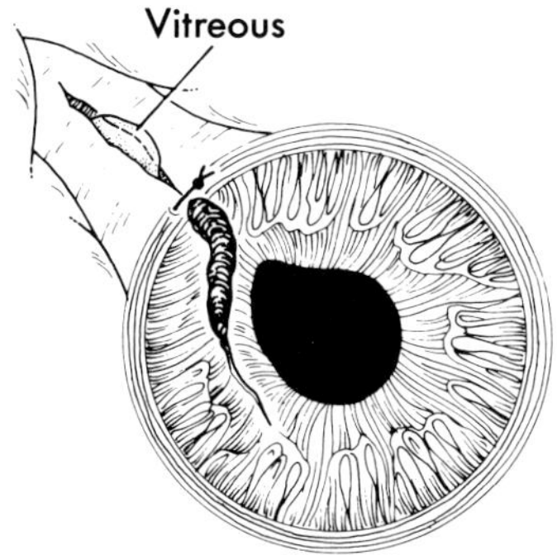

Fig. 13-18. Corneoscleral laceration is first reapproximated with a suture at the limbus to restore correct anatomic relationships.

be placed at the limbus if needed but only if they can be placed without further wound disruption and prolapse of intraocular contents. In other cases, such fixation or rectus bridle sutures may be placed after the globe is initially stabilized.

For large lacerations with an unstable globe, sutures may initially be placed to restore structural integrity before definitive exploration of the wound. At every stage, care must be taken to prevent iatrogenic damage. If possible, the limbus is first reapproximated to restore correct anatomic relationships using nonabsorbable 8-0 nylon or silk sutures (Fig. 13-18). Prolapsed iris is next reposited and the corneal wound closed as previously discussed. The extent of the scleral laceration is then ascertained. For smaller wounds, a localized conjunctival peritomy is made and the wound boundaries explored. For larger injuries, a 360° peritomy is made and all quadrants explored. To progressively stabilize the wound and prevent uveal prolapse during further exploration, it is helpful to place scleral sutures as soon as a new area of laceration is exposed. It is often easier to explore the wound and place scleral sutures using surgical loupes rather than the operating microscope for visualization, because placement of far posterior sutures requires extreme globe positioning and conjunctiva-Tenon's retraction.

For scleral suturing, most surgeons prefer nonabsorbable sutures such as 8-0 nylon or silk; others use absorbable materials such as 7-0 polyglactin 910 (Vicryl, Ethicon). For gaping wounds, it is sometimes helpful to pass the needle completely through one end of the wound before making the second pass, thus avoiding undue globe distortion.

The sclera surrounding the laceration as well as remote quadrants should be completely explored to rule out unsuspected injury. The quadrants are cleaned of overlying Tenon's, and retractors are used to expose the sclera. To facilitate globe manipulation and exploration, sutures of 4-0 silk or 2-0 cotton may be used to isolate the rectus muscles. Because the sclera is thin behind muscle insertions, exploration should be performed carefully in these areas. A laceration extending behind the muscle may be sutured while the assistant retracts the muscle with the bridle suture or muscle hook. Frequently, two instruments are useful to elevate the muscle during exploration and suture placement (Fig. 13-19). If the full extent of the laceration cannot be ascertained or suture placement is difficult, the muscle may be disinserted after being secured with a double-armed 6-0 polyglactin 910 suture, which is subsequently used to reattach the muscle at its insertion. Occasionally, the laceration extends quite far posteriorly, sometimes to the optic nerve. In these poor-prognosis cases, it is probably better to leave the most posterior extent of the wound unsutured than to distort the globe with unwitting delivery of intraocular contents.

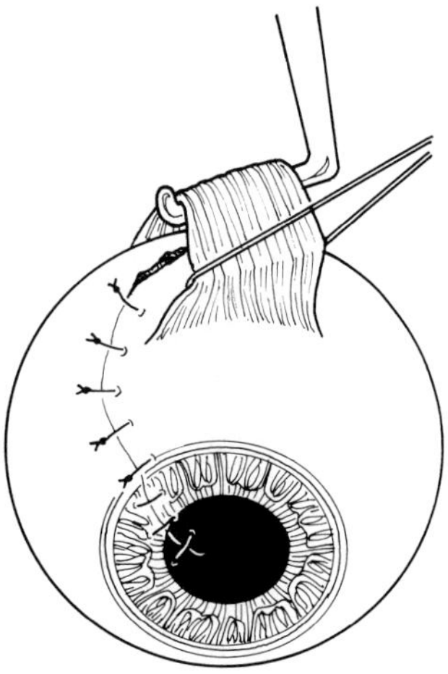

Fig. 13-19. Rectus bridle suture and muscle hook used to elevate the muscle during exploration and suture placement.

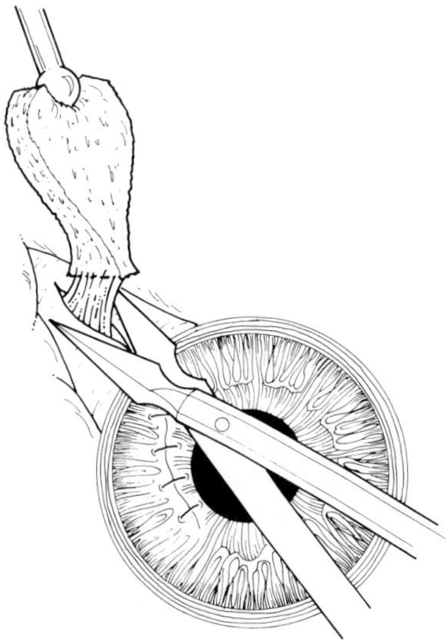

Fig. 13-20. Dry cellulose sponges gently withdraw vitreous, which is cut flush with the wound. Traction on the vitreous should be minimized.

Corneoscleral Lacerations with Uveal and Vitreous Prolapse

Vitreous prolapsing through a scleral wound is secured and gently withdrawn with dry cellulose sponges and cut flush with the sclera (Fig. 13-20). As always, care is taken to avoid traction on the vitreous. If visualization is good, a vitrectomy instrument may be used to excise vitreous at the wound (Fig. 13-21). Moreover, if the wound is through the pars plana and intraocular

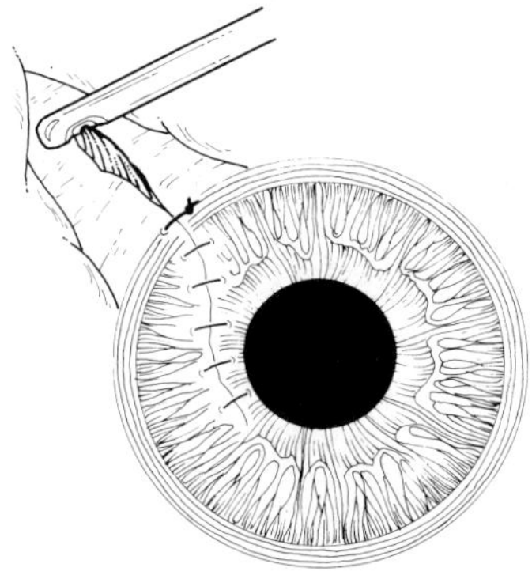

Fig. 13-21. Prolapsed vitreous is excised at the wound with a vitrectomy instrument under direct visualization.

visualization is adequate, the vitrector may be placed intraocularly. However, posterior to the pars plana and in any case in which visualization is poor, to avoid further damage to intraocular structures the tip should not be placed through the wound and into the eye.

As in corneal wounds, one goal of surgery is to clear the wound of vitreous incarceration. This is, of course, much more difficult for posterior wounds because of poor visualization and inability to sweep the wound mechanically. More important in initial surgery is secure, watertight closure of the globe, since posterior vitreous prolapse and incarceration are usually accompanied by severe retinal damage, which will require subsequent vitreous surgery in any case.[14]

Uveal tissue often prolapses from gaping scleral lacerations. If possible, such tissue is reposited because excision may be accompanied by severe bleeding. Furthermore, there is a risk of cutting retinal tissue if the laceration extends posterior to the pars plana. In some severe cases, however, prolapsed uveal tissues must be excised to allow for wound closure. In this event, cauterization before dissection may minimize resultant bleeding. Any tissues removed from the eye should be identified histopathologically. Evidence of retina in the excised specimens indicates an extremely poor prognosis.

The preferred method of scleral closure over prolapsed uvea is a "zippering" technique (Fig. 13-22). The wound is closed from the anterior (limbal) end with interrupted sutures placed successively proceeding posteriorly. The sutures are relatively closely spaced with the goal of oversewing the uveal tissue with the sclera. Suture

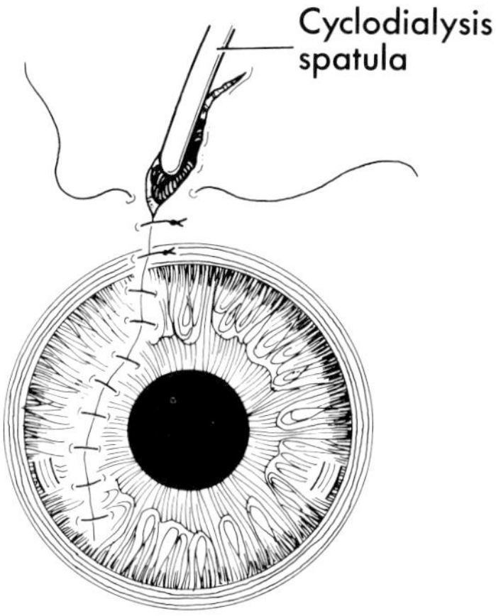

Fig. 13-22. Zippering technique of scleral wound closure. Assistant depresses prolapsed tissue while the sclera is progressively closed proceeding posteriorly. Suture placement may be facilitated by passing the needle completely through one end of the sclera before the second pass. The sclera is then closed over the repositioned uveal tissue.

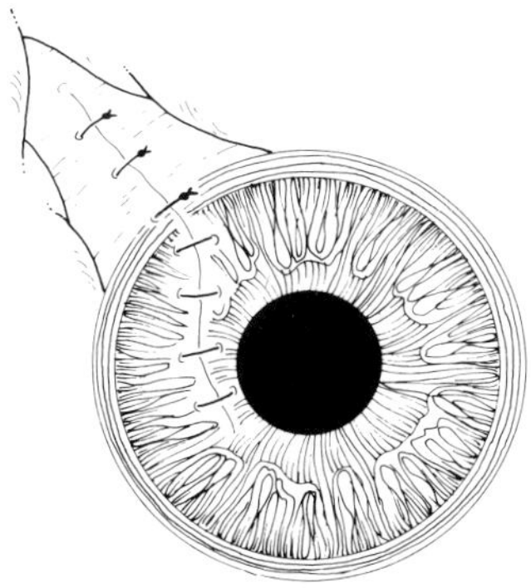

Fig. 13-23. Properly repaired corneoscleral laceration. The wound is watertight, all tissue incarceration has been relieved, and the pupil is round.

placement may be facilitated by passing the needle completely through one end of the gaping sclera before the second pass. Tightening the suture then closes the sclera over the uveal tissue. The assistant may depress the uvea into the eye with a spatula during suture tightening to allow appositional scleral closure without tissue incarceration. Successively passing such sutures will zipper the sclera over the uvea, pushing the prolapsed tissue back into the eye. Alternatively, the wound may be successively bisected, with the assistant using a spatula to press the prolapsed tissue into the eye as sutures are secured (Fig. 13-23).

Posterior Scleral Lacerations

Scleral lacerations without corneal involvement may occur in a variety of settings. Although many blunt scleral ruptures occur at or near the limbus, a number occur posterior to the rectus muscle insertions where the sclera is thin and intrinsically weak.[15] Likewise, although most blunt ruptures are found at or anterior to the equator, approximately 10% to 20% are located more posteriorly.[16] Posterior scleral lacerations may also occur with direct lacerating trauma and as a result of double perforating projectile injuries. Signs of posterior rupture include poor visual acuity, a shallow or unusually deep anterior chamber, low intraocular pressure, hyphema, pupillary distortion, bullous subconjunctival hemorrhage and chemosis, and a brownish subconjunctival coloring caused by prolapsed uvea.[16]

In dealing with posterior scleral lacerations, the globe should be explored completely after 360° conjunctival peritomy as described above. Finding one laceration should not abbreviate a thorough search for a second occult laceration, a double perforation by a foreign body, or contrecoup injury. Lacerated sclera may be repaired as it is uncovered, however, to avoid progressive prolapse of intraocular contents as exploration of the globe proceeds. For specific surgical techniques, see the previous sections on corneoscleral lacerations. The complete management of posterior segment trauma is reviewed in Chapter 20.

Corneoscleral Lacerations with Tissue Loss

Corneoscleral lacerations with tissue loss may be addressed in a number of ways. If necessary with puncture wounds and small avulsive injuries, the cornea or sclera may simply be sutured tightly. This is less than optimal, however, because resultant tissue distortion will stress the wound, causing excessive postoperative scarring and astigmatism.

Puncture wounds and central leaks with stellate lacerations are amenable to closure with tissue adhesive. For larger tissue loss, replacement techniques such as full-thickness and lamellar patch grafting are more appropriate. Such methods are preferable to direct suturing of poorly apposed tissue with its astigmatism-inducing distortion of the ocular architecture. Patch grafting will achieve restoration of structural integrity while maintaining the anatomic relationships that will improve the ultimate outcome of an-

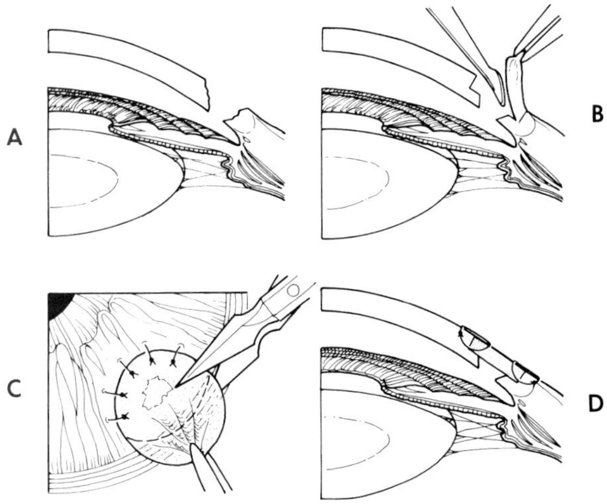

Fig. 13-24. Technique of lamellar inlay grafting. **A,** Full-thickness loss of corneal tissue. **B,** A partial-thickness groove is made around the perforation site with a trephine or sharp blade. Dissection is carried along a lamellar plane at the desired depth. **C,** The graft is partially sutured into position before trimming to final size and shape. **D,** Lamellar graft sutured in place.

terior segment reconstructive surgery. Either viable (fresh) or nonviable (frozen or glycerin-preserved) corneal or scleral tissue may be used.

Both lamellar and full-thickness patch grafts are indicated for perforating corneal injuries with tissue loss. Full-thickness grafts require a healthy recipient tissue in which to suture. Lamellar grafts are more appropriate in situations where irregular wound margins, stromal necrosis, or both make full-thickness dissection and suturing more difficult.

Lamellar Inlay Grafting

To perform a lamellar inlay graft, a partial-thickness groove is trephined or hand-fashioned around the perforation site with a corneal trephine or sharp blade (Fig. 13-24). To facilitate trephination, the anterior chamber may be reformed with viscoelastic, or tissue adhesive may be applied to support the globe tectonically during manipulations. A partial-thickness lamellar bed is then carefully fashioned with a scarifier type of blade.

Donor tissue is prepared in standard fashion as for lamellar keratoplasty (Fig. 13-25). Nonviable donor epithelium is removed by scraping with a dry cellulose sponge or scarifier. Next, a small partial-thickness incision is fashioned at the limbus with a scalpel. A Martinez dissector is introduced through the incision and the plane of dissection carried from limbus to limbus. If a circular lamellar bed of a given diameter has been fashioned in the recipient, a donor button is typically trephined 0.5 mm larger than the recipient bed. If the recipient bed is irregularly shaped, the graft may be hand-fashioned to the appropriate size and shape directly on the recipient eye (Fig. 13-24).

The graft is positioned and secured with interrupted 10-0 nylon sutures. The sutures should extend for approximately 0.5 mm in the donor tissue and 1 mm in the recipient tissue. They should be placed through a 90% thickness of the donor tissue and through the deepest portion of the exposed recipient wound. After suture placement, all knots are trimmed and buried on the recipient side of the wound.

Full-Thickness Patch Grafting

To perform a full-thickness patch graft, the wound margins are debrided to form a rim of healthy tissue into which the graft can be anchored securely (Fig. 13-26). As in lamellar patch grafting, the donor epithelium is removed if nonviable tissue is used. The graft is hand-fashioned or trephined to be slightly larger than the defect. It is helpful to place the donor tissue over the recipient site while cutting to the appropriate size.

The graft is secured with interrupted 10-0 nylon sutures. An alternative mattress-suture closure is described in Chapter 14. Suturing is facilitated by keeping the anterior chamber formed with viscoelastic. After the graft has been securely sutured, the anterior chamber is reformed through the wound or the paracentesis site.

Penetrating Keratoplasty

Penetrating keratoplasty is rarely indicated in primary repair after trauma. Although primary penetrating keratoplasty and anterior segment reconstruction are definitive treatments of complicated anterior segment injury, keratoplasty is usually delayed until the eye is uninflamed and free of infection to optimize graft survival. In the acute setting, it is probably better to use temporizing measures such as patch grafting before undertaking definitive surgical treatment. Even a severely traumatized cornea may heal with remarkably little stigmata of the original injury, giving better vision than initially expected.

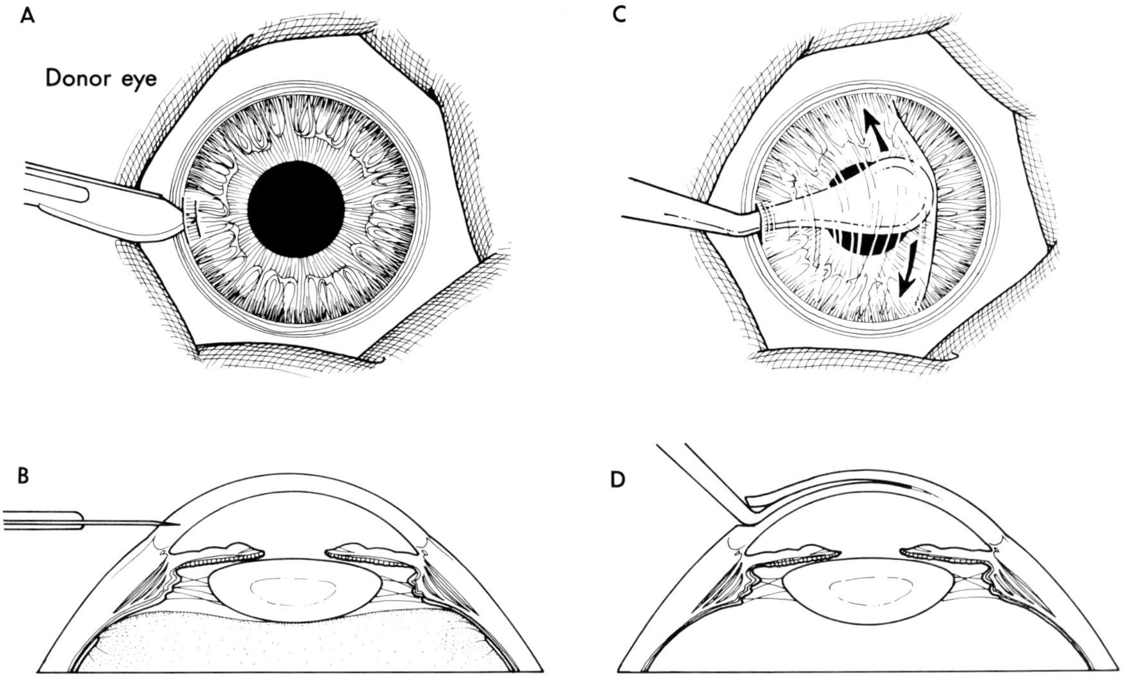

Fig. 13-25. Preparation of donor lamellar tissue. **A,B,** A partial thickness incision is made at the limbus with a scalpel. **C,D,** A Martinez dissector is used to separate the cornea along a lamellar cleavage plane, and the graft is then cut to size from the anterior stromal tissue.

In selected cases, however, particularly those involving extensive corneal tissue loss and anterior segment disruption, penetrating keratoplasty and anterior chamber reconstruction may be performed. A full discussion of the techniques is presented in Chapter 16.

Irreparable Penetrating Injury

Some severe corneoscleral lacerations are beyond repair. These cases include patients with severe loss of retinal tissue and those with profound destruction of the eye. As discussed in Chapter 3, repair of the globe should be attempted if at all possible. However, some cases are clearly irreparable and require primary enucleation. With appropriate informed consent, such a course may be preferable to attempting repair of an unsalvageable eye only to require a second surgery and general anesthetic days later. The technique of enucleation is discussed in Chapter 33.

POSTOPERATIVE MANAGEMENT

After surgical management of acute anterior segment penetrating trauma, appropriate medical

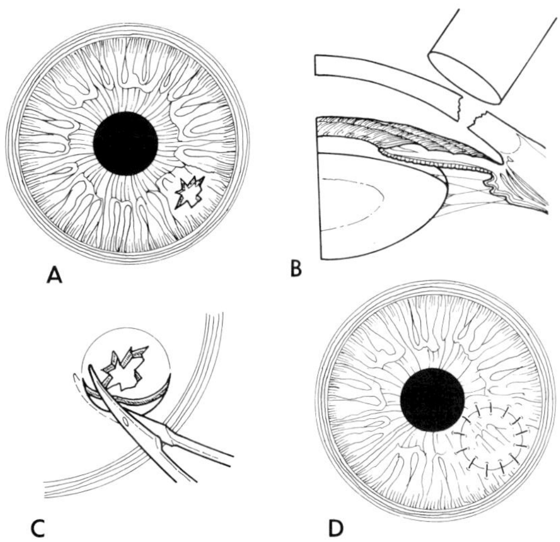

Fig. 13-26. Technique of full-thickness patch grafting. **A,** Full-thickness loss of corneal tissue. **B,** With a trephine or sharp blade, a partial-thickness groove circumscribes the perforation site. **C,** A scissors or blade completes excision of damaged tissue. **D,** Full-thickness patch graft sutured in place.

therapy should be instituted to control infection, suppress inflammation, and stabilize the ocular surface.

At the conclusion of surgery, antibiotics are injected subconjunctivally (e.g., cefazolin 100 mg and gentamicin 40 mg). For "routine" penetrating injuries we currently recommend a 4-day course of intravenous antibiotics, usually combining a cephalosporin and aminoglycoside (see the section on preoperative management). In cases in which injuries are contaminated by vegetable matter, clindamycin may be added to cover *Bacillus* species that may be particularly devastating.[17] Topical fortified antibiotics (e.g., cefazolin [133 mg/ml] and gentamicin [14 mg/ml]) are administered approximately every 2 hours for 4 days and then dosage is reduced. Regular-strength topical antibiotics may be used in cases in which risk of infection is low. Antibiotic therapy is changed as dictated by culture results, and any sign of new infection is promptly cultured. The prevention and treatment of posttraumatic endophthalmitis are described in Chapter 23.

Topical corticosteroids may be useful to minimize scarring and new-vessel ingrowth, but these advantages must be balanced against the theoretical risk of predisposition to infection, especially in eyes contaminated with wood or vegetable foreign matter. Moreover, intensive corticosteroid use early in the wound healing process may diminish the rate of stromal healing and the tensile strength of the wound.[18] In general, then, unless the eye is significantly inflamed, topical corticosteroid dosage is minimized during the early posttrauma phase. Steroids in moderate dosage (e.g., prednisolone acetate 1% 4 times daily) are added after the potential for infection diminishes and are increased if untoward scarring or neovascularization arises. Oral corticosteroids may have a place in treatment of selected severely inflamed eyes, especially those with posterior segment injury. For intraocular pressure control, beta blockers and carbonic anhydrase inhibitors are used as necessary.

The ocular surface is treated as required to promote reepithelialization. Lubricants, bandage soft contact lenses, patching, and tarsorrhaphy all help support and stabilize the ocular surface. These interventions and others are discussed in Chapter 6.

REFERENCES

1. Refojo MF et al: Evaluation of adhesives for corneal surgery, Arch Ophthalmol 80:645-656, 1968.
2. Keates RH and Lichtenstein SB: The management of anterior segment trauma with multiple small incisions, Ophthalmology 87:887-891, 1980.
3. Eisner G: Eye surgery: an introduction to operative technique, New York, 1980, Springer-Verlag.
4. Rowsey JJ and Hays JC: Refractive reconstruction for acute eye injuries, Ophthalmic Surg 15:569-574, 1984.
5. Drews RC: Sodium hyaluronate (Healon) in the repair of perforating injuries of the eye, Ophthalmic Surg 17:23-29, 1986.
6. Thompson JT et al: The use of intravitreal thrombin to control hemorrhage during vitrectomy, Ophthalmology 93:279-282, 1986.
7. McDermott ML, Edelhauser HF, and Mannis MJ: Intracameral thrombin and the corneal endothelium, Am J Ophthalmol 106:414-422, 1988.
8. Mannis MJ et al: Uses of thrombin in ocular surgery, Arch Ophthalmol 106:251-253, 1988.
9. Charles S et al: Bimanual, bipolar intraocular diathermy, Am J Ophthalmol 81:101-102, 1976.
10. Muga R and Maul E: The management of lens damage in perforating corneal lacerations, Br J Ophthalmol 62:784-787, 1978.
11. Eagling EM: Perforating injuries of the eye, Br J Ophthalmol 60:732-736, 1976.
12. Stark WJ et al: Posterior chamber intraocular lens implantation in the absence of capsular support, Arch Ophthalmol 107:1078-1083, 1989.
13. Apple DJ et al: Sutured retropupillary posterior chamber intraocular lenses for exchange or secondary implantation, Ophthalmology 96:1241-1247, 1989.
14. Ryan SJ and Allen AW: Pars plana vitrectomy in ocular trauma, Am J Ophthalmol 88:483-491, 1979.
15. Cherry PMH: Indirect traumatic rupture of the globe, Arch Ophthalmol 96:252-256, 1978.
16. Russell SR, Olsen KR, and Folk JC: Predictors of scleral rupture and the role of vitrectomy in severe blunt ocular trauma, Am J Ophthalmol 105:253-257, 1988.
17. Brinton GS et al: Posttraumatic endophthalmitis, Arch Ophthalmol 102:547-550, 1984.
18. McDonald TO et al: Corneal wound healing. I. Inhibition of stromal healing by three dexamethasone derivatives, Invest Ophthalmol 9:703-709, 1970.

CHAPTER 14

Corneal laceration repair: topographic considerations and suturing techniques

J. JAMES ROWSEY

Effects of penetrating injury and repair on corneal astigmatism
- Effects of the injury
- Effects of suture placement
  - Compression factors
  - Eversion and inversion effects
  - Splinting and torquing effects
  - Wound override

Suturing techniques
- Suture placement
  - Linear lacerations
  - Tissue loss and stellate lacerations
- Suture tightening
- Suture removal

References

Recognition of the micromechanical effects of penetrating injury on corneal topography has given rise to novel repair strategies designed to optimize structural repair, minimize scarring, and restore the native corneal contour. Such surgical concepts may facilitate primary repair and improve ultimate visual outcome by decreasing corneal scarring and astigmatism following trauma.

EFFECTS OF PENETRATING INJURY AND REPAIR ON CORNEAL ASTIGMATISM

Effects of the Injury

The topographic changes induced both by a corneal laceration itself, as well as its subsequent surgical repair and normal wound healing mechanisms will influence astigmatism following trauma. The longer and more central the laceration, the greater is the potential for significant residual astigmatism.[1] Although corneal lacerations less than 4 mm in length often heal with less than 3 diopters of astigmatism, longer lacerations effect more profound topographic changes.

Corneal incisions routinely produce corneal flattening over the area of the incision because of wound gaping. Radial incisions flatten the cornea along both the axis of the incision and the axis 90° away,[2] whereas circumferential incisions flatten the cornea along the axis of the incision and steepen the cornea 90° away.[3] These insights have been exploited in refractive surgical procedures where spontaneous dehiscence of the incision provides the requisite corneal flattening (Fig. 14-1). A traumatic laceration is associated with even greater corneal flattening when sutures close the incision (as described later in this

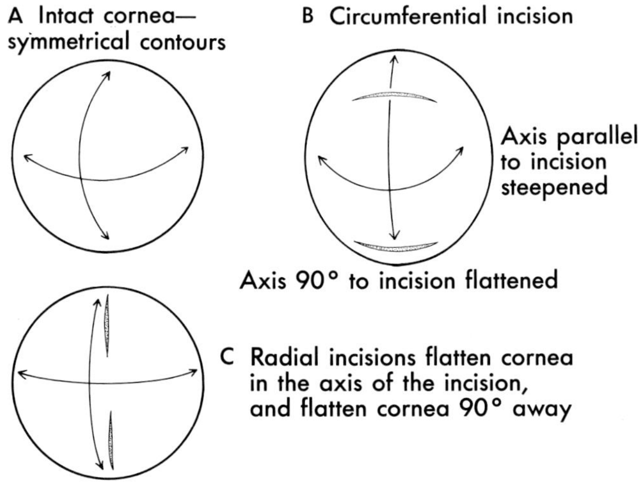

Fig. 14-1. **A,** The intact cornea shows symmetrical contours. **B,** Circumferential incisions flatten the cornea in the axis of the incision and *steepen* the cornea 90° away. **C,** Radial incisions flatten the cornea in the axis of the incision and *flatten* the cornea 90° away.

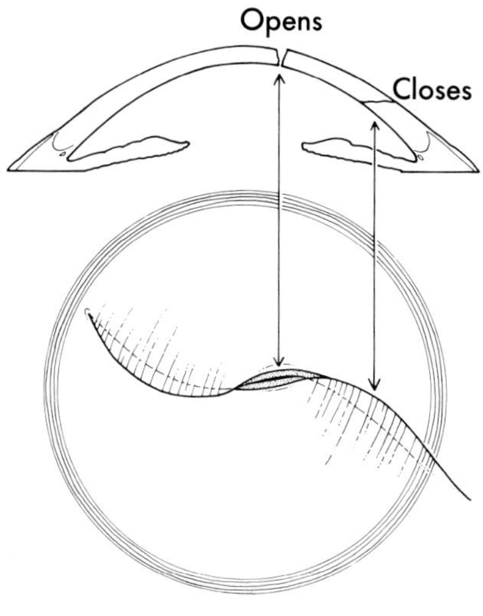

Fig. 14-2. The perpendicular central incision opens spontaneously under the influence of normal intraocular pressure, whereas a shelving incision near the limbus closes spontaneously and therefore requires fewer sutures for coaptation.

chapter). Thus, both laceration orientation and suture placement affect central corneal topography and residual astigmatism.

The physical characteristics of the laceration will also suggest appropriate suture placement for watertight wound closure. Fig. 14-2 demonstrates the valve rule of Eisner, which states that "incisions through the wall of the globe produce valves whose margin of watertightness is equal to the projection of the surface of the incision onto the surface of the globe."[4] Thus, incisions perpendicular to the cornea open spontaneously and require sutures for coaptation. In contrast, incisions that have a shelving effect tend to close spontaneously. For this reason, shelving incisions are preferred for cataract surgery because of the minimal compressive suturing required. Simple inspection of the wound at the time of repair should delineate the areas of perpendicular incisions, which will tend to gape, and oblique incisions, which will close spontaneously because of the valving effect (Fig. 14-2).

Effects of Suture Placement

Unsutured incisions flatten the entire cornea with loss of corneal power. In contrast, sutured incisions—both radial and circumferential—flatten the cornea under the suture but steepen it closer to the visual axis or corneal center (Fig. 14-3). There is also a tendency for the corneal apex to be displaced from the suture site. Obviously, if a sutured incision passes through the visual axis, no residual corneal apex remains, and the entire cornea is flattened during repair.

Suture placement causes both localized and remote corneal topographic shifts. Five components of suture effects should be considered: compression factors, tissue eversion, tissue inversion, torquing, and splinting.[4] Knowledge of

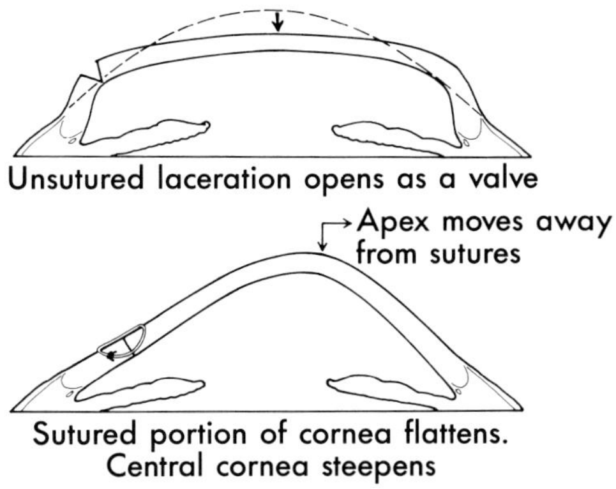

Fig. 14-3. An unsutured incision produces corneal flattening. Sutures coapt the tissue while changing the corneal topography.

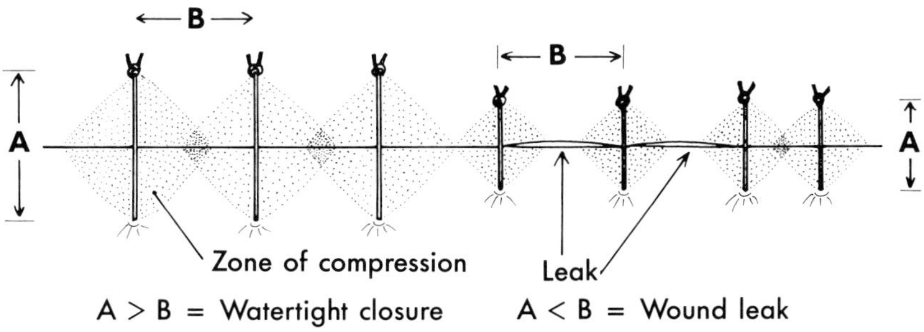

Fig. 14-4. Each suture provides a hypothetical zone of compression approximately equal to the length of the suture along the incision. If these zones of compression overlap, adequate wound coaptation can be expected. If the zones of compression do not overlap, a wound leak is more likely to develop.

each of these factors can assist in accomplishing the goals of corneal laceration repair.

Compression Factors

Simple appositional sutures would be adequate if no intraocular pressure were present to cause wound gaping. However, to overcome the elastic tendency of the globe and prevent wound leaking, tissue compression is required. The zone of tissue compression along the incision is roughly equal to the length of the suture (Fig. 14-4). Therefore, longer sutures have greater lateral zones of tissue compression, and fewer sutures are necessary. Longer and deeper sutures appose the deeper stroma, closing any posterior wound gaping and decreasing the propensity for iris or vitreous to adhere to the raw posterior corneal surface. However, longer sutures are also associated with greater tissue distortion, potential tissue necrosis, and residual corneal astigmatism. Shorter corneal sutures tend to allow wound leakage between the sutures, since the zones of tissue compression are similarly narrower. To avoid wound leakage, therefore, the zones of tissue compression should be in contact or slightly overlap.

Eversion and Inversion Effects

The intrastromal bite of a loop of a single interrupted suture or a running suture produces eversion by elevating the tissue above the suture. Conversely, the overlying portion of an interrupted suture produces posterior tissue pressure and compaction, or inversion of the tissue. For a single interrupted suture, inverting and everting forces are equal, so there is no tendency toward tissue depression or elevation (Fig. 14-5, *A*). However, a nonradial interrupted suture produces tissue torque (Fig. 14-5, *B*). In contrast, a running suture produces an inversion tendency beneath the overlying suture bite with eversion over the intrastromal bite, thus forming

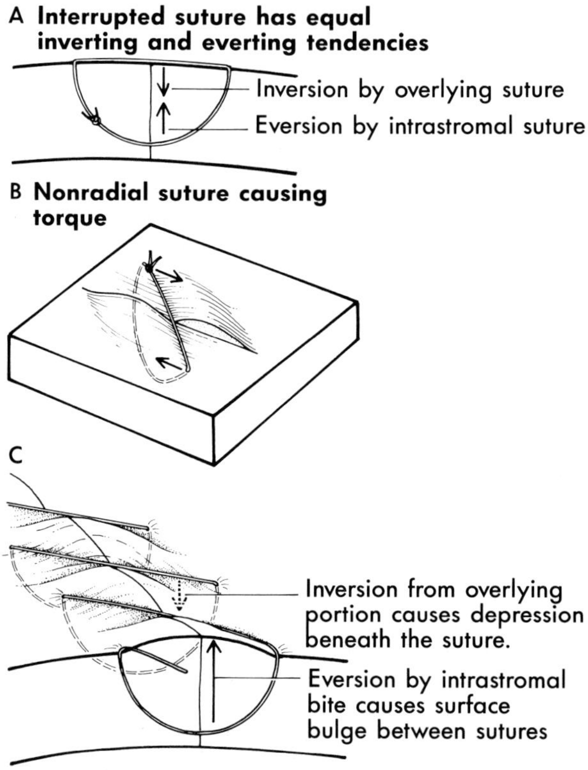

Fig. 14-5. **A,B,C,** The effect of interrupted and running sutures on tissue compression, splinting, and torquing.

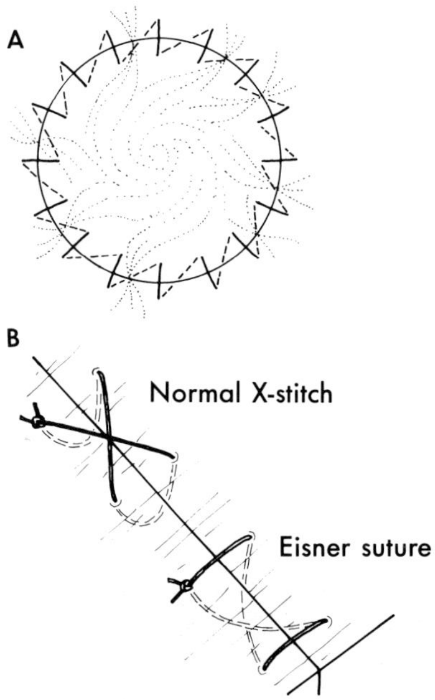

Fig. 14-6. **A,** Deep stromal suture bites can evert the stroma excessively between sutures as shown by a vortex pattern of epithelial sliding. **B,** Superficial or deep stromal compression may be accomplished by appropriate placement of an X stitch. The Eisner X stitch minimizes astigmatism-producing surface compression.

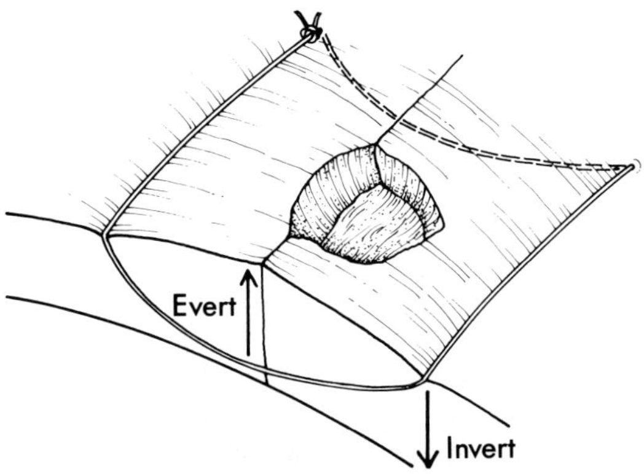

Fig. 14-7. The everting tendency of a deep mattress suture coapts a corneal laceration that is infected, allowing exposure of the stroma to antibiotics.

hillocks of stromal elevation (Fig. 14-5, *C*). These hillocks increase epithelial exposure, predisposing toward localized epithelial drying, erosion, or infection. An epithelial vortex may be visualized by fluorescein staining in these regions, signaling areas of chronic epitheliopathy and epithelial sliding (Fig. 14-6, *A*). Very little tendency toward epithelial breakdown is observed beneath the running suture itself. Eisner[5] has recently demonstrated the value of individual X stitches to minimize the surface compression that induces astigmatism while also minimizing surface eversion (Fig. 14-6, *B*).

The everting tendency of a mattress suture is quite helpful when superficial corneal trauma occurs with tissue loss that would otherwise require gluing. A suture should not be passed through a superficially infected cornea, because it would be a locus of stromal necrosis. It is often possible, however, to suture beneath a traumatized or infected area of the cornea, coapting Descemet's membrane with adequate deep corneal compression and everting the overlying stroma (Fig. 14-7). This also increases stromal access to antibiotics.

Splinting and Torquing Effects

The intrastromal portion of a running suture provides splinting, or resistance to lateral movement of the tissues, in a manner similar to that of the internal fixation rod used during bone fracture repairs. In contrast, the overlying suture in a running technique tends to torque the tissues, the direction of torque eventually providing the shortest distance between neighboring exit and entry sites (Figs. 14-5, *B* and 14-8). Because the overlying torquing effect of the running suture exceeds the intrastromal splinting effect, tissue distortion often results. By placing the intrastromal bite in an oblique fashion, this tissue torquing may be reduced. The advantage of a running suture in corneal laceration repair is the tendency toward equal suture tension along the wound. The major disadvantage is that astigmatism is more difficult to modulate by suture placement and selective suture removal as compared with interrupted suture repair.

It is also important to place interrupted sutures precisely perpendicular to the corneal laceration itself (Fig. 14-5). An oblique interrupted suture tends to move the tissue because of torquing, producing wound gaping and leakage and

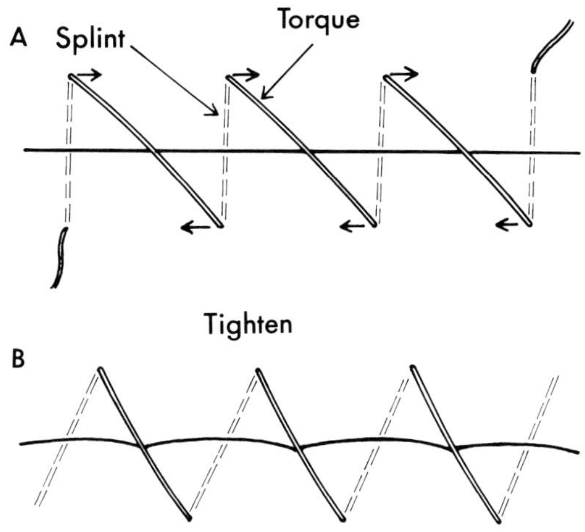

Fig. 14-8. **A,** The intrastromal bite of a suture produces more splinting, whereas the overlying suture produces more torquing effects on the tissues. **B,** When tightened, the wound edges shift. Placing the intrastromal bite in an oblique fashion reduces this subsequent torquing effect and tissue distortion upon tightening.

requiring excessive tightening of the suture to close the wound. Excessive compression accentuates corneal flattening and consequent corneal astigmatism.

Wound Override

The greatest difficulty in suture placement for an irregular corneal laceration is assessing the residual tissue and placing the first interrupted suture with the least torquing and compression that will provide a watertight closure without wound override (Fig. 14-9). Wound override produces an irregular corneal surface, potential epithelial healing problems, and a microwedge resection effect. Moreover, tissue override or gaping is associated with white corneal "stromal outgrowth" onto the stromal surface, producing a false sense of wound healing and excessive scarring.[6] In Fig. 14-9, *A*, the suture needle entrance and exit sites are equidistant from a perpendicular corneal incision with no tendency toward surface movement. In Fig. 14-9, *B*, however, the exit distance of the suture from the incision is shorter than the entry distance. This has a tendency to produce tissue override, with the shorter suture pulling the tissue down and the longer suture elevating it. It is also important to place suture bites at equal depth on both sides of the corneal laceration, for unequal placement will again cause tissue override, with the more

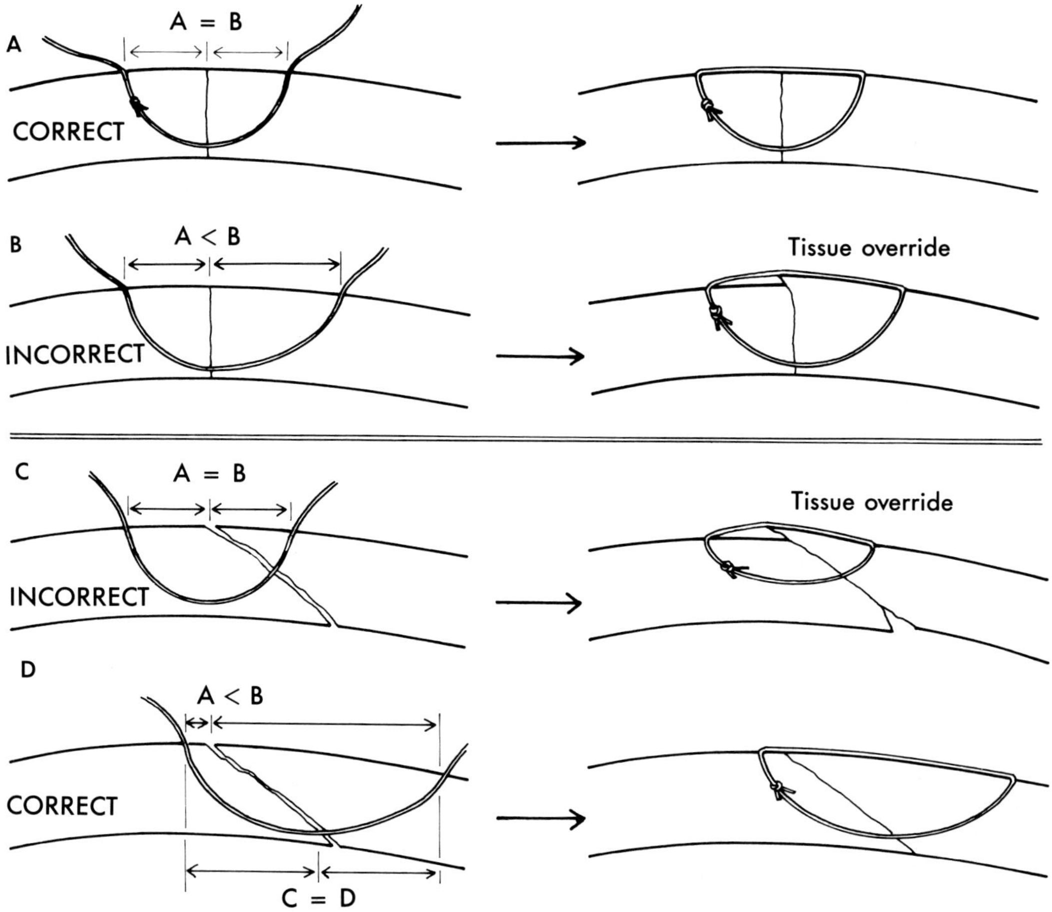

Fig. 14-9. **A** and **B,** In nonshelving lacerations, tissue override is produced if the entry and exit suture sites are unequal. **C** and **D,** An oblique incision should be closed with the deepest passage of the suture of equal lengths, not the superficial portion of the suture. The distance from the needle entry to the posterior edge of the oblique incision is gauged, and the needle is passed to exit the stroma this additional distance past the anterior chamber entry site. This technique allows for minimal tissue override and minimal induced astigmatism.

superficial suture bite causing that side to underride.

An override tendency is also observed when closing oblique wounds (Figs. 14-9, *C* and *D*). Accepted wisdom dictates that the suture entrance and exit sites be equidistant from the wound. However, in this circumstance the upper half of the valve incision tends to override the lower half when the suture is tightened. By observing the obliquity of the incision at the time of surgery, one can place the suture deeply to close Descemet's membrane and exit the stroma at a distance that equalizes the intrastromal bite on both sides of the wound (Fig. 14-9, *D*). This closes the oblique incision with minimal tissue compression and wound override.

SUTURING TECHNIQUES

Suture Placement

Linear Lacerations

As mentioned previously, it is recommended[4] that the surgeon inspect the corneal laceration for perpendicular and shelving portions.[7] The perpendicular incisions are closed first with interrupted sutures to allow for reformation of the anterior chamber. Peripheral compression sutures are then placed to compress and flatten the peripheral cornea while conversely steepening the central cornea. Finally, appositional sutures are placed in the central cornea while observing the corneal reflex with an intraoperative keratometer or a safety pin for optimal cen-

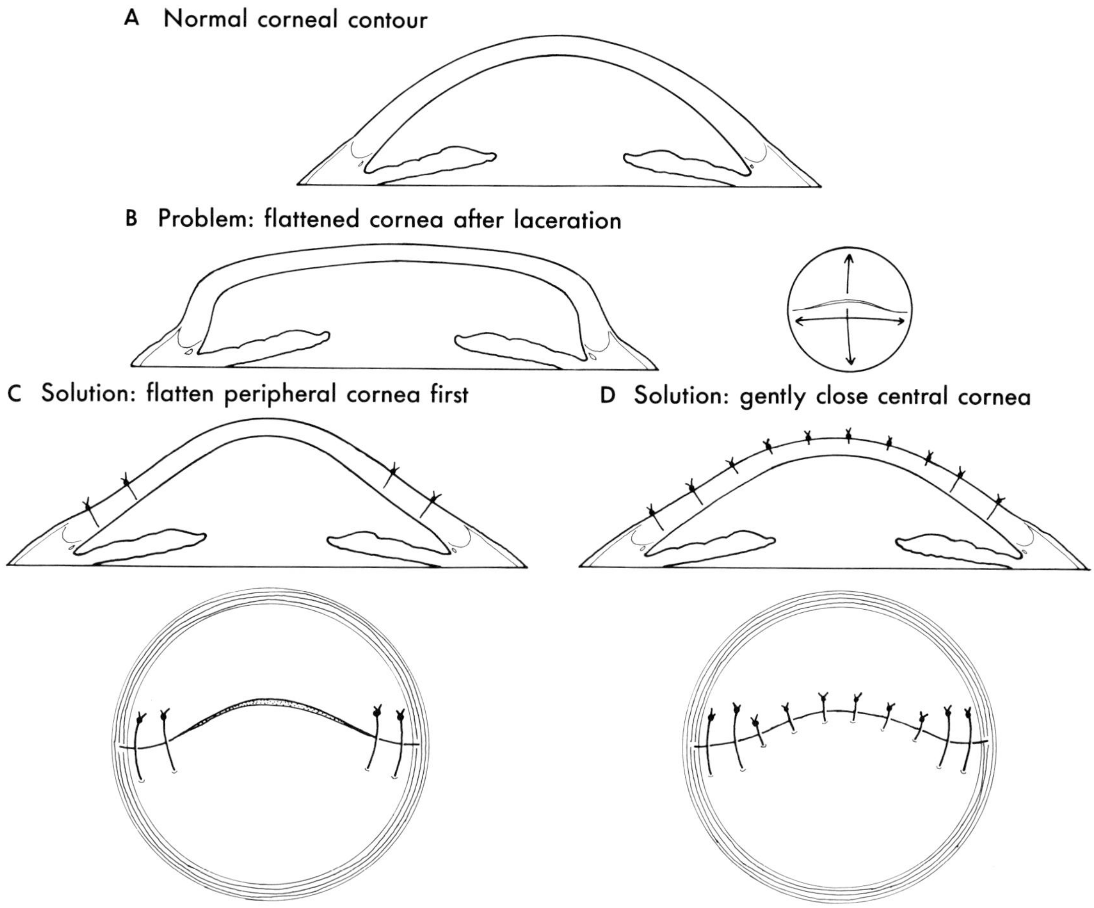

Fig. 14-10. **A,** Normal corneal contour. **B,** Corneal flattening as a result of laceration. **C** and **D,** Placing longer compressing sutures near the limbus and shorter appositional sutures centrally over the visual axis avoids apical flattening and restores the native central corneal contour.

tral corneal sphericity.[8] Fig. 14-10, *A* shows the normal corneal contour. Fig. 14-10, *B* demonstrates the corneal flattening that occurs after laceration. Most suture techniques will exacerbate this flattening effect. In Fig. 14-10, *C*, tight peripheral corneal sutures have been placed in a corneal laceration to flatten the peripheral cornea and steepen the central cornea. In Fig. 14-10, *D*, the central cornea is closed with gentle appositional sutures just sufficient to close the anterior surface. The tight peripheral or limbal sutures close Descemet's membrane over a large zone of compression, and therefore minimal suture tension is required of the central sutures, thus preserving the central corneal dome.

The complicated vectors of force required to close any laceration produce numerous pitfalls that may induce astigmatism. In closing a jagged corneal laceration, attention should be directed to each linear aspect of the laceration individually (Fig. 14-11). Although the normal tendency would be to close the apices of the laceration with simple interrupted sutures first, closing the perpendicular areas of the wound (positions 1 and 2) usually allows the chamber to be reformed more readily and prevents additional trauma to the apices of the corneal laceration. Working from the periphery to the center of the laceration in Fig. 14-12, *A*, lacerations 1, 2, and 3 would be closed in that order. Either an interrupted or a running suture technique may be used for each segment. If a running suture is used, it must be tied before an additional linear portion is undertaken. An attempt to turn the corner with a running suture will inevitably lead to tissue override, loose sutures, and additional astigmatism.

Two types of running shoelace sutures are

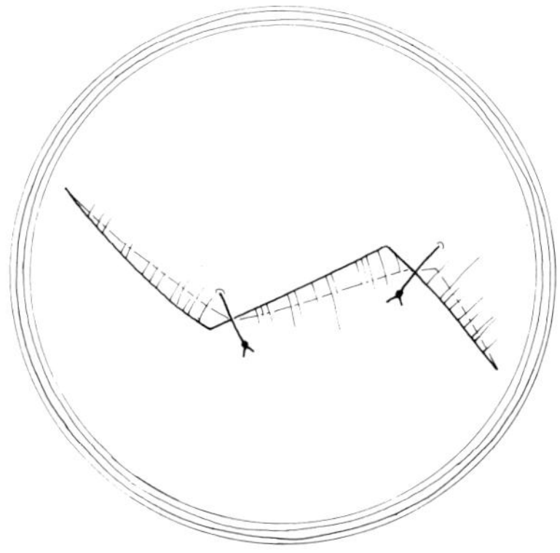

Fig. 14-11. The perpendicular incisions through the cornea are closed first, followed by the valving incisions, which require fewer sutures and less compression.

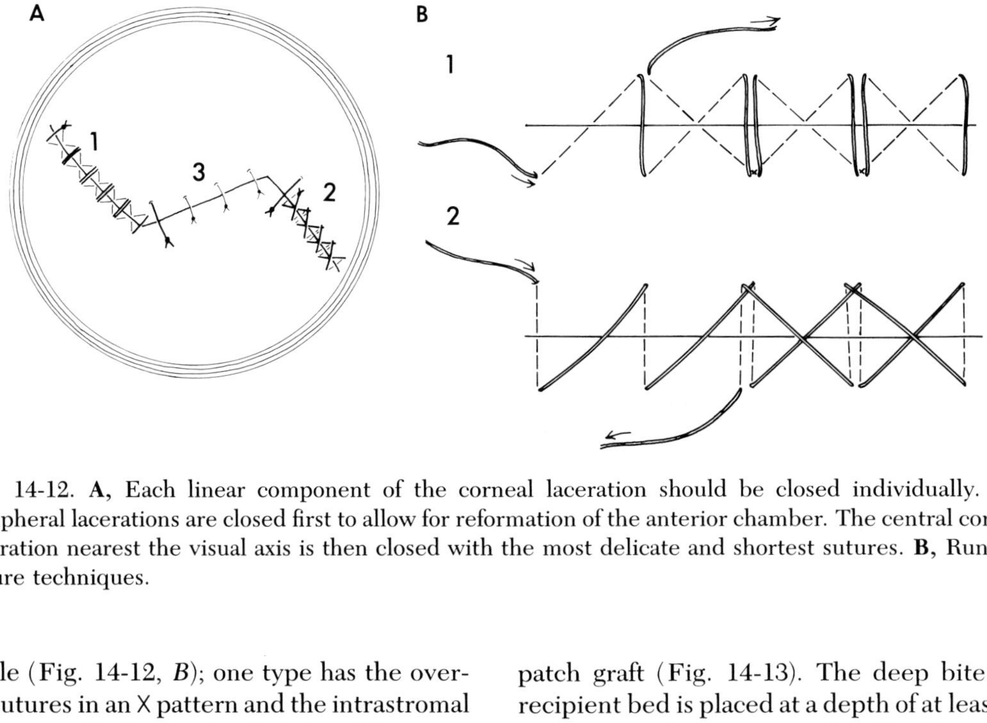

Fig. 14-12. **A,** Each linear component of the corneal laceration should be closed individually. The peripheral lacerations are closed first to allow for reformation of the anterior chamber. The central corneal laceration nearest the visual axis is then closed with the most delicate and shortest sutures. **B,** Running suture techniques.

possible (Fig. 14-12, *B*); one type has the overlying sutures in an X pattern and the intrastromal bites perpendicular to the incision. The more complicated pattern has the intrastromal bites placed obliquely with the overlying bites perpendicular to the incision. This shoelace type of suture splints the cornea and overcomes the torquing effect normally seen with an overlying suture bite. In addition, the deep stromal X maximizes Descemet's membrane closure while minimizing the surface compression required (see Fig. 14-6, *B*).

Tissue Loss and Stellate Lacerations

When corneal trauma or infection removes stromal tissue, Paton's method for closing a corneal hole can be used to suture in a small corneal patch graft (Fig. 14-13). The deep bite of the recipient bed is placed at a depth of at least three quarters and then superficially through the patch graft just beneath Bowman's membrane. The suture is then repassed in the recipient bed at 75% depth and exits the corneal stroma. Both the posterior wound compression afforded by this type of double mattress suture and the anterior-to-posterior pull of the superficial suture close the wound quite readily. All debris must be removed from around the corneal incision so that no aqueous leaks through the edematous stroma. In the presence of appreciable stromal loss, this technique appears to be more effective than direct or pursestring suture closure. Sutures can be removed within a month.

Eisner[4] has suggested the technique dem-

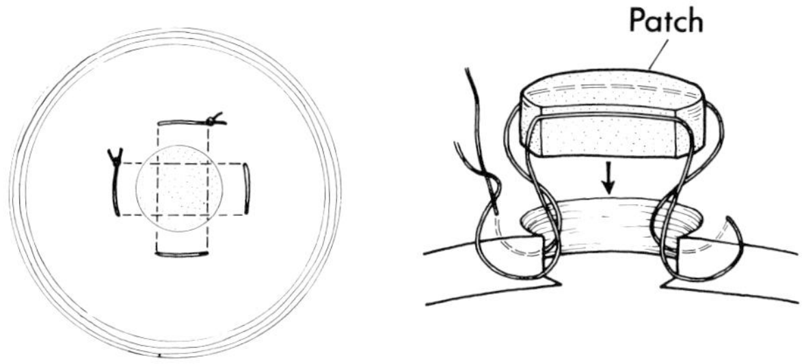

Fig. 14-13. A 2- to 3-mm corneal hole, too large to glue and too small for numerous interrupted sutures, can be closed with a patch graft. The patch is pulled posteriorly by the superficial sutures. The walls of the graft and hole can be tapered posteriorly so that a smaller inside diameter provides maximum tissue compression.

onstrated in Fig. 14-14 for a pursestring suture of a marked stellate laceration when undue tissue compression may be required to reconstitute the anterior chamber. In this instance, the stellate laceration is surrounded by five apices that cannot be adequately closed without distorting the adjacent wounds. A diamond knife incision is made in the normal corneal stroma peripheral to the laceration apices to approximately half stromal depth. A 10-0 nylon suture is then serially passed from the depth of these incisions, through the adjacent stroma and laceration and out through the neighboring incision. Tightening the suture apposes the central stroma, and the entire suture and knot are buried.

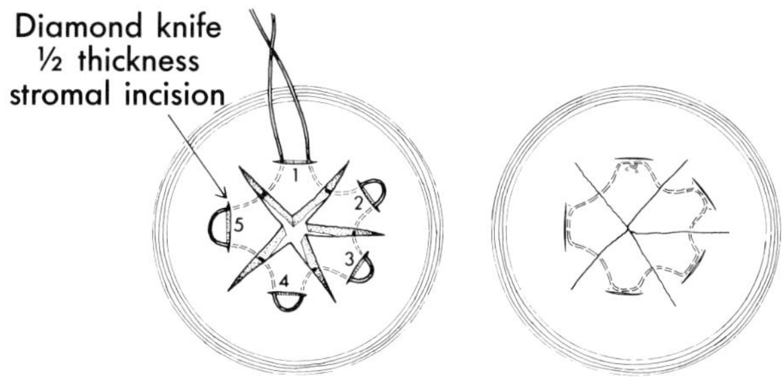

Fig. 14-14. Eisner's recommended technique for closing a stellate laceration with maximum deep stromal compression and minimum overlying tissue necrosis.

Suture Tightening

Locking and slipknots are invaluable in the repair of corneal lacerations. Although a square knot provides good closure, control of astigmatism may be optimized by the use of slipknots. A double half-hitch slipknot is used to adjust wound tension optimally, followed by a square knot to secure closure (Fig. 14-15).

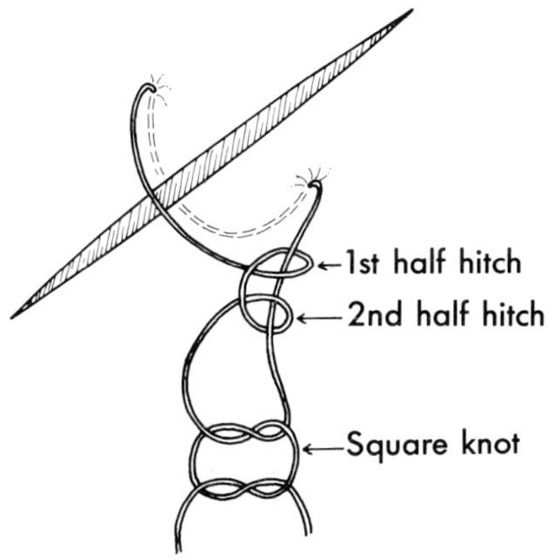

Fig. 14-15. Wound tension is adjusted using a double half-hitch slipknot followed by a square knot to secure closure.

Suture Removal

To maintain corneal integrity, sutures can only be removed from the corneal laceration when adequate interface fibrosis has been attained. This fibrosis is generally observed by oblique illumination with a slit lamp, retroillumination against a red reflex, or marginal retroillumination with the slit beam adjacent to the corneal laceration itself. Sutures that loosen spontaneously because of wound contraction are providing no further tensile strength to the cornea and should be removed before corneal melting, epithelial breakdown, or infection occurs. Corneal vascularization is also generally indicative of adequate wound healing. If iris is attached to the posterior wound and inadvertently incarcerated in the laceration, wound healing may be markedly delayed. If iris touches the posterior corneal laceration without incarceration, wound healing may actually be hastened. If possible, iris should not remain in contact with the corneal laceration because the endothelial cells may slide off the cornea onto the adjacent iris with eventual corneal edema around the corneal laceration site. Keratometry, Placido disc imagery, and corneoscopy are valuable for observing sutures that are producing excess tissue compression and, therefore, corneal astigmatism. When adequate wound healing occurs, the compressive sutures can be selectively removed to correct this induced astigmatism and speed visual recovery.

References

1. Barr CC: Prognostic factors in corneoscleral lacerations, Arch Ophthalmol 101:919-924, 1983.
2. Rowsey JJ: Ten caveats in keratorefractive surgery, Ophthalmology 90:148-155, 1983.
3. Lundergan MK and Rowsey JJ: Relaxing incisions: corneal topography, Ophthalmology 92:1226-1236, 1985.
4. Eisner G: Eye surgery: an introduction to operative techniques, New York, 1980, Springer-Verlag.
5. Eisner G: Personal communication, 1980.
6. Girard LJ et al: Corneal stromal outgrowth, Am J Ophthalmol 76:445-450, 1973.
7. Rowsey JJ and Hays JC: Refractive reconstruction for acute eye injuries, Ophthalmic Surg 15:569-574, 1984.
8. Rowsey JJ, Reynolds AE, and Brown R: Corneal topography: corneascope, Arch Ophthalmol 99:1093-1100, 1981.

CHAPTER 15

Anterior segment intraocular foreign bodies

WILLIAM E. SMIDDY
WALTER J. STARK

Preoperative evaluation
- History
- Physical examination
- Ultrasound and radiography

Treatment
- IOFB composition
- IOFB without lens involvement
- IOFB with lens injury
- Complications

References

Most intraocular foreign bodies (IOFBs) are magnetic[1] and are associated with activities involving striking metal against metal[2] or the use of motorized machines.[3] A minority are nonmagnetic substances such as glass, plastic, vegetable material, or copper.[2] In most cases it is necessary to remove the IOFB, although a glass, stone, sand, or plastic foreign body may be inert and well tolerated.[4,5] Modern microsurgical techniques and instrumentation have lessened the operative risks and increased the efficacy of IOFB removal.

Intraocular foreign bodies are usually associated with less acute eye damage than are other eye injuries.[6,7] IOFBs are usually small and frequently sharp, thereby leaving a relatively small entry site that may be self-sealing. All intraocular structures may be traumatized by even the smallest projectile, however. Larger objects such as BBs may also cause severe, irreparable ocular damage through blunt shock effects.[6] This chapter addresses the diagnosis and management of the patient with an anterior segment IOFB. Posterior segment IOFBs are discussed in Chapter 21.

PREOPERATIVE EVALUATION

History

An accurate and detailed history is essential for proper diagnosis and management of IOFBs. The key to diagnosis is a high index of suspicion based on the history. The critical historical feature is the identification of patient involvement in a high-risk activity such as hammering metal on metal. Patients frequently remember an incident where they felt a speck enter their eye, but symptoms of the IOFB entry may be mild or nonexistent and so may be dismissed as inconsequential. Symptoms may include only minor ocular irritation, possibly with some conjunctival injection, but this may take several hours to develop. Vision is often unaffected in the acute stages, and delayed or minimal symptoms may delay presentation to the physician.

An understanding of the nature of the activity being pursued during IOFB implantation is important for medicolegal purposes but also may aid in determining the composition of the IOFB and hence the need for and urgency of removal. The magnetic characteristics of the IOFB are of critical importance in determining the technique of surgical removal. The possibility of multiple foreign bodies may be suspected from the history (e.g., blast injury) and may guide subsequent confirmatory diagnostic and therapeutic measures.

Physical Examination

The physical examination of a patient with a suspected IOFB differs little from a routine examination. A complete examination of the fellow eye should not be overlooked, because associated or unassociated pathology may be present. It is important for the examining ophthalmologist to document visual acuity, because a mild degree of decreased vision may have escaped attention, especially if the fellow eye is completely normal. The most important step in the physical examination of the patient with an anterior chamber IOFB is the slit-lamp examination; most anterior segment IOFBs are directly visible with the slit lamp.

Associated signs, such as the presumed entry site, hemorrhage, or other injury, may be the key to detecting the IOFB. An entry site in the cornea may be associated with a positive Seidel's test, or it may be detectable only by associated localized edema.

Intracorneal foreign bodies generally do not require removal if they are not easily accessible and cannot be removed without damage to adjacent tissue. They may require removal if they span the full thickness of the cornea or prevent reepithelialization. Usually nonvegetable matter intracorneal foreign bodies are well tolerated (Color Plate 15-1).

Foreign bodies lodged in the anterior chamber angle, within the iris or lens, or in the posterior chamber or anterior vitreous may be more difficult to detect. Through careful examination of the configuration of the entry site, it may be possible to infer the trajectory of the IOFB as a guide to the meridian or region of the hidden IOFB. The peripheral cornea in the area of the anterior chamber angle foreign body may show localized edema. Involvement of other anterior segment structures may be helpful in diagnosing the IOFB and may determine the therapeutic approach. The iris may demonstrate a localized hemorrhage, distortion, or transillumination defect due to the presence or passage of the IOFB. Examination of the iris in the undilated position and the lens after dilation yields maximal information. The lens is usually clear in the acute stage despite localized anterior capsule disruption. There may be surprisingly little progression of lenticular opacities, and it may be possible to retain the lens, as it may still remain clear. If not acutely necessary, lens removal may be performed later under more controlled conditions.

Gonioscopy may be a critical means of localizing an anterior segment IOFB (Color Plate 15-2). The meridian of its location may be inferred from the configuration of the entry site. It is important not to place excessive posterior pressure on the cornea with the contact lens to avoid anterior chamber collapse. The Zeiss four-mirror lens with a handle minimizes pressure on the eye. Gonioscopy can also be helpful in visualizing IOFBs posterior to the iris. The meridian in which the foreign body is seen is important; it should be analysed carefully and diagramed preoperatively.

Factors governing the necessity and timing of foreign-body removal include its mobility and composition. The degree of inflammation depends upon the extent of tissue disruption, the time elapsed since the injury, and the composition of the foreign body. Acutely, there is frequently minimal inflammation, but if the patient comes for evaluation later because of a lack of early symptoms, the degree of inflammation may be moderate or severe and may mimic infective endophthalmitis.[7,8] Prompt preoperative administration of intravenous antibiotics is advisable and should include broad-spectrum coverage with an aminoglycoside and a penicillin or cephalosporin with activity against staphylococci (see Chapters 3 and 23). If the IOFB is vegetable matter, the additional use of clindamycin should be considered to prevent *Bacillus* infection. To avoid delay, this may be initiated by the primary care physician when possible.

Ultrasound and Radiography

Most anterior segment foreign bodies can be visualized using ultrasound and radiography, although glass or plastic fragments might be shaped or situated so as to escape ready detection. Ultrasonographic and radiologic techniques are most useful for posterior segment IOFBs, but they have a role in selected cases of anterior segment IOFBs (see Chapter 2). Computerized tomography (CT) scanning is preferred for identification and localization of sus-

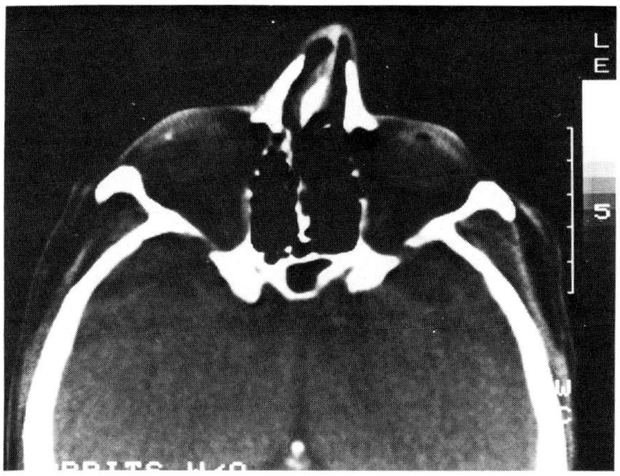

Fig. 15-1. CT scan demonstrates radiodense, nonmagnetic foreign body (possibly a stone fragment) in the inferior anterior chamber angle. Obliquely oriented entry site in cornea directed suspicion to this region.

pected but as yet undetected anterior segment IOFBs (Fig. 15-1). Most glass contains sufficient lead to allow detection through radiologic examination. Once the foreign body has been diagnosed and localized, refining the clinical history may yield more information regarding the possibility of multiple IOFBs and the composition, size, and shape of the foreign body.

Techniques are available to elucidate the magnetic properties of an IOFB but are most useful for posterior segment IOFBs.[3] Magnetic resonance imaging (MRI) is generally contraindicated for metallic IOFBs, although the risk of injurious movement is small.[9,10] MRI may be effective for detecting and localizing nonmetallic IOFBs, especially when CT scanning fails to reveal a suspected IOFB.[11]

TREATMENT

IOFB Composition

Because most IOFBs are metallic, they should be removed to avoid the risk of toxicity. Iron-containing IOFBs result in siderosis.[4] Pure copper usually produces a suppurative response, and alloys of 80% copper or less may subsequently lead to chalcosis. Zinc and aluminum IOFBs are toxic and should be removed.

It is urgent and mandatory to remove vegetable IOFBs because they usually contain microorganisms that can lead to endophthalmitis and cause excessive inflammation. As with other IOFBs, it may be possible to wait several hours if that would yield optimal instrumentation, personnel, and operating room circumstances.

Glass and plastic IOFBs are often well tolerated, and if not mobile or if other structures have not been damaged, they may be retained indefinitely in many cases.[4] In some cases, stone fragments may be well tolerated, but the risk of seeding with microorganisms merits their prompt removal.

IOFB without Lens Involvement

If the IOFB spares the lens and remains anterior to the pupillary plane, the patient should not undergo further pharmacologic dilation preoperatively. In fact, an intracameral miotic injection to constrict the pupil provides an iris shield to protect the lens from subsequent damage during removal. If the fundus cannot be visualized preoperatively or intraoperatively, it should be examined postoperatively.

General anesthesia is preferred for all patients with penetrating injuries, although patients with small, self-sealing corneal lacerations and no other associated intraocular damage may be exceptions and may tolerate retrobulbar anesthesia. However, because most patients suffering IOFBs are young and healthy, the risks associated with general anesthesia are minimal (see Chapter 4).

A stabilizing rectus stay-suture or episcleral suture may facilitate subsequent surgical maneuvers. If there is chemosis or a suspected entry site posterior to the limbus, the conjunctiva is dissected away to allow definitive inspection and treatment.

A shelved, small-caliber incision is made into the anterior chamber at the limbus, and balanced salt solution or a viscoelastic substance is injected to maintain anterior chamber depth. We prefer to remove the viscoelastic substance, when possible, to avoid postoperative intraocular pressure rises.

Attention is next directed toward the IOFB entry site. In many cases a corneal entry site is small and self-sealing and may not require surgical therapy. However, if the wound is large or leaking or if other surgery is required, placement of 10-0 nylon sutures is recommended. This allows more control over the anterior chamber depth during subsequent manipulations. Tissue adhesive may be useful for closing puncture wounds. A postoperative bandage contact lens may also be helpful (see Chapter 13).

The surgical incision depends on the location and size of the IOFB and other associated intraocular damage. Usually the anterior chamber is entered through a limbal conjunctival incision. A foreign body lodged in or attached to the iris can usually be peeled loose by using viscoelastic dissection or by using a needle or hooked instrument to dissect and liberate it, taking care not to traumatize the lens.

When it is anticipated that the IOFB is metallic and can be removed using a magnet, the size of the incision can be minimized. An 18- or 20-gauge rare earth magnet is often useful in this situation. If the foreign body is not magnetic, intraocular forceps or Sheets forceps may be effective in grasping it for its removal (Fig. 15-2). A 3-clock hour superior incision is generally necessary in this instance. Viscoelastic helps prevent damage to the corneal endothelium during intracameral maneuvers.

If an IOFB is lodged in the anterior chamber angle recess, the incision is centered at that meridian (Fig. 15-3). A 3- to 4-clock hour incision is often required. Localization of the exact meridian can be difficult, and intraoperative gonioscopy may facilitate this, especially if the operating microscope has a slit-beam attachment. One technique of further localizing the foreign body is applying external diathermy at the limbus while looking through the gonioscopy lens and monitoring the location of the internal appearance of the burn relative to the IOFB. An anterior chamber angle IOFB may be removed most easily using forceps or a magnet with direct visualization. Because the incision may need to be placed in an awkward location, special care must be directed toward creating and closing the wound to avoid a subsequent inadvertent filtering bleb.

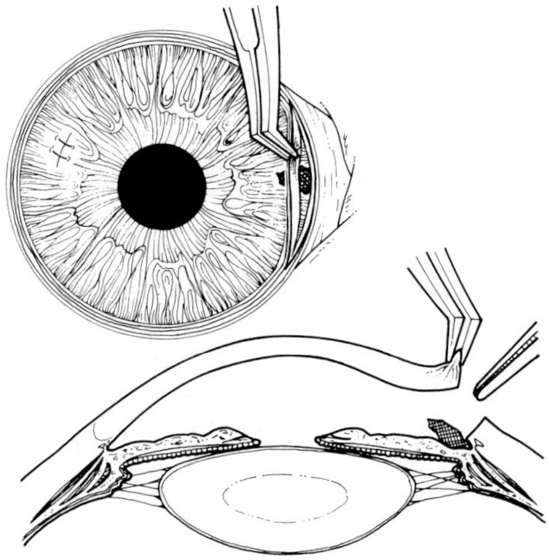

Fig. 15-3. Limbal incision for direct removal of foreign body in the angle.

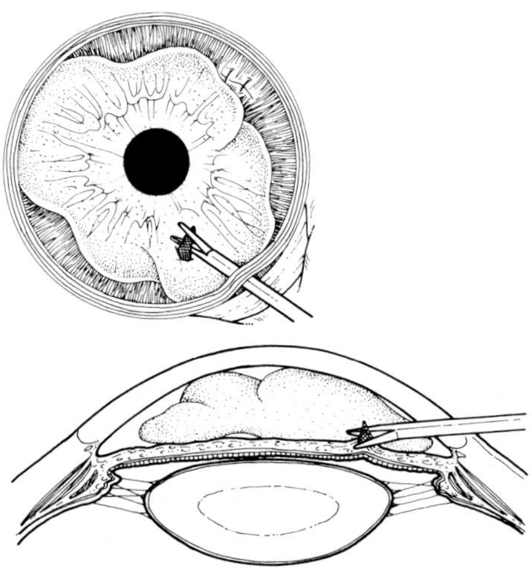

Fig. 15-2. Forceps extraction of anterior chamber foreign body. The chamber is maintained with viscoelastic.

IOFB with Lens Injury

If the lens has become disrupted and the foreign body is accessible (Fig. 15-4), the foreign body is removed and then routine extracapsular cataract surgery is performed at the same session. In some cases, this can be done using phacoemulsification through a 3-mm incision. Because most IOFB patients are young, the nucleus is usually soft and very little sonication is necessary. Planned extracapsular extraction with nuclear delivery can also be considered. If the posterior capsule has been ruptured and vitreous is present, automated microvitrectomy instrumentation may be used. Primary placement of a posterior chamber intraocular lens is not routinely recommended, but one may be placed in selected patients.[12]

If the IOFB is intralenticular and the posterior capsule is intact, an intracapsular technique may be considered for lens removal (Fig. 15-5). Intralenticular metallic foreign bodies often do not result in siderosis[4,13] and may either be observed or removed in toto by intracapsular surgery. Intracapsular surgery requires a much larger incision, which may be undesirable in

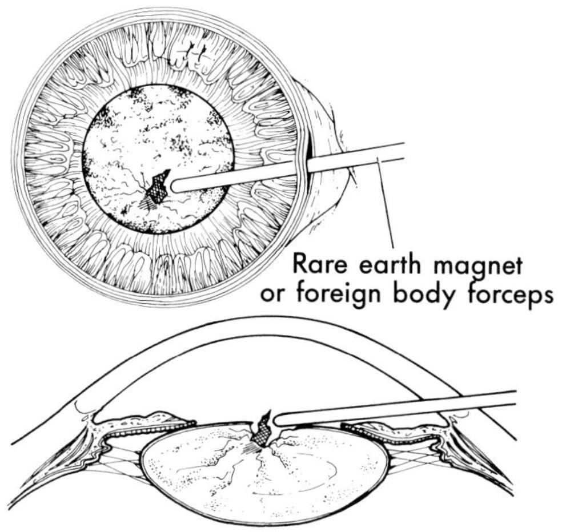

Fig. 15-4. Lenticular foreign body removal with magnet or forceps.

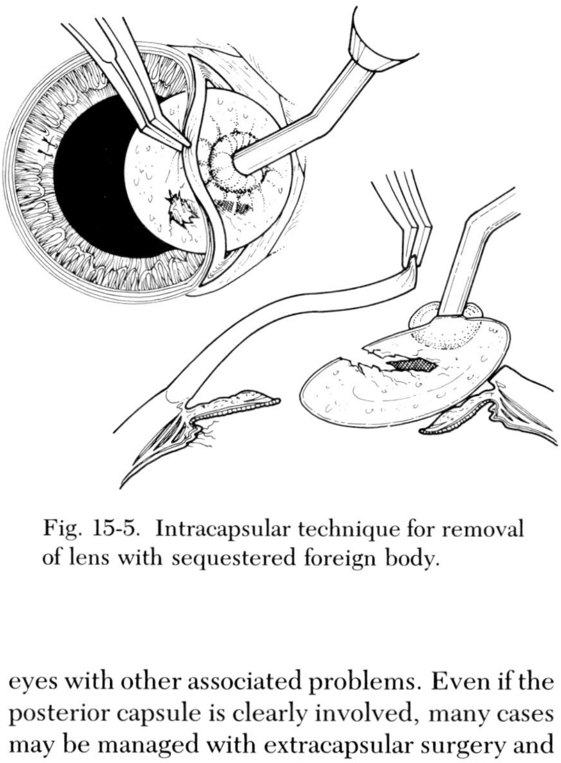

Fig. 15-5. Intracapsular technique for removal of lens with sequestered foreign body.

eyes with other associated problems. Even if the posterior capsule is clearly involved, many cases may be managed with extracapsular surgery and anterior vitrectomy combined with IOFB removal. As much of the posterior capsule as possible is preserved to allow for primary or subsequent secondary posterior chamber lens implantation. Even if intracapsular surgery is necessary or if there is not adequate capsular support, a scleral fixated posterior chamber implant can be placed as a primary or secondary procedure in selected cases.[12,14]

Excessive iris sphincter damage may leave the iris flaps mobile and liable to anterior synechiae. For this reason a pupilloplasty may be advantageous, especially in an aphakic or pseudophakic eye, because the risk of lens damage with the repair is avoided. Iridodialyses do not require repair unless the iris flap obscures the pupillary space. This problem can be repaired by sewing the peripheral edge of the iris to the internal edge of the posterior lip of a limbal incision (see Chapters 8 and 16).[15]

Complications

Intraoperative complications may include corneal endothelial damage, intraocular bleeding, unintentional involvement of the lens, and iridodialysis. The anterior chamber depth can usually be maintained with a viscoelastic substance. Intraocular bleeding may be controlled through the use of bimanual bipolar diathermy.[16] This is not usually necessary, however, because most anterior segment bleeding stops readily. However, if necessary, diathermy leads can be attached to an intraocular probe such as a Ziegler blade, Sinsky hook, or intraocular infusion cannula, and a second lead affixed to an external probe for treating anterior chamber angle bleeding. The diathermy may be attached to the coaptation forceps and applied to bleeding sites directly through the limbal incision if it is peripherally located. If necessary, bimanual bipolar diathermy can be applied to the iris through the use of two intraocular instruments (see Chapter 13).

Postoperatively, intravenous antibiotics are administered for 3 to 5 days for endophthalmitis prophylaxis (see Chapter 23). The anterior and posterior segments are monitored daily during this time for signs of endophthalmitis, wound leak, cataract formation, excessive inflammation, and other complications.

References

1. Smith VH: The incidence of intraocular foreign bodies, Int Ophthalmol Clin 8:137-146, 1968.
2. Percival SPB: A decade of intraocular foreign bodies, Br J Ophthalmol 56:454-461, 1972.
3. Coleman DJ et al: Management of intraocular foreign bodies, Ophthalmology 94:1647-1673, 1987.
4. Barry DR: Effects of retained intraocular foreign bodies, Int Ophthalmol Clin 8:153-170, 1968.
5. Neubauer H: Management of nonmagnetic intraocular foreign bodies. In Freeman HM, edi-

tor: Ocular trauma, New York, 1979, Appleton-Century-Crofts.

6. Sternberg P et al: Multivariate analysis of prognostic factors in penetrating ocular injuries, Am J Ophthalmol 98:467-472, 1984.
7. Williams DF et al: Results and prognostic factors in penetrating ocular injuries with retained intraocular foreign bodies, Ophthalmology 95:911-916, 1988.
8. Brinton GS et al: Posttraumatic endophthalmitis, Arch Ophthalmol 102:547-550, 1984.
9. Williams S et al: Ferrous intraocular foreign bodies and magnetic resonance imaging, Am J Ophthalmol 105:398-401, 1988.
10. Kelly WM et al: Ferromagnetism of intraocular foreign body causes unilateral blindness after MR study, Am J Neurorad 7:243-245, 1986.
11. Lo Bue TD et al: Detection and localization of nonmetallic intraocular foreign bodies by magnetic resonance imaging, Arch Ophthalmol 106:260-261, 1988.
12. Smiddy WE et al: Contact lenses for visual rehabilitation after corneal laceration repair, Ophthalmology 96:293-297, 1989.
13. Cridland N: Magnetic extraction, Int Ophthalmol Clin 8:213-229, 1986.
14. Malbran ES, Balbran E, and Negri I: Lens guide suture for transport and fixation in secondary IOL implantation after intracapsular extraction, Int Ophthalmol Clin 9:151-160, 1986.
15. Michels RG: Vitreous surgery: St. Louis, 1981, The CV Mosby Co, 158.
16. Michels RG and Rice TA: Bimanual bipolar diathermy for treatment of bleeding from the anterior chamber angle, Am J Ophthalmol 84:873-874, 1977.

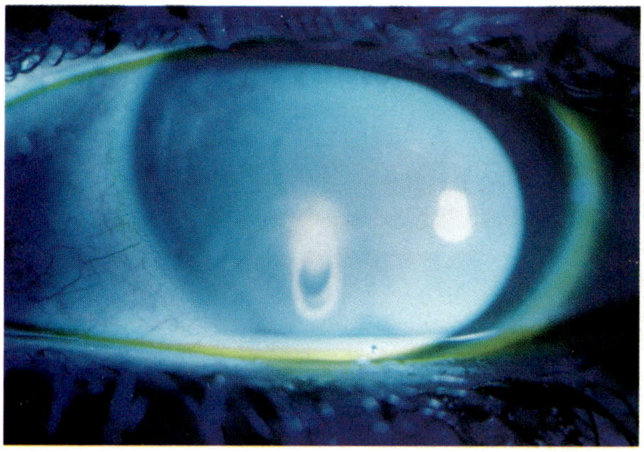

Color Plate 13-1. Positive Seidel's test using 2% fluorescein following corneal puncture wound with wire.

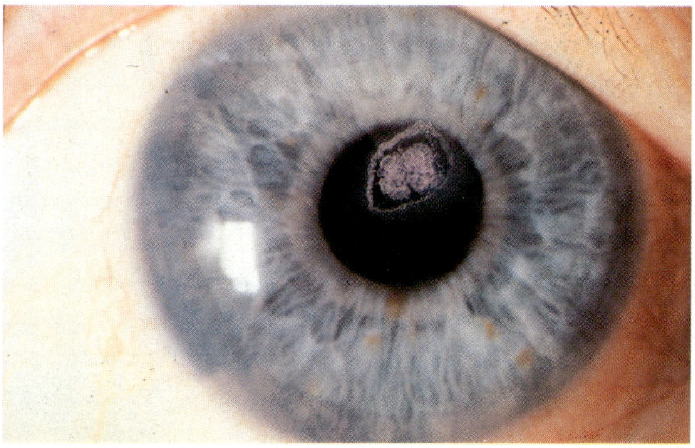

Color Plate 13-2. Small puncture wound near the visual axis sealed with cyanoacrylate tissue adhesive.

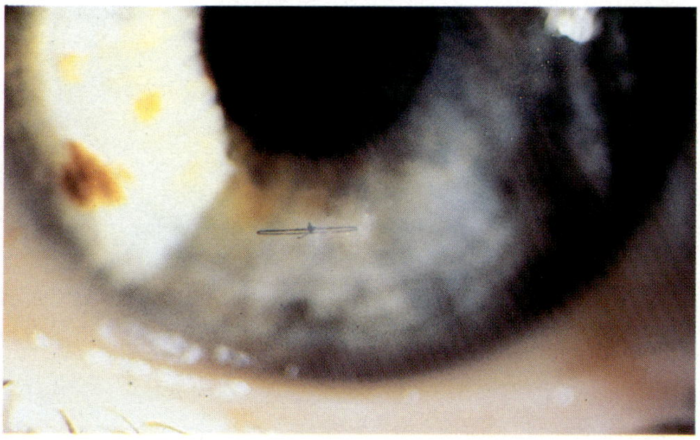

Color Plate 13-3. Small laceration inferior to the visual axis was closed with a single interrupted 10-0 nylon suture.

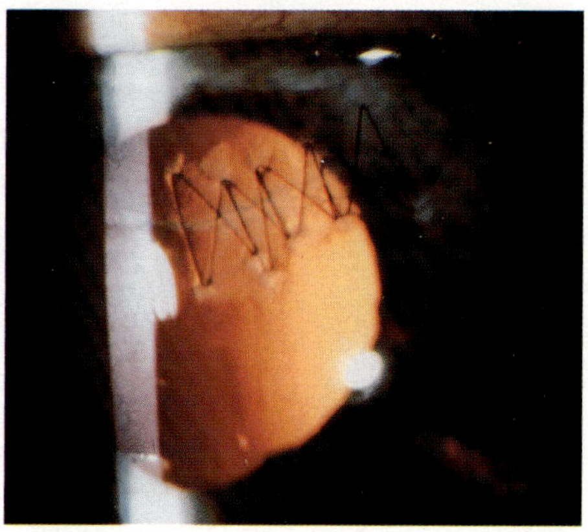

Color Plate 13-4. Clinical example of shoestring suture closure.

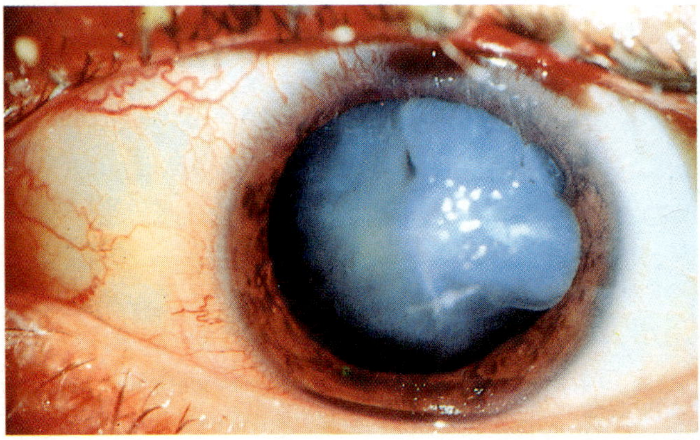

Color Plate 13-5. Cornea laceration with rupture of anterior lens capsule. The flocculent lens material was aspirated with preservation of the posterior capsule during primary repair.

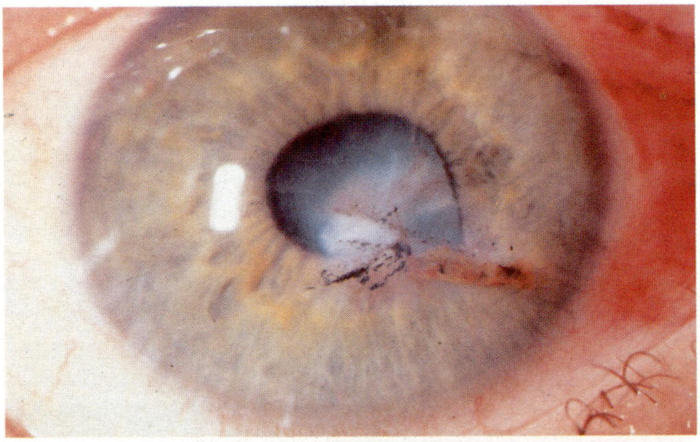

Color Plate 13-6. **A,** Corneal laceration with iris incarceration and lens involvement.

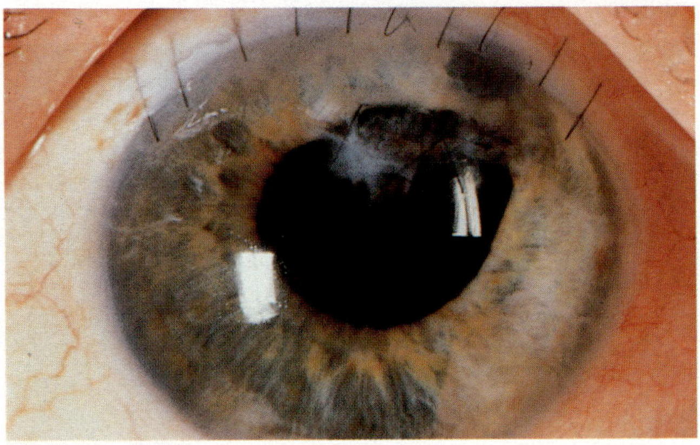

B, After repair of corneal laceration, repositioning of iris, and extracapsular cataract extraction. Postoperative visual acuity was 20/30 with a rigid aphakic contact lens.

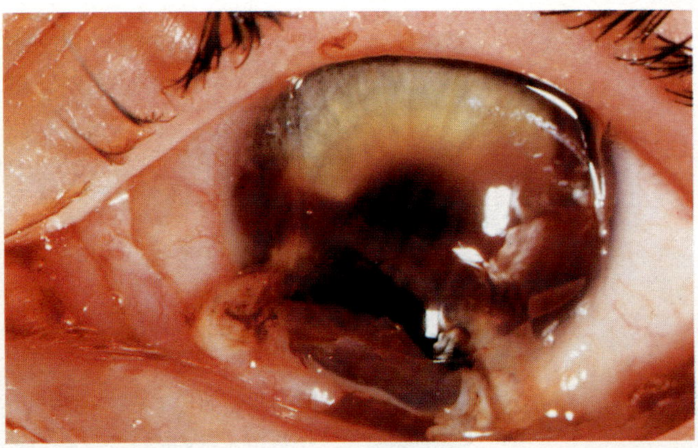

Color Plate 13-7. Lacerating eye trauma with cornea, iris, lens, and vitreous involvement.

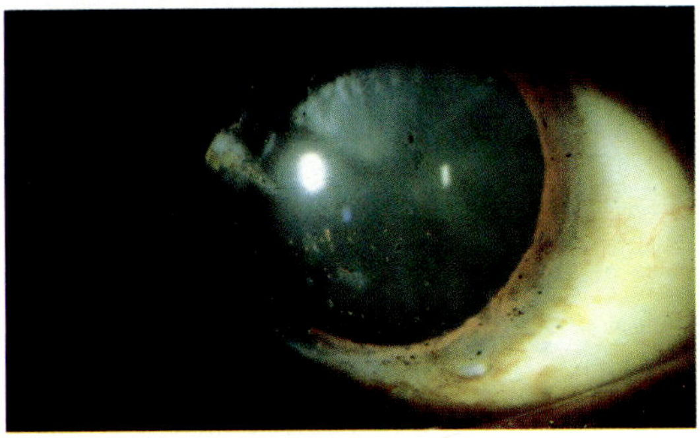

Color Plate 15-1. Patient 20 years after blast injury with multiple corneal foreign bodies. Visual acuity is 20/20 and there is no ocular irritation.

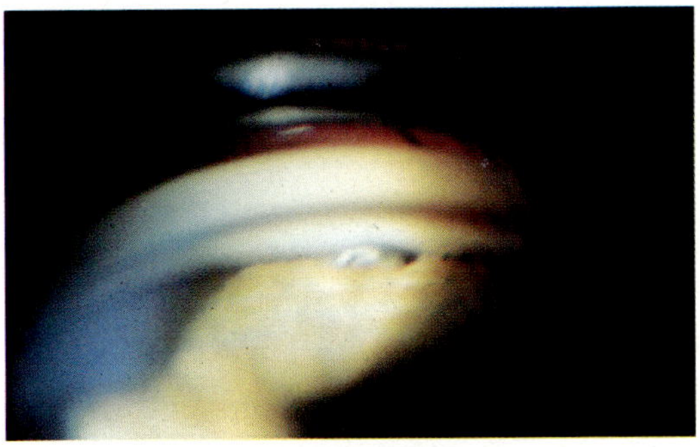

Color Plate 15-2. Gonioscopic appearance of glass intraocular foreign body in the anterior chamber angle.

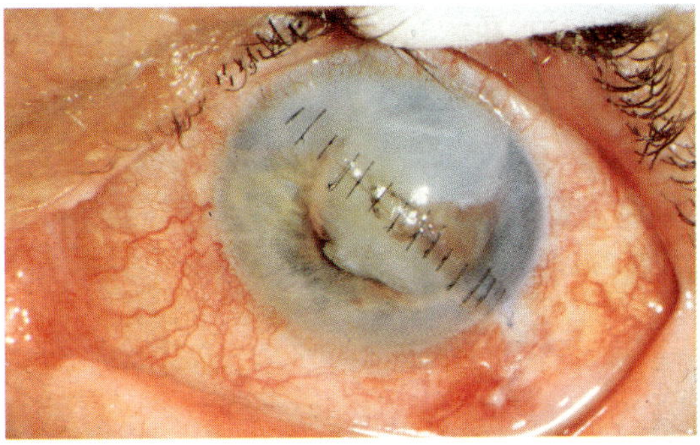

Color Plate 16-1. **A,** Repaired corneal laceration with lens cortical material in anterior chamber and extensive iris loss.

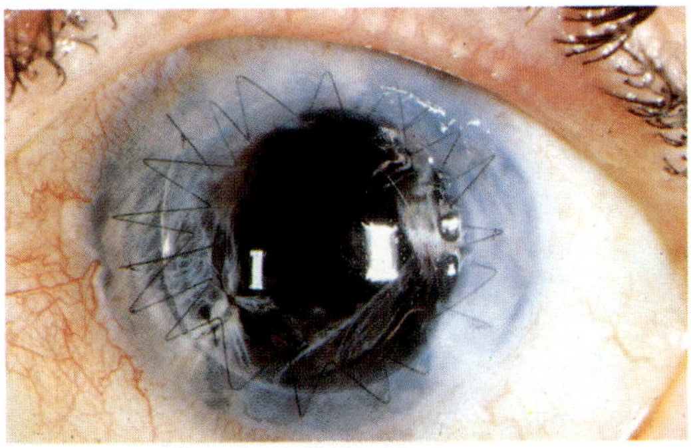

B, Following penetrating keratoplasty, removal of lens remnants and anterior vitrectomy, iris reconstruction, and placement of anterior chamber intraocular lens, visual acuity is 20/70.

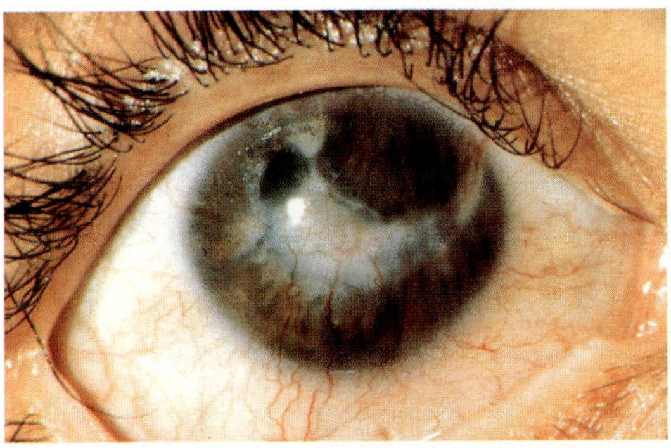

Color Plate 16-2. **A,** Corneal scar with iris and vitreous incarceration, cataract remnants, and peripheral anterior synechiae.

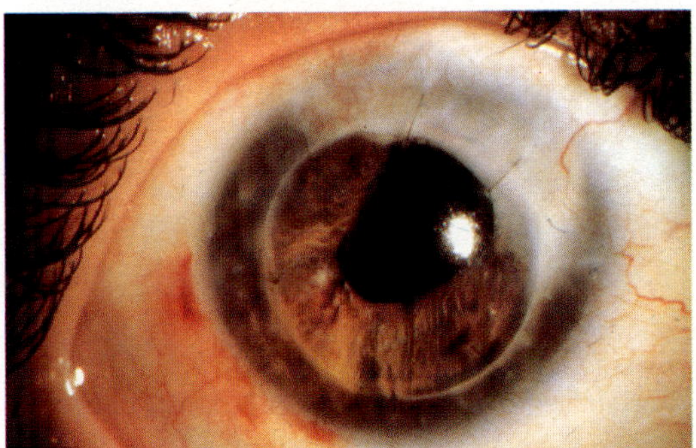

B, Following penetrating keratoplasty, goniosynechialysis, removal of lens remnants and anterior vitrectomy, and iris reconstruction, visual acuity is 20/40 with normal intraocular pressure.

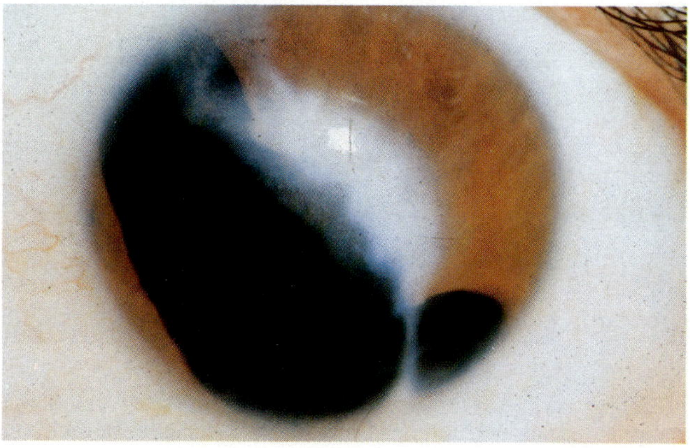

Color Plate 16-3. **A,** Central corneal scar with iris to the wound. Lens remained clear despite the severe injury.
B, Following penetrating keratoplasty and extensive iridoplasty following liberation of retracted iris tissue, visual acuity is 20/80.

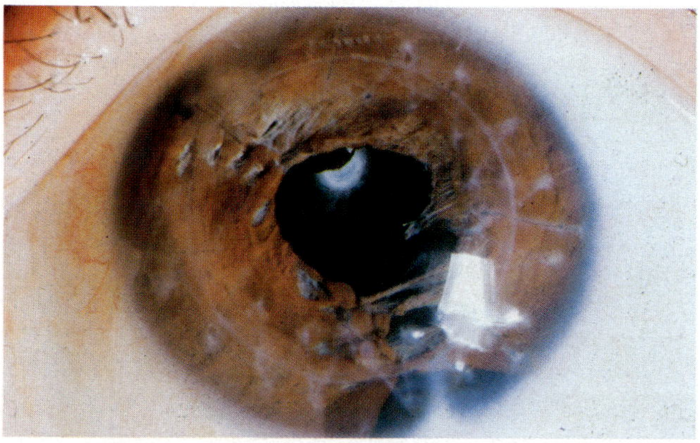

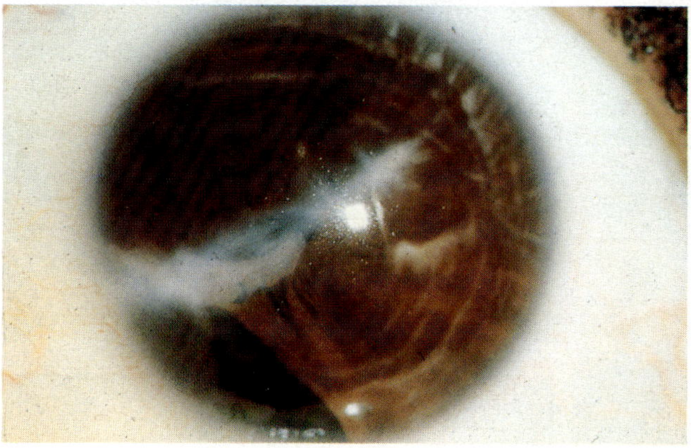

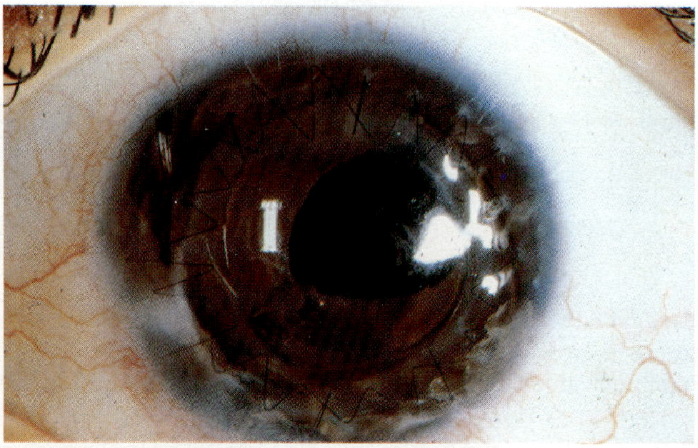

Color Plate 16-4. **A,** Pupil secluded by adherent leukoma following penetrating injury with a knife. A large iridodialysis is present.
B, Following penetrating keratoplasty, goniosynechialysis, iris resuspension and iridoplasty, removal of cataract remnants and anterior vitrectomy, and implantation of anterior chamber intraocular lens, visual acuity is 20/70.

CHAPTER 16

Anterior segment reconstruction following ocular trauma

PETER S. HERSH
KENNETH R. KENYON

Preparatory and adjunctive procedures
- Preliminary considerations
- Ocular surface stabilization
- Tissue adhesive and lamellar keratoplasty
- Superficial keratectomy

Anterior segment reconstruction techniques
- Penetrating keratoplasty
- Lens removal
- Anterior vitrectomy
- Goniosynechialysis
- Removal of anterior segment membranes
- Intraocular lens placement
- Iridoplasty

Results of anterior segment reconstruction

References

Despite meticulous primary repair of a penetrating corneoscleral injury, normal wound-healing mechanisms may result in secondary complications that can be devastating to long-term ocular health and vision. Such sequelae in the anterior segment include (1) corneal scarring, fibrovascular pannus, and astigmatism; (2) glaucoma secondary to either peripheral anterior synechiae, pupillary block, or lens-induced inflammation; (3) vitreous incarceration within ocular wounds and associated chronic inflammation, cystoid macular edema, retinal detachment, and infection; (4) pupillary or cyclitic membranes; (5) conjunctival scarring and symblepharon; and (6) ocular surface epithelial damage with long-term consequences including persistent epithelial defects, stromal vascularization, sterile stromal ulceration, and poor prognosis for penetrating keratoplasty (Fig. 16-1). A number of surgical techniques, when used alone, in combination, or as staged procedures, may restore the normal ocular architecture,

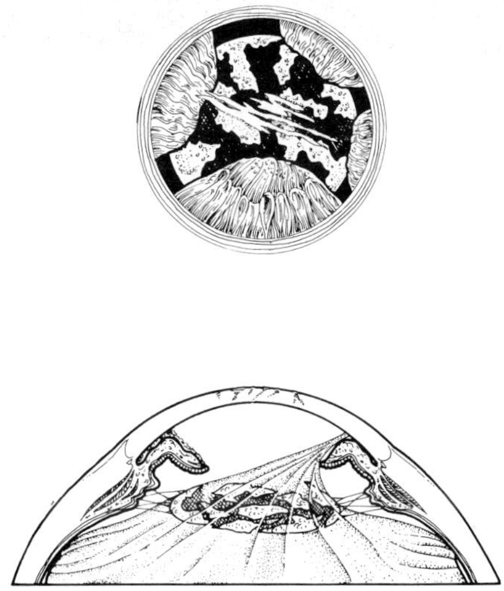

Fig. 16-1. Schematic of traumatized eye showing scarred cornea, disrupted iris, peripheral anterior synechiae, inflammatory membranes over iris, vitreous incarceration, and disrupted lens.

thereby ameliorating adverse sequelae, circumventing further complications, and improving ultimate visual rehabilitation.[1]

The surgical interventions used to reconstruct the traumatized anterior segment are applicable to both closed-chamber and open-sky techniques. This chapter will concentrate on the latter. Chapters 8 and 11 discuss closed-chamber repair of the damaged iris and management of traumatic lens injuries.

PREPARATORY AND ADJUNCTIVE PROCEDURES

Preliminary Considerations

The prognosis for a successful definitive reconstructive effort is optimized by appropriate preoperative preparation of the eye. Intraocular inflammation should be controlled with topical corticosteroids. Penetrating keratoplasty and other intraocular manipulations usually should be withheld until the eye has been quiet for several months. In the presence of an ongoing inflammatory insult—for instance, retained lens material—earlier intervention may be required to remove the offending agent. In addition, intraocular pressure should be controlled before surgery.

Ocular Surface Stabilization

Damage to the lids and ocular adnexa occurs frequently in the eye trauma patient. Ongoing insults such as corneal exposure and trichiasis should be definitively managed before performing complex intraocular surgery. Furthermore, stabilization of the ocular surface is an important concomitant of reconstructive penetrating or lamellar keratoplasty. A variety of lubricants, patching, bandage soft contact lenses, and tissue adhesive help to support, stabilize, and renew the ocular surface.[2] In cases of severe and chronic damage to the ocular surface, pannus stripping and limbal or conjunctival autografting are indicated to improve surface healing, decrease corneal vascularization, and improve the prognosis for subsequent penetrating keratoplasty.[3,4] Chapter 6 discusses these interventions in detail.

Tissue Adhesive and Lamellar Keratoplasty

Tissue adhesive, patch grafting, and lamellar keratoplasty all have a role in providing tectonic support to a cornea severely thinned or persistently leaking after injury. If stromal scarring is located anteriorly, a lamellar keratoplasty with viable epithelium may be of value in providing a more satisfactory stromal bed for future transplant surgery and in improving visual acuity without the potential complications of penetrating keratoplasty. These techniques are discussed in Chapter 13.

Superficial Keratectomy

If corneal surface irregularity and scarring are confined to a superficial fibrovascular pannus, only superficial keratectomy may be required to clear the visual axis, thus obviating penetrating keratoplasty. This procedure may also facilitate intraoperative visualization before closed-chamber reconstructive techniques. Moreover, stripping, or peeling, of corneal pannus is a frequent concomitant of limbal autograft transplantation in the chemical-burned eye (see Chapter 7).

If superficial keratectomy is the only intervention planned, the procedure may be performed in the minor operating room under topical or local anesthesia. The corneal epithelium overlying the involved area is removed with a dry cellulose sponge and, if necessary, careful scraping with a scarifier, avoiding sharp dissection. Preliminary application of cocaine 4% or absolute alcohol with a pledget may be useful to loosen epithelial adhesion. Care should be taken to avoid denuding the entire cornea and damaging the peripheral corneal and limbal epithelium since these represent the source of cells for subsequent reepithelialization.

A distinct cleavage plane is typically present between pannus and relatively normal stroma. To identify this plane atraumatically, the tip of a dry cellulose sponge is insinuated beneath an edge of the fibrovascular tissue (Fig. 16-2). The abnormal tissue is then peeled, or stripped, using the dry sponges and fine tissue forceps. Often the pannus may be removed in toto with relative ease. If sharp dissection with a scarifier or other blade is necessary to mobilize firmly adherent tissue, extreme care should be taken to remain parallel to the cleavage plane, avoiding sharp incision of the corneal stroma with consequent increased scarring.

ANTERIOR SEGMENT RECONSTRUCTION TECHNIQUES

Penetrating Keratoplasty

As discussed in Chapter 13, penetrating keratoplasty is rarely indicated in primary repair af-

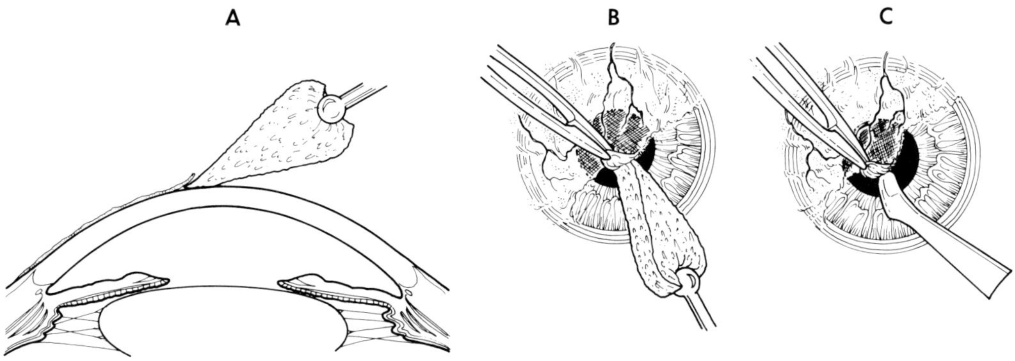

Fig. 16-2. Technique of superficial keratectomy. **A,** A dry cellulose sponge is used to identify a cleavage plane beneath fibrovascular tissue. **B,** The pannus is stripped using a dry sponge and tissue forceps. **C,** A scarifier may be used for firmly adherent tissue, remaining parallel to the cleavage plane to avoid stromal damage.

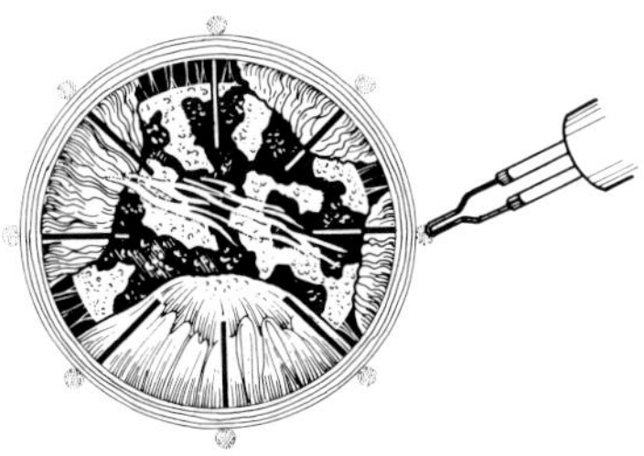

Fig. 16-3. An eight-blade radial keratotomy marker coated with gentian violet is used to delineate the meridians for placement of cardinal sutures. A disposable cautery is used to mark these meridians at the limbus.

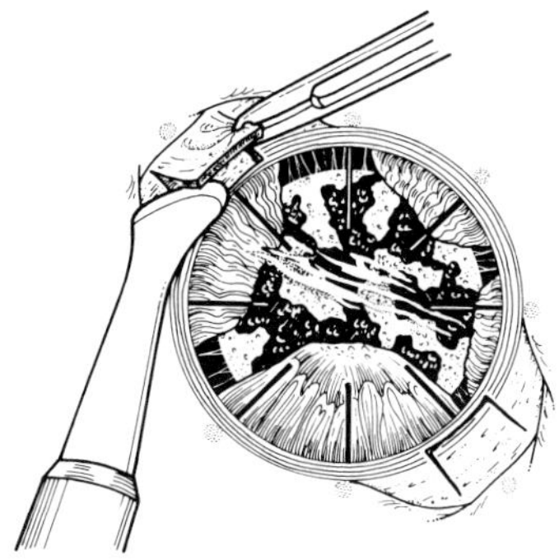

Fig. 16-4. Preparation of scleral flaps for placement of scleral sutured posterior chamber lens.

ter ocular trauma but is used frequently in secondary anterior segment reconstruction. Although penetrating keratoplasty and anterior chamber reconstruction are definitive treatments for complicated anterior segment injury, keratoplasty usually is delayed until the eye is free of infection and inflammation to optimize ultimate graft survival. Although the general surgical principles of penetrating keratoplasty obtain in anterior segment reconstruction as well, additional specialized maneuvers and instrumentation are helpful.

Generally, a Flieringa ring is unnecessary, because the principal meridians of cardinal suture placement may be delineated with an eight-blade radial keratotomy marker. The edges of the marker are coated with a gentian violet tissue-marking pen to clarify the impressions made on the cornea. The eight cardinal suture meridians are then marked at the limbus with disposable cautery (Fig. 16-3). Alignment of the donor tissue and proper suture placement are thereby ensured even in the event of anterior segment and scleral distortion. If preferred, a Flieringa ring may be placed to minimize scleral collapse after trephination, especially in aphakic or highly myopic eyes and in children.

If it is anticipated that a posterior chamber intraocular lens (IOL) will be sutured through the ciliary sulcus, conjunctival peritomy and scleral flaps are prepared in the appropriate meridians. These flaps are subsequently used to cover the anchoring polypropylene suture, thereby preventing erosion through the conjunctiva, which could cause discomfort and supply a conduit for microbial invasion of the globe. A scarifier blade is used to outline and dissect a half-scleral-thickness flap approximately 4 mm at its base (Fig. 16-4). To facilitate subsequent observation of the needle as it is passed, the flap may be triangular or rectangular and limbus-, fornix-, or side-based, depending on its location on the globe. The flap must span the limbus, because the exit point of the suture from the ciliary sulcus should be only 0.5 to 1 mm posterior to the limbus.

A donor cornea button is trephined 0.5 mm larger than the host bed. Such oversizing may aid in preventing peripheral anterior synechiae and glaucoma postoperatively.[5,6] For recipient trephination, an instrument allowing for good visualization and precise trephine placement should be used. Particularly valuable are vacuum and motorized trephines. These designs also make trephination safer in the setting of a flat anterior chamber, corneal perforation, or extensive iridocorneal adhesion.

In the presence of hypotony or corneal perforation, trephination may be facilitated by restoration of the anterior chamber with viscoelastic placed directly through the wound or through a limbal stab incision.[7,8] Application of cyanoacrylate tissue adhesive to the wound may further stabilize the globe for easier trephination.

In eyes with a formed anterior chamber, the chamber may be entered directly with the trephine or sharp microsurgical blade. If the anterior chamber cannot be reformed, a shallow trephination groove is made (avoiding distortion of the globe, if possible), the groove deepened and the eye entered with a blade, and the corneal button removed with Vannas or corneal scissors.

In eyes with a flat chamber, synechiae, and other adhesions involving cornea, iris, lens, and vitreous, forceps, dry cellulose sponges, and Vannas scissors are used to carefully separate the cornea from its posterior adhesions (Fig. 16-5).

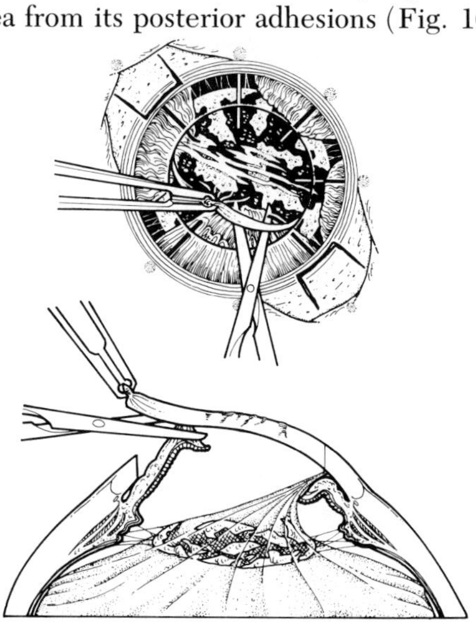

Fig. 16-5. Removal of recipient cornea. After trephination, the cornea is separated from any posterior adhesions by blunt dissection with Vannas scissors or cellulose sponges.

Great care is taken to preserve and not excise or damage any iris tissue along with the corneal button, because this tissue may be used for subsequent iridoplasty.

Rarely, rotating autografts may be used to move a focal scar from the visual axis. Such a procedure is particularly useful in patients at high risk of graft rejection, such as children.[9]

In posttrauma eyes requiring vitreoretinal surgery, a scarred cornea may preclude satisfactory intraocular visualization. In such cases, penetrating keratoplasty may be combined with open-sky vitrectomy, especially in cases with anterior vitreoretinal pathology.[10] Alternatively, a temporary keratoprosthesis may be used to allow a traditional closed-vitrectomy approach.[11] A number of keratoprosthesis designs have been described. The Landers-Foulks lens remains the most popular and gives good visualization of the posterior retina and vitreous.[12] However, its long central cyclinder makes visualization near the pars plana and vitreous base difficult. The Eckardt lens provides a better view of the anterior fundus and may be more useful in patients with anterior proliferative vitreoretinopathy.[13] After vitreoretinal intervention, the prosthesis is removed and keratoplasty completed. Because the keratoprosthesis dilates the trephination opening by about 0.5 mm, the donor cornea should be appropriately oversized.

Lens Removal

The state of the lens dictates the method by which it is managed surgically. The rare lens that remains clear after trauma is, of course, left untouched during surgery. If the lens is cataractous but the posterior capsule appears intact, a standard extracapsular cataract extraction is performed and a posterior chamber IOL may be placed. In many cases of eye trauma, the anterior and posterior capsules have been ruptured, the zonules disrupted, and the vitreous violated.

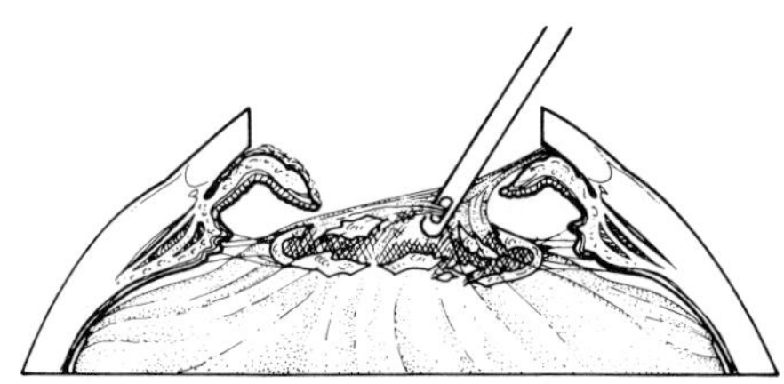

Fig. 16-6. Open-sky lensectomy and anterior vitrectomy performed with microvitrectomy instrumentation.

In such cases, the lens material is often flocculent, and lensectomy and anterior vitrectomy may be performed using microvitrectomy suction and cutting instrumentation (Fig. 16-6 and Color Plate 16-1). Hard nuclear remnants may be removed with a lens loop.

Anterior Vitrectomy

Fibrotic and incarcerated vitreous should be excised to prevent the well-recognized complications of chronic inflammation, cystoid macular edema, intraocular fibrosis, and retinal detachment. All vitreous should be removed from the anterior chamber to prevent vitreous from touching or adhering to the donor cornea, which would predispose toward graft failure. Anterior vitrectomy also facilitates iris reconstruction and IOL placement.

Microvitrectomy suction and cutting instrumentation is used to perform the anterior vitrectomy atraumatically and to lyse iridovitreal and other adhesions (Fig. 16-6). When using an open-sky technique, irrigation is not necessary. In some instances, cellulose sponges may be used to gently identify and isolate vitreous strands that may then be excised with Vannas scissors (Fig. 16-7). Such sponges may also be used to verify the complete removal of vitreous from the anterior chamber, iris, and angle. At the completion of the vitrectomy, the iris diaphragm should spontaneously fall back into its physiologic position.

Goniosynechialysis

Goniosynechialysis is performed with two major goals. The first is to lyse peripheral anterior synechiae in the hope of improving aqueous outflow, thus minimizing postoperative glaucoma.[14] Careful synechialysis may also mitigate postoperative reformation of peripheral anterior synechiae (PAS) with progressive closure ("zippering") of the angle, a dreaded complication of penetrating keratoplasty. The second goal of goniosynechialysis is to liberate incarcerated and scarred iris tissue for subsequent reconstructive iridoplasty.

When performing open-sky goniosynechialysis, extreme caution must be exercised to avoid damaging iris remnants, creating an iatrogenic iridodialysis and causing excessive bleeding from the iris, fibrovascular scar tissue, or ciliary body. To prevent cutting or tearing remaining iris, blunt dissection with dry cellulose sponges is preferred. Adherent iris is pushed posteriorly while supplying anterior countertraction on the keratoplasty wound margin with tissue forceps (Fig. 16-8). If the proper plane of dissection cannot be obtained in this manner or the adhesion is too tenacious, a blunt cyclodialysis spatula may be used with a similar technique. It is important, however, to avoid lateral sweeping with metal instruments that may tear tissue or induce bleeding.

Alternatively, smooth forceps may be used to hold the pupillary edge of the iris. The adherent iris is pulled down posteriorly, applying countertraction on the wound margin. In rare circumstances in which the iris is tightly adherent to posterior cornea, Vannas scissors may be used in a spreading fashion to dissect bluntly

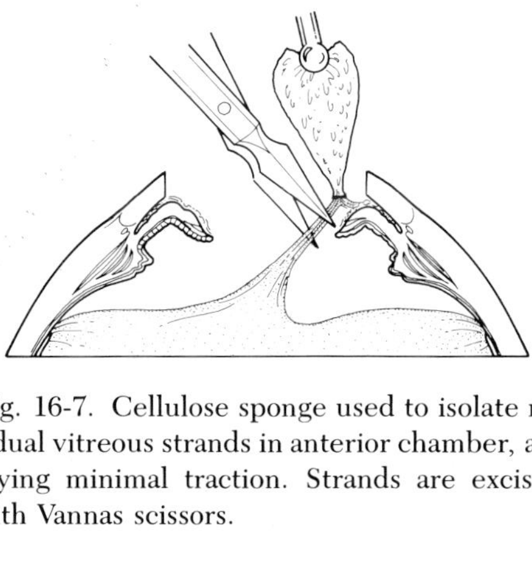

Fig. 16-7. Cellulose sponge used to isolate residual vitreous strands in anterior chamber, applying minimal traction. Strands are excised with Vannas scissors.

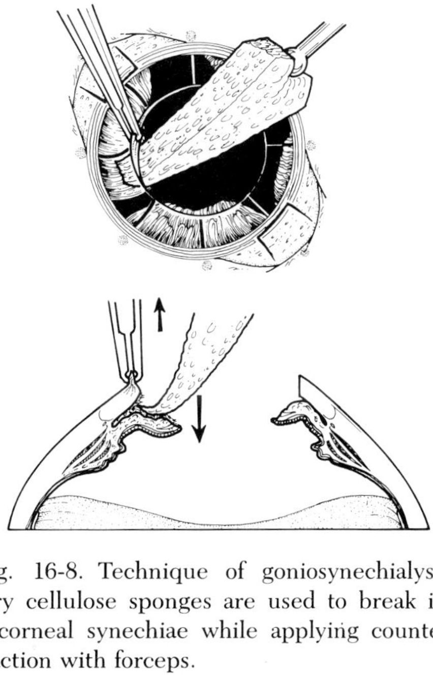

Fig. 16-8. Technique of goniosynechialysis. Dry cellulose sponges are used to break iridocorneal synechiae while applying countertraction with forceps.

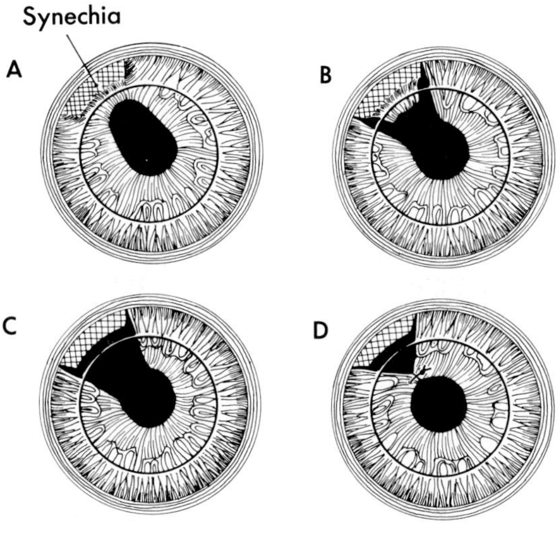

Fig. 16-9. Technique of goniosynechialysis in cases with extensive peripheral anterior synechiae (PAS). **A,** Iris with firmly adherent PAS from the 9 o'clock to the 11:30 position. **B,** Iris is cut radially at each side of the PAS. **C,** The included sector of iris is excised. **D,** Iridoplasty performed to restore taut iris diaphragm without synechiae.

within the appropriate plane. Cellulose sponges and smooth forceps may then be used to peel back the iridocorneal adhesions. A pupil drawn toward the wound can usually be freed by similar synechialysis techniques (Color Plate 16-2).

When synechiae cannot be lysed despite meticulous effort, the iris may be cut radially on each side of the PAS and the included sector of iris excised[15] (Fig. 16-9). This leaves a sector iris defect that may be closed by iridoplasty techniques. More importantly, the risk of zippering new synechiae adjacent to the original PAS is reduced.

The success of the goniosynechialysis maneuvers may be visualized intraoperatively with an angled dental mirror. If bleeding is encountered, viscoelastic should be placed into the anterior chamber to isolate the blood and prevent leakage posteriorly into the vitreous. Other methods of hemostasis include the direct application of epinephrine 1:10,000, thrombin-soaked cellulose sponges or Gel-foam (100 U/ml), or direct cauterization of the bleeding site with underwater microcautery.

Goniosynechialysis techniques also may be used in closed-chamber reconstructive efforts. Entering the eye through small paracentesis sites and filling the anterior chamber with viscoelastic will maintain chamber depth during the procedure. For phakic eyes, a special curved cyclodialysis spatula has been devised to vault the lens, thereby preventing damage.[16] Intraocular scissors may be used in some instances to lyse synechiae directly through the small incision. Early intervention, before irreversible scarring of PAS with the trabecular meshwork occurs, may be rewarded with improved postoperative intraocular pressure control.

In cases with long-standing synechiae, high intraocular pressure despite maximally tolerated glaucoma therapy, and optic nerve damage, filtration surgery usually should be performed before penetrating keratoplasty and anterior segment reconstruction. This allows intraocular pressure to be stabilized before extensive intraocular surgery. Only in rare cases are combined trabeculectomy and penetrating keratoplasty appropriate.[17]

Removal of Anterior Segment Membranes

Following trauma, organized fibrovascular membranes and Descemet's-like hyalinized membranes frequently form over the anterior iris, angle structures, and posterior cornea. These membranes should be identified and peeled to avoid further fibrosis, synechiae, angle compromise, and ciliary body detachment. A dry cellulose sponge may be used to identify the cleavage plane between membrane and normal iris tissue. The edge is elevated with fine tissue forceps and the membranes gently peeled from the anterior chamber angle, exercising extreme care to avoid tearing the fragile iris tissue (Fig. 16-10).

Intraocular Lens Placement

The placement of an intraocular lens and selection of IOL type and implantation technique must be tailored to the individual case. Patient

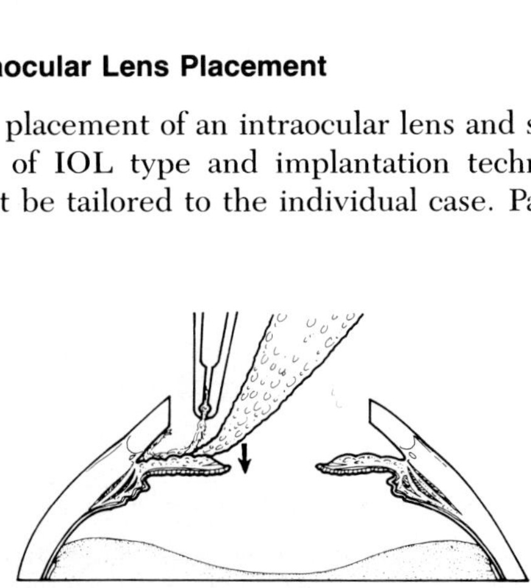

Fig. 16-10. Removal of hyalinized membranes from anterior chamber.

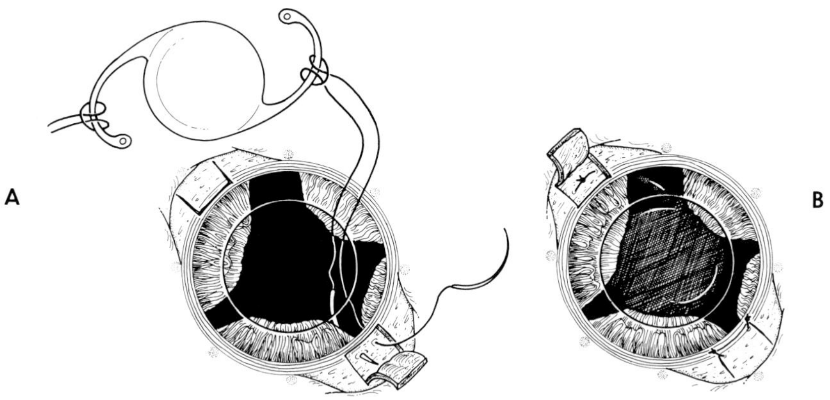

Fig. 16-11. Placement of scleral-sutured posterior chamber intraocular lens in absence of capsular support. **A,** After anterior vitrectomy, a girth-hitch knot is used to secure IOL haptics with double-armed polypropylene sutures. The needles are brought under the iris and through the ciliary sulcus, exiting approximately 0.5 to 1 mm posterior to the limbus. **B,** Sutures are tied in mattress fashion, and the scleral flap is repositioned over the knot and secured with sutures.

age, optical and physical status of the other eye, and architectural state of the injured eye will all be factors in decisions regarding the advisability of IOL implantation. Some younger patients, for instance, may be able to wear an aphakic contact lens postoperatively and not require an IOL.[18] Contact lens correction may, in fact, neutralize irregular astigmatism caused by a corneal scar. Other patients may require IOL insertion for optimal visual rehabilitation.

If an anterior chamber IOL is chosen, a flexible uniplanar lens may be preferred to prevent forward vaulting toward the graft endothelium. Moreover, the splinting action of an anterior chamber IOL may actually be helpful in maintaining an open angle postoperatively. In selected cases where the angle seems especially prone to postoperative synechia formation, a flexible tripod type of implant with slightly angled haptics (e.g., Allergan #AC21) may be placed in a reversed position (haptics angled anteriorly) so that the optic is concave to the haptics. This configuration will mechanically push the angle open and displace the optic posteriorly from the graft. If an anterior chamber IOL is used, it should be placed after iris reconstruction is completed (as described later in this chapter).

The potential benefits of a posterior chamber IOL include less compromise of the filtration angle and corneal endothelium, the anatomical structures most often damaged after trauma. Clearly, if an extracapsular cataract extraction has been performed, it is preferable to place a posterior chamber IOL. Recently, posterior chamber IOLs sutured directly to the posterior surface of the iris or into the ciliary sulcus in the absence of posterior capsular support have been successful in nontraumatic cases.[19,20] When such a technique is used, adequate anterior vitrectomy must be verified before lens placement.

If sulcus fixation is desired, IOL implantation should be performed before iridoplasty to allow for better visualization (Fig. 16-11). Each haptic is secured respectively with one double-armed 10-0 polypropylene suture. We prefer the Ethicon BV100-4 needle because of its sharpness and fine caliber, which prevent tissue trauma. A standard spatula needle (e.g., Ethicon TG160 or Alcon CU-5) may also be used. Occasionally, the longer Ethicon CIF-4 needle (generally most valuable for secondary posterior chamber IOL implantation without keratoplasty) may be used if the ciliary sulcus is difficult to reach with a short needle. The haptic may be secured by the suture either through a control hole at its tip or by a girth-hitch knot tied around the haptic itself.[18] The two sutures should be symmetrically positioned 180° apart to ensure lens centration. The needles are then brought under the iris, through the ciliary sulcus, and out through the previously dissected scleral beds. The suture exit is approximately 0.5 to 1 mm posterior to the limbus. The lens optic is positioned, the anchoring sutures tied, and the scleral flaps brought over the knot and secured at their corners with 10-0 nylon or 8-0 absorbable suture.

Alternatively, the posterior chamber IOL may be sutured directly to the iris.[21] This procedure should be performed after partial iris reconstruction, thereby allowing the ultimate position of the iris segments to be appreciated but still permitting admission of the IOL to the posterior chamber. Two double-armed mattress sutures of 10-0 polypropylene on fine needles are placed through opposing positioning holes on the optic or around the optic-haptic junctions and brought up through the underside of the iris. The 2-inch Ethicon BV100-4 suture is specially tailored for this purpose. Each suture is tied over the iris and the ends are trimmed close to the knot.

Although sutured posterior chamber IOLs have some theoretical advantages over anterior chamber designs, their long-term propriety is as yet unclear.

Iridoplasty

Iridoplasty is undertaken when the iris is free of all adhesions, membranes and other scar tissues have been cleared from the anterior chamber, and anterior vitrectomy has been performed. The goals of such iris reconstruction are (1) restoration of a tight iris diaphragm to lessen the risk of further synechia formation and secondary glaucoma, (2) improvement in graft survival by preventing iridocorneal adhesions and glaucoma, (3) reconstruction of the pupil to prevent glare and improve appearance, and (4) formation of a stable iris diaphragm for support of an anterior or posterior chamber IOL.[22]

In performing iridoplasty, thorough goniosynechialysis must first be achieved. The more iris adhesions that can be freed, the more tissue is available for reconstructive efforts (Color Plate 16-3). Simple interrupted sutures of 10-0 nylon or polypropylene are then placed from iris edge to iris edge to reform the iris diaphragm (Fig. 16-12). Polypropylene is preferred for sutures placed under tension, as in the resuspension of dialyzed iris. Although polypropylene is also an excellent suture material for iris surgery in general, we have not encountered long-term degradation or separation of iris repair performed with nylon sutures. This is, of course, contrary to the fate of nylon used to fixate IOLs or corneal grafts. As described, a fine, round, tapered needle is preferable to a spatula or cutting needle to minimize tissue trauma.

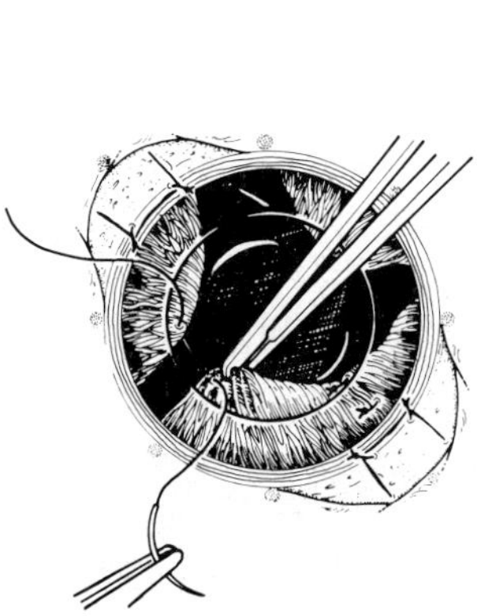

Fig. 16-12. Interrupted sutures of 10-0 nylon or polypropylene used to perform iridoplasty.

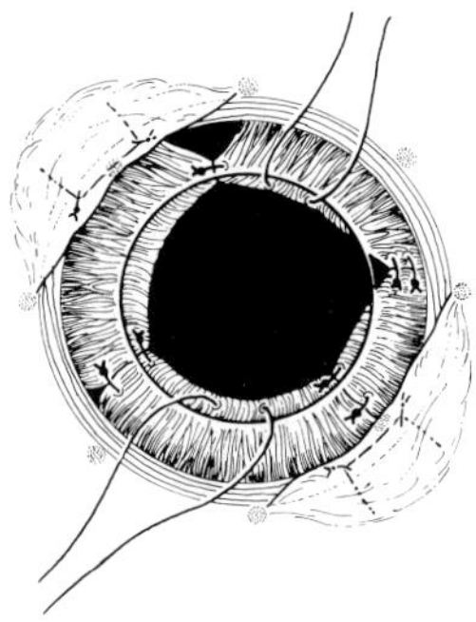

Fig. 16-13. Tucking sutures placed near the pupil to tighten flaccid iris.

The suture needle should be passed completely through one edge of the iris, regrasped with the needle holder, and then passed through the other edge of the iris. This maneuver prevents excessive traction and possible tearing of fragile iris tissue during the second needle pass. Any sector iridectomies created during goniosynechialysis should be closed with interrupted sutures (Fig. 16-12). Flaccid irides with excessively large pupils can be made more taut by "tucking" with one or more broad interrupted sutures placed tangentially near the iris sphincter (Fig. 16-13).

Despite the extraordinary plasticity of the iris, additional tissue mobilization may be necessary. For instance, relaxing incisions and sphincterotomies may aid in forming a rounder pupil after preliminary iridoplasty sutures are placed. In the event of traumatic loss of large areas of tissue with only small pieces remaining, iris pedicle flaps may be mobilized that can then be used to form an adequate pupillary aperture. Such mobilization can be achieved by judiciously cutting relaxing incisions in the remaining iris tissue. The freed tissue is then recon-

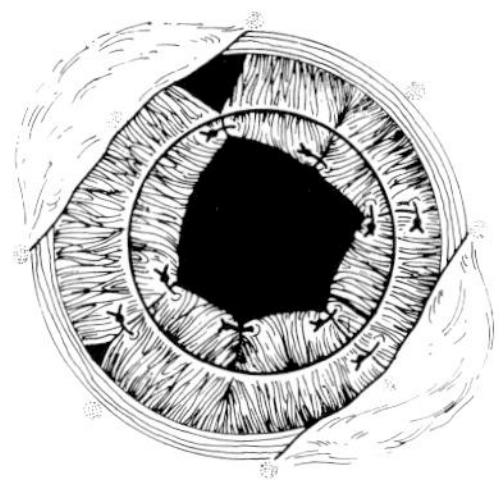

Fig. 16-14. At the completion of iridoplasty, the iris architecture has been restored, the anterior chamber is deep, and the angle is open.

A

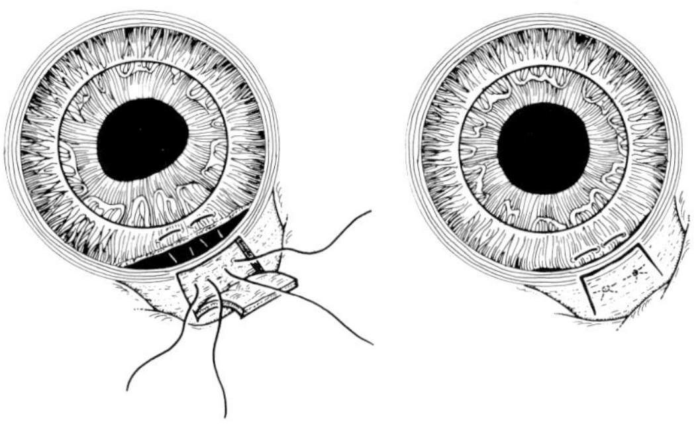

B

Fig. 16-15. Repair of iridodialysis. **A,** A conjunctival peritomy and scleral flap has been prepared. Mattress sutures of 10-0 polypropylene are placed through the iris and passed through the ciliary sulcus. **B,** The sutures are tied and the scleral flap repositioned over the knots and secured.

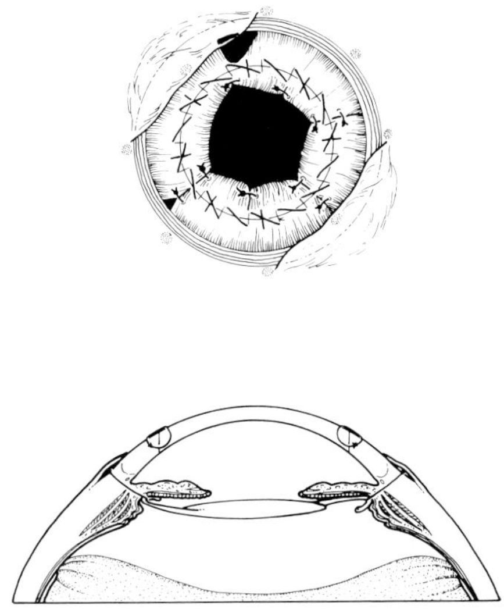

Fig. 16-16. Corneal graft sutured with eight interrupted sutures and one running suture. Vitreous is behind the iris, posterior chamber lens in place, anterior segment free of inflammatory membranes, chamber deep, angle open, and iris diaphragm restored.

structed using standard iridoplasty techniques (Fig. 16-14).

If an iridodialysis is present or only small amounts of iris remain, iris remnants and pedicle flaps may be anchored with one or more mattress sutures passed through the angle just anterior to the ciliary sulcus and secured through the limbus (Color Plate 16-4). Polypropylene suture material is preferred, using either a fine tapered needle or a longer needle (e.g., Ethicon CIF-4) if necessary to reach through the sclera. A conjunctival peritomy and scleral flap should first be prepared as for sulcus-sutured posterior chamber IOLs to allow for easier needle penetration and for subsequent coverage and protection of the suture knot. Sutures are then placed in mattress fashion through the iris tissue, passed through the sclera, and finally exit the sclera through the premade bed (Fig. 16-15). Scleral depression with a cotton-tipped applicator may aid in direct visualization of the ciliary sulcus during suture placement. These techniques may also be adapted to closed-chamber iris repair[23] (see Chapter 8).

If the preceding maneuvers have resulted in a complete, stable iris diaphragm but the pupil is overly small and misshapen, the pupil may be trimmed with Vannas scissors to form a rounder central opening. At the completion of the procedure, the pupil should be central, the iris posterior, the angle open with a deep anterior chamber, and the vitreous behind the iris with a clear visual axis. The corneal donor graft may then be sutured by the surgeon's preferred technique (Fig. 16-16). We have seen few intraoperative or postoperative complications with the iridoplasty techniques described.

RESULTS OF ANTERIOR SEGMENT RECONSTRUCTION

A review of penetrating eye trauma cases that have undergone secondary anterior segment reconstruction has revealed encouraging results.[24] In a series of 40 consecutive patients, 90% of whom started with a visual acuity of 20/200 or worse (70% <20/400), 50% attained postoperative vision of 20/100 or better. Visual acuity improved by at least two Snellen lines in 70% of the cases. At 2-year follow-up, 80% of the corneal grafts remained clear. Goniosynechialysis anatomically corrected approximately 65% of the preoperative synechiae. Postoperative glaucoma was generally restricted to those patients with preoperative glaucoma and persistent synechiae. Severe complications were rare.

References

1. Mackenson G and Faulborn J: Primary and secondary reconstruction of the eyeball after extensive lacerations, Ophthalmic Surg 5:43-49, 1974.
2. Kenyon KR: Decision-making in the therapy of external eye disease: noninfected corneal ulcers, Ophthalmology 89:44-51, 1982.
3. Kenyon KR and Tseng SCG: Limbal autograft transplantation for ocular surface disorders, Ophthalmology 96:709-723, 1989.
4. Thoft RA: Conjunctival transplantation, Arch Ophthalmol 95:1425-1427, 1977.
5. Zimmerman T et al: Transplant size and elevated intraocular pressure, Arch Ophthalmol 96:2231-2233, 1978.
6. Heidemann DG et al: Oversized donor grafts in penetrating keratoplasty, Arch Ophthalmol 103:1807-1811, 1985.
7. Drews RC: Sodium hyaluronate (Healon) in the repair of perforating injuries of the eye, Ophthalmic Surg 17:23-29, 1986.
8. Stegmann R and Miller D: Use of sodium hyaluronate in severe penetrating ocular trauma, Ann Ophthalmol 18:9-13, 1986.
9. Bourne WM and Brubaker RF: A method for ipsilateral rotational autokeratoplasty, Trans Am Acad Ophthalmol Otolaryngol 85:1312-1316, 1978.
10. Schepens CL: Clinical and research aspects of subtotal open-sky vitrectomy, Am J Ophthalmol 91:143-171, 1981.
11. Gelender H et al: Temporary keratoprosthesis for combined penetrating keratoplasty, pars plana vitrectomy, and repair of retinal detachment, Ophthalmology 95:897-900, 1988.
12. Landers MB et al: Temporary keratoprosthesis for use during pars plana vitrectomy, Am J Ophthalmol 91:615-619, 1981.
13. Eckardt C: A new temporary keratoprosthesis for pars plana vitrectomy, Retina 7:34-37, 1987.
14. Chandler PA and Simmons RJ: Anterior chamber deepening for gonioscopy at time of surgery, Arch Ophthalmol 74:177-190, 1965.
15. Cohen EJ, Kenyon KR, and Dohlman CH: Iridoplasty for prevention of post-keratoplasty angle closure and glaucoma, Ophthalmic Surg 13:994-996, 1982.
16. Campbell DG and Vela A: Modern goniosynechialysis for the treatment of synechial angle-closure glaucoma, Ophthalmology 91:1053-1060, 1984.
17. Barraquer J et al: Penetrating keratoplasty combined with trabeculectomy, cataract extraction and, occasionally, vitrectomy, An Inst Barraquer 18:13-53, 1985.
18. Smiddy WE et al: Contact lenses for visual rehabilitation after corneal laceration repair, Ophthalmology 96:293-298, 1989.
19. Cowden JW and Hu BV: A new surgical technique for posterior chamber lens fixation during penetrating keratoplasty in the absence of capsular or zonular support, Cornea 7:231-235, 1988.
20. Price FW and Whitson WE: Visual results of suture-fixated posterior chamber lenses during penetrating keratoplasty, Ophthalmology 96:1234-1240, 1989.
21. Soong HK et al: Implantation of posterior chamber intraocular lenses in the absence of lens capsule during penetrating keratoplasty, Arch Ophthalmol 107:660-665, 1989.
22. Troutman RC: Microsurgery of the anterior segment of the eye, vol II, St Louis, 1977, The CV Mosby Co.
23. Pallin SL: Closed chamber iridoplasty, Ophthalmic Surg 12:213-214, 1982.
24. Kenyon KR, Starck T, and Hersh PS, Unpublished data, 1990.

PART 3

Posterior segment trauma

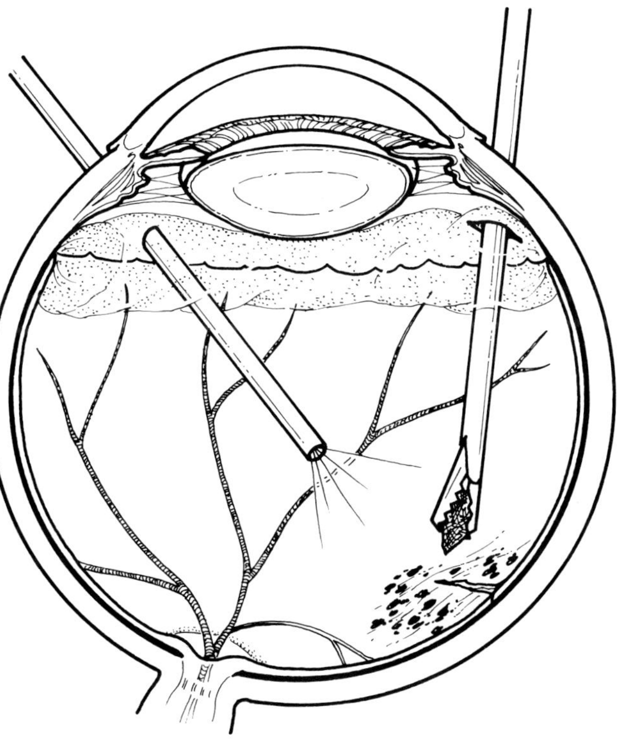

CHAPTER 17

Traumatic maculopathies

SUSAN B. BRESSLER
NEIL M. BRESSLER

Commotio retinae (Berlin's edema, concussion edema)
Purtscher's retinopathy
Choroidal rupture
Retinitis sclopetaria
Traumatic macular hole
References

Several posterior pole retinopathies may result from blunt injury. Direct injury to the globe, lid, or orbit may result in commotio retinae, choroidal rupture, retinitis sclopetaria, or macular hole. Remote trauma, such as a compressive or crush injury to the chest or long bones, may result in Purtscher's retinopathy.

Blunt trauma delivered to the ocular, periocular, or cranial region may produce ocular damage by one or any combination of the following mechanisms: coup, contrecoup, or direct ocular compression.[1] A coup injury is one that is produced by local trauma directly at the site of blunt impact. A contrecoup mechanism explains contusive damage that appears at a site opposite to the site of the blunt impact: a line of force is created that traverses the eye, creating contusive damage at tissue interfaces. Because one such interface is between the chorioretinal tissues and the dense sclera, the retina is particularly vulnerable to a contrecoup injury.[1] Blunt ocular injuries often compress the eye along its anteroposterior axis. Because the volume of the eye is fixed, this anteroposterior compression results in horizontal displacement of the eye's fluid volume. As the eye expands in its horizontal plane, several posterior segment structures are severely stretched and may tear, producing, for example, choroidal ruptures.

Blunt ocular trauma may create many types of injuries, and a traumatized eye must be examined thoroughly so as not to overlook damage in any structure. However, associated injuries such as hyphema or vitreous hemorrhage may hinder the examiner's ability to evaluate the retinal structures. Sequential retinal examinations may be necessary as the media clear. Furthermore, the effects of the trauma on the visual prognosis may not be realized in the acute setting. For instance, maculopathies may arise as a delayed consequence and ultimately contribute to visual disability. Therefore, an injured eye should be observed periodically, for an indefinite period to search for late complications of the initial injury.

Little is known regarding effective therapeutic intervention for fundus lesions resulting from blunt trauma, but it is important to recognize these injuries to help formulate a prognosis.[2] The long-term prognosis is based on the immediate anatomic derangement, the immediate functional performance, and the potential effects of long-term sequelae.[3]

COMMOTIO RETINAE (BERLIN'S EDEMA, CONCUSSION EDEMA)

Commotio retinae (Latin for retinal contusion) was first described by Berlin in 1873. This clinical entity was characterized by (1) an immediate diminution in central vision regardless of the location of visible retinal opacification, (2) ophthalmoscopically visible retinal clouding that ultimately resolved without visible sequelae, and (3) return of visual function to pretrauma levels. At present, the term commotio retinae is used in a broader sense to include cases of Berlin's edema, as well as cases of contrecoup concussive damage in which vision may not return to prior levels and in which fundus morphology may be affected permanently.

Blunt trauma to the anterior portion of the globe may produce commotio retinae anywhere in the posterior segment. Typically, the injury occurs opposite the site of direct impact. It may take several minutes or hours for the ophthalmoscopic features to be manifest. The lesion consists of a geographic pattern of gray-white cloudy opacification of the outer retina (Color Plate 17-1). The margins of the lesion are frequently ill defined. On contact lens biomicroscopy, the inner retinal blood vessels are clearly seen and undisturbed, and the hazy edematous swelling appears localized to the outer retina. The edema may be confined to the macula, posterior pole, or peripapillary region or involve more extensive and peripheral areas of retina. If the entire posterior pole is involved, a pseudo–cherry red spot may arise, and the condition may be confused with a central retinal artery occlusion.[2] Other associated injuries, such as subretinal, intraretinal, or preretinal hemorrhages, choroidal rupture, and serous macular detachment, may be present.

The patient may be asymptomatic if the commotio is limited to the peripheral retina. If the macular region is involved, the patient may experience acute visual loss. The visual acuity, which may range from 20/20 to 20/400, does not always correlate with the degree of retinal opacification.[4]

In most cases, fluorescein angiography performed within hours or days of the original injury fails to show any alteration of retinal or choroidal vascular permeability in the affected area.[5] The opaque retina may block background choroidal fluorescence. On occasion, transient retinal arteriolar dye leakage has been demonstrated on angiography, but these patients also may have had Purtscher's retinopathy.[6] Hyperfluorescent staining at the level of the retinal pigment epithelium (RPE) has also been reported on angiography obtained early in a patient's course. In such instances, the staining probably represents necrosis of the RPE sustained from the same injury.[7]

The retinal whitening gradually subsides within several weeks following the trauma. Generally speaking, the prognosis for central vision is excellent but guarded, particularly if other injuries are present. The ophthalmoscopically visible lesion may clear entirely with complete restoration of visual function, or there may be permanent loss of visual function with or without visibly apparent fundus changes. Patients may progress to varying degrees of retinal abnormality. The RPE may appear mottled, with areas of distinct atrophy or hyperplasia or both. In these cases, subsequent angiography may demonstrate hyperfluorescent window defects and hypofluorescent areas corresponding to the areas of RPE atrophy and RPE hyperplasia, respectively. Pigment migration into the retina may be so severe that a pseudo–retinitis pigmentosa syndrome is noted.[7] If significant areas of photoreceptors are destroyed, localized visual field defects may result.[4] A partial or full-thickness macular hole may develop. The absence of fluorescein angiographic abnormalities early in the course may help in assessing the long-term prognosis.[5]

The etiology of commotio retinae is controversial. Sipperley, Quigley, and Gass[8] produced an experimental model of commotio retinae in the monkey eye in which a contrecoup posterior pole injury followed blunt corneal trauma. The model had ophthalmoscopic and angiographic features identical to those of acute traumatic retinal opacity in humans. Within 4 hours of the trauma, all histologic abnormalities were limited to the photoreceptors, with disorganization and pyknosis of their nuclei. The retinal blood vessels, choroidal blood vessels, and RPE were normal. Within the first day posttrauma, progressively increasing photoreceptor degeneration was seen. By the second day, RPE cells had begun to migrate into the retina. Several weeks to months later, RPE cells were found at all levels of the sensory retina, and there was generalized thinning of the outer plexiform and outer nuclear layers. No intracellular or extracellular edema was found.

This model suggests that the visual outcome of an eye with commotio retinae is dependent on the number and location of damaged photoreceptors. If the damage is limited to the outer segment, this portion of the cell may be regenerated and normal function returned. If more extensive photoreceptor destruction occurs at the nuclear level, the cell is more apt to die.

Blight and Hart[9] produced traumatic retinopathy in pigs following blunt trauma. This model produced a coup injury. Photoreceptor fragmentation occurred within minutes of the injury, followed by loss of the photoreceptor outer segments and absence of extracellular edema. However, they also found intracellular edema of the RPE. Perhaps the RPE of the pig responds differently from the RPE of primates, including humans.[9]

Histopathologic study of human eyes subjected to blunt injury has demonstrated edema in the outer plexiform layer, nuclear layers, and subretinal space. Whether this edema represents a primary or secondary event is not known. The macula may contain cystoid areas that coalesce to produce a large cyst. The walls of the macular cyst may degenerate and create a partial or full-thickness macular hole. Photoreceptor loss is evident, as is generalized atrophy of the neuronal and supporting elements. RPE degeneration, hyperplasia, and migration are also present.

PURTSCHER'S RETINOPATHY

In 1912 Purtscher described traumatic retinal angiopathy in five patients who had suffered severe head injuries. A retinopathy developed that was characterized by inner retinal white spots, superficial retinal hemorrhages, and papillitis.

In its classic form, Purtscher's retinopathy consists of marked generalized retinal edema, macular edema, multiple patches of peripapillary superficial retinal whitening, intraretinal hemorrhages, and disc edema (Color Plate 17-2). The nerve fiber layer infarcts follow the distribution of the major temporal vessels, are 1 disc diameter or smaller in size, and are accompanied by a few intraretinal or preretinal hemorrhages or both. The intraretinal hemorrhages are found predominantly in the posterior pole.[10] These ocular findings may be either unilateral or bilateral and asymmetric. In cases of apparent unilateral involvement, very subtle findings on biomicroscopy or angiography may be present in the contralateral eye.[11]

In Purtscher's retinopathy, the setting is one of severe head trauma or chest compression in the absence of direct trauma to the globe. The frequency of this condition is unknown, but it is generally considered rare. The fundus changes begin immediately following the injury, may progress for 1 to 2 days, and are not accompanied by systemic disease other than that directly related to the injury. Visual acuity is variably affected and may range from 20/20 to finger-counting. Dense paracentral or central scotomas and an afferent pupillary defect may be present. The fundus changes typically resolve over a 4-month period.[12] Visual acuity and fundus appearance may return to normal, or there may be permanent visual loss associated with various fundus findings. Often there is some degree of optic atrophy, alteration of the RPE (particularly in the macula), and residual paracentral or central scotoma or arcuate field defects.[6,12] Any afferent pupillary defect may persist. The fundus may also show attenuation of the retinal vessels and nerve fiber bundle atrophy.[12]

In the acute stages of Purtscher's retinopathy, the following fluorescein angiographic findings have been demonstrated: normal choroidal filling with some blockage of background choroidal fluorescence, impaired or occluded retinal arteriolar flow or leakage of small arterioles, areas of retinal capillary nonperfusion or leakage, late perivenous staining and/or partial vein obstruction, and optic disc edema.[6,11-13]

The fundus features of Purtscher's retinopathy may also appear as the result of other traumatic injuries or disease states, such as post-traumatic fat embolism, compression cyanosis, minor chest compression associated with seat-belt injury, acute pancreatitis with fat embolism, ophthalmological hydrostatic pressure syndrome, lupus erythematosus, dermatomyositis, air embolism, scleroderma, and amniotic fluid embolism.[7] However, a few clinical features—such as precipitating events, associated systemic disease, and the interval between injury and onset of visual signs and symptoms—may serve to distinguish between classic Purtscher's retinopathy and other conditions.

A similar fundus picture may result as a rare and delayed complication following fracture or crush injury of one or several long bones, most commonly the tibia and femur. The fracture may result in liberation of intramedullary fat emboli, which escape into the venous circulation, circumnavigate the pulmonary circulation, traverse the left side of the heart, and eventually reach the retinal vessels.[2] Ophthalmoscopically, these emboli may be recognized as hard, yellow-white exudates. These fat emboli may also lodge within the pulmonary, cerebral, and cutaneous circulations. Therefore, the ocular disturbance is often accompanied by other systemic pathology, such as increased respiratory rate, cough, cyanosis, restlessness, disorientation, seizure, coma, and cutaneous petechial hemorrhages.[10] Additional distinguishing features of the retinopathy associated with fat embolization are mild delay in onset of the visual disturbance following the initial trauma (often 2 to 3 days following the trauma rather than immediately, as in Purtscher's retinopathy), progressive increase in number of retinal exudates for a few days after the initial appearance of retinal findings, and widespread posterior pole edema giving a pseudo–cherry red macular appearance.[10]

Acute pancreatitis may be accompanied by a fundus picture similar to that of Purtscher's retinopathy. Digestive enzymes released from the inflamed pancreas are believed to degrade omental fat, once again liberating into the general circulation free fat emboli that may eventually lodge in the retinal circulation.[12] A complement cascade may be activated by the release of pancreatic proteases, and this may lead to leukoembolic retinal arteriolar occlusion.[14]

In compression cyanosis or traumatic asphyxia, the identical fundus picture is accompanied by bluish discoloration of the chest, neck, face, and upper extremities. The sudden increase in intrathoracic pressure is transmitted to the head and neck veins because of incompetent venous valves. The suddenly increased pressure in the cerebral venous system presumably ruptures capillaries, producing massive subconjunctival and retinal hemorrhages.[10]

Air embolization is a rare complication of chest or jugular vein surgery or injury. Distinguishing fundus features include a uniformly gray appearance of the fundus, pale optic nerve, and direct visualization of intraarterial air appearing as glistening white lines interrupting the blood column.[10]

The ophthalmologic hydrostatic pressure syndrome occurs when a person is ejected from an aircraft traveling at a very high speed. The high decelerating forces drive blood toward the head, creating mental confusion, temporary loss of vision, periocular edema, ecchymosis of the lids, and subconjunctival and retinal hemorrhage.[10]

Thus, a variety of causes (head trauma, long bone fracture, chest compression) may lead to a similar retinopathy on clinical examination. Nevertheless, the pathophysiologic mechanism responsible for Purtscher's retinopathy is poorly understood. Limited pathologic material has been available for study. In 1936, Savitsky and Gross reviewed the eye of a patient who had suffered multiple traumatic skull fractures and had premortem evidence of Purtscher's retinopathy (discussed by Pratt and de Venecia[15]). The white intraretinal lesions stained positively for fat. Possible mechanisms for the pathogenesis of Purtscher's or Purtscher's type of retinopathy include (1) arteriolar occlusion from embolization such as air or fat, (2) retinal venous wall trauma from increased intravenous hydrostatic pressure, (3) arteriolar endothelial damage as a consequence of sudden increase in retinal arterial and venous pressure,[6] (4) local retinal vascular coagulopathy or granulocytic aggregation leading to multiple arteriolar occlusions,[14] and (5) retinal angiospastic response following sudden increase in venous pressure.[10]

CHOROIDAL RUPTURE

Severe concussive injury to the globe may result in anteroposterior compression and horizontal expansion of the ocular contents. When the globe suddenly changes its configuration, the relatively elastic retina and tough sclera resist rupture, but the relatively inelastic Bruch's membrane is prone to rupture under these mechanical forces. If it does, the overlying RPE and underlying choriocapillaries also tend to tear, and the fundus lesion is referred to as a choroidal rupture (Color Plate 17-3). Patients with ocular conditions associated with increased fragility of Bruch's membrane, such as angioid streaks, are especially vulnerable to choroidal rupture in the presence of blunt ocular trauma (Color Plate 17-4).

Because direct choroidal rupture may occur at the site of contusive impact, direct ruptures tend to be anterior and oriented parallel to the ora.[2] Direct ruptures are thought to be due to compression necrosis of tissues. Indirect choroidal ruptures are located away from the site of blunt impact and tend to be posterior, crescent-shaped, and oriented concentric to the optic disc (Color Plate 17-3). Indirect ruptures are attributed to mechanical forces arising from the ocular compressive event. Typically these ruptures are in the macular region, occur singly, and are curvilinear; however, they may be nasal to the optic nerve, multiple, and occasionally oriented radially. The rupture of the choriocapillaris may result in intrachoroidal, subretinal pigment epithelial, subretinal, intraretinal, or even vitreous hemorrhage (Fig. 17-1). Often the choroidal rupture itself is obscured by the overlying hemorrhage, and serial examinations are necessary to diagnose the presence and extent of the choroidal rupture as the hemorrhage resorbs. As the hemorrhage and associated retinal and choroidal edema resolve, a yellow-white scar is seen at the level of Bruch's membrane. The RPE immediately surrounding the rupture maybe hyperpigmented or hypopigmented. Unless late complications are encountered, the choroidal rupture's appearance is stable over time.

Initial visual acuity may be severely affected. Factors influencing initial visual acuity include location of the rupture with reference to the fovea, accompanying intraocular hemorrhage (extent and location), and accompanying retinal edema. In a prospective study of 10 patients with indirect posterior pole choroidal ruptures, visual acuity was initially reduced to 20/200 or worse in every case.[16] The immediate visual impairment was attributed to retinal dysfunction. Of the 10 patients, 6 regained visual acuity of 20/30 or better. If the rupture transects the fovea or extensive pigmentary changes result within the posterior pole, central acuity will probably be permanently impaired. Dense, subfoveal hemorrhage may be a poor prognostic sign for vision, but some eyes continue to do well despite this complication.[4,16]

A variety of visual field defects, including dense central scotomas, cecocentral scotomas, and sector field loss, have been associated with acute choroidal ruptures. The actual size, shape, and location of the defect usually fail to correspond to the ophthalmoscopically visible pathology.[16,17] This decrease in retinal sensitivity is often more extensive than the rupture site and gradually recovers, to a variable degree, over a period of weeks to months.[16] However, most patients are left with a residual defect.

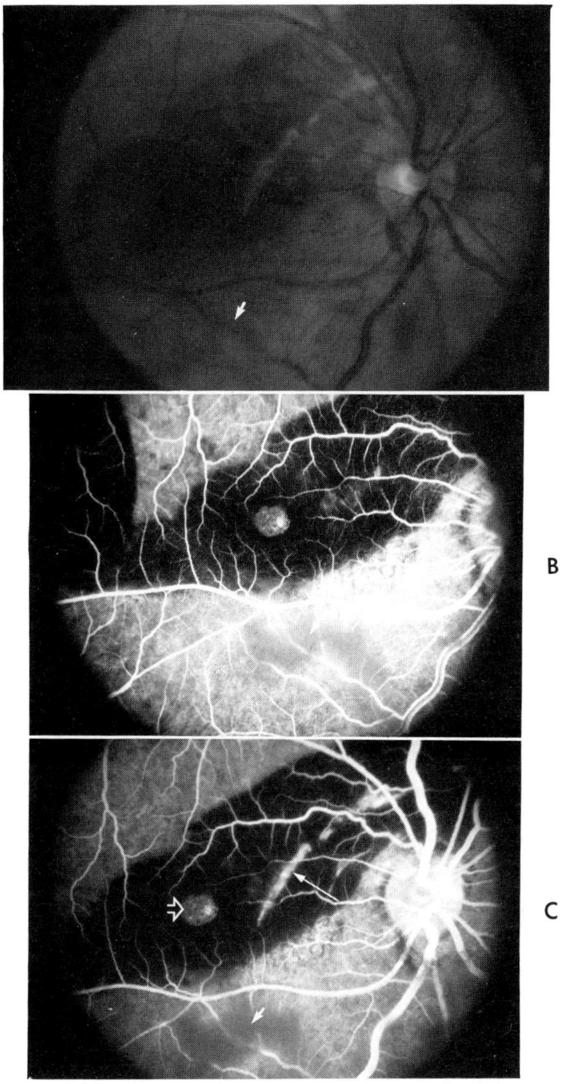

Fig. 17-1. **A,** Fundus photograph demonstrating choroidal rupture and traumatic macular hole with associated subretinal hemorrhage and vitreous hemorrhage *(small arrow)*. **B, C,** Fluorescein angiogram demonstrating blocked fluorescence from subretinal blood in early frames, and areas of staining concentric to the optic nerve in late frames, corresponding to choroidal rupture *(large arrow)*. Staining in foveal center corresponds to macular hole with surrounding cuff of fluid *(open arrow)*.

Fluorescein angiography is particularly useful to detect small choroidal ruptures, ruptures obscured by hemorrhage, and the precise localization of the rupture with reference to the foveal center (Fig. 17-2). Immediately following the trauma, the angiogram demonstrates the un-

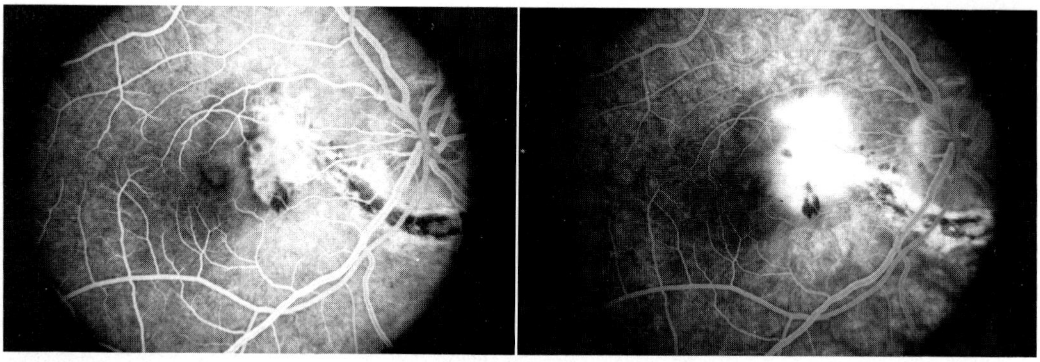

A B

Fig. 17-2. Early and late phase fluorescein angiogram demonstrating **A**, lacy net of choroidal neovascularization with late leakage, **B**, associated with a choroidal rupture.

affected retinal vascular system and a local disturbance in the choroidal vessels within the ruptured area. In some patients, fluorescein dye may leak from the site of the rupture into the outer retinal layers.[16] This defect resolves within a few days. On subsequent angiograms, the local disruption of the choriocapillaris within the rupture creates a hypofluorescent streak in the early transit period. However, filling of the large-caliber intact choroidal vessels is often undisturbed. In the late transit phase, the rupture site is hyperfluorescent because fluorescein diffuses into the area from the surrounding intact choriocapillaris. The intensity of the hyperfluorescence is greatest in the venous phase but may persist into the recirculation phase.

Histopathologic study of enucleated eyes with choroidal rupture has demonstrated tears in the choroid, Bruch's membrane, and RPE. Fibroblastic activity has been seen as early as 4 days following the injury and is usually present between 6 and 14 days after the event. Within 4 weeks of the trauma, a well-developed scar forms at the rupture site. In all cases, choroidal vessels participate in the healing and scarring process. In most cases, these choroidal new vessels regress and do not cause exudation as the scar evolves. Typically, the RPE becomes hyperplastic at the margins of the healed lesions. The retina overlying the rupture may be normal or variably atrophic, with differing degrees of fibroglial scarring.[16,18]

Funduscopically, the choroidal rupture assumes a stable appearance at the time of scar formation, but patients must be reevaluated periodically for the development of secondary choroidal neovascularization (Fig. 17-2). Patients should monitor central vision and field and report any sudden changes in acuity, metamorphopsia, or scotoma. Clinical signs of choroidal neovascularization include the presence of subretinal fluid, subretinal hemorrhage, subretinal lipid, or a subretinal pigmented lesion. Fluorescein angiography will demonstrate a lacy subretinal network of vessels associated with late extravasation of dye into the subretinal space (Fig. 17-2). Treatment of choroidal neovascularization in the setting of choroidal rupture is somewhat controversial. Several small series of patients retained good acuity with spontaneous regression of neovascularization; other patients retained central vision following successful photocoagulation of the neovascularization.[16,19-22] To date, there has not been a controlled clinical trial evaluating the efficacy of laser photocoagulation for choroidal neovascularization in this setting.

Theoretically, the focal nature of the pathology in this condition is similar to that in choroidal neovascularization associated with the ocular histoplasmosis syndrome. Therefore, the favorable results of photocoagulation for histoplasmosis-related choroidal neovascularization that does not extend through the foveal center may be helpful in deciding whether treatment is indicated for a particular patient with neovascularization associated with a choroidal rupture. Although retention of good acuity with spontaneous regression of neovascularization associated with choroidal rupture has been reported, the visual prognosis with treatment may be even better.

RETINITIS SCLOPETARIA

Retinitis sclopetaria, chorioretinitis sclopetaria, and chorioretinitis proliferans are all names that have been applied to a distinct fundus picture that may follow high-velocity missile injury to the orbit. Classically, this condition is seen following a gunshot wound to the orbit, but any other high-velocity missile, such as a BB pellet, may produce the same injury. This concussive, nonpenetrating ocular injury is attributed to shock waves produced in the orbit by the missile.[4] Two areas of the globe are injured: the area directly adjacent to the path of the missile, and the macula.[23] These two traumatized areas often become confluent, producing one large, ophthalmoscopically visible lesion (Color Plates 17-5 and 17-6). The missile's proximity to the globe, its velocity, and its size are believed to determine the extent of ocular damage.[23]

The fundus lesion of retinitis sclopetaria includes choroidal and retinal rupture in the presence of an intact sclera. Immediately following the injury there is extensive intraocular hemorrhage, including subretinal and vitreous hemorrhage. As the hemorrhage resorbs or organizes, extensive retinal destruction and proliferation become apparent. The proliferation appears to fuse the choroid and retina. The lesion has irregular borders, sometimes with a clawlike configuration. There may also be an associated pigment disturbance.

The extensive fibrous tissue proliferation probably results in fusion of the retina to the eye wall and greatly reduces the likelihood of future retinal detachment. However, vision is almost invariably poor, especially if the optic nerve is involved.

TRAUMATIC MACULAR HOLE

In 1869 Knapp described a macular hole that followed a contusive ocular injury. Subsequent reports have identified traumatic macular holes in association with the following postcontusion injuries: commotio retinae, subretinal hemorrhage and choroidal rupture, whiplash maculopathy, and cystoid macular edema.[1,7]

Pathogenic mechanisms for production of a full-thickness hole in the exquisitely thin foveola following trauma include any one or a combination of (1) postcontusion necrosis of tissues, (2) subfoveal hemorrhage, and (3) vitreous traction.[7] Postcontusion necrosis may result in cystoid macular edema. Rupture of the inner layer of a larger macular cyst may produce a lamellar hole. If both the inner and outer walls of a macular cyst disappear, a full-thickness hole may develop. This sequence of macular edema progressing to a full-thickness macular hole may take months to years. Differentiation of lamellar holes from full-thickness macular holes is assisted by biomicroscopic recognition of an intact outer retinal layer and the absence of any subretinal fluid in the lamellar hole. Fluorescein angiography is less likely to demonstrate an RPE window defect in a lamellar hole.[24] Acute vitreofoveal traction may be involved in production of a traumatic macular hole, because there is a zone of special adherence of the vitreous to the retina in the macular region. This adhesion appears to be greatest at the foveal crest.[7] Sudden complete or partial separation of the posterior vitreous face, such as may be produced in a whiplash injury, may extend through this area and tear a macular hole.[25] In select cases, a retinal operculum may be seen immediately anterior to the macula.

In the presence of a full-thickness macular hole, one would expect the visual acuity to be reduced to the 20/80 to 20/200 range, as seen in idiopathic macular holes. A central scotoma should be present, and there may be associated metamorphopsia. The size of the hole may vary, but the margins are usually sharp and regular (Fig. 17-1). A surrounding zone of subretinal fluid and intraretinal cystic damage often accompanies the hole.

Fluorescein angiography of traumatic and idiopathic macular holes gives identical results (Fig. 17-1 and Color Plate 17-7). During early transit, an RPE window defect is seen in the base of the hole, and this gradually fades in the late phase. A lighter halo of fluorescence may surround the hole in the midphase.

The macular hole and its localized detachment may remain stationary; however, progressive detachment of the posterior pole and peripheral retina have been known to occur with a traumatic macular hole.[24] Prophylactic laser photocoagulation to the margins of the hole may not be necessary in the vast majority of patients, nor is there any evidence to suggest that this decreases the risk of progressive retinal detachment.[3] Conservative management consists of periodic reevaluation, with deferment of treatment until progressive enlargement of the detachment is noted. Meticulous examination of the peripheral retina is required to rule out additional sites of pathology. Treatment may ultimately consist of laser photocoagulation with or without air/fluid exchange, scleral buckle, and vitrectomy, singly or in combination. The intent of treatment is to maintain peripheral vision rather than correct the central deficit.

References

1. Wolter JR: Coup-contrecoup mechanism of ocular injuries, Am J Ophthalmol 56:785-796, 1963.
2. Deutsch T: Paton and Goldberg's ocular injuries, ed 2, Philadelphia, 1985, WB Saunders, 207-212.
3. Pruett RC: Traumatic maculopathies. In Freeman HM, editor: Ocular trauma, New York, 1979, Appleton-Century-Crofts.
4. Benson WE, Shakin J, and Sarin LK: Blunt trauma. In Duane TE, editor: Clinical ophthalmology, vol 3, Philadelphia, 1988, JB Lippincott.
5. Hart JCD and Frank HJ: Retinal opacification after blunt nonperforating concussional injuries to the globe, Trans Ophthalmol Soc UK 95:94-100, 1975.
6. Beckingsale AB and Rosenthal AR: Early fundus fluorescein angiographic findings and sequelae in traumatic retinopathy: case report, Br J Ophthalmol 67:119-123, 1983.
7. Gass JDM: Stereoscopic atlas of macular diseases: diagnosis and treatment, ed 3, St Louis, 1987, The CV Mosby Co, 552-555.
8. Sipperley JO, Quigley HA, and Gass JDM: Traumatic retinopathy in primates: the explanation of commotio retinae, Arch Ophthalmol 96:2267-2273, 1978.
9. Blight R and Hart JCD: Structural changes in the outer retinal layers following blunt mechanical nonperforating trauma to the globe: an experimental study, Br J Ophthalmol 61:573-587, 1977.
10. Marr WG and Marr EG: Some observations on Purtscher's disease: traumatic retinal angiopathy, Am J Ophthalmol 54:693-705, 1962.
11. Kelley JS: Purtscher's retinopathy related to chest compression by safety belts: fluorescein angiographic findings, Am J Ophthalmol 74:278-283, 1972.
12. Burton TC: Unilateral Purtscher's retinopathy, Ophthalmology 87:1096-1105, 1980.
13. Fischbein F and Safir A: Monocular Purtscher's retinopathy: a fluorescein angiographic study, Arch Ophthalmol 85:480-484, 1971.
14. Jacob HS et al: Complement-induced granulocyte aggregation: an unsuspected mechanism of disease, N Engl J Med 302:789-794, 1980.
15. Pratt MV and de Venecia G: Purtscher's retinopathy: a clinico-histopathological correlation, Surv Ophthalmol 14:417-423, 1970.
16. Hart JCD et al: Indirect choroidal tears at the posterior pole: a fluorescein angiographic and perimetric study, Br J Ophthalmol 64:59-67, 1980.
17. Maberley AL and Carvounis EP: The visual field in indirect traumatic rupture of the choroid, Can J Ophthalmol 12:147-152, 1977.
18. Aguilar JP and Green WR: Choroidal rupture: a histopathologic study of 47 cases, Retina 4:269-275, 1984.
19. Fuller B and Gitter KA: Traumatic choroidal rupture with late serous detachment of macula: report of successful argon laser treatment, Arch Ophthalmol 89:354-355, 1973.
20. Hart CD and Raistrick R: Indirect choroidal tears and late onset serosanguineous maculopathies, Graefes Arch Clin Exp Ophthalmol 218:206-210, 1982.
21. Hilton GF: Late serosanguineous detachment of the macula after traumatic choroidal rupture, Am J Ophthalmol 79:997-1000, 1975.
22. Smith RE, Kelley JS, and Harbin TS: Late macular complications of choroidal ruptures, Am J Ophthalmol 77:650-658, 1974.
23. Richards RD, West CE, and Meisels AA: Chorioretinitis sclopetaria, Am J Ophthalmol 66:852-860, 1968.
24. Aaberg TM, Blair CJ, and Gass JDM: Macular holes, Am J Ophthalmol 69:555-562, 1970.
25. Kelley JS, Hoover RE, and George T: Whiplash maculopathy, Arch Ophthalmol 96:834-835, 1978.

CHAPTER 18

Traumatic retinal tears and detachments

JOHN T. THOMPSON

Pathophysiology of traumatic retinal tears from blunt trauma
Traumatic retinal tears: clinical setting
Clinical manifestations of trauma to the eye
  Vitreous base avulsion
  Retinal dialysis without retinal detachment
  Retinal dialysis with rhegmatogenous retinal detachment
  Traumatic retinal tears without retinal detachment
  Traumatic retinal tears with retinal detachment
  Giant retinal tears without retinal detachment
  Giant retinal tears with retinal detachment
References

Ocular trauma accounts for approximately 10% to 12% of rhegmatogenous retinal detachments and is the most frequent cause of retinal detachment in children.[1-3] Retinal tears resulting from trauma are usually the result of damage to the retina at the vitreous base, although some tears may result from either direct blunt damage or indirect contrecoup injuries. Recognition of the location and types of tears associated with trauma is important, because prompt treatment can often prevent a rhegmatogenous retinal detachment. This chapter will review the pathophysiology of blunt trauma on the retina, the types of retinal tears produced by trauma, and the treatment of retinal tears and detachments produced by blunt trauma.

PATHOPHYSIOLOGY OF TRAUMATIC RETINAL TEARS FROM BLUNT TRAUMA

Retinal tears due to trauma are the result of transmission of an external force to the globe with resultant distortion. The shape of the eye may change markedly when deformed by a direct blow. Since sclera and cornea are relatively inelastic, the globe cannot stretch in response to deformation. This inelasticity, in combination with the low compressibility of the fluid-filled eye, has important implications in a blunt injury to the globe. When a force is suddenly applied to the globe, the volume of the eye must remain essentially constant since the aqueous outflow cannot increase rapidly enough to absorb the volume displacement. If one portion of the globe is compressed by the force, a corresponding volume of fluid must be displaced elsewhere within this closed container. The net effect is to change the shape but not the volume of the globe. The sudden change in shape may exert tractional forces on a number of ocular structures, including the vitreous base, where the vitreous is normally firmly adherent to the peripheral retina. Vitreous base traction from blunt trauma most frequently creates retinal dialyses at the ora ser-

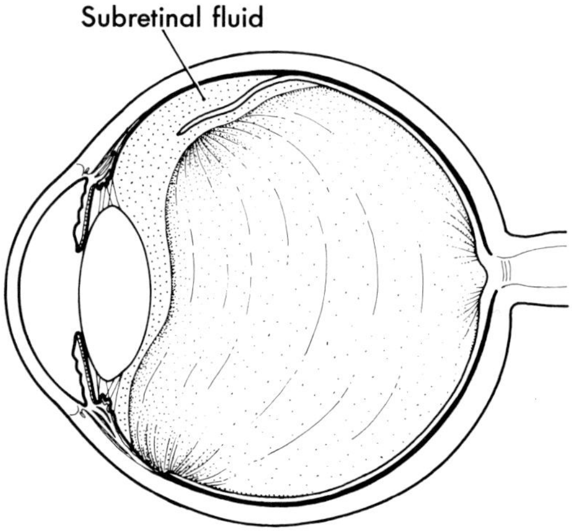

Fig. 18-1. Retinal dialysis and rhegmatogenous retinal detachment caused by avulsion of the vitreous base from the ora serrata.

rata or peripheral retinal tears at the posterior edge of the vitreous base insertion (Fig. 18-1).

The effect of blunt trauma on the peripheral retina has been studied in a laboratory model using high-velocity projectiles.[4,5] Pellets were fired from a modified air rifle at an animal cadaver eye. The effects were evaluated histologically and with high-speed cinematography. A pellet fired at the center of the cornea frequently caused lens damage and tenting of the peripheral retina and pars plana nasally with possible nasal retinal dialysis. A pellet fired at the temporal limbus often caused temporal retinal dialyses.[4] These peripheral retinal changes resemble those seen in human eyes after blunt trauma. High-speed cinematography in a similar model defined four phases of globe deformation after being hit by a high-speed pellet.[5] The type of ocular damage produced by the projectile can be understood by examining the globe deformation during these four phases of (1) compression, (2) decompression, (3) overshooting, and (4) oscillation,[5] as shown in Fig. 18-2. Retinal

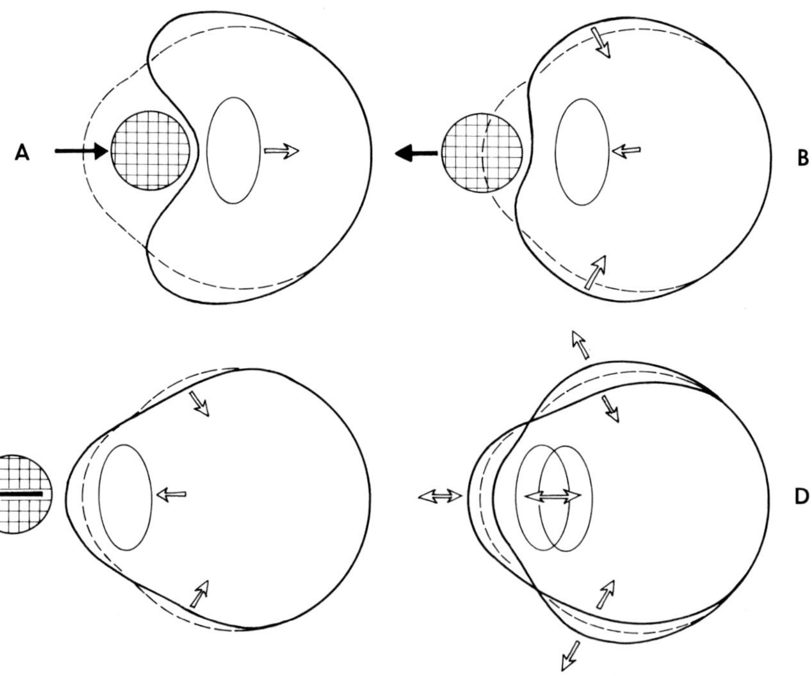

Fig. 18-2. Four phases of globe deformation by a high-speed projectile. **A,** Phase 1. Compression of the globe by the projectile with a decrease in axial length and expansion of the equatorial diameter of the globe. **B,** Phase 2. Decompression when the projectile recoils from the cornea with an increase in axial length back to normal and a decrease in equatorial diameter of the globe. **C,** Phase 3. Overshooting with a rebound increase in axial length over the normal length and a decrease in equatorial diameter below the normal diameter. **D,** Phase 4. Oscillation with cyclical small increases and decreases in the axial length and equatorial diameter, which dampen until the eye is stationary.

dialyses and peripheral retinal tears appeared to be produced by tractional forces on the peripheral retina by the vitreous base as the equatorial diameter of the globe increased. The distribution of retinal tears in these eyes was similar to that in human eyes with blunt trauma.

Two major mechanisms may lead to retinal tears after blunt trauma. The first results from changes in the shape of the globe with secondary tractional effects on the vitreous base (Fig. 18-3); this mechanism appears to produce the majority of traumatic retinal tears. Such traction on the vitreous base is transmitted to the retina, leading to retinal tears at the anterior or posterior border of the vitreous base. The exact pathogenic mechanism for the retinal tear or dialysis is unknown but probably involves inertial and shearing forces by the vitreous base, leading to traction on the peripheral retina. Retinal breaks may also occur at a site of focal vitreoretinal attachment such as the edge of lattice degeneration or a chorioretinal scar. A second type of retinal tear results from fragmentation and necrosis of the retina at the site of direct trauma to the sclera. These tears usually occur in the relatively unprotected temporal retina. Retinal tears associated with direct trauma are often associated with intraretinal hemorrhages and retinal edema, producing large, irregular retinal tears.

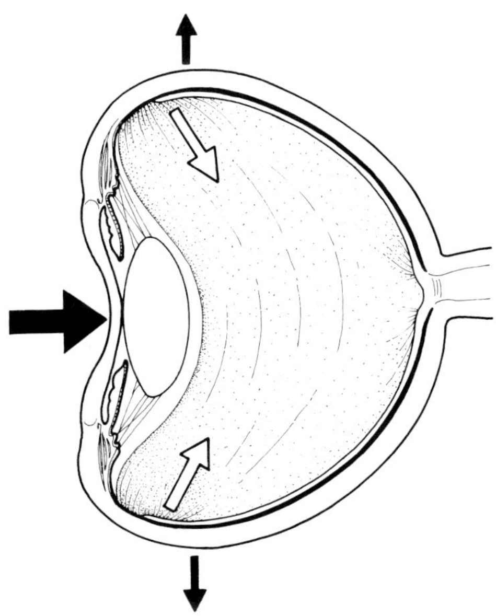

Fig. 18-3. Traumatic deformation of the globe induces tractional forces on the vitreous base and peripheral retina. Indentation of the cornea produces a decrease in axial length and an increase in equatorial diameter of the globe *(solid arrows)* with secondary tractional forces on the peripheral retina by the vitreous base *(open arrows)*.

TRAUMATIC RETINAL TEARS: CLINICAL SETTING

Traumatic retinal tears may occur after many different types of ocular injuries. The vast majority of traumatic retinal tears and detachments result from direct trauma to the globe. The patient may perceive that indirect trauma to the head or body has contributed to a retinal tear or detachment, but actually it is an infrequent cause. Approximately 40% of traumatic retinal detachments related to nonpenetrating ocular contusion are caused by an injury at home, 35% are caused by an athletic injury, and 8% are work related.[6] The trauma usually produces a retinal tear immediately, although the tear may be delayed if it results from cellular proliferation on the retina or necrosis of the traumatized retina. The interval between the ocular contusion and discovery of the retinal tear or detachment may be prolonged. In one study the mean interval between the injury and discovery of a detachment was 5 years, with a range of 1 day to 27 years.[2] In other studies, 12% to 20% of traumatic retinal detachments were detected within 24 hours of injury, 30% to 46% within 1 month, 50% to 60% within 8 months, and 80% to 82% within 2 years.[7,8] Traumatic retinal detachments tend to occur in younger individuals, 80% before age 40.[8] Males with traumatic retinal detachments tend to outnumber females, by 87% to 13% in one study[7] and 78% to 22% in another.[8] Myopic eyes appear more likely than emmetropic eyes to develop a retinal tear or detachment after trauma.[7]

Trauma to the retina and vitreous base may be manifested by one of several different types of retinal tears. The prevalences in traumatic as compared with apparently nontraumatic detachments are as follows: dialyses, 53% versus 5%; giant retinal tears, 16% versus 2%; tears related to abnormal vitreoretinal adhesion, 11% versus 45%; and lattice degeneration, 8% versus 38%.[8] Another study evaluating only eyes with traumatic retinal detachment found that 84% had a dialysis, 8% had giant retinal tears, 3% had horseshoe tears, and 5% had round holes.[2]

CLINICAL MANIFESTATIONS OF TRAUMA TO THE EYE

Vitreous Base Avulsion

Avulsion of the vitreous base from the peripheral retina is pathognomonic of ocular trauma, because the vitreous base is normally firmly adherent to the peripheral retina and pars plana. Trauma to the globe may disinsert the vitreous base from the peripheral retina and pars plana. Avulsion of the vitreous base results in minimal ocular symptoms, although the patient may complain of floaters associated with a partial vitreous detachment. Fragments of nonpigmented pars plana epithelium often remain adherent to the avulsed vitreous base, giving the appearance of an arcuate pigmented band draped over the peripheral retina (Fig. 18-4). Vitreous base avulsion alone does not have to be treated, but examination must be performed for associated traumatic ocular damage such as retinal dialysis, giant retinal tear, angle recession, or subluxed crystalline lens.

Retinal Dialysis Without Retinal Detachment

Retinal dialysis is characterized by separation of the retina from the border of the nonpigmented pars plana epithelium at the ora serrata. The vast majority of retinal dialyses are related to trauma,[9] although some authors have postulated a developmental anomaly[10] or genetic predisposition[11] in some eyes. Many retinal dialyses are "silent," which accounts for the delay in detection of traumatic retinal detachments. Patients with a retinal dialysis may complain of mild blurring of vision, possibly with floaters or photopsia. Most retinal dialyses occur at the time of trauma, although some related to vitreoretinal traction may not develop until weeks or months later. To check for retinal dialysis, the peripheral retina must be examined by scleral depression in an eye with blunt trauma as soon as it is safe to do so. Occult perforation or rupture of the globe may need to be ruled out, however, before a scleral depressed examination can be performed. Most dialyses resemble a slit at the ora serrata and are best highlighted by scleral depression.

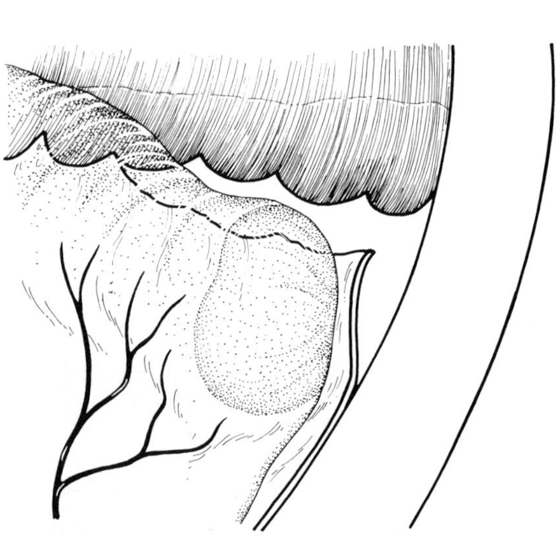

Fig. 18-4. Avulsion of the vitreous base with a retinal dialysis. The contour of the ora serrata appears to bifurcate at the edge of the dialysis.

The normal serrated contour of the ora serrata will appear to deviate at the site of the dialysis, with blunting of the serrations within the dialysis. Pigment may be visible at the previous line of attachment of the peripheral retina, giving the appearance of a bifurcation at the border of the dialysis and normal ora serrata (Fig. 18-4). Associated signs may include avulsion of the vitreous base or retinal detachment posterior to the dialysis. Some dialyses do not lead to retinal detachment but become surrounded by pigmentary changes with a spontaneous chorioretinal adhesion. The quadrant distribution of retinal dialyses with or without retinal detachment is 66% inferotemporal, 14% superonasal, 10% superotemporal, 4% inferonasal, and 6% in more than one quadrant.[10] Most dialyses in the absence of retinal detachment should be treated with cryopexy or laser photocoagulation. Photocoagulation using a three-mirror contact lens is usually not possible because of the peripheral location, but a laser indirect ophthalmoscope delivery system may be used with scleral depression to surround the dialysis with laser photocoagulation. Most traumatic dialyses should be treated prophylactically to try to prevent a rhegmatogenous retinal detachment. Occasional dialyses with extensive chorioretinal reaction surrounding the dialysis and without associated retinal detachment may simply be followed.

Retinal Dialysis with Rhegmatogenous Retinal Detachment

Rhegmatogenous retinal detachments secondary to dialyses often progress slowly and may be detected incidentally months or years later. The symptoms of mild blurring, diplopia, floaters, or photopsia are similar to those of dialysis without detachment. The symptoms of a retinal detachment due to retinal dialysis may be accompanied by visual field changes when the detachment progresses posterior to the equator or by loss of vision if the detachment involves the macula. The location and extent of the detachment are determined by the topology of the retinal dialysis and vitreoretinal interface. A retinal detachment caused by a dialysis in the absence of extensive vitreous detachment or liquefaction is often limited in extent, with minimal elevation of the retina. The detachment is more likely to develop a bullous configuration when there is extensive posterior vitreous detachment, avulsion of the vitreous base, a large dialysis, or a superior dialysis (Color Plate 18-1). One or more demarcation lines may be present in long-standing posttraumatic retinal detachments (Color Plate 18-2). Such lines were present in 46% of one series of eyes with traumatic retinal detachment related to dialyses.[9] A chronic detachment may cause the retina to become very thin and can be confused with retinoschisis if not examined carefully. Retinal macrocysts are found within the detached retina in 14% of traumatic retinal detachments secondary to dialyses,[9] avulsion of the vitreous base in 12% to 26%,[7,9] and detachment of the pars plana in 40%.[9] Preretinal or subretinal fibrous proliferation may develop, producing a combined traction-rhegmatogenous retinal detachment.

Table 18-1 summarizes the distribution of dialyses associated with traumatic retinal detachment in seven studies. The descending order of frequency is inferotemporal, superonasal, superotemporal, and inferonasal. The varied distribution emphasizes the importance of scleral depressed examination in all quadrants of eyes with blunt trauma.

Rhegmatogenous retinal detachments secondary to traumatic dialyses are generally treated with cryopexy and placement of a circumferential scleral buckle to support the dialysis. Some surgeons prefer to use a segmental circumferential scleral buckle; others, an encircling buckle. The former has the advantage of less surgical manipulation of the eye, and the latter of more extensive support of the vitreous base. Drainage of subretinal fluid can be avoided in many circumstances but may need to be performed if there is bullous detachment or vitreoretinal traction on the dialysis or if the intraocular pressure must be lowered for placement of a broad scleral buckle. Traumatic dialysis and minimal retinal detachment may be managed by cryopexy or laser photocoagulation alone. Some eyes with a localized superior dialysis can be treated with pneumatic retinopexy.[16]

The surgical results of repair of traumatic retinal detachment secondary to dialyses are generally excellent. The rate of retinal reattachment with one operation has been reported as 87% to 94% and overall, with one or more operations, as 96% to 98%.[9,15] The final postoperative visual acuity depends in large part on whether the macula was attached or detached preoperatively. The visual acuity may also be limited by concurrent damage to the macula such as choroidal rupture, commotio retinae, or macular holes. In one series the visual acuity was 20/40 or better in 44% of eyes, 20/50 to 20/100 in 24%, and 20/200 or worse in 32%.[9]

Table 18-1. Percentage quadrant distribution of dialyses associated with traumatic retinal detachment

Author	Inferotemporal	Superonasal	Superotemporal	Inferonasal
Ross[9]	72	16	8	4
Tasman[12]	48	20	14	18
Assaf[13]	73	2	8	6
Dumas[2]	69	3	3	3
Malbran, Dodds, and Hulsbus[14]	34	29	31	2
Hagler[15]	30	46	11	13
Cox, Schepens, and Freeman[7]	27	38	22	13

The percentages in a series may not total 100% because some studies classified dialyses occurring in more than one quadrant as a separate category.

Traumatic Retinal Tears without Retinal Detachment

Traumatic retinal tears due to contusion-induced retinal necrosis or traction at a site of vitreoretinal adhesion occur less frequently than dialyses following blunt trauma. Three basic types of retinal tears are found as a result of direct ocular trauma: (1) Round holes without apparent vitreoretinal traction may vary from one or more peripheral small round holes to larger irregular holes with apparent disintegration of the retina. The large irregular holes are usually located at the site of direct ocular contusion and are most often inferotemporal because of decreased orbital protection there. Vitreous or intraretinal hemorrhage and damage to the retinal pigment epithelium and choroid may be associated with large breaks. (2) A macular hole usually results from contrecoup damage, which exerts traction on the normal attachment of the vitreous gel to the macula. Traumatic macular holes are discussed in Chapter 17. (3) Tractional retinal tears typically show attachment of the vitreous to the edge of the tear, producing a horseshoe configuration or other signs of vitreoretinal traction such as an operculated hole. It may be difficult to determine whether a tractional retinal tear was related to trauma unless there are other associated signs of trauma. Traumatic retinal tears are often associated with symptoms that include floaters, photopsia and decreased vision from commotio retinae, and vitreous and retinal hemorrhage. Traumatic retinal breaks are generally more likely than dialyses to progress to a detachment. Prophylactic treatment to prevent a retinal detachment is indicated in most traumatic retinal breaks with the exception of macular holes. Some large retinal breaks cannot be visualized immediately after trauma because of opacities in the ocular media and may only be detected weeks or months later. Some large tears show extensive chorioretinal scarring and have developed a chorioretinal adhesion by the time they are visible. If a traumatic retinal break is discovered more than 1 month after trauma and is surrounded by a chorioretinal adhesion, treatment may not be necessary. However, these eyes must be followed carefully, because some tears will progress to a retinal detachment as a result of persisting vitreoretinal traction. Most traumatic tears should be treated with cryopexy or laser photocoagulation and then followed for possible progression to a rhegmatogenous retinal detachment.

Traumatic Retinal Tears with Retinal Detachment

Rhegmatogenous retinal detachments generally develop more rapidly from traumatic retinal tears than from traumatic dialyses. The retinal detachments are also more likely to become bullous if there is persisting vitreoretinal traction on the retinal break. The symptoms are similar to those of traumatic retinal tears, with the addition of visual field changes from progression of the detachment and loss of vision from macular involvement. The configuration of the detachment is determined by the location of the retinal breaks, the presence of posterior vitreous detachment, and the presence of vitreoretinal traction on the breaks. Traumatic retinal tears without and with apparent vitreoretinal traction are inferotemporal in 54% versus 8% of eyes, superotemporal in 28% versus 20%, superonasal in 10% versus 60%, and inferonasal in 8% versus 13%.[7]

Rhegmatogenous retinal detachments from traumatic tears are usually treated with cryopexy and a scleral buckle. The location and type of buckle is determined by the location of the tears and whether vitreoretinal traction is present. An encircling buckle is used when there are multiple retinal tears or when additional support to the vitreous base is required. Drainage of subretinal fluid may be necessary if the retina is bullously detached or to obtain adequate intraocular volume displacement for a broad scleral buckle. Occasional limited retinal detachments related to traumatic retinal tears can be managed by cryopexy or laser photocoagulation alone. Pars plana vitrectomy with injection of an intraocular gas bubble may be preferable in eyes with large areas of contusion-induced retinal necrosis that would be difficult to support on a scleral buckle. The surgical results for repair of rhegmatogenous retinal detachments from traumatic retinal tears are variable, depending on the preoperative pathology, but the success rate is still in excess of 80%.[7]

Giant Retinal Tears without Retinal Detachment

Giant retinal tears are defined as retinal tears extending for 90° or more of the circumference of the globe. They are frequently related to blunt trauma. Patients often notice floaters immediately following the trauma, caused by bleeding from the retinal tear. This may be followed by decreased peripheral and central vision as the detachment progresses into the macula. Retinal detachments from giant tears usually show rapid progression because of the size of the tear and the presence of vitreoretinal traction, which may hold the mouth of the tear open. Eyes with high myopia appear to be at greater risk than emmetropic eyes of developing a giant retinal tear as a result of ocular trauma. Giant retinal tears usually occur circumferentially at the borders of the vitreous base but may develop radial extensions posteriorly. Some giant tears result from contusion-induced necrosis of the retina at the site of blunt trauma to the sclera. These tears may be associated with extensive retinal necrosis, making their repair difficult. Giant retinal tears resulting from retinal disintegration most often develop in the inferotemporal quadrant. Giant tears without retinal detachment may be treated successfully by cryopexy or laser photocoagulation, although some will progress to retinal detachment despite therapy. A prophylactic scleral buckle should be considered in eyes with vitreoretinal traction on an elevated flap of a giant tear because of the risk of progression to a rhegmatogenous retinal detachment before the chorioretinal adhesion from cryopexy or laser photocoagulation has adequately formed. Eyes with giant retinal tears are also at increased risk of developing proliferative vitreoretinopathy (PVR) because of possible dispersion of cells from the large areas of retinal pigment epithelium exposed by the tear.[17]

Giant Retinal Tears with Retinal Detachment

The management of rhegmatogenous retinal detachment resulting from giant retinal tears varies depending on the preoperative features. Some eyes with a tear of 90° to 120° can be treated with a broad scleral buckle alone if there is no evidence of PVR. The presence of an inverted retinal flap (Color Plate 18-3), a tear of 120° or greater, PVR, or failure of the repair of a previous giant retinal tear necessitates pars plana vitrectomy with fluid-gas exchange in addition to a broad circumferential scleral buckle.

The lens must be removed in many eyes with giant retinal tears of 120° or greater and in some eyes with tears between 90° and 120°. Lens removal allows more complete removal of the peripheral anterior vitreous, mobilization of the retinal flap, and facilitation of postoperative fluid-gas exchange, if needed. Eyes with PVR and giant retinal tears almost always require lens removal to facilitate removal of cellular proliferation from the anteroperipheral vitreous and peripheral retina.

The basic surgical technique for the repair of giant retinal tears includes the placement of cryopexy, diathermy, or endolaser photocoagulation surrounding the tear.[18] A chorioretinal adhesion for 360° is desirable in eyes with larger giant tears, because the instability of the vitreous base that produced the tear may allow it to expand beyond its original borders. A broad circumferential scleral buckle is placed to support the retinal tear and vitreous base. A fluid-gas exchange is then performed to unfold the retina before tightening the circumferential buckle. The retina is best unfolded by an intraocular gas bubble if the patient is rolled over to a prone position before the fluid-gas exchange.[19] The exchange is then performed with the patient in the prone position, the bubble first accumulating over the optic nerve. As the bubble fills the globe, its buoyancy unfolds the retina. The surface tension between the unfolded retina and retinal pigment epithelium in the gas-filled eye will hold the retina against the eye wall if there is no persisting traction on the retina. The patient is then rolled back to the supine position, and the scleral buckle is tightened to create an indentation of the peripheral retina. A long-acting gas bubble such as a mixture of air and sulfur hexafluoride (SF_6) or perfluoropropane (C_3F_8) is injected to tamponade the giant tear for at least 1 week to allow formation of chorioretinal adhesion. Some surgeons do not use a circumferential buckle if other means of internal retinal fixation such as silicone oil are used.[20]

Several ancillary techniques for retinal fixation may be necessary in treating rhegmatogenous retinal detachments resulting from giant retinal tears with inverted retinal flaps, very extensive giant retinal tears, or PVR. These include the use of retinal sutures to fixate the retina against the retinal pigment epithelium and intentional incarceration of the retina into the sclera.[18,21] Retinal tacks may also be used to fixate the retina against the retinal pigment epithelium.[22,23] Cyanoacrylate tissue adhesive may serve to glue the edges of torn retina to the retinal pigment epithelium.[24] Perfluorocarbon liquids, which are more dense than saline, can be used instead of an intraocular gas bubble to help unroll the retina with the patient in the supine instead of the prone position.[25] The use of intravitreal silicone oil can provide temporary or permanent intraocular tamponade in eyes with traumatic giant retinal tears.[20,26]

The success rate in repair of giant retinal tears secondary to trauma has gradually increased with improvements in techniques of vitreoretinal surgery. The success rate depends in large part on the extent of the tear and whether PVR is present. Rhegmatogenous retinal detachments produced by giant retinal tears of more than 180° have a lower success rate than tears of less than 180°. The presence of PVR also lowers the success rate regardless of the extent of the tear. Although earlier studies[19,27] reported retinal reattachment in 39% to 43% of eyes 6 months postoperatively, more recent studies have reported reattachment in 78% to 87%, depending on the preoperative characteristics.[20,28,29] The visual prognosis depends on many factors. In one series, 74% of eyes with giant retinal tears and inverted retinal flaps achieved a visual acuity of 20/400 or better, and 70% of eyes with giant retinal tears treated with silicone oil had a visual acuity of 20/200 or better at 6 months.[29] In the same group of patients, the percentage of eyes with a visual acuity of 20/200 or better decreased to 57% at 18 months.[23] In another study, 44% of eyes with giant retinal tears and PVR treated with silicone oil had a postoperative visual acuity of 5/200 or better.[20]

The treatment of retinal tears and rhegmatogenous retinal detachments related to ocular trauma is successful in most eyes. The visual results are variable and often determined more by the retinal damage caused by the trauma than by the retinal tear or detachment itself. Despite surgical advances that have improved the success rate in treatment of traumatic retinal detachments, many tears or detachments are not detected until months or years after the trauma. Therefore, improved awareness of the possible retinal complications of blunt trauma may result in a more timely and thorough retinal examination, with earlier detection and treatment.

References

1. Haimann MH, Burton TC, and Brown CK: Epidemiology of retinal detachment, Arch Ophthalmol 100:289-292, 1982.
2. Dumas JJ: Retinal detachment following contusion of the eye, Int Ophthalmol Clin 7:19-38, 1967.
3. Tasman W: Retinal detachment in children, Trans Am Acad Ophthalmol Otolaryngol 71:455-460, 1967.
4. Weidenthal DT and Schepens CL: Peripheral fundus changes associated with ocular contusion, Am J Ophthalmol 62:465-477, 1966.
5. Delori F, Pomerantzeff O, and Cox MS: Deformation of the globe under high-speed impact: its relation to contusion injuries, Invest Ophthalmol 8:290-301, 1969.
6. Cox MS and Freeman HM: Traumatic retinal detachment. In Freeman HM, editor: Ocular trauma, New York, 1979, Appleton-Century-Crofts, 285-293.
7. Cox MS, Schepens CL, and Freeman HM: Retinal detachment due to ocular contusion, Arch Ophthalmol 76:678-685, 1966.
8. Goffstein R and Burton TC: Differentiating traumatic from nontraumatic retinal detachment, Ophthalmology 89:361-368, 1982.
9. Ross WH: Traumatic retinal dialyses, Arch Ophthalmol 99:1371-1374, 1981.
10. Zion VM and Burton TC: Retinal dialysis, Arch Ophthalmol 98:1971-1974, 1980.
11. Levy J: Inherited retinal detachment, Br J Ophthalmol 35:626-636, 1952.
12. Tasman W: Retinal dialysis following blunt trauma. In Freeman HM, editor: Ocular trauma, New York, 1979, Appleton-Century-Crofts.
13. Assaf A: Traumatic retinal detachment, J Trauma 25:1085-1089, 1985.
14. Malbran E, Dodds R, and Hulsbus R: Traumatic retinal detachment, Mod Probl Ophthalmol 10:479-489, 1972.
15. Hagler WS: Retinal dialysis: a statistical and genetic study to determine pathogenic factors, Trans Am Ophthalmol Soc 78:686-733, 1980.
16. Hilton GF et al: Pneumatic retinopexy: a collaborative report of the first 100 cases, Ophthalmology 94:307-314, 1987.
17. Campochiaro PA et al: Cryotherapy enhances intravitreal dispersion of viable retinal pigment epithelial cells, Arch Ophthalmol 103:434-436, 1985.
18. Michels RG, Rice TA, and Blankenship G: Surgical techniques for selected giant retinal tears, Retina 3:139-153, 1983.
19. Freeman HM and Castillejos ME: Current management of giant retinal breaks: results with vitrectomy and total air fluid exchange in 95 cases, Trans Am Ophthalmol Soc 79:89-102, 1981.
20. Glaser BM: Treatment of giant retinal tears combined with proliferative vitreoretinopathy, Ophthalmology 93:1193-1197, 1986.
21. Federman JL, Shakin JL, and Lanning RC: The microsurgical management of giant retinal tears with trans-scleral retinal sutures, Ophthalmology 89:832-838, 1982.
22. de Juan E Jr, Hickingbotham D, and Machemer R: Retinal tacks, Am J Ophthalmol 99:272-274, 1985.

23. Ando F and Kondo J: A plastic tack for the treatment of retinal detachment with giant tear, Am J Ophthalmol 95:260-261, 1983.
24. McCuen BW II, Hida T, and Sheta SM: Transvitreal cyanoacrylate retinopexy in the management of complicated retinal detachment, Am J Ophthalmol 104:127-132, 1987.
25. Chang S et al: Perfluorocarbon liquids in the management of traumatic retinal detachments, Ophthalmology 96:785-792, 1989.
26. Billington BM and Leaver PK: Vitrectomy and fluid/silicone-oil exchange for giant retinal tears: results at 18 months, Graefes Arch Clin Exp Ophthalmol 224:7-10, 1986.
27. Machemer R and Allen AW: Retinal tears 180° and greater: management with vitrectomy and intravitreal gas, Arch Ophthalmol 94:1340-1346, 1976.
28. Vidaurri-Leal J, de Bustros S, and Michels RG: Surgical treatment of giant retinal tears with inverted posterior retinal flaps, Am J Ophthalmol 98:463-466, 1984.
29. Leaver PK et al: Vitrectomy and fluid/silicone-oil exchange for giant retinal tears: results at six months, Br J Ophthalmol 68:432-438, 1984.

CHAPTER 19

Pathophysiology of posterior segment trauma

RAYMOND F. WONG
COLIN MA
STEPHEN J. RYAN

Pathophysiology of injury
- Blunt trauma
- Penetrating trauma

Animal models
- Natural history
- Histopathology of penetrating injury
- Histopathology of contusion injury

Factors influencing the healing response
- Blood
- Retinal laceration
- Vitreous-lens admixture

Rationale for surgical treatment
- Efficacy of vitrectomy
- Timing of vitrectomy

References

Although modern surgical techniques have greatly improved the prognosis for patients with anterior segment injury, the advances in treatment of trauma to the posterior segment have been less dramatic. In several recent series, functional vision was attained in approximately half of the patients with posterior segment trauma.[1-3] Blindness is frequently due to fibrovascular and glial proliferation within the vitreous causing complex retinal detachment and to ciliary body damage leading to hypotony. Several studies of experimental injury in animals have demonstrated the importance of the topologic relationships of the vitreous and retina and have shown that mechanical alteration of these relationships by vitrectomy can prevent retinal detachment. Animal models and in vitro cell cultures have permitted examination of the substrates and cellular mechanisms of the wound-healing response, which is the basis for post-traumatic vitreoretinal traction. It is to be hoped that our growing understanding of the mechanism of fibroblast proliferation, the role played by the retinal pigment epithelium, and the effects of macrophages and tissue growth factors will eventually enable modification of these biologic processes.

PATHOPHYSIOLOGY OF INJURY

An extremely broad spectrum of sequelae may result from ocular trauma, reflecting the numerous causes of injury. It is useful to consider blunt contusion and laceration separately as they have different effects, although in practice any injury will include both components. Blunt injuries, however, appear to carry a worse prognosis than penetrating injuries due to sharp objects.[2]

Blunt Trauma

An object striking the eye causes a complex deformation of the globe that varies depending on the kinetic energy of the object and the site of

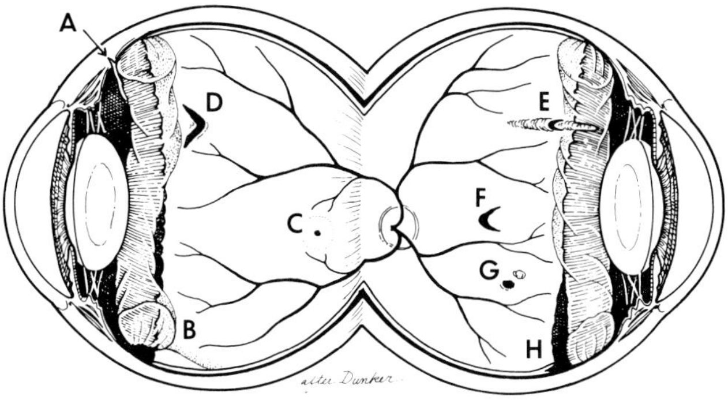

Fig. 19-1. Retinal lesions following blunt trauma. *A*, Pars plana tear at anterior border of vitreous base. *B*, Avulsion of vitreous base. *C*, Macular hole. *D*, Horseshoe tear at posterior border of vitreous base. *E*, Horseshoe tear at meridional fold. *F*, Horseshoe tear at equator. *G*, Operculated hole. *H*, Retinal dialysis at vitreous base. (Modified from Green WR: Vitreoretinal juncture. In Ryan SJ, editor: Retina, St Louis, 1989, The CV Mosby Co.)

impact. Initially, the eye is compressed anteroposteriorly and stretched equatorially, but before it recovers its normal shape, there is an overshoot during decompression, with equatorial shortening and anteroposterior elongation.[4] The resulting rapid deformation of the posterior pole and vitreous can lead to injury remote from the impact site. Commotio retinae, ophthalmoscopically visible as retinal whitening, is commonly seen peripherally and in the macula (see Chapter 17). This has been attributed to extracellular edema or swelling of glial cells and to damaged photoreceptors.

Acute vitreoretinal traction may cause retinal breaks (Fig. 19-1), dialyses being the most common after blunt trauma (see Chapter 18). The vitreous base is occasionally elevated and is seen as a "bucket-handle" in the vitreous cavity if the dialysis forms at both the anterior and posterior borders of the vitreous base. Horseshoe tears may develop at the posterior border of the vitreous base or at other sites of abnormal vitreoretinal relationships, such as meridional folds, and are found most frequently in the upper nasal quadrant.[5]

Contusive injury posterior to the vitreous base occasionally leads to large, irregular retinal holes overlying the site of impact and may be accompanied by disruption of the pigment epithelium and hemorrhage in the vitreous and choroid. These holes appear to develop almost immediately after trauma. Animal studies suggest that they are due to mechanical fragmentation of the retina.[6]

Penetrating Trauma

Large penetrating injuries that result in hypotony and expulsive choroidal hemorrhage with extensive prolapse of ocular contents clearly have little potential for visual recovery. Smaller wounds, which are sealed by uveal or vitreous prolapse or both, carry a better prognosis, but the normal mechanisms of wound repair may result in intraocular fibrosis and complex retinal detachment.

In a series of 74 eyes with retinal detachment following penetrating injury, the most common pathogenesis was contraction of the vitreous membranes that radiated from a site of vitreous incarceration in the laceration of the ocular wall.[5] These membranes first became ophthalmoscopically visible 2 or 3 weeks after injury. In 23 of these eyes the progressive contraction of the fan-shaped membranes created a dialysis opposite the site of vitreous incarceration. In six eyes in which retina was also incarcerated in the wound, a dense white mass of tissue proliferated into the cavity, and fixed retinal folds radiated out from the wound. Traction bands developed in the track of a foreign body in 1 eye. Retinal lacerations caused rhegmatogenous detachments in 12 eyes. In this series, reported in 1966, 70% of the detachments were reattached. Failure was attributed mostly to "relentless traction from shrinking vitreous membranes."

Winthrop et al[7] reviewed the histopathologic findings in 34 eyes enucleated between 1 day and 3 years after penetrating injury. Fibrous ingrowth was present in limbal and scleral wounds despite good surgical closure, although such eyes often showed vitreous incarceration, lens damage, and vitreous hemorrhage. The vitreous was posteriorly detached in 6 of 13 eyes removed 2 weeks after injury. Blood was loculated in the gel in 18 of the 22 eyes with vitreous detachment. Vitreous fibrils radiated from incarceration sites at limbal or scleral wounds and stretched between entry and exit sites in eyes with perforating injuries. Inflammatory cells, mainly monocytes, were present in the wound and in incarcerated tissues. Macrophages were found at the margins of blood clots within the vitreous, in areas of subretinal hemorrhage, and lining the posterior vitreous separation. Fibroblastic proliferation within the vitreous emanated from the nonpigmented ciliary epithelium or from the uvea and episclera at wound sites and often resulted in the incorporation of lens material and detached retina into a cyclitic membrane. Fibroblasts appeared to extend along a scaffold formed by vitreous fibrils and posteriorly over the surface of the retina. By 4 to 6 weeks after injury, multilayered epiretinal membranes containing pigmented cells and macrophages were present on the posterior retina. Subretinal membranes were prominent 2 weeks after injury and were associated with areas of subretinal hemorrhage and areas of proliferation of the retinal pigment epithelium. Traction retinal detachment was present in 27 of the 34 eyes.

Clinical series of patients undergoing surgical repair of penetrating ocular injuries indicate that final visual outcome depends upon initial acuity, mechanism of injury, location and size of wound, and presence or absence of vitreous hemorrhage, all of which reflect the severity of the injury.[1,2] The wide variability of ocular trauma makes it difficult to study the influence of each of these factors and the effects of different treatment strategies. Accordingly, these issues have been approached by studying several animal models, which permit the controlled variation of individual factors.

ANIMAL MODELS

Natural History

Standardized models in animal eyes have enabled the effects of posterior penetrating trauma to be studied. Traction retinal detachments, the most common cause of vision loss in this type of trauma, have been reproduced in rabbit, monkey, and pig eyes. The rabbit model was produced by making a full-thickness 8-mm incision through the pars plana and injecting autologous blood (0.5 ml) through the wound.[8] Retinal detachment developed by 12 to 15 days. Condensed vitreous strands extended from the wound to both the posterior retina and the peripheral retina at the vitreous base. Retinal detachment posteriorly was attributable to anteroposterior traction along the vitreous strands. Contraction of the peripheral elements caused a forward rolling of the anterior retina over the pars plana. With further contraction and fibrosis, a total retina detachment developed, and eventually the retina was drawn up into a cyclitic membrane formed by fibrous ingrowth originating at the wound.

Because the primate eye does not have the strong posterior vitreoretinal adhesions found in the rabbit eye, it allows study of the effects of posterior vitreous detachment, which typically develops 2 weeks after injury (Color Plate 19-1).[9] In a rhesus monkey model, the posterior retina was completely free of vitreous attachments by 8 days, although there was vitreous strand formation as in the rabbit model. Retinal detachment most commonly occurred at 7 to 11 weeks following injury. Two mechanisms appeared to contribute to this development. Fibrous ingrowth along the vitreous scaffold that was created by the incarceration of vitreous in the wound resulted in the formation of a cyclitic membrane. Because the vitreous remained attached at the base, traction caused a retinal detachment beginning at the periphery. In addition, the contraction of epiretinal membranes, formed on the peripheral retinal surface and extending posteriorly to the equator, caused shortening of the retina and posterior detachment (Fig. 19-2).

Because the monkey sclera is too thin to permit much ocular contusion without resulting in rupture, the pig eye has been used to investigate the role of the contusion effects that often accompany penetrating trauma.[10] Following the standard penetrating injury, the response of the pig eye resembles that of the rabbit, rather than the monkey or human. Transvitreal strands form between the wound and the posterior retina, but posterior vitreous detachment does not develop. Although retinal folds form at the posterior pole, extensive retinal detachment does not occur.

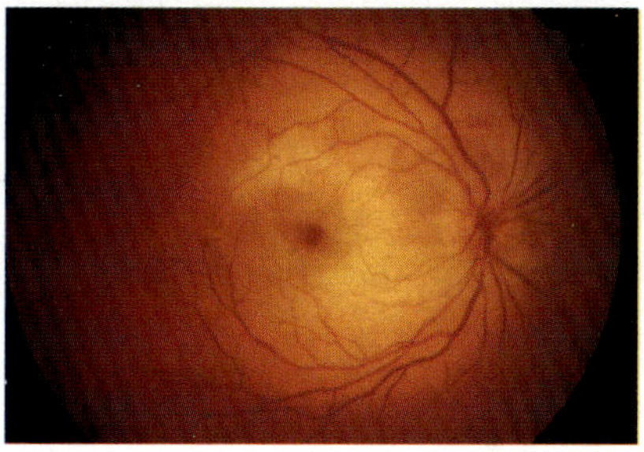

Color Plate 17-1. Fundus photograph demonstrating commotio retinae in the posterior pole with gray-white opacification of the outer retina due to disorganization of the photoreceptor outer segments following blunt trauma.

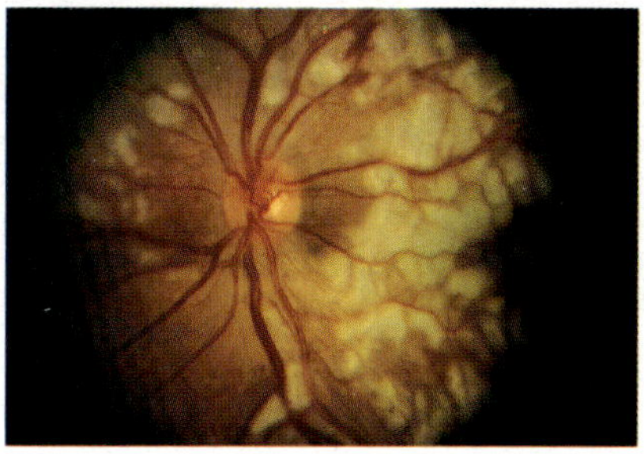

Color Plate 17-2. Fundus photograph demonstrating Purtscher's retinopathy with nerve fiber layer infarcts in a peripapillary distribution.

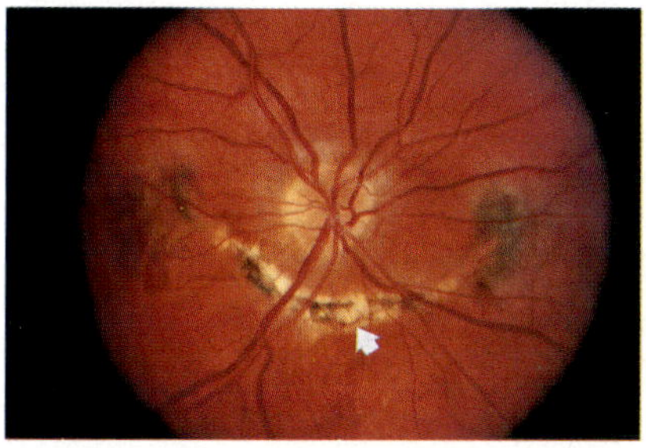

Color Plate 17-3. Fundus photograph demonstrating choroidal rupture *(arrow)* that developed concentric to the optic nerve.

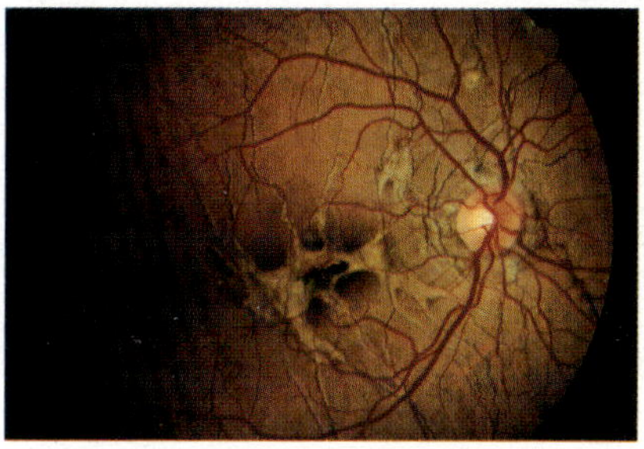

Color Plate 17-4. Fundus photograph of extensive choroidal rupture and scarring in macula following blunt trauma to an eye with angioid streaks associated with pseudoxanthoma elasticum.

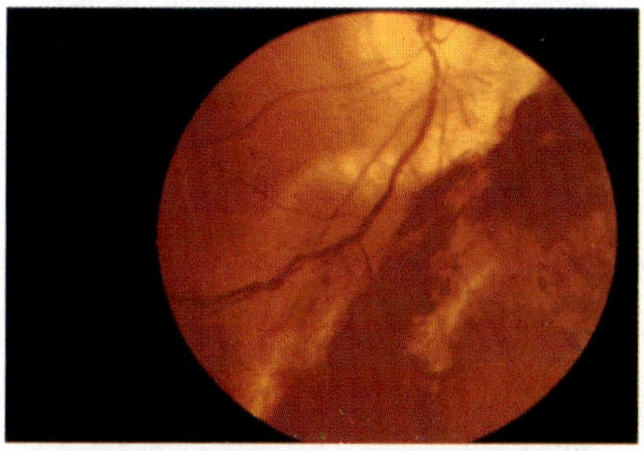

Color Plate 17-5. Fundus photograph demonstrating retinitis sclopetaria with rupture of retina and choroid inferonasally and intraretinal and preretinal hemorrhage.

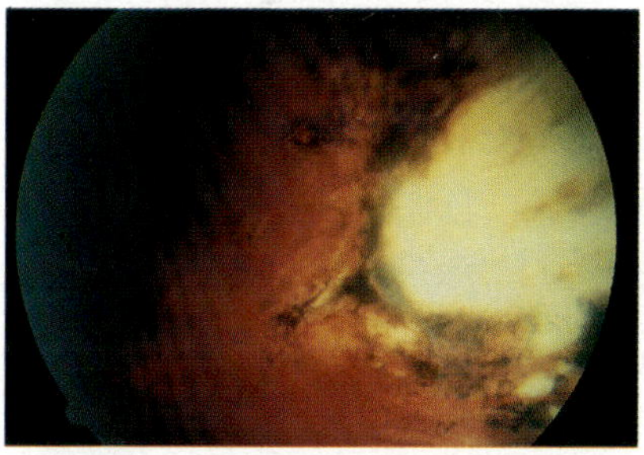

Color Plate 17-6. Fundus photograph of eye in Color Plate 17-5 taken 2 years later. Hemorrhage has resolved, and extensive zone of choroidal and retinal rupture (retinitis sclopetaria) is more apparent.

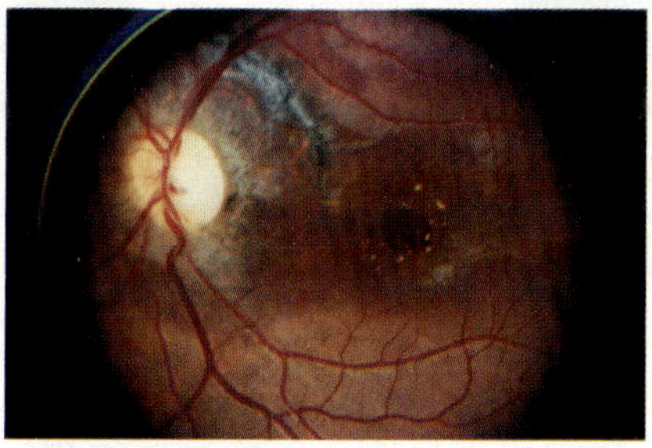

Color Plate 17-7. Fundus photograph demonstrating traumatic macular hole.

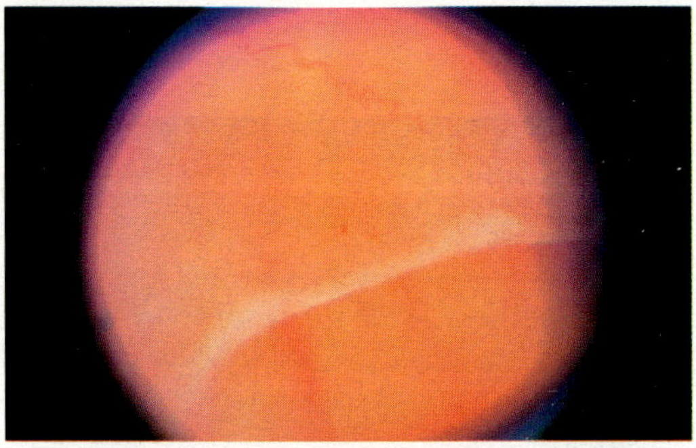

Color Plate 18-1. Traumatic inferotemporal retinal dialysis producing a bullous rhegmatogenous retinal detachment. The mouth of the dialysis appears to be held open by the vitreous base.

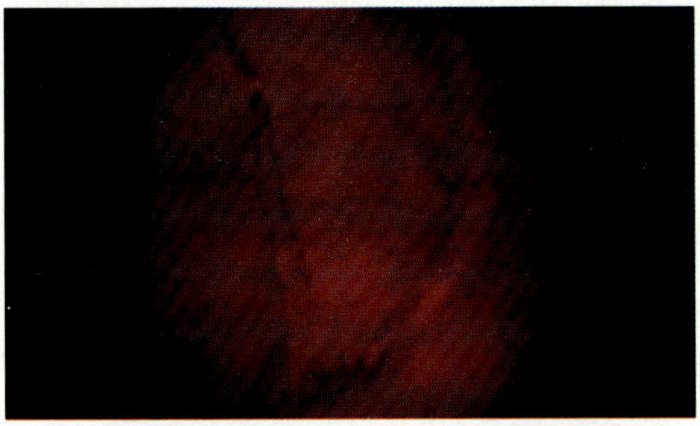

Color Plate 18-2. Two arcuate pigmented demarcation lines corresponding to the two previous posterior margins of a chronic rhegmatogenous retinal detachment.

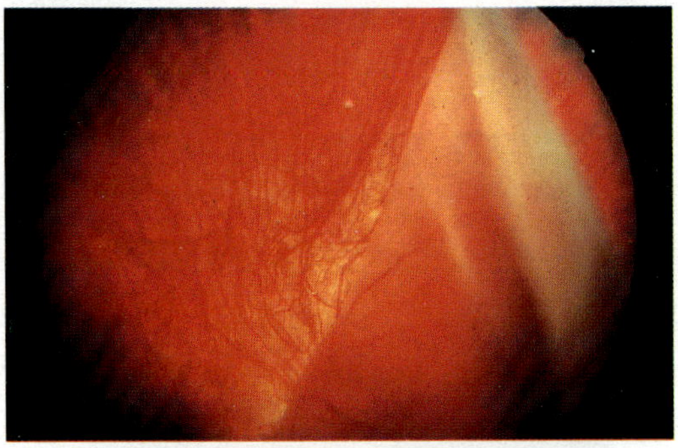

Color Plate 18-3. Giant retinal tear (180°) with inverted retinal flap.

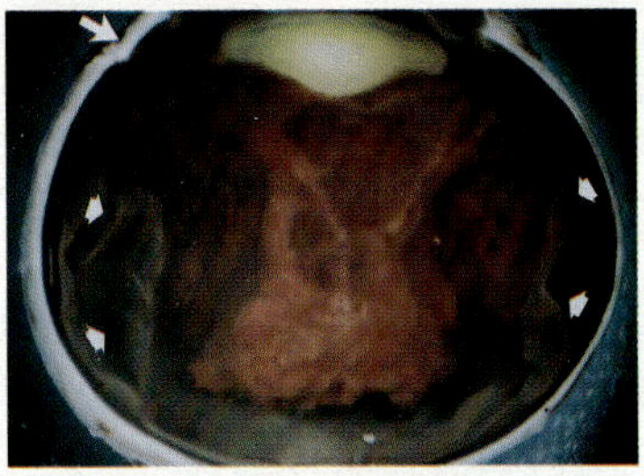

A, At 4 days, blood in the vitreous cavity is surrounded by clear vitreous; vitreoretinal attachments are intact. *Single arrow:* entry site. *Double arrows:* artifactitiously detached retina.

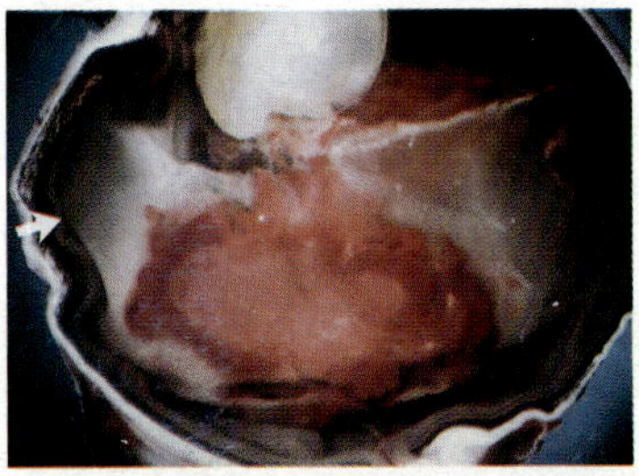

B, At 8 days, a posterior vitreous detachment has occurred; the vitreous is opacified.

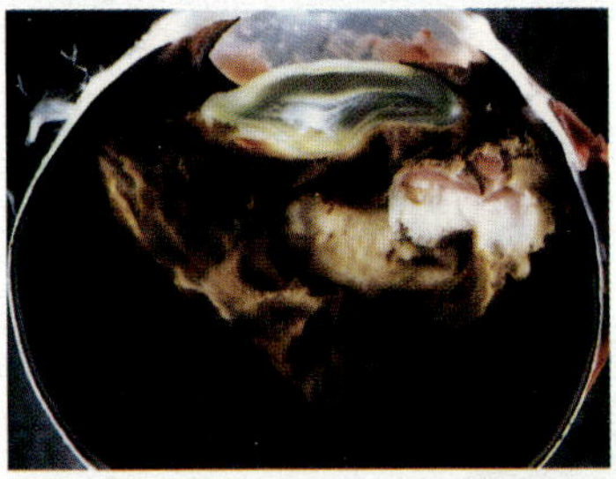

C, At 5 weeks, a complete posterior vitreous detachment, appearing as a yellow ochre membrane, is present.

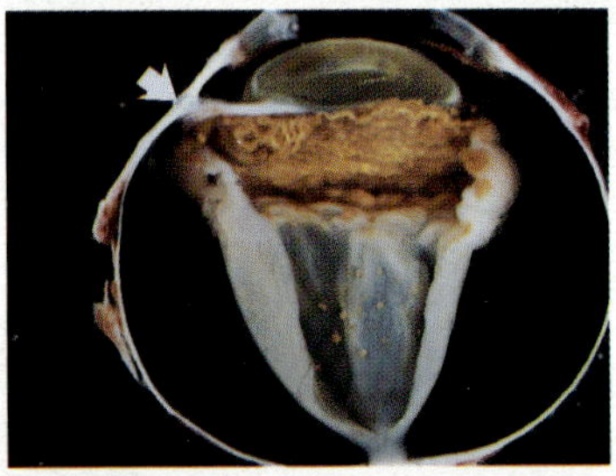

D, At 3 months, a total funnel-shaped retinal detachment shows peripheral retinal folds caused by epiretinal membranes; note the cyclitic membrane formed from fibrous ingrowth originating at the wound. (From Cleary PE and Ryan SJ: Am J Ophthalmol 88:212-220, 1979.)

Color Plate 19-1. Natural course following posterior segment penetrating injury with blood injection in the rhesus monkey eye.

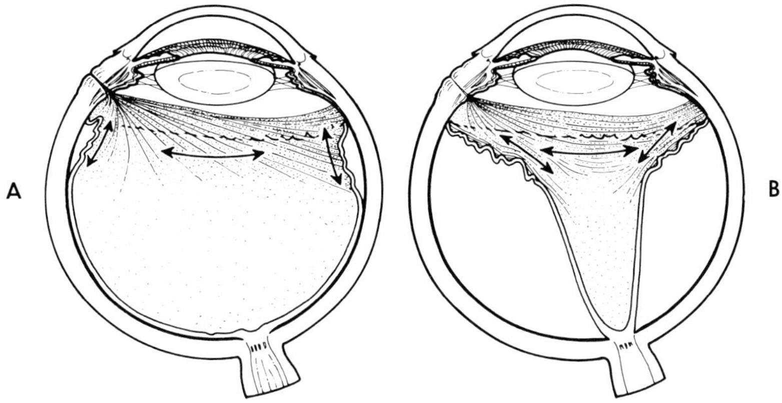

Fig. 19-2. Mechanism of traction retinal detachment in the rhesus monkey eye following posterior penetrating trauma. **A,** Peripheral retinal detachment is caused by traction from fibrous ingrowth along the vitreous scaffold formed with incarceration of vitreous in the wound site. **B,** Posterior retinal detachment results from shortening of the retina caused by contraction of epiretinal membranes extending posteriorly on the retinal surface. (Modified from Cleary PE and Ryan SJ: Am J Ophthalmol 88:212-220, 1979.)

In these studies, contusion injuries were created by firing lead pellets from a pistol held perpendicular to the sclera at a point 2.5 cm from the limbus. Retinal whitening and wrinkling were immediately noted posterior to the impact site. Anterior hemorrhagic retinal detachments developed in the form of circumferential retinal folds concentric with the impact site, with overlying vitreous hemorrhage at the ora serrata. The retinal detachments resolved after 2 weeks, and the vitreous hemorrhage cleared 1 week later. The posterior retina remained normal.

In eyes subjected to both contusion and penetrating trauma, similar findings evolved but in two distinct phases. Initially, retinal opacification and anterior hemorrhagic retinal detachments developed. As these resolved over the ensuing 2 to 3 weeks, full-thickness radial folds of the posterior retina, due to anteroposterior traction, were noted beginning at 8 days. These posterior folds persisted throughout the follow-up period (4 months), in contrast to the anterior folds resulting from contusion. Later, a forward rolling of the anterior retina onto the pars plana was noted. The effects of contusion were thus largely confined to the first 2 weeks, whereas those of penetrating injury became clinically evident after 2 weeks.

Histopathology of Penetrating Injury

In the first 3 days after penetrating injury to the rabbit eye, the inner aspect of the wound is infiltrated with leukocytes and macrophages.[11] Wound healing begins with proliferation from the episclera, but by 6 days there is fibroblastic proliferation from the uvea and nonpigmented ciliary epithelium as well. Fibroblasts proliferate along the vitreous strands incarcerated in the wound and form membranes that result in retinal detachment at 12 days. Fibroblastic proliferation originates also from the optic nerve head. The blood clot within the vitreous cavity gradually disperses and is absorbed. Hemosiderin-laden macrophages are present within the clot and the inner retina. In the late stages (18 days to 3 months) there is hyperplasia of the retinal pigment epithelium. A total retinal detachment develops, with the retina drawn up into a cyclitic membrane extending from the wound. Ultimately, the eye becomes phthisical.

Although the initial response of the monkey eye to penetrating injury is similar to that of the rabbit, subsequent events differ in several respects.[12] After 8 days, the monkey vitreous is no longer attached to the posterior retina but does remain attached anteriorly. With detachment of the posterior vitreous during the second week, the posterior hyaloid forms a yellow-brown membrane behind the blood clot that is loculated in midvitreous. The clot undergoes hemolysis, fibrinolysis, and organization by fibroblasts derived from the ciliary body, choroid, and optic nerve head and is usually absorbed after 10 weeks. Fibroblasts also invade the anterior hyaloid along vitreous strands, reaching the lens equator at 4 weeks and the midline at 6 to 8 weeks. At 10 weeks, a cyclitic membrane extends from the wound to the ciliary body and peripheral retina opposite the wound. Ultrastructural studies revealed myofibroblasts embedded in a matrix of collagenlike fibrils within the vitreous at 2 to 6 weeks following injury.[13] These cells have features of both fibroblasts and smooth muscle cells. Contributing to the fibrous ingrowth from the wound are proliferating pigmented and nonpigmented cells from the ciliary epithelium. These cells extend into the vitreous cavity and along the surface of the detached posterior hyaloid.

As early as two days following injury, perivascular mononuclear cells containing granules staining positive for iron are found in the monkey retina. These cells migrate into the nerve fiber and ganglion cell layers at 8 to 10 days. Hemosiderin-laden macrophages initially line the internal limiting membrane and optic nerve head but are subsequently found in the inner retina by 14 days. Epiretinal membranes are present over the peripheral retina at 4 to 6 weeks following injury. These membranes, composed of fibroblasts and myofibroblastlike cells, are only a few cell layers thick, whereas at 3 months much thicker epiretinal membranes are seen in association with retinal detachments and full-thickness folds. The predominant cell type here has features characteristic of myofibroblasts but lacks the cytoplasmic filaments. In addition, cells apparently derived from retinal glial cells are present. These cells extend cytoplasmic processes through breaks in the internal limiting membrane to form bridges between the retina and epiretinal membrane. Finally, macrophages are found also in the epiretinal membranes.

The presence of these various cell types, particularly the myofibroblasts, in intravitreal membranes formed after penetrating injury in both monkey and rabbit eyes suggests that the development of traction retinal detachment is pathophysiologically related to the normal cellular processes of wound healing and contraction. An inflammatory reaction induced by injury is followed by cellular proliferation with membrane formation and ultimately by fibrosis with collagen formation. The contractile property of intravitreal membranes in rabbit eyes has been measured using microstrain gauges.[14] Forces of 30 to 100 mg were generated by the membranes in the presence of serotonin, norepinephrine, prostaglandin F1-alpha, angiotensin II, bradykinin, and vasopressin. An electrical stimulus and depolarizing solutions also induced contraction. The effect of norepinephrine was blocked by phentolamine mesylate, implicating adrenergic receptors. Relaxation was achieved with papaverine, diphenhydramine hydrochloride, cytochalasin B, and diltiazem, but acetylcholine and histamine had no effect. These pharmacologic responses simulated those of granulation tissue but differed from those of smooth or skeletal muscle.

Histopathology of Contusion Injury

The immediate response of the pig eye to contusion injury is hyperemia at the impact site with dilation of the anterior choroidal vessels and infiltration of polymorphonuclear leukocytes.[15] However, by the end of 1 week these changes resolve, and the macrophage is the predominant cell type. Rupture of choroidal vessels leads to subretinal hemorrhage that extends into the vitreous through areas of disrupted retina. At the end of 2 weeks, the subretinal blood is replaced by a fibrocellular membrane resulting from proliferation of the underlying retinal pigment epithelium. Thus the histologic appearance corresponds to the transient changes seen ophthalmoscopically.

In eyes that have undergone both contusion and penetrating injury, intravitreal fibrous proliferation develops from the wound, and these membranes become continuous with the subretinal membranes at the contusion site. With development of intravitreal fibrous proliferation, posterior retinal folds appear 8 days after injury.

FACTORS INFLUENCING THE HEALING RESPONSE

Blood

Blood appears to be an important element in the pathogenesis of traction retinal detachment following posterior segment trauma. In the three animal models described, the presence of blood was essential for the development of intravitreal traction membranes. Following the standard incision in rabbit eyes, 28 of 34 eyes developed retinal detachment if autologous blood was injected, compared with only 1 of 15 eyes if balanced salt solution was injected.[8] Vitreous strands extended from the wound to the posterior retina in both groups, but fibrous ingrowth developed only in eyes injected with blood.

Histopathologic studies showed proliferation from the episclera in the saline-treated group, but this led only to uncomplicated wound healing and scar formation.[12,16] Similar results were obtained in the monkey and pig models. Specifically, no histologic evidence of epiretinal fibrous proliferation or retinal detachment was found in monkey eyes after injection of balanced salt solution, despite the presence of vitreous strands and incarceration.

Serum-derived proteins may play a major role in the stimulation of intravitreal proliferation by blood. Fibronectin is a high–molecular weight glycoprotein found in serum and within the extracellular matrix. It is chemotactic for retinal pigment epithelial cells, fibroblasts, and glial cells and is an important mediator in the interaction between collagen and retinal pigment epithelial and other cells.[17,18] Using immunochemical staining, fibronectin was identified in epiretinal membranes obtained from human eyes undergoing vitrectomy for traction retinal detachment following trauma.[19] Indeed, a peptide analog of the cell-binding site of fibronectin, which has been shown in vitro to disrupt retinal pigment epithelial cell–collagen adhesion, may have therapeutic value.[18]

Platelet-derived growth factor (PDGF), another serum chemotactic agent for retinal pigment epithelial cells, fibroblasts, and monocytes, is found in relatively high concentration in wounds.[20] It is also mitogenic for glial cells and fibroblasts. Other serum components that may play a role in the stimulation of intravitreal fibrosis include complement and interleukin-1.

Retinal Laceration

The effect of retinal laceration was studied in the rabbit by making incisions that involved the retina and pars plana to a varying extent.[21] Incisions 8 mm long were made at the equator (slanted incision 3 to 6 mm from the limbus), along the ora, or within peripheral retina and pars plana (slanted incision 0.5 to 3 mm from the limbus). Retinal detachment occurred in 16%, 78%, and 14% of these eyes, respectively. It therefore appears that retinal laceration alone (in the absence of blood) is not sufficient to cause detachment. Only lacerations with rolled edges, indicating vitreoretinal traction, proceeded to detachment. This occurred most commonly in lacerations along the ora, because traction due to the vitreous base was applied only to the posterior edge. In contrast, this asymmetric traction would occur at only one point along the peripheral retinal laceration, where it crossed the ora. Similarly, equatorial penetrating injuries in the monkey eye did not lead to retinal detachment.[22]

Vitreous-Lens Admixture

The effect of lens rupture in posterior penetrating injury was investigated by injecting autologous lens material from the fellow eyes of five monkeys that had undergone standard incision through the pars plana without blood injection into the vitreous.[23] Fibrous ingrowth from the wound varied from minimal to moderate along the vitreous scaffold. However, no clinical or histologic evidence for epiretinal membrane formation or retinal detachment was found. Therefore, vitreous-lens admixture appears much less important than blood in stimulating intravitreal proliferation.

RATIONALE FOR SURGICAL TREATMENT

Histopathologic studies of clinical specimens and experimentally injured animal eyes have demonstrated the importance of vitreous fibrils that serve as a scaffold for alignment and contraction of fibroblasts.[7,12] Clinical reports suggest that vitrectomy would prevent traction retinal detachment by mechanically removing this scaffold and by removing any blood that would stimulate inflammation and fibrosis. However, the wide variation in ocular trauma makes it impossible to obtain clinical data sufficient to determine statistical significance. Therefore, the scientific basis for much of the treatment of ocular trauma rests upon the models of standardized penetrating injuries in animal eyes.[24-27]

Efficacy of Vitrectomy

Cleary and Ryan[24] performed vitrectomy, lensectomy, and conventional reattachment procedures in the rhesus monkey at intervals of 1, 14, or 70 days after injury. Surgery at 1 or 14 days prevented retinal detachment, but the operation was technically easier at 14 days because of the development of posterior vitreous detachment. Retinal detachment developed in eyes left untreated for 70 days, and these detachments could not be repaired. In the same model, core vitrectomy was also ineffective in preventing traction retinal detachment.[26,27]

Timing of Vitrectomy

The optimal timing of vitrectomy is controversial and depends on many factors. There is evidence that vitrectomy is ineffective if delayed much more than 2 to 3 weeks after injury. The time sequence of vitreous fibroplasia was studied in the rabbit eye after perforating injury and intravitreal implantation of a polyvinyl sponge. The production of collagen (assayed as the hydroxyproline content of the sponge) showed a rapid increase during the second week after injury.[28] In the rhesus monkey, traction detachment developed at 4 to 16 weeks after injury and could not be repaired at 10 weeks. In addition to the animal models, there is also some clinical evidence that vitrectomy is more successful if performed within 2 weeks of injury.[1]

Very early vitrectomy carries some disadvantages. Complete vitreous removal is more difficult before posterior vitreous detachment, and there is a greater risk of iatrogenic tears.[26,27] In the rhesus monkey, posterior vitreous detachment developed at 1 to 3 weeks. Moreover, early vitrectomy in the clinical setting is occasionally complicated by expulsive choroidal hemorrhage.

In actual injuries, contusion, causing choroidal and subretinal hemorrhage, usually occurs along with the penetrating trauma.[7] Such combined injury in the pig eye model results in resolution of the hemorrhagic sequelae of blunt trauma in the 2 weeks following injury, but vitreoretinal traction due to the penetrating injury develops after 2 weeks. In the same model, vitrectomy performed on the first day after combined injury was often complicated by severe bleeding from the contusion site. In contrast, this rarely occurred when surgery was performed 2 weeks or more after injury, suggesting that the optimal timing for vitrectomy would be 2 weeks following the injury.[25]

In perforating injuries of the globe, where a posterior exit wound is not accessible to primary closure, it may be necessary to delay vitrectomy until physiologic wound repair has sealed the exit site. In a rabbit eye model, both entry and exit scleral wounds are sealed at 2 weeks.[29]

In summary, vitrectomy can effectively prevent traction retinal detachment if performed within 2 weeks of injury. Although equally effective within a few days of injury, there is a greater risk of intraoperative complications, such as bleeding, when such surgery is performed in the immediate posttraumatic period. Chapter 20 details the surgical management of penetrating injuries of the posterior segment.

References

1. Brinton GS et al: Surgical results in ocular trauma involving the posterior segment, Am J Ophthalmol 93:271-278, 1982.
2. De Juan E, Sternberg P, and Michels RG: Penetrating ocular injuries: types of injuries and visual results, Ophthalmology 90:1318-1322, 1983.
3. Hutton WL and Fuller DG: Factors influencing final visual results in severely injured eyes, Am J Ophthalmol 97:715-722, 1984.
4. Delori F, Pomerantzeff O, and Cox MS: Deformation of the globe under high speed impact: its relation to contusion injuries, Invest Ophthalmol 8:290-301, 1969.
5. Cox MS, Schepens CL, and Freeman HM: Retinal detachment due to ocular contusion, Arch Ophthalmol 76:678-685, 1966.
6. Cox MS: Retinal breaks caused by blunt nonperforating trauma at the point of impact, Trans Am Ophthalmol Soc 78:414-465, 1980.
7. Winthrop SR et al: Penetrating eye injuries: a histopathological review, Br J Ophthalmol 64:809-817, 1980.
8. Cleary PE and Ryan SJ: Experimental posterior penetrating eye injury in the rabbit. I. Method of production and natural history, Br J Ophthalmol 63:306-311, 1979.
9. Matsumoto B, Blanks JC, and Ryan SJ: Topographic variations in the rabbit and primate internal limiting membrane, Invest Ophthalmol Vis Sci 25:71-82, 1984.
10. Gregor Z and Ryan SJ: Combined posterior contusion and penetrating injury in the pig eye. I. A natural history study, Br J Ophthalmol 66:793-798, 1982.
11. Cleary PE and Ryan SJ: Experimental posterior penetrating eye injury in the rabbit. II. Histology of wound, vitreous and retina, Br J Ophthalmol 63:312-321, 1979.
12. Cleary PE and Ryan SJ: Histology of wound, vitreous and retina in experimental posterior penetrating injury in the rhesus monkey, Am J Ophthalmol 88:221-231, 1979.
13. Cleary PE, Minckler DS, and Ryan SJ: Ultrastructure of traction retinal detachment in rhesus monkey eyes after a posterior penetrating ocular injury, Am J Ophthalmol 90:829-845, 1980.

14. Kirmani M and Ryan SJ: In vitro measurement of contractile force of transvitreal membranes formed after penetrating ocular injury, Arch Ophthalmol 103:107-110, 1985.
15. Gregor Z and Ryan SJ: Combined posterior contusion and penetrating injury in the pig eye. II. Histological features, Br J Ophthalmol 66:799-804, 1982.
16. Cleary PE and Ryan SJ: Method of production and natural history of experimental posterior penetrating eye injury in the rhesus monkey, Am J Ophthalmol 88:212-220, 1979.
17. Campochiaro PA, Jerdan JA, and Glaser BM: Serum contains chemoattractants for human retinal pigment epithelial cells, Arch Ophthalmol 102:1830-1833, 1984.
18. Glaser BM, Cardin A, and Biscoe B: Proliferative vitreoretinopathy: the mechanism of development of vitreoretinal traction, Ophthalmology 94:327-332, 1987.
19. Weller M, Heimann K, and Wiedemann P: Immunochemical studies of epiretinal membranes using APAAP complexes: evidence for macrophage involvement in traumatic proliferative vitreoretinopathy, Int Ophthalmol 11:181-186, 1988.
20. Compochiaro PA and Glaser BM: Platelet derived growth factor is chemotactic for human retinal pigment epithelial cells, Arch Ophthalmol 103:576-579, 1985.
21. Hsu H-T and Ryan SJ: Experimental retinal detachment in the rabbit: penetrating ocular injury with retinal laceration, Retina 6:66-69, 1986.
22. Hsu H-T and Ryan SJ: Natural history of penetrating ocular injury with retinal laceration in the monkey, Graefes Arch Clin Exp Ophthalmol 224:1-6, 1986.
23. Cleary PE, Jarus G, and Ryan SJ: Experimental posterior penetrating eye injury in the rhesus monkey: vitreous-lens admixture, Br J Ophthalmol 64:801-808, 1980.
24. Cleary PE and Ryan SJ: Vitrectomy in penetrating eye injury: results of a controlled trial of vitrectomy in an experimental posterior penetrating eye injury in the rhesus monkey, Arch Ophthalmol 99:287-292, 1981.
25. Gregor Z and Ryan SJ: Combined posterior contusion and penetrating injury in the pig eye. III. A controlled treatment trial of vitrectomy, Br J Ophthalmol 67:282-285, 1983.
26. Gregor Z and Ryan SJ: Complete and core vitrectomies in the treatment of experimental posterior penetrating eye injury in the rhesus monkey. I. Clinical features, Arch Ophthalmol 101:441-445, 1983.
27. Gregor Z and Ryan SJ: Complete and core vitrectomies in the treatment of experimental posterior penetrating eye injury in the rhesus monkey. II. Histological features, Arch Ophthalmol 101:446-450, 1983.
28. Pilketon AR et al: Experimental vitreous fibroplasia following perforating ocular injuries, Arch Ophthalmol 97:1707-1709, 1979.
29. Topping TM, Abrams GW, and Machemer R: Experimental double-perforating injury of the posterior segment in rabbit eyes: the natural history of intraocular proliferation, Arch Ophthalmol 97:735-742, 1979.

CHAPTER 20

Surgical management of posterior segment injuries

TREXLER M. TOPPING

Management options
- Timing of surgery
- Management of nonpenetrating injuries without rupture
- Management of penetrating injuries and globe rupture

Surgical methods
- Infusion port location
- Lensectomy
- Vitrectomy
- Vitreous bands
- Preretinal membranes
- Subretinal blood
- Retinal incarceration
- Retinal reattachment
- Scleral buckling
- Temporary keratoprosthesis

References

MANAGEMENT OPTIONS

Timing of Surgery

Current techniques of vitreoretinal surgery enable the surgeon to clear media opacities, identify and treat retinal abnormalities, and remove vitreous scaffolds to prevent later fibrocellular proliferation. Timing for surgical intervention remains a matter of controversy. Immediate intervention, usually at the time of primary repair of the serious injury or within the first 3 days, has the advantage of preceding development of significant intraocular fibrosis and membrane formation.[1] Delayed vitrectomy, usually performed 10 to 14 days after injury and primary repair, may have the advantages of less intraoperative hemorrhage and generally easier surgery because posterior vitreous separation has often occurred spontaneously.[2] The 10- to 14-day postinjury interval, therefore, is generally selected by most vitreoretinal surgeons. If the eye is deemed irreparable at this time, enucleation may still be performed in the time window of relative safety from sympathetic ophthalmia (see Chapter 24).

Management of Nonpenetrating Injuries without Rupture

Blunt ocular injuries can result in dense vitreous hemorrhage. With severe hemorrhage, prognosis seems to be poor.[3] The source of the hemorrhage may reflect the likelihood of later complications: hyphema that drifts posteriorly may clear spontaneously, but hemorrhage emanating from a large retinal tear is very likely to progress to retinal detachment and further complications. Unfortunately, in the presence of opaque media it is difficult to determine whether there has been significant retinal damage. These patients require close examination and follow-up, with periodic ultrasonography to assure that the retina remains attached. Vitrectomy intervention is required if retinal detachment occurs. Otherwise, the patient may be followed with frequent reassessment. If the media clears, surgery may be avoided. With persistent opacification, vitrectomy intervention is reasonable and is often performed 3 to 6 months later, although earlier surgical intervention is usually preferred because of the high risk of retinal detachment.

Retinal detachment may be seen with blunt injury, commonly from dialyses, peripheral tractional tears, or ragged traumatic breaks (see Chapter 18). Such retinal detachments require immediate repair. Scleral buckling is indicated, although vitrectomy may be required in special cases of giant tear, macular hole, or opaque media.

Management of Penetrating Injuries and Globe Rupture

Penetrating injuries of the posterior segment and perforating (through-and-through) injuries usually require vitrectomy intervention. Commonly a primary repair of both the anterior injury and the scleral laceration is performed acutely. At primary closure, the tissue margins are carefully reapproximated. Uveal tissue that is not devitalized and retinal tissue should be reposited and not be permitted to remain incarcerated in the wound repair. At completion of surgery the wound should be watertight (see Chapter 13).

When indicated, vitrectomy is performed at a later time, usually after 10 to 14 days. Earlier intervention may be required if there is an intraocular foreign body (see Chaper 21), a penetrating injury with associated endophthalmitis, or an acute retinal detachment. Otherwise the eye is monitored following the primary repair and assessed for any intercurrent complications. Eyes with opaque media receive ultrasound evaluation and usually undergo vitrectomy after 2 weeks.

Eyes with penetrating or perforating injuries and fairly clear media may be amenable to conservative follow-up and not require vitreous surgical intervention. For example, a dart injury may cause a posterior segment perforation with a vitreous band extending from an anterior entrance site to a posterior exit wound. Primary management entails closure of the anterior wound. It is usually not necessary to close the posterior wound, which typically will seal with the fibroproliferative healing response in 2 weeks. With relatively clear media, the fundus appearance can be followed. As long as no complication of tractional or rhegmatogenous retinal detachment occurs, vitrectomy is not necessary. Cases in which the fundus appearance can be monitored and, therefore, complications detected early may be followed with frequent examination and assessment. Surgery may be withheld if no complication occurs.

Weeks to months after primary repair, some patients develop late complications such as puckers, retinal detachment, PVR, cyclitic membrane, or persistent vitreous opacification. When surgery is required, the approaches outlined in the following section are used, although the membranes typically are much thicker and more dense and tight than those seen in earlier repair.

SURGICAL METHODS

The surgical goals in cases of posterior segment injury include clearing media opacity, repairing retinal tears and detachment, preventing future complications by removal of vitreous scaffold and posterior hyaloid, and performing prophylactic scleral buckling. Vitreous surgery is usually performed through a three-port system: one for intraocular infusion of a balanced salt solution, one for fiberoptic endoillumination, and one for the vitreous cutter or intraocular forceps or scissors. Currently most vitreoretinal surgeons use 20-gauge instrumentation. The first step is insertion of the infusion port through the sclera, followed sequentially, if needed, by lensectomy, vitrectomy, membrane peeling, air-fluid exchange, endolaser photocoagulation, scleral buckling, and injection of intraocular gas.

Infusion Port Location

Intraocular infusion is critical to the maintenance of intraocular volume during vitrectomy. The infusate enters the eye through the infusion line and the infusion port, which is typically sutured to the sclera externally in the inferotemporal quadrant. The traumatized eye may present a special situation for entrance site selection. The port should be in an area of healthy sclera and should not pass through a previously sutured laceration because the infusion tip may put stress on the incarcerated vitreous, creating retinal tears, and the port may place undue stress on the sutured laceration. Therefore it may be necessary to place the infusion port more inferiorly or superiorly or possibly nasally, to avoid entrance through injured eye wall. The infusion port tip must be situated within the vitreous cavity, so the presence of a large, highly elevated, hemorrhagic choroidal detachment may necessitate placing the infusion on the opposite side of the eye to avoid infusion into the suprachoroidal space.

If the eye is aphakic or the crystalline lens is to be removed, the infusion port is placed 3 to 3.5 mm posterior to the surgical limbus. If the lens is to be retained, a more posterior entrance, 3.5 to 4 mm posterior to the limbus, should be used. Because of the dense opacity usually present in these eyes, visualization of the tip of the infusion port is often difficult. A tip 4 to 6 mm in length will maximize the likelihood that it will lie within the vitreous cavity, although the longer, 6-mm tips are more likely to injure the crystalline lens and cause iatrogenic traumatic cataract. After the port is sutured in place on the sclera, the infusion fluid should not be allowed to enter the eye until the tip of the port has been visualized and found to be within the vitreous cavity with no overlying choroidal, retinal, or pars plana epithelial tissue. It may be necessary to use an auxiliary infusion line, often a small-gauge butterfly needle brought in through either the limbus or the pars plana to serve as a source of infusion until the opaque vitreous is removed from the area overlying the tip of the sutured infusion port (Fig. 20-1). After the tip of the permanent port is visualized and found to be within the vitreous cavity, infusion is switched to the permanent port.

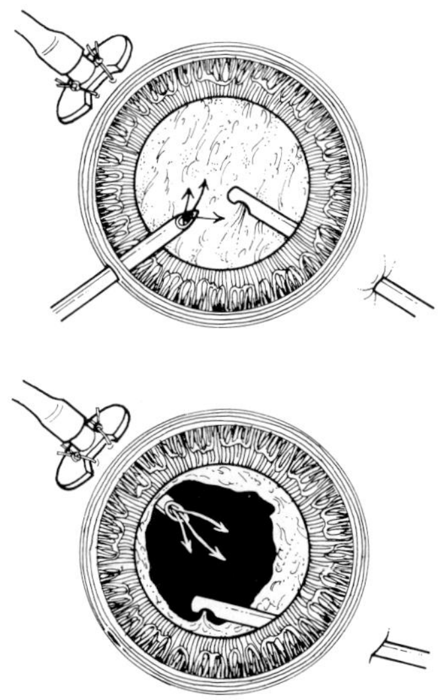

Fig. 20-1. **A,** In opaque media, the tip of the permanent infusion port may not be visible initially. An auxiliary infusion is introduced either through the limbus, as shown here, or through the pars plana, with its tip brought anteriorly where it may be well visualized. The anteriorly located opacities are then removed to permit visualization of the permanent port tip. **B,** After removal of the anterior opacities and anterior peripheral vitreous, the tip of the permanent infusion port is visible within the vitreous cavity.

Lensectomy

Severe injuries of the posterior segment often require surgical removal of the lens. Blood in the anterior chamber will obscure visualization of the posterior pole, so lensectomy may be needed to maintain anterior chamber clarity and permit visibility for posterior surgery. Traumatic cataract is common with serious injuries and of course requires extraction. Completion of extensive anterior retinal repairs frequently requires lensectomy to permit far anterior access with cutting instrumentation. Severe blunt injuries may cause zonular disruption resulting in subluxation or total dislocation of the lens, which may then be removed during vitrectomy.

Removal of traumatic cataract is much like the pars plana removal of cataract performed as part of other vitreous surgery. Traumatized patients tend to be young, and their lenses soft and easily aspirated. If the capsule is ruptured, the lens material may be flocculent. In young patients the vitreous cutter itself may be used to aspirate fluffy lens material. With increasing patient age, there is a concomitant increase of nuclear density and inelasticity, often requiring the use of an ultrasonic lens fragmentation device. The current generation of phacoemulsifiers employ switchable ultrasonic fragmentation and continuously variable suction for aspiration and removal of lens material. Sonication of the hard nucleus is performed first, leaving a large buffer of cortex between the fragmentation device and lens capsule (Fig. 20-2). Rupturing the posterior capsule by zealous overaspiration and fragmentation will create an opening through which lens fragments may drop posteriorly. Creation of an anterior capsular rent will allow transmission of suction forces directly to the anterior chamber, causing anterior chamber flattening. After the nuclear material has been removed, the cortex is aspirated. The periphery of the globe may be indented with a cotton-tipped applicator or other depressor to bring the peripheral lens

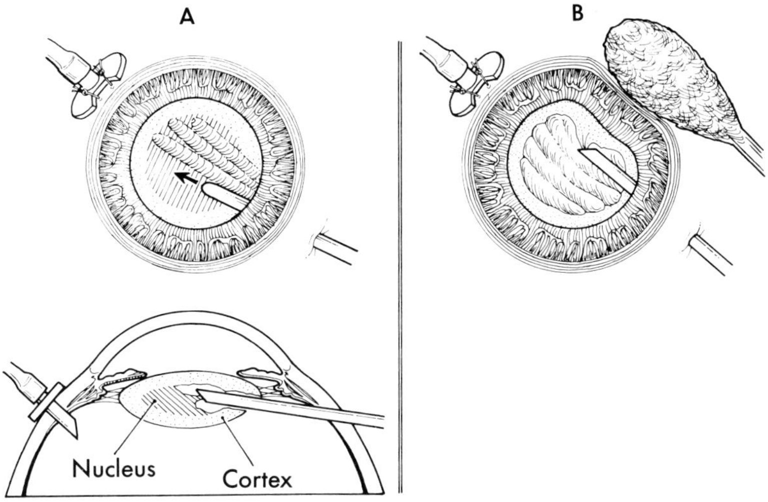

Fig. 20-2. Cataract extraction via the pars plana is a three-stage process. Sequentially the lens nucleus, cortex, and capsule are removed. **A,** Initially, an ultrasonic fragmentation device is introduced to the central portion of the lens within the nucleus. The nucleus is removed using ultrasonic fragmentation to disrupt the lens material and controlled aspiration to remove the debris. Contiguous holes are bored through the nucleus, and with some overlap it is possible to remove the nucleus within a surrounding protective barrier of lens cortex. **B,** Cortical material is aspirated after nuclear extraction. The peripheral material is pulled centrally to remove it from areas hidden by overlying iris. After removal of as much cortex as is easily seen, peripheral indentation may permit the removal of previously hidden lens cortex.

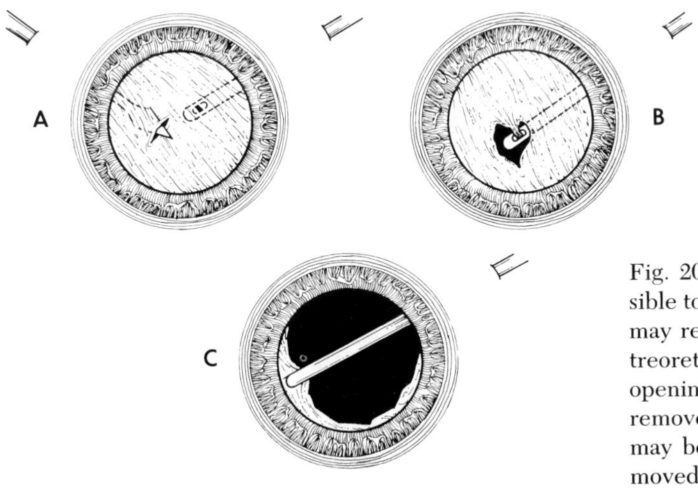

Fig. 20-3. **A,** The lens capsule may be impossible to open with the vitreous cutter alone and may require an initial incision with a microvitreoretinal (MVR) blade. **B,** Once there is an opening in the capsule, it is much easier to remove capsular material. The thin membrane may be brought into the cutting port and removed. **C,** After the capsule is trimmed back close to the pupillary margin, it is important to use a slightly different technique to prevent iris injury. The cutter is brought to the superior border of the capsule, between the capsule and iris, and the cutting port is directed posteriorly. Residual capsular material is then removed without damage to adjacent iris.

remnants into better view and enable removal of hidden cortex.

The vitreous cutting device then removes the residual anterior and posterior capsular material. Engagement of capsular material may be difficult initially. The sclerotomy knife may be required to make a capsular opening. If the capsule cannot be removed easily, it may be useful to place the cutter in aspiration mode, engage the capsule, and then cut after the capsule is incarcerated within the cutting port (Fig. 20-3).

It is important to keep the port turned away from the iris to avoid unintentional iridectomy. Iris trauma should be avoided, as it results in unwanted pupillary miosis and increased postoperative inflammation.

The special cases of subluxated and dislocated lenses may require a second instrument to stabilize the lens and hold it in position for fragmentation and aspiration. When the lens is hinged and subluxated, it falls posteriorly when the patient is in the supine position for surgery. Suction is applied to the lens with the phacofragmentor, and the lens is elevated into the pupillary plane where it may be speared with a microvitreoretinal (MVR) blade to secure it for fragmentation and removal. Similarly, a posteriorly dislocated lens is engaged posteriorly, lifted into the pupillary plane, transfixed with an MVR blade, and removed.[4] Extremely hard nuclei may have to be removed through a limbal incision. With the high quality of current phacofragmentors, this is now rarely necessary (see Chapter 11).

Vitrectomy

The initial goal of vitrectomy is removal of all vitreous opacities. The vitreous cutting device is held in the anterior vitreous with the cutting port directed anteriorly so that material being aspirated may be inspected visually before sectioning and removal (Fig. 20-4). Acutely, the opaque vitreous may be red, yellowish, or slightly green in color and quite hazy. Older blood is often a dirty ocher color. Opaque vitreous should be removed cautiously to minimize the risk of retinal tissue being brought into the cutting port. Helpful techniques include orientation of the vitrectomy tip to keep the cutting port turned anteriorly, maintaining visualization of the cutting port, keeping the cutter in front of the retina and behind the vitreous opacity, and using low suction levels so material is aspirated slowly into the cutting port. During removal of dense hemorrhagic vitreous, pockets of old loose blood may be encountered. Wisps of hazy material swirling throughout the vitreous cavity will hinder visualization. In this case, the cutter should be brought into the more anterior vitreous, where the tip can be seen, and aspiration continued until a clear view is established. If new active bleeding occurs, as from the iris, ciliary body, or a retinal or choroidal location, the infusion bottle should be raised to elevate the intraocular pressure and slow the bleeding. After bleeding stops, the fresh blood may be removed from the vitreous. If bleeding continues, unimanual, bipolar endodiathermy may be required to coagulate the source of bleeding. This is easily done for an anterior source, such as hemorrhage from the iris, but a source of bleeding in the posterior segment may be difficult to visualize because of the haze it creates. If hemostasis cannot be obtained by elevation of the infusion bottle, a rapid air-fluid exchange can be considered. Through the air bubble, the posterior structures can be well visualized and endodiathermy applied to the source of hemorrhage (Fig. 20-5). After bleeding stops, the eye may be refilled with fluid and vitrectomy continued.

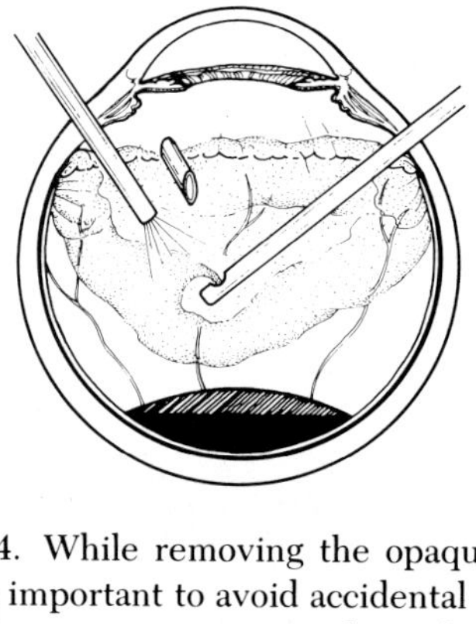

Fig. 20-4. While removing the opaque vitreous, it is important to avoid accidental retinectomy. The cutting port must always be turned anteriorly, which reduces the risk of retina being inadvertently drawn into the cutter. In this illustration one sees both the opaque vitreous more anteriorly and a pool of blood cells lying loosely on the retinal surface posteriorly.

Blood that has been in the eye for days or weeks may be loose and may be aspirated from pools on the retinal surface posteriorly (Fig. 20-6). Conversely, fresh blood tends to clot rapidly and adhere tenaciously to ocular structures. Thus it is important to stop active bleeding before a large amount of blood accumulates, clots, and causes a coagulum cementing fragile intraocular structures together. Thrombin[5] may be added in situations where bleeding is difficult to control; it results in rapid clot formation, but with the attendant problems just described.

Initially, the opaque central vitreous is removed. The posterior hyaloid may have already become detached if significant vitreous hemorrhage has been present several weeks before

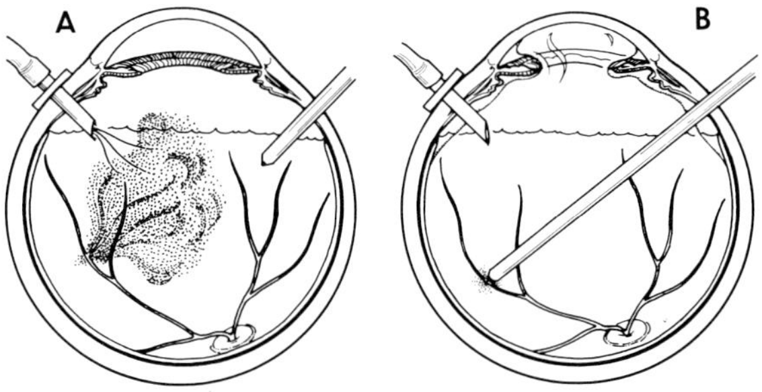

Fig. 20-5. **A,** In the fluid-filled eye, if hemorrhage from a retinal vessel posteriorly is not controlled by elevation of the infusion bottle, the blood may cloud the overlying fluid phase, making visualization and consequent treatment of the source difficult or impossible. **B,** After rapid air-fluid exchange, the surgeon may obtain excellent visualization of the retina and the site of bleeding, permitting application of endodiathermy to the bleeding vessel. After the bleeding stops, the air may again be exchanged with fluid, permitting vitrectomy to continue.

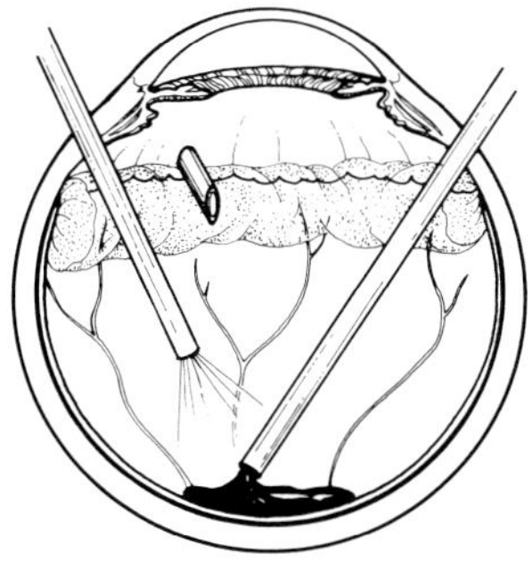

Fig. 20-6. The posterior pool of blood may be aspirated through an extrusion needle after a passageway has been cleared through the vitreous for insertion of instruments.

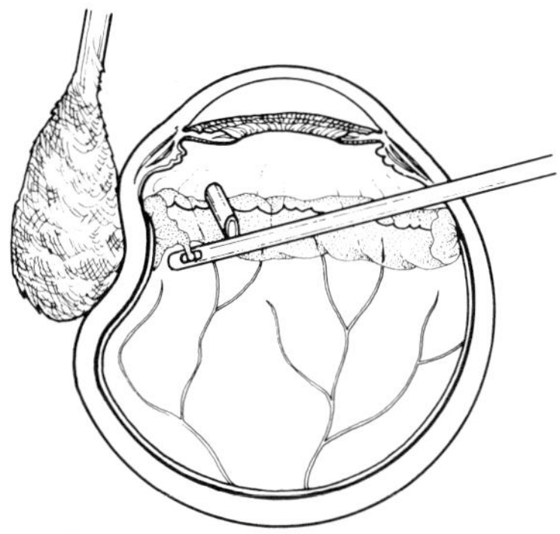

Fig. 20-7. Following removal of the central core of opaque vitreous, a large peripheral band of opacity persists. The vitreous skirt is trimmed back as far as possible with the assistance of scleral depression. While removing the vitreous skirt, the surgeon must point the cutting port directly toward the vitreous, at a right angle to the surgeon. Caution should be exercised to avoid cutting too deeply and removing a portion of retina or pars plana epithelium.

surgery. If the posterior hyaloid is detached, the remaining vitreous anterior to the retina is removed, leaving only the opaque peripheral vitreous skirt. With scleral depression using a cotton-tipped applicator or similar device, peripheral opaque vitreous is depressed centrally and trimmed back with the vitreous cutter (Fig. 20-7). However, it is virtually impossible to remove all of the peripheral vitreous skirt.

It is important to remove posterior hyaloid from the retina posterior to the equator. It may be aspirated into an extrusion needle or vitreous cutter or engaged with a membrane pick. The posterior hyaloid is gently elevated and peeled from the retina until the retina behind the equator is bare (Fig. 20-8). Failure to remove the posterior hyaloid may result in later secondary contracture requiring reoperation.[6]

Pools of old blood visualized behind the detached posterior hyaloid are easily thrown into swirls if suction is applied with the vitreous cutter far from the collection of loose blood cells. It is better to bring the aspiration device, such as an extrusion needle or fluted needle, in close proximity to the superior surface of the blood pool before applying suction. A stream of blood cells can be seen being aspirated directly into the suction device without creation of surrounding haze (Fig. 20-9).

Vitreous Bands

Acutely, vitreous under traction may give an appearance of a white vitreous band.[7] Optically visible bands representing only vitreous incarceration are usually easily sectioned with the vitreous cutting device. In time, the bands become thickened, dense, and elastic following proliferation of cells within the vitreous scaffolding[7] and are the cause of retinal dialyses and detachments.[8] Formed and tense bands may be very difficult to cut using only the vitreous cutter because the bands may be too stiff to be

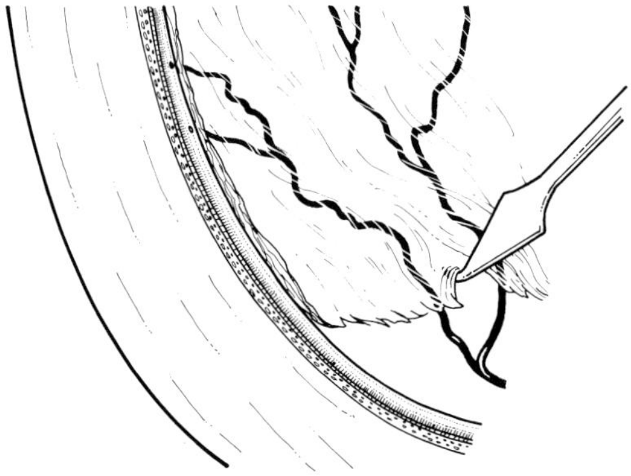

Fig. 20-8. Posterior hyaloid or posterior cortical vitreous may remain adherent to the retina. As it may form a scaffold for cell growth and membrane contraction, it should be peeled forward anterior to the equator. A loose edge is obtained. It may be freely floating, aspirated into a fluted needle, or, as shown, grasped with a barbed MVR blade. The posterior vitreous is stripped forward, using the blade, a forceps, or any device capable of holding the vitreous. The loosened posterior cortical vitreous is then removed with the vitrectomy probe.

A

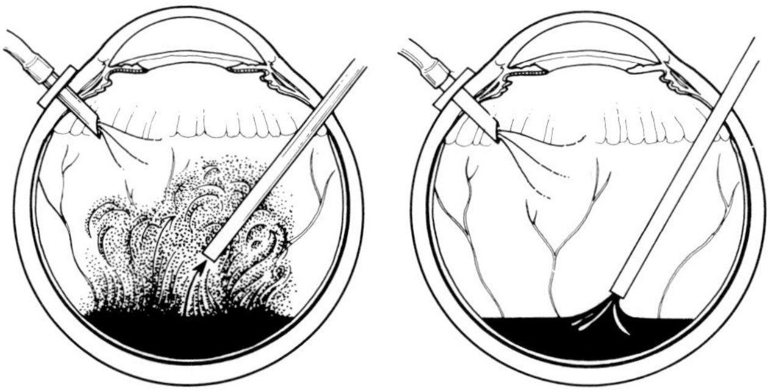

B

Fig. 20-9. **A,** When aspiration of a posterior blood pool is attempted with the extrusion needle or vitrectomy probe far from the blood pool, the blood intermixes with fluid and swirls within the vitreous cavity, obscuring the surgeon's view. **B,** With the extrusion needle or other suction source close to the surface of the blood pool, the blood is evacuated slowly in a column that can be seen ascending from the surface into the lumen of the needle.

aspirated into its small opening. In such instances an intraocular scissors is introduced into the vitreous cavity and the cellular band sectioned (Fig. 20-10). The loose ends of the band may then be aspirated into the vitreous cutter port, sectioned, and removed with relative ease. Bands that extend along the retinal surface may be elevated using membrane picks. If there is a zone of eye wall laceration with vitreous incarceration or retinal laceration, there may be quite dense tissue anchoring the band to the eye wall. In these circumstances the proliferative membrane is trimmed down as close as possible to the eye wall surface. The residual tissue persisting on the retinal surface will usually shrink and is rarely a problem if no traction persists.

Preretinal Membranes

Preretinal membranes may occur as localized puckers or may represent part of a more significant and extensive picture of PVR. Puckers in the macula affect visual acuity and should be peeled and removed. A membrane pick or barbed MVR blade may be brought posteriorly to the margin of such a pucker, and the edge of the peeling instrument insinuated beneath an elevated edge of the pucker or into a thickened, more central region of the pucker. Gently, the

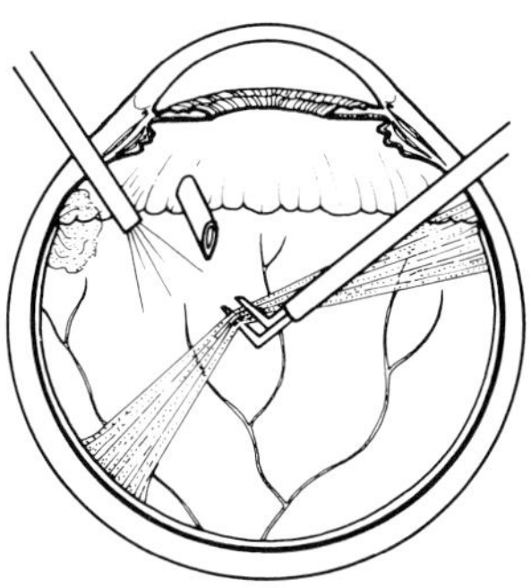

Fig. 20-10. Transvitreous bands that cannot be aspirated and cut with the vitrectomy probe may require sectioning with intraocular scissors. After the band is cut, the band ends retract and are easily engaged and removed with the vitrectomy probe.

preretinal membrane is elevated from the retinal surface. After mobilizing much of a membrane, it is possible to grasp it with an intraocular forceps and apply gentle traction parallel to the retinal surface to peel the membrane from the retina. If it can be peeled free without causing a break, that should be done. If the membrane is too adherent in a certain area, scissors are used to delaminate the membrane from the retinal surface, leaving only a small amount of residual material on the retinal surface.

Preretinal membrane and starfolds, as part of PVR, present serious problems to the traumatized eye. After removal of the overlying vitreous, a membrane pick or barbed MVR blade may be used to peel these extensive membranes from the retinal surface. Membrane peeling should begin near the epicenter of tissue where the epiretinal membrane is thicker, more easily seen, and better engaged with surgical instruments.[9] Most membranes can be stripped by slow peeling in an anterior direction with picks or forceps. After membrane removal, underlying and adjacent retina will become mobile. Membrane peeling is carried out as far anteriorly as possible. The anterior vitreous must also be removed, usually with scleral indentation, to deal with the problems of anterior PVR.[10] Membrane peeling is complete when all areas of visible traction have been released, the retina has become mobile, and the retina lies flat following air-fluid exchange.

Subretinal bands do not present a problem in surgery performed within several weeks of injury, because they take much longer to form. After much longer delays, injuries may exhibit retinal detachment with PVR and sheets and bands of subretinal fibrosis. After completion of all membrane removal from the preretinal surface, air-fluid exchange and retinal reattachment should proceed. Only if the retina fails to flatten is it necessary to remove the subretinal tissue. Through a previous retinal break or a retinotomy, scissors may be placed in the subretinal space and the band cut.[11] The band will usually retract and allow sufficient relaxation of traction. If needed, forceps can be placed through the retinotomy and used to extract the membrane. The membrane will often have attachments to the retina at places remote to the retinotomy. After the bands are removed, it is important to make sure that no retinal breaks develop at sites of previous attachment to the underside of the retina distal to the pulled end.

Subretinal Blood

Severe subretinal hemorrhage may occur with trauma. If there is much blood in the macular area or the blood is subjacent to a retinal break, it may be prudent to remove the blood. Blood has proven toxic to the retina and retinal pigment epithelium,[12] and a large bolus of blood could reduce visual outcome. In addition, the edges of a retinal break may not seal to the choroid below if a thick clot intervenes to prevent the approximation of these tissues. To remove the blood, all vitreous is removed overlying the large elevated clot. An extrusion needle is placed through the retinal break to the surface of the clot. If the break is far from the blood, a cannulated extrusion needle can be used by inserting the silicone hose into the subretinal space through the break and snaking the hose to the blood pool.[13] If there is no break nearby and the clot cannot be aspirated through the cannulated extrusion needle, endodiathermy is used to create a retinotomy in an area that will cause little damage and that will receive a good postoperative gas tamponade. Suction is applied to the surface of the blood. If the blood is loose, it will be evacuated easily. If the clot persists, it is removed by applying suction to the surface with the extrusion needle. The clot is then elevated and rocked back and forth to loosen the adhesions between clot and retina and clot and retinal pigment epithelium (RPE). When the clot is free and mobile, it may be slowly teased through the retinal opening. The process is slow

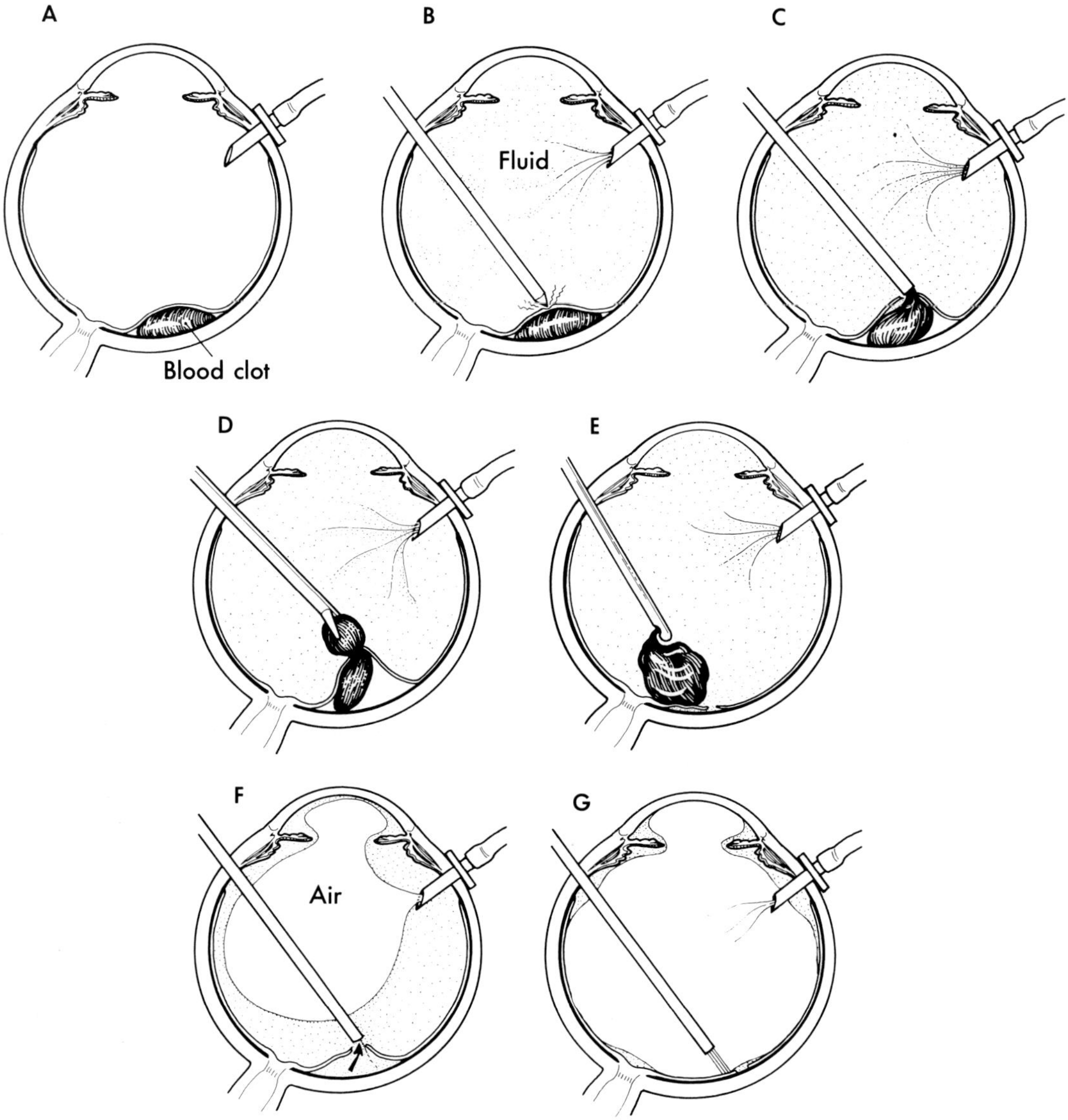

Fig. 20-11. Removal of subretinal clot. **A,** A blood clot in the subretinal space with no nearby retinal break results in elevation of the foveal retina. **B,** Endodiathermy used to create a retinotomy outside the vascular arcades in a zone superiorly. **C,** An extrusion needle aspirates the blood. All loose blood is evacuated. Clotted blood is engaged by suction and gently moved to loosen its adhesion to the retina and RPE. **D,** After the clot is freed from the overlying retina and the subjacent RPE, an intraocular forceps may be placed through the retinotomy to grasp the mobile clot and deliver it gently through the retinotomy. **E,** If the freed clot is too large to pass through the sclerotomy site, the clot may be reposited on the retinal surface and then removed with the vitrectomy probe. **F,** Air-fluid exchange is performed, flattening the retina. **G,** With the retina flat and air under constant infusion, endolaser photocoagulation is applied to the margins of the retinotomy and any retinal breaks.

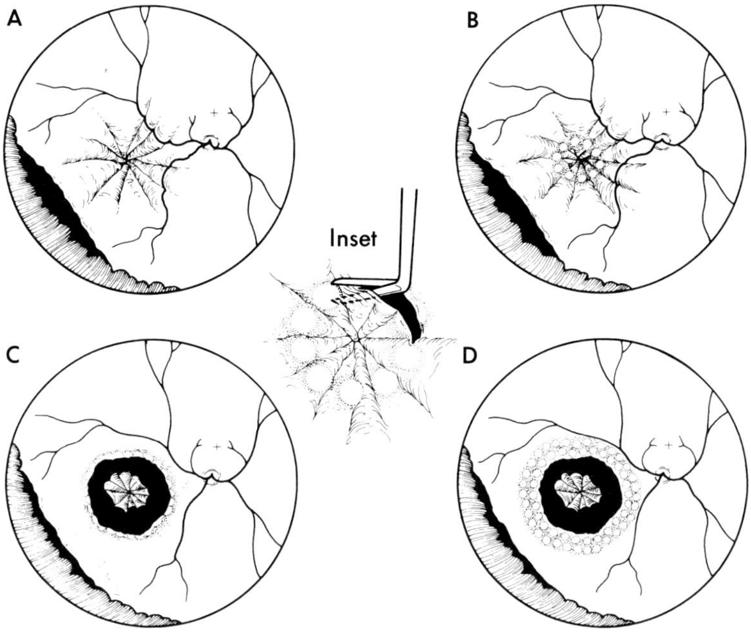

Fig. 20-12. **A,** Major retinal incarceration located posteriorly cannot be relieved entirely by a scleral buckle. It creates traction posteriorly and anteriorly and causes a retinal dialysis. **B,** Endodiathermy marks are placed around the incarceration. *(Inset)* A retinotomy is then created using vitreous scissors. Care is taken to assure that the vessels have been treated heavily with diathermy, or bleeding will ensue. **C,** Following retinotomy, traction is released. **D,** The retina is flattened with air-fluid exchange, and endolaser photocoagulation is applied to the retinal margins.

and tedious, and often the extrusion needle must be exchanged for an intraocular forceps, which may grasp the clot more firmly and enable it to be molded through the retinal opening. The vitreous cutter is used to remove the clot from the vitreous cavity. This maneuver removes the toxic blood products from direct contiguity with the RPE and photoreceptor cells and enables the application of endolaser photocoagulation or cryotherapy to the margins of the retinal break. Occasionally it is necesary to remove a massive clot subjacent to the macula by creating a retinotomy outside the temporal vascular arcade and carrying out the technique described above. The retinotomy is then treated with laser photocoagulation after flattening of the retina with air-fluid exchange (Fig. 20-11).

Retinal Incarceration

If a significant amount of retina is incarcerated in the wound at the time of primary repair, retinal traction with dialyses, tears, and detachment are likely to occur. Very anterior incarcerations may be treated by scleral buckling alone. With more posterior or large incarcerations, it is usually necessary to create a retinotomy to release the traction forces so generated.[14,15] Endodiathermy is applied around the region of incarceration to ensure that the vessels will not bleed when sectioned. Intraocular scissors are used to generate retinal cuts, freeing the retina within the eye from the traction pulling it to the wound. The retinal tissue then tends to slide away from the traction (Fig. 20-12). Air-fluid exchange is performed, and the margins of the retinotomies, well outlined from the diathermy, may be treated under air with several rows of endolaser photocoagulation.

Retinal Reattachment

After the vitreous has been removed and preretinal membranes peeled, the detached retina must be reattached, chorioretinal adhesion developed, internal tamponade instilled, and external buckle applied. The order in which these are accomplished depends upon the treatment modalities being used. Retinal reattachment entails reapproximation of the retina to the RPE,

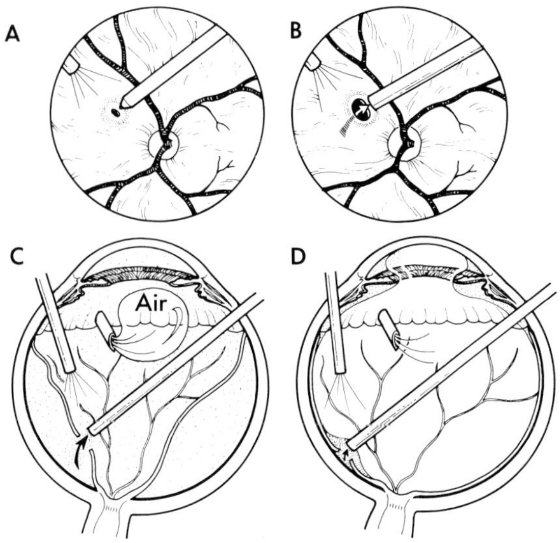

Fig. 20-13. Creation of a retinotomy and transvitreous drainage of subretinal fluid. **A,** A site is selected superior and nasal to the optic disc, and an endodiathermy probe is brought to the bare retinal surface. There can be no intervening residual vitreous. A diathermy spot is placed in the elevated retina and the energy increased until a hole develops in the retinal tissue. The whitening at the margins outlines the site. **B,** The extrusion needle is brought to the area immediately above the retinotomy, and subretinal fluid is exhausted through the retinotomy. **C,** Simultaneously, air is infused into the vitreous cavity. Air fills the vitreous cavity, displacing the vitreous and subretinal fluid into the extrusion needle. **D,** After the retina has flattened, more subretinal fluid slowly trickles to the retinotomy, requiring several more drainages before the subretinal space is dry.

often involving drainage of the subretinal fluid. Drainage can be carried out across either the sclera or the vitreous cavity. External or transscleral drainage is usually performed after placing an external scleral buckling element but before tying the scleral sutures that affix the buckle to the sclera. This may be difficult because of the posterior location of the subretinal fluid or choroidal congestion following injury. Internal or transvitreous drainage of subretinal fluid is easily performed after the vitreous has been fully removed. It may be performed through a preexisting retinal break, especially a posterior one. If there is a peripheral break, the cannulated extrusion needle may be used; a small silicone hose is placed through the break into the subretinal space and its silicone tip is advanced into the posterior pole. Alternatively, a site may be selected for internal drainage of subretinal fluid through an iatrogenic retinotomy, usually at a position superior and nasal to the optic disc. Unimanual, bipolar endodiathermy is then brought down to the retinal surface and an intense burn applied to the dome of retina over the subretinal fluid (Fig. 20-13). With high intensity this will accomplish the goal of developing a full-thickness opening through the retina and simultaneously create a white margin about the opening to permit easy visualization. The extrusion or fluted needle is placed through the retinotomy, around which there must be absolutely no residual vitreous. Any persisting clear vitreous will block the needle lumen, preventing aspiration of fluid. To avoid inadvertent damage to the subjacent choriocapillaris, a reflux fluted needle with a silicone brush tip may be considered. The subretinal fluid is aspirated through the fluted needle while air simultaneously enters the eye[16] through a continuous air infusion system. In an aphakic eye the routine contact lens used during the vitrectomy may still be used, but in a phakic or pseudophakic eye it is necessary to employ a high minus contact lens such as the Landers' lens. In the pseudophakic eye, placement of a viscoelastic substance in the anterior chamber may prevent air from escaping around the intraocular lens if there is an opening in the posterior capsule or a large iridectomy. Air in the anterior chamber totally obscures visualization of the posterior segment. After air-fluid exchange, posterior corneal striae may develop in some aphakic eyes that have had significant corneal trauma. These folds in Descemet's membrane cause a very distorted image of the posterior fundus. A thin layer of viscoelastic substance applied internally will smooth out the internal surface, and after several minutes excellent visualization is reestablished (Fig. 20-14).

After the retina has been initially flattened using the technique of internal drainage and air-fluid exchange, further residual subretinal fluid trickles back to the retinotomy, where it is again aspirated, a process repeated several times over several minutes. With the retina reattached, appropriate treatment is performed to generate a chorioretinal adhesion. If the media are clear and there is no residual opaque peripheral vit-

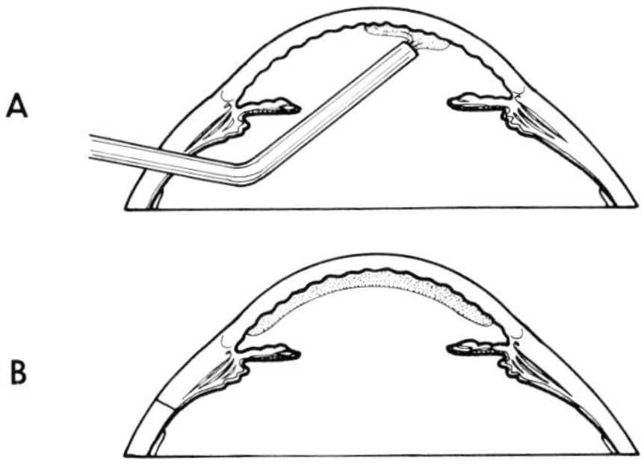

Fig. 20-14. **A,** An irregular corneal endothelial surface due to stromal edema intraoperatively presents a major problem for visualization after air-fluid exchange; multiple blurred images are seen. **B,** Placement of a viscoelastic substance on the corneal endothelial surface restores a smooth optical surface within a few minutes, enabling surgery to continue.

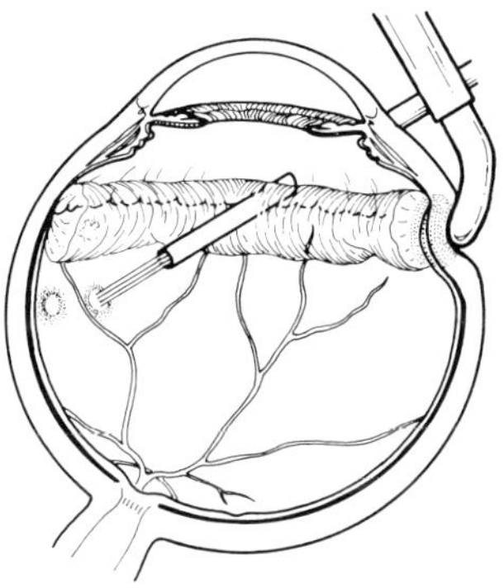

Fig. 20-15. Argon laser endophotocoagulation may be applied peripherally if the media are clear. However, peripheral vitreous skirt opacification can prevent photocoagulation in the periphery. Photocoagulation may still be placed in regions of clear media and is especially useful for posterior tears and retinotomies. Cryotherapy may be used even where the freeze cannot be seen well because of opacity. A cryo spot is first made in a region where the freeze can be monitored visually, and the time for freeze is recorded. Treatment of the same duration is then applied in regions with poor visualization.

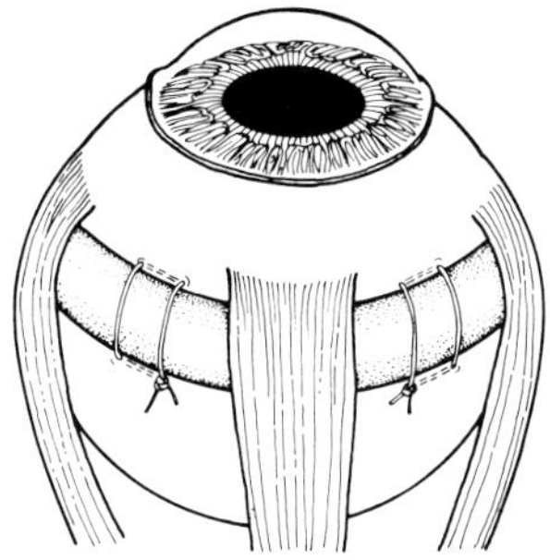

Fig. 20-16. A 360° encircling buckle is placed prophylactically to support the vitreous base. Silicone sponge or solid silicone may be equally effective.

reous skirt, endolaser photocoagulation may be performed in areas of peripheral and posterior retinal abnormalities (including the retinotomy). If the periphery cannot be seen well, so that laser would not penetrate and create the necessary and controlled chorioretinal reaction, external cryopexy is applied (Fig. 20-15). Cryotherapy should be applied first in areas where the retina is easily visible, and the time for a full-thickness white reaction calculated. Several rows of similarly timed freeze applications may then be applied in less visible peripheral areas to treat the most likely areas of trauma. (Note that the time for a full-thickness freeze is considerably shorter in an air-filled than in a fluid-filled eye.)

Scleral Buckling

Scleral buckling indents the eye wall, reduces the internal circumference of the globe, supports the vitreous base, and is useful in preventing and treating traumatic retinal detachment. In eyes where opaque vitreous persists peripherally at the end of the procedure, small retinal breaks or dialyses may be hidden behind the opacity and later progress to retinal detachment. Even in eyes with clear peripheral vitreous, it is possible for later vitreous base contraction to lead to late retinal tears and detachment. Prophylactic scleral buckling in eyes with severe injury to the posterior segment has been shown to reduce significantly this risk of late retinal detachment.[3,17]

An encircling buckle should be placed with an attempt made to support the peripheral vitreous base. Typically, a band, a band with a tire, or an encircling sponge element is used (Fig. 20-16). In a prophylactic buckle, a small buckle or band is appropriate; in situations with more severe abnormalities, such as a giant retinal tear with penetrating trauma, a larger and more extensive buckle is useful. Thus the buckle is tailored to the clinical situation. Although one ideally places retinal breaks on the buckle, this is not absolutely necessary if all traction has been relieved around the retinal breaks, retinal reattachment has been accomplished using air-fluid exchange, laser photocoagulation has been performed, and internal gas tamponade has been applied. If no breaks or detachment are present, the eye is permitted to remain fluid filled. However, internal tamponade is necessary if retinal breaks have occurred in an eye that has been treated with vitrectomy. Air usually lasts 4 to 7 days, sulfur hexafluoride (SF_6) gas at a nonexpanding concentration persists about 2 weeks, and perfluoropropane (C_3F_8) lasts 6 weeks. Air does not usually persist long enough to permit tamponade during development of a chorioretinal adhesion, especially if the breaks are more inferior. SF_6 is quite useful in a 20% mixture (with 80% sterile air), being well suited to the phakic eye requiring tamponade for retinal tears and detachment when the longer duration of C_3F_8 is likely to cause cataract formation. In eyes with early or advanced PVR, the longer duration of tamponade from C_3F_8 (15% in air) is most beneficial.

Silicone oil offers potential as a transparent intraocular tamponade in cases of severe retinal detachment. Although gases are resorbed postoperatively and thereby lose their ability to maintain tamponade, silicone oil persists and acts as a "permanent" tamponade. Because of its long-term toxicity, however, silicone oil cannot be left indefinitely within the vitreous cavity and is usually removed 3 months after placement. Since silicone oil floats on water, it supplies an excellent superior tamponade within the vitreous cavity but poor inferior support. Persistent inferior retinal detachments are often seen beneath the silicone oil bubble. Silicone oil will not flatten a retinal detachment with persistent traction, so it cannot be instilled until all membranes are peeled and all traction released. Its role in trauma management is at this time very limited. Long-acting gas tamponade may be equally effective and does not require a second surgery for removal. Silicone oil is typically not used until long-acting gases have been given an adequate trial.

Temporary Keratoprosthesis

Pars plana vitrectomy is dependent upon the ability to view the posterior segment through the cornea. If the cornea is too scarred, edematous, or disturbed to permit vitrectomy, the cornea may be trephined and replaced with a temporary keratoprosthesis (see Chapter 13). This clear plastic device is placed either as a tight-fitting plug within the corneal trephination site[18] or overlying the cornea and sutured to the anterior surface of the cornea.[19] Such devices allow a clear view to the vitreous cavity, permitting all of the aforementioned surgical techniques, including air-fluid exchange with pneumatic retinal reattachment (Fig. 20-17). After vitreous surgery is completed, the keratoprosthesis is removed and replaced with a corneal graft. If long-acting gas tamponade is needed, the gas is exchanged after the corneal graft is sutured in place but before removal of the infusion port. While placing the donor cornea in place, irrigation should be minimized; otherwise fluids will enter the posterior segment and may detach the retina.

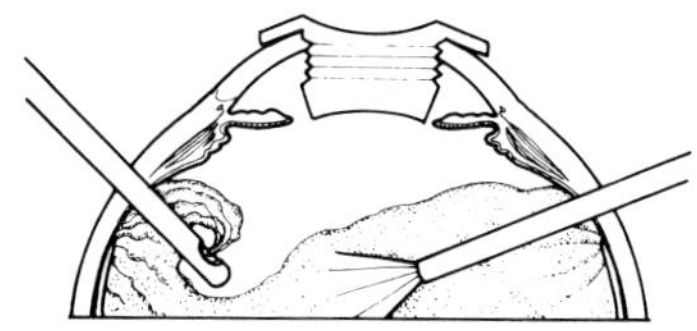

Fig. 20-17. The Landers-Foulks keratoprosthesis inserted through a centrally opaque cornea permits standard vitrectomy repair. At the completion of surgery, the keratoprosthesis is replaced with a donor cornea.

This approach enables surgery with air and pneumatic reattachment, thus extending the capabilities of open-sky vitrectomy alone.

References

1. Coleman DJ: Early vitrectomy in the management of the severely traumatized eye, Am J Ophthalmol 93:543-551, 1982.
2. Cleary PE and Ryan SJ: Method of production and natural history of experimental posterior penetrating eye injury in the rhesus monkey, Am J Ophthalmol 88:212-220, 1979.
3. Brinton GS et al: Surgical results in ocular trauma involving the posterior segment, Am J Ophthalmol 94:271-278, 1982.
4. Michels RG and Shacklett DE: Vitrectomy technique for removal of retained lens material, Arch Ophthalmol 95:1767-1773, 1977.
5. de Bustros S, Glaser BM, and Johnson MA: Thrombin infusion for control of intraocular bleeding during vitreous surgery, Arch Ophthalmol 103:837-839, 1985.
6. Michels RG: Surgical management of nonmagnetic intraocular foreign bodies, Arch Ophthalmol 93:1003-1006, 1975.

7. Topping TM, Abrams GW, and Machemer R: Experimental double-perforating injury of the posterior segment in rabbit eyes: the natural history of intraocular proliferation, Arch Ophthalmol 97:735-742, 1979.
8. Cox MS and Freeman HM: Retinal detachment due to ocular penetration. I. Clinical characteristics and surgical results, Arch Ophthalmol 96:1354-1361, 1978.
9. Charles S: Vitreous surgery. In Ryan SJ, Glaser BM, and Michels RG, editors: Retina, vol III, Surgical retina, St Louis, 1989, CV Mosby Co.
10. Aaberg TM: Management of anterior and posterior proliferative vitreoretinopathy: XLV Edward Jackson memorial lecture, Am J Ophthalmol 106:519-532, 1988.
11. Machemer R: Surgical approaches to subretinal strands, Am J Ophthalmol 90:81-85, 1980.
12. Glatt H and Machemer R: Experimental subretinal hemorrhage in rabbits, Am J Ophthalmol 94:762-773, 1982.
13. Flynn HW Jr et al: Cannulated subretinal fluid aspirator for vitreoretinal microsurgery, Am J Ophthalmol 103:106-108, 1987.
14. Machemer R, McCuen BW II, and de Juan E Jr: Relaxing retinotomies and retinectomies, Am J Ophthalmol 102:7-12, 1986.
15. Han DP et al: Management of traumatic retinal incarceration with vitrectomy, Am J Ophthalmol 106:640-645, 1988.
16. Charles S: Vitreous surgery, ed 2, Baltimore: Williams & Wilkins, 1987.
17. Hutton WL and Fuller DG: Factors influencing final visual results in severely injured eyes, Am J Ophthalmol 97:715-722, 1984.
18. Landers MB III et al: Temporary keratoprosthesis for use during pars plana vitrectomy, Am J Ophthalmol 91:615-619, 1981.
19. Eckardt G: A new temporary keratoprosthesis for vitrectomy, Retina 7:34-37, 1987.

CHAPTER 21

Posterior segment intraocular foreign bodies

SERGE DE BUSTROS

Diagnosis and localization
- History
- Ocular examination
- Radiologic studies
- Ultrasound
- Metal locators
- Transillumination

Pathophysiology of damage
- Siderosis
  - Clinical setting
  - Clinical findings
    - Iris
    - Lens
    - Retina
    - Glaucoma
  - Electroretinogram
  - Explanation of damage
  - Outcome
- Chalcosis
  - Clinical setting
  - Clinical findings
    - Cornea
    - Lens
    - Anterior chamber
    - Iris
    - Retina
  - Explanation of damage
  - Outcome

Management of IOFBs
- Conservative management
- External magnets
  - Case selection
  - Surgical technique
    - Direct approach
    - Indirect approach
- Vitrectomy
  - Case selection
  - Surgical technique
  - Special situations
    - Intraretinal or subretinal IOFB
    - Large IOFB
    - Lensectomy
  - Treatment of retinal breaks
- Results

References

To perforate the eye and reach the posterior segment, a foreign body must have sufficient momentum and energy. Therefore, most posterior segment foreign bodies are metal fragments.[1,2] Vegetable matter such as wood may reach the posterior segment but usually remains confined to the anterior segment.[3] Animal matter such as cilia can be carried along with denser matter to the posterior segment.[3]

Posterior segment intraocular foreign bodies (IOFBs) penetrating through sclera retain the highest momentum. When the foreign body penetrates through cornea, some momentum is lost in the anterior chamber, lens, or iris before reaching the posterior segment.[4] Foreign bodies reaching the posterior segment usually exceed 0.25 mm in length.[3] Metallic foreign bodies usually arise from hammering on a chisel[2] or using machine tools;[5] most metallic foreign bodies are magnetic.[6]

Ocular damage caused by an IOFB occurs by two mechanisms: (1) the penetrating injury with its secondary complications and (2) the presence of the IOFB itself causing damage from microbial endophthalmitis, toxicity, or other inflammatory reactions.

The ocular reaction to the IOFB depends on several factors including the size and shape of the IOFB,[3,7] its intraocular location, and its composition. The larger the IOFB and the more angular or irregular its shape, the greater are the initial damage and tissue reaction. Moreover, the tolerance of different ocular tissues to an IOFB varies. In general, the more vascular the tissue and the higher its metabolic activity, the lower is the tolerance.[3]

The composition of the IOFB is also important in determining the ocular reaction, inert foreign bodies being better tolerated. Chemically inert IOFBs include precious metals such as gold, silver, platinum, and tantalum, and other matter such as stone, glass, plastic, porcelain, rubber, and powder from firearms.[3] Reactive metallic foreign bodies can cause extensive ocular damage known as metallosis bulbi. The mechanism of damage is thought to be electrolytic dissociation of the metal or reaction with tissue fluids, usually by oxidation, causing diffusion and spread of the toxic products to the various ocular structures.[1,3]

This chapter discusses the diagnosis and management of posterior segment IOFBs. The emphasis is on sharp, penetrating ocular injuries with a missile type of IOFB. Blunt penetrating ocular injuries caused by air guns and BB pellets produce more extensive ocular damage and tissue disruption.[8-10] These eyes usually have a double penetrating injury and a worse prognosis.[8,9] The management of such injuries is discussed in Chapter 20. Anterior segment IOFBs are discussed in Chapter 15.

DIAGNOSIS AND LOCALIZATION

The clinical problem of a posterior segment IOFB is approached systematically, starting with the history and followed by an ocular examination and additional tests.

History

A careful history is important in any case of penetrating ocular injury. In addition to its medicolegal and Worker's Compensation purposes, the history can uncover the exact circumstances of the injury, which can shed light on the possible presence of an IOFB.

Ocular Examination

A complete, careful ocular examination is performed in all cases of penetrating ocular injury. Prompt fundus examination is vital since the view may be quickly lost because of the development of cataract or, more commonly, diffusion of vitreous hemorrhage. Direct visualization of the IOFB is by far the best diagnostic method. Bubbles of air introduced into the posterior segment at the time of the injury appear as transient, glistening spheres that gradually disappear as the air is reabsorbed.[3] Retroillumination can show iris defects, and gonioscopy can reveal the presence of a foreign body in the angle.

Radiologic Studies

Radiologic studies represent an important step in the initial evaluation of posterior segment IOFBs. Major advances have been made in recent years in the detection of IOFBs, primarily through the development and improvement of computerized tomography (CT) (see Chapter 2).

Ultrasound

Ultrasound can give a general idea of the presence and relative position of an IOFB and is useful in eyes with opaque media. Ultrasound can occasionally be used for determining the magnetic properties of an IOFB.[11] However, a CT scan is preferred if the IOFB is radio-opaque.

Metal Locators

Electronic locators are sometimes used to detect metallic IOFBs[12,13] but have been largely supplanted by computerized tomography.

Transillumination

Transillumination using an indirect ophthalmoscope and a condensing lens can be a helpful adjunct technique for intraoperative IOFB localization in eyes with opaque media. At surgery, the assistant transilluminates the general area of pathology while the surgeon observes the globe. The IOFB will often cause a shadow over the adjacent sclera.[14]

PATHOPHYSIOLOGY OF DAMAGE

Siderosis

Clinical Setting

Iron, either pure or as an alloy, is the most frequent constituent of a metallic IOFB. Iron contamination of intraocular tissues causes a characteristic clinical picture termed siderosis. The greater the corrosion (the chemical interaction of the metal with surrounding tissues[15]), the higher is the metal toxicity. Alloys in general decrease metal corrosion and therefore decrease metal reactivity.

Clinical Findings

Siderosis affects virtually all ocular structures, but the most characteristic changes involve the iris and lens, causing rusty brown deposits and discoloration and degenerative pigmentary changes of the retina.[3]

Iris. The iris in siderosis assumes a brownish color that is best appreciated by comparing the affected and fellow eyes. Heterochromia is most striking in lightly pigmented irides. The pupil in an affected eye is often middilated and becomes nonreactive to light. In addition, the pupil may lose its miotic response to accommodation. The probable mechanism for mydriasis is damage to the sphincter dilator muscle by iron. These changes are occasionally partially reversible upon removal of the IOFB.

Lens. Iron deposits in the epithelial cells of the anterior capsule form many brownish dots, or rust spots. Eventually the whole lens may take on a deep yellow coloration with large, rusty-brown patches.

Retina. Pigmentary degeneration develops starting in the periphery and gradually extends posteriorly causing concentric visual field loss. The retinal arteries may develop sclerotic changes. In time, fine pigmentary changes can occur in the macula.

Glaucoma. Chronic open-angle glaucoma is an occasional complication of siderosis. The exact mechanism is unclear and is probably related to iron infiltration of the trabecular meshwork.

Electroretinogram

The electroretinogram (ERG) is a very sensitive test for evaluating retinal function in metallosis bulbi in general and siderosis bulbi in particular.[15,16] Since siderosis bulbi affects the peripheral retina first, the ERG is more sensitive than visual acuity measurements in assessing retinal damage. The ERG abnormalities in siderosis are characterized by a decrease in b-wave amplitude. Untreated eyes will gradually develop complete flattening of the ERG curves. Up to 50% b-wave reduction appears to be reversible; more advanced changes with further reduction in b-wave amplitude are permanent.[15]

Explanation of Damage

Damage caused by an iron IOFB (exogenous siderosis) is similar to damage caused by intraocular hemorrhages or systemic causes of iron deposition such as repeated blood transfusions or hypersideremia (endogenous siderosis).[17] Iron interacts with intraocular tissues by electrolytic dissociation causing gradual disappearance of the foreign body and spread of ferric ions throughout the globe. Trivalent ions liberated from the iron foreign body penetrate cells, causing interruption of cellular activity and resultant cell damage.[3]

The mechanism of tissue damage in siderosis appears to be related mainly to cytoplasmic deposition and accumulation of iron leading to alteration of cell membrane permeability, breakdown of lysosomes and liberation of enzymes, and cell degeneration.[18] Iron deposits in cells in the form of ferritin and siderosomes.[18] In the retina, iron is preferentially found in Muller and retinal pigment epithelial cells. Iron may also interact with hyaluronic acid in the vitreous and with acid mucopolysaccharides in perivascular tissue.[17]

Outcome

The outcome in siderosis is related primarily to the amount of free iron gaining access to the intracellular space. Toxic changes are irreversible after a certain stage, and electroretinography is helpful in monitoring retinal damage and determining need for surgical intervention.

Chalcosis

Clinical Setting

Copper or one of its alloys (brass or bronze) is an occasional nonmagnetic constituent of posterior segment IOFBs. This occurs mostly with wire injuries or shell explosions (cartridges are usually made of brass).[3]

Pure copper usually causes a severe acute inflammatory reaction often associated with hypopyon. This violent reaction, if untreated, can lead to phthisis.[3] One important factor in the type of ocular reaction is the intraocular location of the IOFB and the degree of chemical dissociation and tissue reaction. If the IOFB is located in the lens, the eye may remain very quiet, in contrast to the reaction to retinal and choroidal penetration. Similarly, early tissue encapsulation of the IOFB will contain the chemical interaction and subsequent damage.

The ocular reaction to an IOFB of a copper alloy such as bronze or brass is less dramatic and is termed chalcosis.[3] The clinical findings are similar to those encountered with endogenous chalcosis due to hepatolenticular degeneration.

Clinical Findings

The complete clinical picture of chalcosis is "striking in its beauty"[3] and includes a greenish blue ring in the peripheral cornea (Kayser-Fleisher ring), a sunflower anterior subcapsular cataract, metallic refractile particles in the aqueous humor, a greenish coloration of the iris and sometimes the vitreous, and a brilliant and highly refractile deposit on the surface of the retina, usually in the macula.[3,19]

Cornea. Tiny granules deposit near Descemet's membrane in the deep stroma, close to the limbus, and usually involve the entire circumference of the cornea but may be segmental. Visualization is best with the slit-lamp using an indirect light.

Lens. The appearance of sunflower cataract is pathognomonic of chalcosis. It is usually greenish to brownish. The appearance of the sunflower with radial rays mimicking petals is thought to be related to the radial folds on the posterior surface of the iris; the movement of the iris influences the distribution of the particles deposited in the lens.[3] It usually does not impair vision significantly.

Anterior chamber. Brightly refractile microscopic particles can be seen in the anterior chamber.

Iris. The iris may become greenish in color and sluggish in response to mydriatics.

Retina. The appearance in the retina may be striking, with shining particles along the retinal vessels. Occasionally, copper may accumulate in the macula causing highly refractile particles.[19]

Explanation of Damage

Copper has a tendency to be deposited on limiting membranes—Descemet's membrane of the cornea, lens capsule, and internal limiting membrane of the retina.[1,3] This is in contrast to iron, which tends to be deposited inside cells. This fact may partially explain the more benign course of chalcosis as compared with siderosis.

The reason for the predilection of copper for deposition on limiting membranes is unclear. Normally, an electric current is present in the eye; the cornea is positive and the optic nerve negative. Copper interaction with intraocular fluids and tissues causes its ionization, and its subsequent distribution on limiting membranes may be induced by electrostatic factors.

Outcome

The clinical course in chalcosis is variable and depends on several factors, including the copper content of the IOFB, its intraocular location, and the adjacent tissue reaction.[3] A high copper content (over 85%) or pure copper will cause a severe inflammatory reaction and sterile endophthalmitis, dictating immediate removal of the IOFB to prevent phthisis.[20] At the other end of the spectrum is localization of the copper foreign body in the lens nucleus, causing little or no intraocular reaction. Many of the changes in chalcosis are reversible upon removal of the IOFB.[21] ERGs may be helpful in detecting retinal toxicity and deciding on the timing of surgery.

MANAGEMENT OF IOFBs

The management of an acute posterior segment IOFB is an ocular emergency. The goals of surgery for a posterior segment IOFB include optimal wound closure, restoration of the normal ocular architecture, and, in most instances, removal of the IOFB. Prevention or treatment of microbial endophthalmitis is another important component of therapy (see Chapter 23). The surgery is usually performed under general anesthesia.

Conservative Management

The decision to remove an IOFB and the timing of surgery depend on several considerations, including the nature and location of the IOFB, the type of injury, and other factors relating to a particular clinical situation.

In general, IOFBs of reactive substances such as iron or copper are considered toxic and should be removed promptly. Vegetable IOFBs present a high risk of microbial endophthalmitis and should also be removed as soon as possible. A less emergent approach can be used for nonreactive IOFBs; the extraction can be delayed for several days after initial wound closure to permit some healing of the tissues and better evaluation of the injured eye.

Encapsulation of the IOFB often protects against metal dissociation and toxicity, and copper or iron IOFBs have been left in place for years in some instances without evidence of metallosis bulbi.[20,22] A conservative approach is often taken with inert and with chronic IOFBs in the absence of signs and symptoms of toxicity or other problems.

The advent of vitreous surgery and refinements in surgical techniques have introduced new capabilities for removal of IOFBs, resulting in a more aggressive approach toward removal. Still, the therapeutic dilemma persists in certain situations—removal of the IOFB at the risk of causing additional tissue damage versus leaving the IOFB at the risk of additional ocular damage, principally metallosis bulbi. As always in surgery, the benefits are weighed against the risks in each individual situation.

External Magnets

Electromagnets have been used to remove magnetic IOFBs for more than 100 years,[23] and both the understanding and the design of magnets have improved over the years.[5,24-29] Technical progress has resulted in the development of small, hand-held, practical electromagnets.[26] Several tips are available for this magnet, ranging from short blunt tips with more magnetic force to long thin curved tips with less magnetic force to permit extraction of IOFBs in more posterior and less accessible areas. A slender tip has also been developed for intraocular use where the weaker magnetic force is offset by the close proximity of the tip to the IOFB.[30,31]

Parel has developed a 19-gauge permanent magnet for vitreoretinal surgery.[32,33] The magnetic force is at the tip of the instrument and is effective only at a distance of 1 mm or less. The instrument is gold plated, and the magnetic material is made of rare earth elements subjected to intense magnetization. Up to 15% of magnetic power is lost every year, but the instrument can be remagnetized in a few seconds.

Case Selection

Only electromagnets have sufficient magnetic power to remove IOFBs using an external approach. IOFBs suitable for an attempt at external magnetic extraction include small magnetic IOFBs and well-visualized IOFBs located in the vitreous or over the pars plana or retina.

Surgical Technique

Two approaches, direct and indirect, may be used, depending on the situation.

Direct approach. The direct approach refers to application of the electromagnet over the sclera directly adjacent to the IOFB. Ideally, localization is provided by direct visualization using the indirect ophthalmoscope. Alternatively, localization is provided by computerized tomography or transillumination. The IOFB should be located in the intraretinal or subretinal space or over the pars plana, and the location must be accessible for scleral incision. This technique is unsuitable if the IOFB is located too posteriorly (posterior pole).

The procedure is similar in some respects to that used for external drainage of subretinal fluid in surgery for rhegmatogenous retinal detachment. Conjunctival peritomy is performed, and the adjacent recti muscles are isolated and placed on traction sutures to provide adequate exposure and immobilization of the globe when needed. A full-thickness sclerotomy is then performed as close to the IOFB as possible, although some surgeons prefer to prepare a partial-thickness scleral flap first.[14,28] Diathermy is applied to the choroid, and a mattress suture is preplaced in the sclera. The eye is softened by paracentesis to minimize the risk of extrusion of intraocular contents during the IOFB extraction.[34]

The magnet is then applied directly over the choroid between the lips of the sclerotomy (Fig. 21-1). If the magnet is applied in the proper location and the IOFB is magnetic, a tenting of the choroid is often observed (Fig. 21-2). At this point, the electromagnet is pulsed by turning it on and off.[26] Pulsing minimizes heating, which interferes with the magnetic force; in addition, pulsing will gradually magnetize a feebly magnetic IOFB. Sometimes the IOFB will be extruded through the choroid under the force of magnetization. However, incision of the choroid may be necessary to remove the IOFB. In cases of good visualization with clear media, it is sometimes helpful to monitor movements of the IOFB with the indirect ophthalmoscope.

As soon as the IOFB is extracted, the sclerotomy site is closed and additional scleral sutures placed if necessary. Any extruding vitreous

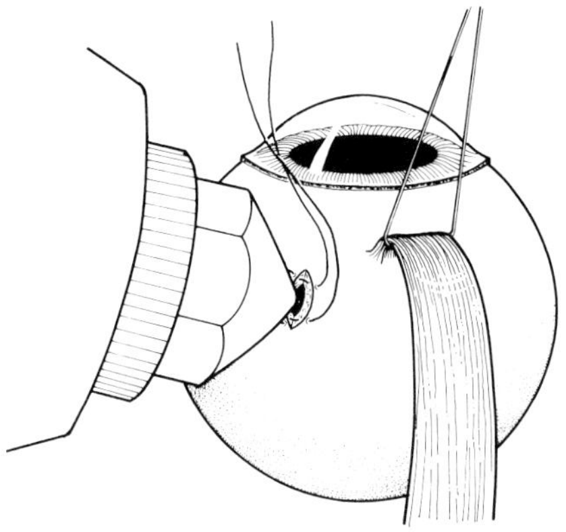

Fig. 21-1. Magnetic extraction of IOFB (direct approach). Hand-held external electromagnet is applied over the choroid adjacent to the IOFB. Note preplaced mattress suture at the sclerotomy site. The eye is stabilized by traction sutures around the rectus muscles.

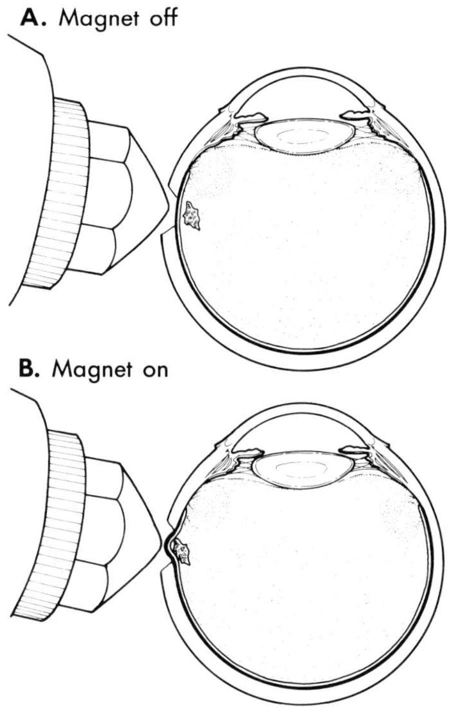

Fig. 21-2. **A,** The electromagnet is applied as close as possible to the IOFB to increase the traction force. **B,** When the magnet is turned on, a choroidal bulge will often be observed. Pulsing of the magnet is helpful, and choroidal incision may be required.

is cut with sharp scissors. Retinal tears are then treated appropriately, as described later.

Extrusion of intraocular contents with hemorrhage and retinal incarceration is the main complication with the direct approach, but softening of the eye will minimize this risk. Another occasional problem is inability to remove the IOFB. This usually occurs when there is a delay between the injury and surgery and the IOFB becomes encapsulated or anchored in the eye wall by fibrosis.[14] Alternative techniques are used in these situations as described later.

Indirect approach. The indirect approach refers to application of the electromagnet above the pars plana at a distance from the IOFB. This is done when the IOFB is located in the vitreous, over the retina without evidence of retinal penetration, or posteriorly (when a preretinal or intraretinal location is inaccessible to extraction through adjacent sclera).

An extraction site is selected over the pars plana of the same or opposite side of the eye (Fig. 21-3). An appropriately sized circumferential sclerotomy is performed over the pars plana, and diathermy is applied to the choroid as in the direct method. The electromagnet is then applied over the pars plana, aligned in the proper axis, and activated. The choroid may have to be incised to allow extrusion of the IOFB.

Simultaneous ophthalmoscopic monitoring of the magnetic extraction is particularly useful

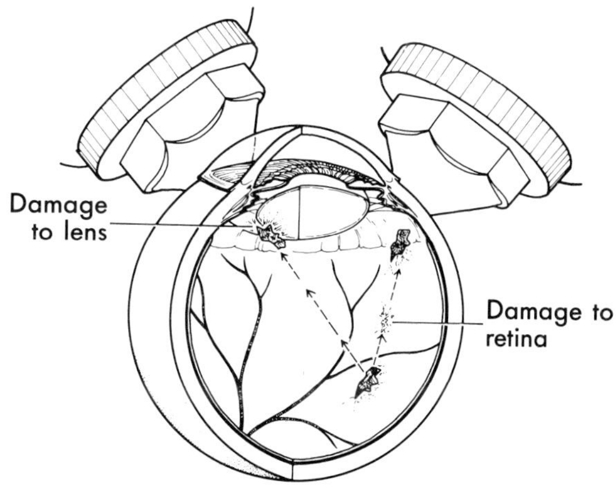

Fig. 21-3. Magnetic extraction (indirect approach). Electromagnet is applied over the pars plana. Placement of magnet on opposite side increases risk of lens damage, whereas placement on the same side increases risk of retinal damage. Magnet is used only for small IOFBs.

in this situation to monitor the progress of the extraction and take the appropriate corrective steps when necessary.

The main complication of this procedure is lens or retinal damage caused by the rapid displacement of the magnetized IOFB during extraction.[35] The larger the IOFB, the greater the risk, and therefore magnetic extraction is avoided in cases of large IOFBs. In general, the risk of lens damage is greater when the magnet is applied from the opposite side, whereas the risk of retinal damage is greater when the magnet is applied to the adjacent side (Fig. 21-3).

The electromagnet provides a quick, effective, and relatively noninvasive method for IOFB extraction. The disadvantage is that there is little control over the actual extraction process in terms of speed and precise direction of IOFB displacement, which may result in retinal or lens damage. There is also a need for nonmagnetic instruments, including a speculum, forceps, and a few other selected instruments. After the surgery, magnetized instruments are placed in a demagnetizer for a few seconds.

Vitrectomy

Case Selection

Vitreous surgery has introduced new capabilities into the management of posterior segment IOFBs.[36,37] Vitrectomy is used in cases of nonmagnetic, large, or subretinal IOFBs, eyes with opaque media, or more generally, whenever IOFBs cannot be removed by a magnet. Vitrectomy offers the advantage of clearing the media and operating under the microscope with good visualization and full control over the extraction process.

Surgical Technique

Pars plana vitrectomy proceeds in the usual manner from anterior to posterior. The goals of surgery are to clear the media opacities, remove the IOFB, and repair any posterior segment damage such as retinal tear or detachment. In addition, an attempt is made to remove as much vitreous as possible, including the posterior cortical vitreous since it may act as a scaffold for growth of fibrovascular tissue.[14]

Special attention is directed to removing the vitreous around the IOFB and relieving all adhesions. The goal is to free the IOFB from all vitreous attachments so that when it is grasped with forceps, no traction is transmitted to the retina with consequent iatrogenic retinal tear or break.

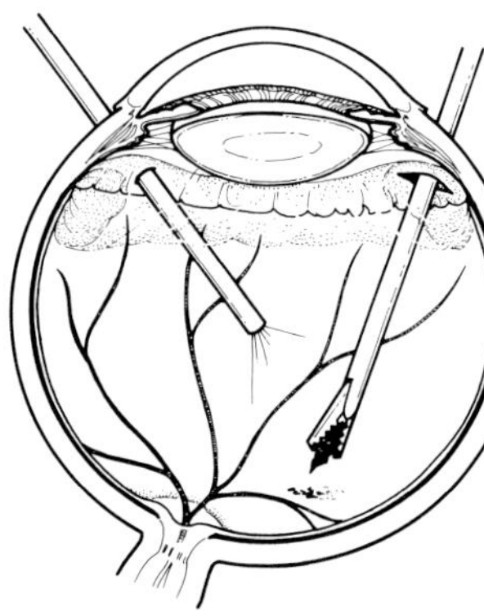

Fig. 21-4. Vitrectomy for IOFB extraction. When vitrectomy is completed and IOFB is mobilized, it is grasped with serrated forceps along its long axis and extracted under direct visualization. There should be full control over the extraction process. The sclerotomy may have to be enlarged to accommodate the IOFB.

To prevent the IOFB from falling farther posteriorly, its movements should be observed as the surrounding vitreous is removed. When judged to be sufficiently mobile, it is grasped with intraocular forceps, of which several styles are available (Fig. 21-4).[28,29] Alternatively, an intraocular rare earth magnet may be used to retrieve the foreign body.[32,33]

Special Situations

Intraretinal or subretinal IOFB. IOFBs usually gain access to the intraretinal or subretinal space through an anterior penetration site. In most instances, the IOFB is metallic. Fibrous tissue reaction starts at the time of the injury, and the IOFB becomes anchored in its location or encapsulated by fibrous tissue in a period of days. This fibrous tissue reaction progresses over a period of weeks, and the IOFB becomes tightly adherent to the ocular tissues. At this stage the IOFB is often invisible and can be detected only by radiologic investigation. Accurate localization is important in planning the surgical approach.

The use of an external magnet is not recommended for subretinal IOFBs because it is often ineffective and can cause further retinal damage from displacement of the IOFB induced by the magnet. Removal is accomplished by vitreous surgery. Vitrectomy is performed in the usual manner, and vitreous opacities are cleared. The IOFB is then exposed and grasped with intraocular forceps.

Exposure of the IOFB often requires incision

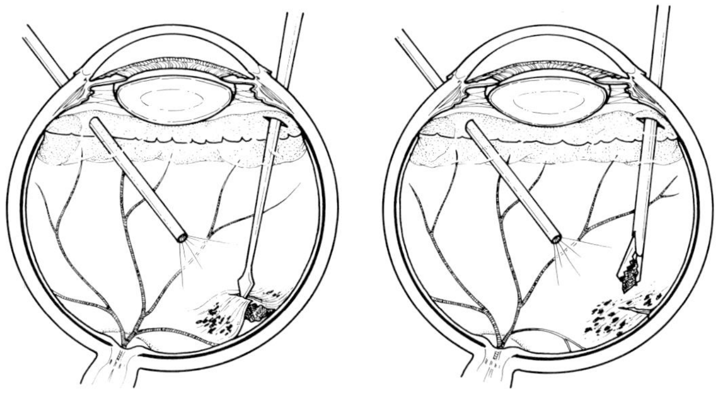

Fig. 21-5. Removal of subretinal IOFB. **A,** Fibrous capsule is incised with a sharp instrument to expose subretinal IOFB. **B,** IOFB is then grasped with serrated intraocular forceps. Retinal tears, when present, are treated appropriately.

of the capsule using a knife or other sharp instrument (Fig. 21-5).[38,39] A subretinal IOFB can sometimes be retrieved through the retinal tear produced during the initial injury. In other situations, however, a retinotomy adjacent to or overlying the IOFB is performed. This is done using a sharp instrument, with avoidance of retinal vessels to minimize bleeding. Retinal tear or detachment is treated as described later.

The main complications of this procedure are enlargement of a retinal tear and uncontrolled bleeding. Delicate manipulation of retinal tissue will minimize the risk of further retinal damage. Bleeding is usually controlled by temporary elevation of the infusion bottle or addition of thrombin to the infusion solution.[40]

Large IOFB. Once the IOFB is exposed, mobilized, and ready for extraction with intraocular forceps, a decision is made regarding the route of extraction. In general, one of the superior sclerotomies is used for extraction, and it may have to be enlarged circumferentially to accommodate the size of the IOFB. If a large pars plana incision is required, a double Flieringa ring is sutured to minimize collapse of the globe.[41]

Large IOFBs, however, are best removed through a limbal incision.[42] Usually in these situations the lens will have been damaged and removed at the beginning of surgery. Otherwise, a lensectomy is performed at this time.

A limbal incision of appropriate size is made similar to incisions performed for cataract surgery (Fig. 21-6). The IOFB is grasped with the forceps, brought into the anterior chamber, and extracted through the incision. The infusion may

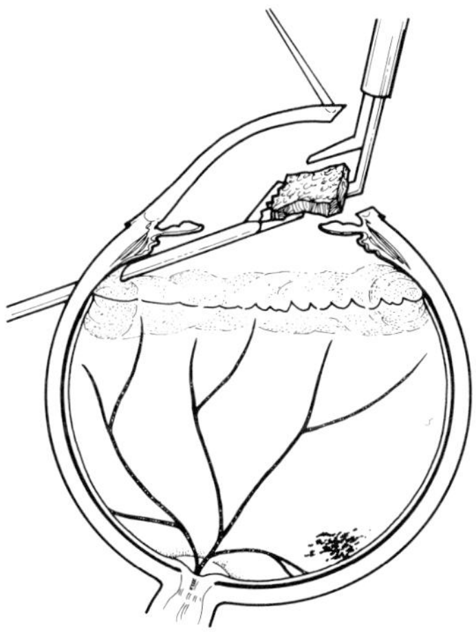

Fig. 21-6. Extraction of large IOFB using limbal approach. IOFB is grasped with intraocular serrated forceps, brought into the anterior chamber, and extracted through the limbus with the help of a second forceps, while the assistant retracts the cornea with a preplaced suture.

be turned off during the extraction to minimize iris prolapse. The limbal wound is then sutured.

On rare occasions, the IOFB can be extracted through the corneoscleral or scleral laceration, if the extraction is performed at the time of initial repair.[5] The IOFB extraction is performed toward the end of surgery, after the scleral laceration has been sutured and the vitrectomy has been performed. This extraction route is used when the scleral laceration has sharp edges and when it is in a convenient location, anterior to the ora serrata. The sutures are cut, the foreign body extracted, and the corneoscleral or scleral laceration resutured in a watertight fashion.

Lensectomy. The lens is often damaged by the penetrating ocular injury, and a cataract often develops, precluding visualization of the posterior segment. In other situations, the IOFB may be located over the pars plana, and the presence of the lens may interfere with its surgical removal. The indication for lensectomy, therefore, is the inability to complete the surgical objective.

The lensectomy is usually performed at the beginning of the vitrectomy procedure using the vitrectomy probe or ultrasonic fragmentation. Many trauma patients are young, and the lens is often soft and easily removed with these methods. A careful attempt is made at removing all lens material to avoid fibrous tissue proliferation over a residual lens capsule.

Treatment of Retinal Breaks

Retinal breaks and rhegmatogenous retinal detachments are sometimes associated with posterior segment IOFBs. The breaks can be caused by direct retinal injury from the IOFB or by secondary complications such as intraocular fibrosis and proliferation. In other situations, retinal breaks are associated with extraction of the IOFB.

Regardless of the origin and location of the breaks, treatment involves creation of a chorioretinal adhesion around the retinal break and relief of traction caused by vitreous or epiretinal membranes.

In general, anterior retinal breaks are treated by external cryotherapy and supported by an external scleral buckle. In some cases, despite vitrectomy sufficient vitreous is left anteriorly in the vitreous base area to provide a scaffold for growth and contraction of fibrovascular tissue, sometimes causing a recurrent retinal detachment and proliferative vitreoretinopathy. Therefore, in case of sufficient posterior segment damage, and especially in the presence of vitreous hemorrhage, a broad encircling scleral buckle should be placed to support the vitreous base.[36]

Posterior retinal tears are usually treated with endolaser photocoagulation or endocryotherapy, although on occasion a chorioretinal adhesion will form spontaneously because of the inflammation and scarring caused by the original penetrating injury. A posterior radial scleral buckle is used to support the posterior retinal break in cases of persistent traction adjacent to the break. The traction can be caused by epiretinal proliferation and is often present when posterior cortical vitreous was not removed at the time of the vitrectomy. In cases of posterior retinal tears where the IOFB was removed by an external magnet without vitrectomy, the retinal tears may be treated by external laser photocoagulation.

All vitrectomized eyes with retinal tears are treated with intraocular tamponade and postoperative prone positioning. Sterile air is usually adequate, although longer-acting gases can be used in cases of inferior retinal tears or whenever longer-acting tamponade is necessary.

Results

It is difficult to assess treatment methods and accurately compare surgical results and visual acuity outcomes in penetrating ocular injuries in general and IOFBs in particular because of the number of variables involved. These include the type and extent of injury, the size, shape, type, and location of IOFBs, the extent of initial irreversible ocular damage and secondary ocular complications, the time interval between injury and surgery, the treatment methods, and the methodology of the various studies and reports of results.

With these limitations in mind, the following approximations and generalizations can be made. The visual results after magnetic extraction of IOFBs are fairly good, with approximately two thirds of eyes recovering a final visual acuity of 20/50 or better and three fourths a final acuity of 20/200 or better.[2,5,28,34,43-47] These results have remained fairly constant over the past 30 years, primarily because the surgical methods have undergone little change. Magnetic extraction is a fairly safe, noninvasive surgical procedure.

This favorable outcome is due primarily to the selection criteria for magnetic extraction of IOFBs, which include small, magnetic IOFBs, eyes with clear media, and an IOFB location usually in the vitreous or overlying the retina or pars plana (Fig. 21-7). These eyes usually have little associated ocular damage.

In contrast, IOFBs selected for vitrectomy constitute a more heterogeneous group and are often associated with more ocular damage and secondary complications (Fig. 21-8). These include eyes in which magnetic extraction has failed, eyes with large IOFBs, nonmagnetic IOFBs, or IOFBs in the subretinal space, eyes

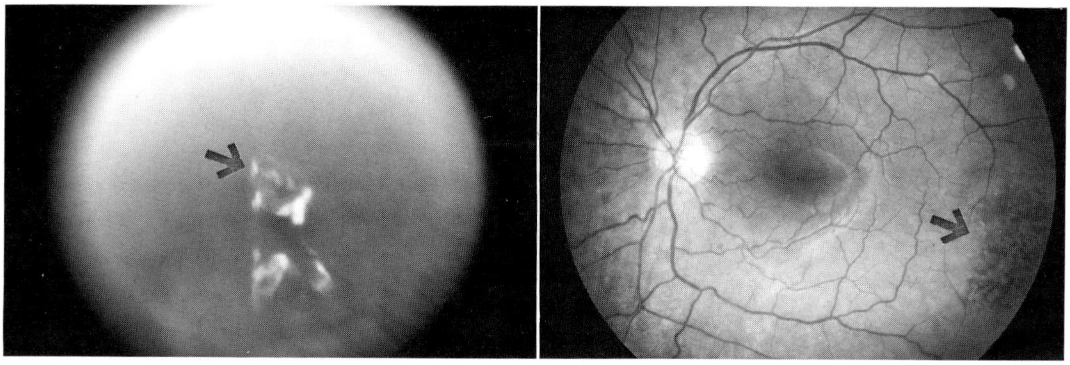

A B

Fig. 21-7. A 26-year-old carpenter injured his left eye while hammering metal on metal. **A,** Preoperative fundus appearance showing metallic IOFB *(arrow)* in the posterior vitreous overlying the retina. Some vitreous strands are present inferior to the IOFB. Visual acuity is 20/25. **B,** Postoperative fundus appearance 1 month after magnetic extraction of IOFB. Visual acuity is 20/25. Note the pigmentary changes *(arrow)* appearing in an area of previous retinal edema adjacent to the site of impact.

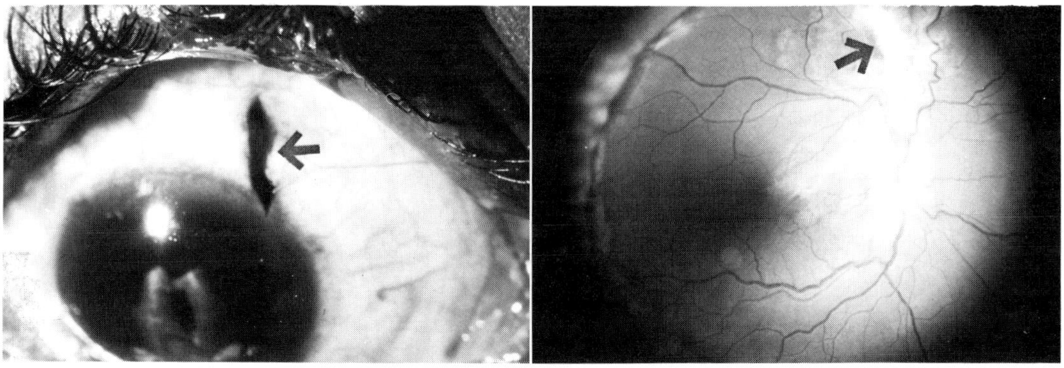

A B

Fig. 21-8. A 27-year-old construction worker injured his right eye while activating a jackhammer. **A,** Preoperative external appearance *(arrow)* shows the corneoscleral laceration with a prolapse of uveal tissue. Note the presence of total hyphema. Visual acuity is light perception. CT scan showed posterior segment IOFB, and ultrasound showed a vitreous hemorrhage. **B,** Postoperative appearance after pars plana lensectomy, vitrectomy, and scleral buckling showing chorioretinal scarring at the site of impact superior to the optic nerve *(arrow)*. The retina is reattached, but there is residual dragging on the macula. Visual acuity is 20/80. Note the edge of an encircling buckle effect temporally.

with opaque media including vitreous hemorrhage and cataract formation, eyes with retinal detachment, and eyes with bacterial endophthalmitis.

Keeping in mind the limitations, the results of modern vitreous surgery are such that approximately one third of these injured eyes recover visual acuity of 20/40 or better, two thirds recover to 20/200 or better, and three fourths have ambulatory vision (5/200 or better).[36,39,44,46,48-55] Furthermore, the advent of vitreous surgery has decreased the rate of enucleations. All in all, these results compare favorably with those of penetrating ocular injuries without IOFBs (see Chapter 22).

References

1. Barry DR: Effects of retained intraocular foreign bodies, Int Ophthalmol Clin 8:153-170, 1968.
2. Percival SPB: A decade of intraocular foreign bodies, Br J Ophthalmol 56:454-461, 1972.
3. Duke-Elder SS and MacFaul PA: In Duke-Elder SS, editor: System of ophthalmology, vol XIV, part 1, Mechanical injuries, St Louis, 1972, The CV Mosby Co.
4. Brown IAR: Nature of injury, Int Ophthalmol Clin 8:147-152, 1968.

5. Coleman DJ et al: Management of intraocular foreign bodies, Ophthalmology 94:1647-1653, 1987.
6. Smith VH: The incidence of intraocular foreign bodies, Int Ophthalmol Clin 8:137-146, 1968.
7. Potts AM and Distler JA: Shape factor in the penetration of intraocular foreign bodies, Am J Ophthalmol 100:183-187, 1986.
8. DeJuan E, Sternberg P Jr, and Michels RG: Penetrating ocular injuries: types of injuries and visual results, Ophthalmology 90:1318-1322, 1983.
9. Sternberg P Jr et al: Ocular BB injuries, Ophthalmology 91:1269-1277, 1984.
10. Sternberg P Jr, De Juan E Jr, and Michels RG: Penetrating ocular injuries in young patients: initial injuries and visual results, Retina, 4:5-8, 1984.
11. Penner R and Pasmore JW: Magnetic vs nonmagnetic intraocular foreign bodies: an ultrasonic determination, Arch Ophthalmol 76:676-677, 1966.
12. Roper-Hall MJ: An intra-ocular foreign body locator, Trans Ophthalmol Soc UK 77:239-250, 1957.
13. Shaylor HR and Whitaker PD: Electronic localization, Int Ophthalmol Clin 8:193-198, 1968.
14. Michels RG: Vitreous surgery, St Louis, 1981, The CV Mosby Co.
15. Knave B: Electroretinography in eyes with retained intraocular metallic foreign bodies: a clinical study, Acta Ophthalmol (suppl) 100:1-63, 1969.
16. Knave B: The ERG and ophthalmological changes in experimental metallosis in the rabbit. II. Effects of steel, copper and aluminum particles, Acta Ophthalmol 48:159-173, 1970.
17. Cibis PA, Yamashita T, and Rodriguez F: Clinical aspects of ocular siderosis and hemosiderosis, Arch Ophthalmol 62:46-53, 1959.
18. Tawara A: Transformation and cytotoxicity of iron in siderosis bulbi, Invest Ophthalmol Vis Sci 27:226-236, 1986.
19. Delaney WV Jr: Presumed ocular chalcosis: a reversible maculopathy, Ann Ophthalmol 14:378-380, 1975.
20. Rao NA, Tso MOM, and Rosenthal R: Chalcosis in the human eye: a clinicopathologic study, Arch Ophthalmol 94:1379-1384, 1976.
21. Felder KS and Gottlieb F: Reversible chalcosis, Ann Ophthalmol 16:638-641, 1984.
22. Rosenthal AR et al: Chalcosis: a study of natural history, Ophthalmology 86:1956-1969, 1979.
23. Hirschberg J: Der Electromagnet in der Augenheilkunde, Leipzig, 1885, Veit, 88-91.
24. McCaslin MF: An improved hand electromagnet for eye surgery, Trans Am Ophthalmol Soc 56:571-605, 1958.
25. Robinson A: Powerful new magnet material found, Science 223:920-922, 1984.
26. Bronson NR II: Practical characteristics of ophthalmic magnets, Arch Ophthalmol 79:22-27,1968.
27. Lancaster WB: Stronger eye magnets, Trans Am Ophthalmol Soc 14:168-183, 1915.
28. Neubauer H: Intraocular foreign bodies, Trans Ophthalmol Soc UK 95:496-501, 1975.
29. Parel JM and Machemer R: Diamond-coated all-purpose foreign-body forceps, Am J Ophthalmol 91:267-268, 1981.
30. Coleman DJ: A magnet tip for controlled removal of magnetic foreign bodies, Am J Ophthalmol 85:256-258, 1978.
31. May DR, Noll F, and Munoz R: A 20-gauge intraocular electromagnetic tip for simplified intraocular foreign-body extraction, Arch Ophthalmol 107:281-282, 1989.
32. Crock GW, Janakiraman P, and Reddy P: Intraocular magnet of Parel, Br J Ophthalmol 70:879-885, 1986.
33. Parel JM: Progress in foreign body extractors. In Blankenship GW et al, editors: Basic and advanced vitreous surgery, Padua, 1986, Liviana Press, 321-328.
34. Ross WH and Tasman WS: The management of magnetic intraocular foreign bodies, Can J Ophthalmol 10:168-173, 1975.
35. Amalong RJ: Retinal detachment after manipulation of magnetic foreign body, Am J Ophthalmol 70:10-13, 1970.
36. Benson WE and Machemer R: Severe perforating injuries treated with pars plans vitrectomy, Am J Ophthalmol 81:728-732, 1976.
37. Michels RG: Vitrectomy methods in penetrating ocular trauma, Ophthalmology 87:629-645, 1980.
38. Charles S: Vitreous microsurgery, ed 2, Baltimore, 1987, Williams & Wilkins, 182-194.
39. Slusher MM, Sarin LK, and Federman JL: Management of intraretinal foreign bodies, Ophthalmology 89:369-373, 1982.
40. de Bustros S and Michels RG: Intraoperative and postoperative control of hemorrhage. In Ryan SJ, editor: Retina, St Louis, 1989, The CV Mosby Co, 541-549.
41. Michels RG: Surgical management of nonmagnetic intraocular foreign bodies, Arch Ophthalmol 93:1003-1006, 1975.
42. Hanscom TA and Landers MB III: Limbal extraction of posterior segment foreign bodies, Am J Ophthalmol 88:777-778, 1979.
43. Heimann K, Paulmann H, and Tavakolian U: The intraocular foreign body, Int Ophthalmol 6:235-242, 1983.
44. Shock JP and Adams D: Long-term visual acuity results after penetrating and perforating ocular injuries, Am J Ophthalmol 100:714-718, 1985.
45. Roper-Hall MJ: Review of 555 cases of intraocular foreign body with special reference to prognosis, Br J Ophthalmol 38:65-99, 1954.

46. Williams DF et al: Results and prognostic factors in penetrating ocular injuries with retained intraocular foreign bodies, Ophthalmology 95:911-916, 1988.
47. Bronson NR II: Management of intraocular foreign bodies, Am J Ophthalmol 66:279-284, 1968.
48. Conway BP and Michels RG: Vitrectomy techniques in the management of selected penetrating ocular injuries, Trans Am Acad Ophthalmol Otolaryngol 85:560-583, 1978.
49. Peyman GA et al: Vitrectomy in the management of intraocular foreign bodies and their complications, Br J Ophthalmol 64:476-482, 1980.
50. Brinton GS et al: Surgical results in ocular trauma involving the posterior segment, Am J Ophthalmol 93:271-278, 1982.
51. Han DP et al: Vitrectomy for traumatic retinal incarceration, Arch Ophthalmol 106:640-645, 1988.
52. Hutton WL, Snyder WB, and Vaiser A: Vitrectomy in the treatment of ocular perforating injuries, Am J Ophthalmol 6:733-739, 1976.
53. Malbran ES, Dodds R, and Caride F: Vitreous surgery in the treatment of intraocular foreign bodies, Mod Probl Ophthalmol 20:237-243, 1979.
54. Ounnas N et al: Indications de la vitrectomie pour l'extraction des corps etrangers intra-oculaires, J Fr Ophtalmol 6:815-823, 1983.
55. Peyman GA and Schulman JA: Intravitreal surgery: principles and practice, Norwalk, CT, 1986, Appleton-Century-Crofts, 239-278.

CHAPTER 22

Prognosis and outcomes for penetrating ocular trauma

PAUL STERNBERG, JR.

Historical perspective
Prognostic features
Initial visual acuity
Afferent pupillary defect
Size of laceration
Location of laceration
Vitreous hemorrhage
Presence of intraocular foreign body
References

HISTORICAL PERSPECTIVE

Ocular trauma remains a leading cause of visual loss in the world, although many authors have pointed to an improved prognosis over the last two decades. For example, in Snell's review of penetrating injuries repaired between 1935 and 1942,[1] only 30% of patients regained visual acuity of 20/40 or better. By the time of Roper-Hall's 1959 report,[2] the percentage had improved to 45%. The decade of the 1960s witnessed the introduction of the operating microscope and microsurgery, and in her 1976 review of 228 patients managed between 1971 and 1974, Eagling[3] reported that 62% of those with penetrating injuries attained 20/40 visual acuity. Vitreoretinal surgery was introduced into the management of ocular injuries in the 1970s, and de Juan, Sternberg, and Michels[4] noted in 1983 that 71% of patients with penetrating injuries had final visual acuity of 20/50 or better.

Despite these advances in management, certain aspects of the injured eye have long been known to carry a poor prognosis. Snell[1] listed severe intraocular hemorrhage, endophthalmitis, severe prolapse of ocular contents, double perforating injuries, and blunt injuries as factors associated with a decreased likelihood of good visual function. Noting that most of these factors implied damage to the posterior segment, Eagling[5] subsequently separated penetrating injuries into those affecting primarily the anterior or posterior segment. In an era before vitreoretinal surgery, she found that 85% of the eyes with anterior segment injuries and 40% with posterior segment injuries regained 20/40 vision.[3,5] Moreover, when Cherry[6] reviewed the subgroup of blunt ruptured globes managed at Johns Hopkins Hospital in the 1960s, he found that only 6% recovered visual acuity of 5/200. Comparison of Eagling's[3] findings in 1976 with those of de Juan, Sternberg, and Michels[4] does not reveal a significant improvement in the prognosis for anterior segment injuries, but 31% of patients with blunt ruptured globes now regain 5/200 vision.[4]

Patients requiring vitrectomy for management of penetrating ocular injuries involving the posterior segment have a greater than 50% chance of obtaining vision of 5/200 or better. Of

74 eyes with trauma involving the posterior segment and treated with vitrectomy, Brinton et al[7] found that 52% achieved functional success and an additional 15% attained anatomic success but were functional failures. Of 191 patients treated by pars plana vitrectomy for severe injury with posterior segment involvement, Hutton and Fuller[8] reported 114 (60%) with final visual acuity of 5/200 or better. Most recently, Meredith and Gordon[9] reviewed 50 consecutive eyes with penetrating injuries and vitreous hemorrhage; 31 (62%) were functional successes, including 17 with retinal detachment.

PROGNOSTIC FEATURES

In any review of trauma patients, it is clear that certain types of injuries carry a better prognosis than others. Many of the anatomic and sensory features of the injured eye that carry either a good or bad prognosis have remained unchanged through the years, despite major advances in surgical techniques. However, a greater percentage of eyes obtain 20/40 visual acuity and fewer are enucleated.

Snell[1] identified endophthalmitis as a poor prognostic factor, finding 26 cases (15%) in a series of 172 eyes. Of these, 21 were enucleated and 1 lost light perception; only 4 (19%) were functional successes. Today traumatic endophthalmitis is seen less frequently (2% to 7% of penetrating injuries)[10] but still carries a grave prognosis, owing largely to the difficulties in making an early diagnosis and in effectively treating the injury, despite the use of vitrectomy. Affeldt et al[11] reported 27 cases of traumatic endophthalmitis seen in Miami from 1969 to 1985; only 7 eyes (26%) regained vision of 5/200 or better.

Initial Visual Acuity

Visual acuity at the time of presentation appears to be the single most important factor in predicting final visual acuity in patients with penetrating eye injuries, perhaps because acuity is a cumulative measurement of the sensory status of the eye. In a review of 453 patients with penetrating injuries seen at the Wilmer Institute over a 12-year period, de Juan, Sternberg, and Michels[4] found that 97% of patients with initial acuity of 5/200 or better regained final acuity of 5/200 or better. When initial acuity was worse than 5/200, there was only a 36% chance of a final acuity of 5/200 or better. When these data were subjected to multivariate statistical analysis comparing initial acuity to other prognostic factors, initial visual acuity was found to be the most important factor.[12] Eyes with initial acuity of 5/200 or better were 28 times more likely to have final acuity at that level than eyes with initial acuity worse than 5/200. In addition, these eyes were 8 times more likely to have final acuity of 20/50 or better.

These findings were confirmed in Barr's[13] review of corneoscleral lacerations. He found initial visual acuity to be one of the best predictors of final vision; of 43 eyes with initial vision of finger-counting or better, only 2 (5%) had final vision worse than finger-counting. On the other hand, of 61 eyes with initial vision worse than finger-counting, 33 (54%) had final vision at that level. Although Hutton and Fuller[8] found visual evoked potential to be the best predictor of postoperative vision, they also found preoperative acuity to be a statistically significant prognostic factor.

The importance of preoperative vision was noted in several earlier reports. For example, Moncreiff and Scheribel[14] reviewed 185 penetrating injuries in their 1945 paper. Of 35 eyes with initial acuity of finger-counting or better, only 1 (3%) was lost; of 155 with worse initial vision, 96 (62%) were lost.

Afferent Pupillary Defect

Although the concept of an afferent pupillary defect has been ascribed to Marcus Gunn[15] in 1904, Levatin, Prasloski, and Collen[16] introduced the swinging flashlight test into clinical examination in 1973. The importance of the reverse afferent pupillary defect has been emphasized, so that one can check for an afferent pupil even if one pupil is mechanically or pharmacologically nonreactive or cannot be visualized because of corneal damage or hyphema.[17]

Because the presence of an afferent pupillary defect implies optic nerve or retinal dysfunction, this test theoretically should be useful in predicting visual outcome in a traumatized eye. Whether dense media opacities can produce an afferent pupillary defect remains controversial. Miller[17] has never seen a patient with unilateral vitreous hemorrhage and an afferent pupillary defect in the absence of retinal or optic nerve damage, but he refers to Thompson and Loewenfeld as supporters of the concept of dense vitreous hemorrhage causing an afferent pupil.

In de Juan, Sternberg, and Michel's study,[4] the presence of an afferent pupillary defect was associated with a poor visual outcome: only 2 of 13 eyes (14%) with an afferent pupil regained vision of 5/200 or better, as opposed to 59 of 84 eyes (74%) specifically noted not to have an afferent pupil. Unfortunately, only 97 of the 453 records noted the findings of the pupillary examination.

Hutton and Fuller[8] did not evaluate the importance of the pupillary examination, but they did emphasize the value of the bright-flash visual evoked potential. The response in this electrophysiological test is reduced in the presence of damage to the macula or optic nerve. The test does not require contact with the eye being tested and can be done in the presence of opaque ocular media. The pupillary examination has similar advantages and can also determine damage to the macula or optic nerve; it is the "poor-man's" visual evoked potential.

Size of Laceration

Several investigators have evaluated the importance of the size of the ocular laceration in determining the visual outcome. Snell[1] felt that the length of the laceration was important but was unable to prove it, because eyes with lacerations of 9 mm or greater were felt not to be salvageable and were enucleated primarily. Johnston[18] reviewed 295 penetrating injuries and found that the prognosis worsened as the laceration length increased. In his series, only 3 of 61 eyes (5%) with wounds greater than a corneal diameter in length (approximately 10 mm) recovered vision of 20/40 or better. When the wound was less than one corneal diameter in length, 199 or 223 eyes (51%) gained good final vision.

More recent studies have confirmed these findings. Hutton and Fuller[8] showed that lacerations greater than 12 mm in length carried a grave prognosis; de Juan, Sternberg, and Michels[4] used 10 mm as the indicator of a "large" laceration and also found the longer lacerations to be a predictor of poor visual ouctome. However, in both series, factors describing the sensory status of the eye were more important than those related to anatomic factors such as laceration length.

Location of Laceration

Location of the laceration is also an important prognostic feature, with posterior injuries generally carrying a graver prognosis. Presumably, this is because lacerations involving the sclera are more likely to violate the integrity of the vitreous, damage the retina and ciliary body, and cause intraocular hemorrhage. Since the ultimate cause of permanent visual loss in eyes with penetrating injury is frequently retinal detachment or loss of ciliary body function, eyes with posterior segment injuries should not do as well as those with injuries limited to the anterior segment.

De Juan, Sternberg, and Michels[4] found that lacerations limited to the cornea carried the best prognosis (83% 5/200 or better), followed by corneoscleral lacerations (48%), and scleral lacerations (40%). When lacerations involved the sclera, the prognosis worsened as the wounds extended more posteriorly. If the posterior extent of the wound was anterior to the rectus muscle insertions, 60% of the eyes regained ambulatory vision as opposed to 28% if the laceration extended posterior to the insertions and 4% if posterior to the equator. Gilbert, Soong, and Hirst[19] found similar figures in their 2-year prospective study of penetrating ocular trauma. Brinton et al[7] combined length and location and found that 27 eyes with scleral lacerations greater than 5 mm in length carried a poorer visual prognosis than 79 other eyes. However, the differences were not statistically significant.

Vitreous Hemorrhage

Since the 1970s, vitrectomy surgery has played an integral role in the management of penetrating injuries. The justification for its use stems from laboratory work by Cleary and Ryan[20] who reported an experimental model of penetrating ocular injury, finding that retinal detachment was much more likely to develop following an ocular laceration in the presence of vitreous hemorrhage than when hemorrhage was absent. They also demonstrated that vitrectomy decreased the risk of developing retinal detachment.[21] The importance of vitreous hemorrhage had been noted by Snell[1] and confirmed more recently by de Juan, Sternberg, and Michels,[4] Cinotti and Maltzman,[22] Barr,[13] and others. Several studies have also emphasized the importance of the severity of the hemorrhage; Brinton et al[7] demonstrated that eyes with moderate to severe vitreous hemorrhage had a 48% functional success rate as opposed to 67% in eyes with mild or no hemorrhage.

Presence of Intraocular Foreign Body

Several investigators have studied the importance of the presence of an intraocular foreign body (IOFB) on the prognosis of eyes with penetrating injuries. In Snell's[1] 1945 report, the presence of an IOFB carried a poor prognosis. However, a variety of surgical advances have led to improved capabilities for managing most foreign bodies so that eyes with IOFBs now seem to carry a good prognosis. The better prognosis appears to be related to the finding that most eyes with foreign bodies have anterior entry sites, small lacerations, and relatively good initial visual acuity. In Brinton et al's[7] series, functional success was achieved in 63% of the eyes with an IOFB but in only 46% of eyes without an IOFB. In de Juan, Sternberg, and Michels' study,[4] 65% of eyes with an IOFB had a good visual result as opposed to 58% without an IOFB.

In contradistinction, larger foreign bodies such as BBs carry a grave prognosis. Of the 12 eyes with BB gun injuries in de Juan, Sternberg, and Michels'[4] series, none gained final vision of 5/200. When these eyes were eliminated from the IOFB group, 75% of eyes with IOFBs retained good vision. Hutton and Fuller[8] confirmed this finding, noting a statistically significant difference between foreign body injuries with BB pellets and with other foreign bodies.

As late as 1971, nonmagnetic foreign bodies were considered to carry a poor prognosis because of inability to extract the foreign body unless it rested in the anterior segment.[18] With the advent of vitrectomy instrumentation, nonmagnetic foreign bodies carry a much improved prognosis.

References

1. Snell AC: Perforating ocular injuries, Am J Ophthalmol 28:263-281, 1945.
2. Roper-Hall MJ: The treatment of ocular injuries, Trans Ophthalmol Soc UK 79:57-69, 1959.
3. Eagling EM: Perforating injuries of the eye, Br J Ophthalmol 60:732-736, 1976.
4. de Juan E, Sternberg P, and Michels RG: Penetrating ocular injuries: types of injuries and visual results, Ophthalmology 90:318-322, 1983.
5. Eagling EM: Perforating injuries involving the posterior segment, Trans Ophthalmol Soc UK 95:335-339, 1975.
6. Cherry PMH: Indirect traumatic rupture of the globe, Arch Ophthalmol 96:252-256, 1978.
7. Brinton GS et al: Surgical results in ocular trauma involving the posterior segment, Am J Ophthalmol 93:271-278, 1982.
8. Hutton WL and Fuller DG: Factors influencing final visual results in severely injured eyes, Am J Ophthalmol 97:715-722, 1984.
9. Meredith TA and Gordon PA: Pars plana vitrectomy for severe penetrating injury with posterior segment involvement, Am J Ophthalmol 103:549-554, 1987.
10. Brinton GS el al: Post-traumatic endophthalmitis, Arch Ophthalmol 102:547-550, 1984.
11. Affeldt JC et al: Microbial endophthalmitis resulting from ocular trauma, Ophthalmology 94:407-413, 1987.
12. Sternberg P et al: Multivariate analysis of prognostic factors in penetrating ocular injuries, Am J Ophthalmol 98:467-472, 1984.
13. Barr CC: Prognostic factors in corneoscleral lacerations, Arch Ophthalmol 101:919-924, 1983.
14. Moncreiff WF and Scheribel KJ: Penetrating injuries of the eye: a statistical survey, Am J Ophthalmol 28:1212-1220, 1945.
15. Gunn RM: Discussion on retro-ocular neuritis, Lancet 4:412, 1904.
16. Levatin P, Prasloski PF, and Collen MF: The swinging flashlight test in multiphasic screening for eye disease, Can J Ophthalmol 8:356-359, 1973.
17. Miller NR: Walsh and Hoyt's clinical neuro-ophthalmology, vol 2, ed 4, Baltimore, 1985, Williams & Wilkins.
18. Johnston S: Perforating eye injuries: a five-year survey, Trans Ophthalmol Soc UK 91:895-921, 1971.
19. Gilbert CM, Soong HK, and Hirst LW: A two-year prospective study of penetrating ocular trauma at the Wilmer Ophthalmological Institute, Ann Ophthalmol 19:104-106, 1987.
20. Cleary PE and Ryan SJ: Method of production and natural history of experimental posterior penetrating eye injury in the rhesus monkey, Am J Ophthalmol 88:212-220, 1979.
21. Cleary PE and Ryan SJ: Vitrectomy in penetrating eye injury: results of a controlled trial of vitrectomy in an experimental posterior penetrating eye injury in the rhesus monkey, Arch Ophthalmol 99:287-292, 1981.
22. Cinotti AA and Maltzman BA: Prognosis and treatment of perforating ocular injuries, Ophthalmic Surg 6(4):54-61, 1975.

CHAPTER 23

Traumatic endophthalmitis

MARC R. LEVIN
DONALD J. D'AMICO

Microbiology
Diagnosis
Antibiotic prophylaxis and therapy
Traumatic fungal endophthalmitis
Vitrectomy
Corticosteroids
Subsequent management
Prognosis
References

Despite recent advances in the treatment of endophthalmitis, infection resulting from penetrating ocular trauma continues to present a clinical challenge. It remains an important cause of visual failure following open globe injuries and may complicate seemingly benign injuries such as small, self-sealing corneal lacerations without associated intraocular damage. Nonsurgical trauma is involved in 25% of cases of endophthalmitis,[1] and 2% to 7% of all penetrating injuries result in culture-proven endophthalmitis.[2,3] These cases include injuries with and without a retained intraocular foreign body (IOFB). The great majority (approximately 62%) of all cases of endophthalmitis occur following intraocular surgery, 10% are associated with planned or inadvertent filtering blebs, and the remainder are caused by metastatic spread from other infected foci.[4]

Although the prognosis has been greatly improved by recent refinements in diagnosis, intravitreal antibiotic therapy, and vitreous surgery, the overall prognosis in traumatic endophthalmitis remains poor compared to that in cases occurring after intraocular surgery. The reasons for the poorer prognosis include associated damage to vital ocular structures, infection with organisms of greater virulence, and delay in diagnosis and treatment.

MICROBIOLOGY

The type and relative frequency of the pathogenic organisms encountered in traumatic endophthalmitis and in other clinical settings for endophthalmitis differ (Table 23-1). Postoperative endophthalmitis is most frequently caused by gram-positive cocci, *Staphylococcus epidermidis* accounting for about half of these cases. Most of the gram-negative organisms are *Proteus; Pseudomonas* are less common.[5] Fungi are an uncommon cause, with fewer than 100 culture-proven cases having been reported. Moreover, recent studies are skewed in the di-

Table 23-1. Causative organisms of traumatic and postoperative endophthalmitis (%)

Traumatic*		Postoperative†	
S. epidermidis	24	*S. epidermidis*	41
Bacillus species	22	*S. aureus*	19
Streptococcus species	13	Gram-negative organisms	16
Gram-negative organisms	11	*Streptococcus* species	6
Mixed flora	10	Fungi	5
S. aureus	8	Misc. gram-positive organisms	9
Fungi	8	Anaerobes	2
Anaerobes	3	Mixed flora	2
Other	1	*Bacillus* species	0

*Pooled data from Parrish CM and O'Day DM: Traumatic endophthalmitis, Int Ophthalmol Clin 27:112-119, 1987.

†Pooled data from Puliafito CA et al: Infections endophthalmitis: review of 36 cases, Ophthalmology 89:921-929, 1982; Rowsey JJ et al: Endophthalmitis: current approaches, Ophthalmology 89:1055-1066, 1982; and Driebe WT et al: Pseudophakic endophthalmitis: diagnosis and management, Ophthalmology 93:442-448, 1986.

rection of fungal endophthalmitis owing to two epidemics involving contaminated intraocular irrigating solutions and intraocular lenses, which accounted for 25 of these cases.[6,7] More than 50% of filtering bleb-related cases are caused by streptococci and another 25% by *Hemophilus*, with the remainder caused by staphylococci and gram-negative organisms.[8] Metastatic endophthalmitis is most commonly fungal but can also involve streptococci, gram-negative bacilli, gram-positive bacilli, and anaerobes.[9]

Traumatic endophthalmitis is unique in having a high incidence of *Bacillus* species (Table 23-1), in particular *B. cereus*. In pooled series, these organisms are encountered in approximately 20% of cases. Clostridia are uncommon after trauma and essentially nonexistent in other forms of endophthalmitis.[2,10,11]

B. cereus is probably the single most destructive organism encountered in the eye. It elaborates several enzymes and exotoxins that typically cause infections to advance explosively to an unsalvageable state within 24 hours of diagnosis. Only one reported case of an eye with *B. cereus* endophthalmitis retained useful visual acuity after treatment.[12] There appears to be a strong association between *B. cereus* infection and retained metallic IOFBs, especially when associated with farm- and soil-related injuries.[2] Because of their predominance and virulence, *Bacillus* species have important implications for prophylaxis and therapy, as will be discussed later. This organism and clostridia are typically the only endophthalmitis-causing agents that produce constitutional signs and symptoms such as fever, sweat, and leukocytosis.[13]

As in postoperative cases, fungi are a relatively uncommon cause of traumatic endophthalmitis. Only 20 cases of posttraumatic fungal endophthalmitis have been reported. In the recent literature, pooled series implicate fungi in approximately 8% of trauma-related endophthalmitis cases. These fungi are invariably filamentous and not yeast forms, and the worst prognosis is typically encountered in cases involving *Fusarium solanae* and similarly virulent species.[14]

DIAGNOSIS

The diagnosis of traumatic endophthalmitis depends on a high index of suspicion followed by the application of appropriate diagnostic procedures and culture techniques. The recognition of endophthalmitis following trauma may be obscured by the consequences of the trauma itself, such as pain, swelling, redness, media opacity, and loss of vision. These can make the usual signs and symptoms difficult to distinguish from an appropriate inflammatory response to the injury. These difficulties in diagnosis often contribute to delay in treatment, an important factor in the poorer prognosis in traumatic endophthalmitis compared with postoperative cases. Although the mean interval beween the injury and onset of clinically detectable endophthalmitis is difficult to determine, recent series have addressed the interval from the time of injury to the start of treatment for suspected endophthalmitis. According to Affeldt et al,[10] this interval was 4 days for bacterial cases and 57 days for fungal cases. An injury-to-treatment interval of 4 days was observed from gram-negative bacteria, 3.6 days for *S. epidermidis*, 2 days for streptococci, and 1.4 days for *Bacillus* species, consistent with the fulminating character of the latter. Brinton et al[2] found a mean interval of 3 days (range, 1 to 14 days) in their failure group and 8 days in the success group. They concluded that this time interval difference reflected the better prognosis with organisms of lower virulence; with such organisms, endophthalmitis may develop more slowly and remain treatable for a longer period after injury.

Given the varying complexity of the antecedent trauma, the symptoms of endophthalmitis may dominate or be difficult to elicit. The typical symptoms may include pain and visual loss inappropriate for the injury, purulent discharge, headache, and photophobia.

Clinical signs may include fever; proptosis; eyelid swelling and ecchymosis; elevated intraocular pressure; decrease or absence of the red reflex; corneal edema; corneal ring abscess;[13] anterior chamber reaction including flare, cells, fibrin, or frank hypoyon; intraocular gas bubbles; vitreous puff balls; and retinal periphlebitis.[15] Contrary to popular notions, intraocular gas bubbles are not absolutely diagnostic of clostridia; *B. cereus* has also been reported to cause this sign.[16]

Features diagnostic of *B. cereus* include very rapid and explosive onset, usually within 24 hours after the injury, accompanied by ecchymosis, periorbital swelling, extreme proptosis, low-grade fever, and polymorphonuclear leukocytosis. A peripheral corneal ring infiltrate,[12,13] which may progress to an abscess within hours, may also be present (Figs. 23-1 and 23-2). When *B. cereus* infections reach this stage, the eye has already suffered severe and irretrievable visual loss.

If there is any suspicion of a retained IOFB, the appropriate radiologic and ultrasonographic studies must be obtained. They are especially indicated with injury resulting from metal striking on metal. Although IOFB films are successfully employed in many cases, computerized tomography (CT) scan is perhaps the single most sensitive technique available. In addition, CT does not require contact with the globe. It is performed with the patient in supine position, permitting sedation or anesthesia if necessary. Because a high incidence of the devastating *B. cereus* infection is associated with IOFBs,

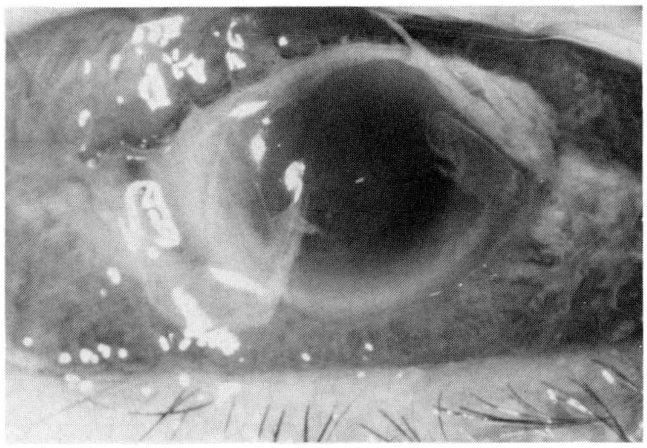

Fig. 23-1. Anterior segment photograph of *Bacillus cereus* endophthalmitis displaying extreme eyelid edema, chemosis, corneal ring abscess, and intraocular inflammation.

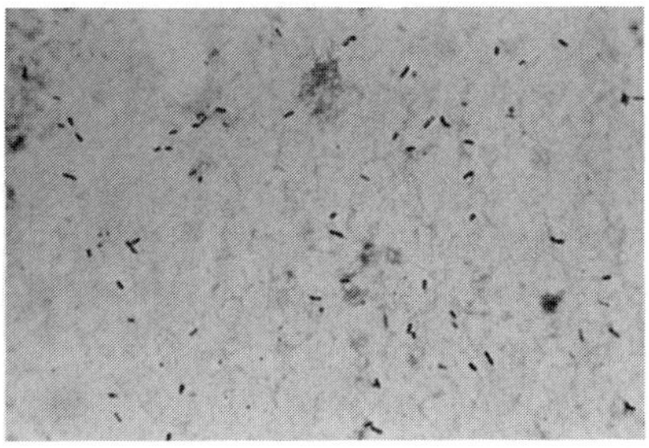

Fig. 23-2. Gram stain of vitreous from eye in Fig. 23-1 showing the gram-positive rods of *Bacillus cereus*.

knowledge of the presence of an IOFB is essential. In a study of penetrating trauma, Brinton et al[2] noted endophthalmitis in 10.7% of cases with an IOFB and 5.2% without an IOFB. Ultrasound evaluation may show anterior and posterior vitreous opacities and thickening of the retinochoroidal layer in endophthalmitis and may detect an occult IOFB. Ultrasound is especially important in cases where an IOFB may not be radio-opaque, and it may also delineate an occult retinal detachment. The combination of retinal detachment and endophthalmitis carries an extremely poor prognosis.

Diagnosis ultimately rests with the demonstration of infectious organisms in the eye by appropriate cultures and stains. If the examination raises serious concerns that endophthalmitis is present, vitreous and aqueous samples must be obtained for culture before therapy. Although vitreous is a much better culture medium for microorganisms than is aqueous, and the rate of recovery of organisms from vitreous is much higher, in some instances aqueous cultures are positive and vitreous cultures negative; both cultures, therefore, should be obtained routinely.

The culture procedure is most conveniently performed in the operating room; an office setting may be used on rare occasions if the patient is cooperative and the trauma well defined and limited. The choice of anesthesia will vary depending on the severity of trauma, but a preference for general anesthesia in the management of ocular trauma is recommended. Aqueous can be obtained by a simple anterior chamber tap with a 25- or 27-gauge needle on a tuberculin syringe, aspirating 0.10 ml of fluid. Vitreous can be obtained by needle aspiration or vitrectomy instrumentation, the latter limited to the operating room setting. Needle aspiration is performed in aphakic eyes by inserting a 22-gauge needle at the limbus and through the pupil and aspirating 0.2 to 0.3 ml into a 3-ml syringe. If the eye is phakic or pseudophakic or has an intact posterior capsule, the needle can be introduced through the pars plana into the anterior vitreous with the use of the operating microscope to visualize the needle tip before aspirating. Vitreous sampling with vitrectomy instrumentation can be done by a variety of procedures, ranging from limited vitreous biopsy without infusion to standard pars plana vitrectomy. The complexity will depend on the need for vitrectomy for endophthalmitis and the manifestations of the trauma itself, as described later.

The samples should be examined by gram stain, but because a gram stain is positive in only 60% of culture-positive cases, presumptive therapy for suspected bacterial endophthalmitis is not withheld solely because of a negative gram stain. The use of fungal stains and, in particular, Calcofluor white stain on fresh vitreous and aqueous specimens is important in determining initial therapy and is routinely recommended. These stains can be obtained within minutes, and the direct demonstration of fungi in the samples will alter the selection of initial therapy (see the boxes on pp. 245 and 246). Samples should be promptly plated on fresh petri dishes containing blood agar, chocolate agar, and thioglycolate broth and incubated at 37° C. A separate blood agar plate and a Sabouraud's plate should be incubated at room temperature for fungi. One plate containing cooked meat medium should be incubated anaerobically. If the vitreous sample has been obtained in the setting of a pars plana vitrectomy with infusion, the most effective culture yield is obtained by concentrating the sample with a membrane filtering system.[23] The use of such a system remains the best method for recovering organisms from the vitreous, but Joondeph et al[24] have recently described the direct inoculation of blood culture bottles with aqueous and vitreous samples and documented a 90% recovery rate with this sim-

RECOMMENDED DRUG THERAPY IN SUSPECTED TRAUMATIC ENDOPHTHALMITIS

Intravitreal administration

Foreign body absent
  Vancomycin 1 mg[17] and amikacin 400 μg[18]
Foreign body present
  Clindamycin 250 μg and gentamicin 100 μg[13,19]
  (Vancomycin 1 mg and amikacin 400 μg are currently under investigation)[20]
Dexamethasone 200 to 400 may be considered for *all* cases with severe inflammation, but strict guidelines for intravitreal steroid use have not been determined; its use must be considered experimental.[21]

Subconjunctival administration

Foreign body absent
  Vancomycin 25 mg* and gentamicin 20 mg[22]
Foreign body present
  Clindamycin 34 mg[2] and gentamicin 20 mg

Topical administration

Foreign body absent
  Cefazolin 133 mg/ml or vancomycin 25 mg/ml drops administered q4h alternated with fortified gentamicin 14 mg/ml drops q4h†
Foreign body present
  Clindamycin 20 mg/ml q4h alternated with fortified gentamicin 14 mg/ml drops q4h†
In cases with severe inflammation, prednisolone acetate 1% drops may be added after initiation of antibiotic therapy.

Systemic administration

Foreign body absent
  Vancomycin and gentamicin
Foreign body present
  Clindamycin and gentamicin
In cases with severe inflammation, prednisone may be given orally after initiation of antibiotic therapy.

* Under investigation.
† Massachusetts Eye and Ear Infirmary protocol, under investigation.

RECOMMENDED DRUG THERAPY FOR TRAUMATIC FUNGAL/ ENDOPHTHALMITIS*

Intravitreal administration†

Amphotericin B 5 μg
(Miconazole 25 μg may be used in addition or given as a subsequent injection after failure of treatment with amphotericin B)

Subconjunctival administration‡

Miconazole 5-10 mg *or* amphotericin B 1 mg

Topical administration‡

Natamycin 5% *or* amphotericin B 0.15% *or* miconazole 1% drop qlh

Systemic administration§

Ketaconazole 400-600 mg daily by oral administration

These recommendations are derived in their entirety from the article by Pflugfelder et al,[14] to which the reader is referred.
*Therapy for fungi is administered if the vitreous or aqueous specimen displays fungal elements on fresh smear or a positive fungal culture is obtained.
†Intravitreal injections are not repeated except in cases with a positive repeat culture or smear.
‡Pflugfelder et al[14] reserve adjunctive subconjunctival and topical therapy for cases with significant anterior segment involvement.
§Ketaconazole therapy appears to be well tolerated and may be used orally as sensitivities indicate. Systemic therapy with amphotericin B has a high incidence of toxicity, and its use in fungal endophthalmitis may be questioned. If intravenous therapy with amphotericin B is selected, careful attention to systemic toxicity is essential.

ple and easily available technique. All foreign bodies removed from the eye should be submitted for culture.

Once the appropriate specimens have been obtained for culture, presumptive antibiotic treatment for endophthalmitis may be offered by intravitreal, periocular, topical, and systemic routes, as described later.

Approximately 64% of eyes with the clinical diagnosis of infectious endophthalmitis will display a positive culture; this is an overall figure and includes postoperative, traumatic, and metastatic series.[4] Culture results establish the diagnosis, determine the suitability of ongoing antibiotic therapy based on the sensitivities of the offending organism, and are strongly correlated with prognosis. For endophthalmitis in general, poor results are obtained with *B. cereus,* fungi, and gram-negative organisms. Staphylococci and other gram-positive organisms have a better prognosis, and culture-negative eyes have the best prognosis. In one series of postoperative endophthalmitis, 94% of culture-negative eyes achieved visual acuity of 20/400 or better.[25] The 36% culture-negative in pooled series[4] undoubtedly includes a percentage of anaerobic and other organisms that were not recovered. It is important to note that anaerobic *Propionibacterium acnes* endophthalmitis has also been reported in the specific setting of traumatic endophthalmitis.[26,27]

ANTIBIOTIC PROPHYLAXIS AND THERAPY

The management of traumatic endophthalmitis includes three clinical settings: prophylaxis of endophthalmitis, initial management of suspected endophthalmitis (presumptive treatment), and subsequent management of culture-positive cases. The specific elements of management include antibiotics (selection, route of administration), vitrectomy, and steroids (route of administration, timing). These clinical settings and elements of management are highly interrelated; specific recommendations for drug therapy are summarized in the boxes on p. 245 and this page. Guidelines are summarized in the box on p. 247.

The routine use of intravenous, periocular, and topical antibiotics is indicated in virtually all cases of penetrating ocular trauma, encompassing the clinical settings of prophylaxis, presumptive treatment, and ongoing management of traumatic endophthalmitis. Despite numerous experimental and clinical studies documenting the poor intraocular penetration of commonly used antibiotics, the breakdown of the blood/ocular barrier by inflammatory processes in the setting of trauma improves antibiotic penetration. Thus, the actual intraocular drug levels may reach therapeutic levels. In series including postoperative and traumatic cases of endophthalmitis some authors have advocated intravenous antibiotic course of differing duration ranging from 3 to 5 days[28] to 10 to 14 days.[11] The routine use of systemic antibiotics for postoperative endophthalmitis has recently been questioned, and successful management of both bacterial and fungal postoperative cases without

GUIDELINES FOR THE MANAGEMENT OF SUSPECTED TRAUMATIC ENDOPHTHALMITIS

1. Prompt collection of vitreous and aqueous specimens for culture, stain, and smear in all suspected cases.
2. Evaluation for intraocular foreign bodies by CT, X ray, and ultrasound where indicated.
3. Systemic, periocular, and topical antibiotic prophylaxis in all cases of globe laceration, rupture, or penetration (see the boxes on pp. 245 and 246). These eyes may be carefully followed in a hospital setting without intravitreal drug therapy if a foreign body is not involved and signs of endophthalmitis are absent.
4. Intravitreal antibiotic therapy (in addition to systemic, periocular, and topical therapy) in all cases of suspected traumatic endophthalmitis and all cases of intraocular foreign body or soil-related injury.
5. Vitrectomy (often dictated by management of specific trauma such as intraocular foreign body) offered to cases of suspected traumatic endophthalmitis that display loss of red reflex, severe inflammation, or intraocular gas. Limited vitrectomy is preferred to minimize the risk of iatrogenic retinal detachment.
6. Consideration of intravitreal steroid therapy for cases with severe inflammation.
7. Reculture of vitreous and aqueous in 48 to 72 hours in cases with a positive initial culture and clinical deterioration following initial therapy.
8. Avoidance of repeat intravitreal injections, except in cases with a positive *repeat* culture or stain.

adjunctive systemic antibiotic therapy has been reported.[14,22] Nevertheless, in the setting of penetrating trauma, the potential benefits of systemic, periocular, and topical antibiotics appear to outweigh the risks. Furthermore, the toxicities of intravenously administered antibiotics are well characterized, and appropriate monitoring of blood levels will minimize potential adverse effects. A recent experimental study has documented excellent penetration of orally administered rifampin into the vitreous and aqueous.[29] The broad spectrum of this drug coupled with its excellent penetration into the eye after oral administration may establish a role for it in the prophylaxis and therapy of endophthalmitis if its initial promise is confirmed.

Because of its ability to bypass the blood/ocular barrier, intravitreal antibiotic injection has assumed a major and successful role in treating infectious endophthalmitis. The infrequent mechanical complications include trauma to ocular tissues and hemorrhage due to the injection procedure. Of greater concern is the development of drug-related retinal toxicity. Numerous studies establishing the safety and efficacy of a variety of intravitreally injected drugs, including vancomycin, clindamycin, aminoglycosides, penicillin, cephalosporins, and amphotericin B, have permitted the formulation of guidelines for clinical use.

Antibiotics selected to cover a broad spectrum of gram-positive and gram-negative organisms typically include vancomycin or a cephalosporin for gram-positive coverage and an aminoglycoside for gram-negative coverage. These choices, however, continue to be modified by ever-changing clinical experience and experimental evidence. For gram-positive coverage, many isolates of *S. epidermidis*—a common organism encountered in traumatic endophthalmitis—and other organisms have been found to be resistant to semisynthetic penicillins and cephalosporins.[17] These organisms are uniformly sensitive to vancomycin, and intravitreal vancomycin may be considered the drug of choice for gram-positive coverage. However, a report of vancomycin-resistant gram-positive organisms,[30] although not yet observed in the setting of endophthalmitis, indicates the need for continued surveillance of current recommendations for intravitreal drugs of choice. Similarly, although most gram-negative organisms remain sensitive to gentamicin, the superior antibacterial coverage of amikacin and its somewhat lower retinal toxicity have suggested it be considered the aminoglycoside of choice for gram-negative coverage.[18] Specific studies have established that the doses recommended in Box 6-1 can be given safely in combination.

Despite the similarities between prophylaxis and presumptive treatment, however, differences emerge on two important questions: Are intravitreal antibiotics necessary in every case of globe rupture? Are intravitreal antibiotics indicated in every case of IOFB, even in the absence of other inflammatory signs?

Several authorities advocate the use of intraocular antibiotics routinely after penetrating trauma. Peyman, Carroll, and Raichand[28] inject antibiotics in the anterior chamber if the lens is not involved in the injury, and in the vitreous if the lens or vitreous is violated. However, clinical experience suggests that most ocular lacerations (without IOFB) do not develop endophthalmitis. Although there are no controlled trials to date, it is possible that the risks of intravitreal drug injection, including mechanical trauma and dosage errors, would be greater than the benefits of prophylaxis. In addition, cases of penetrating trauma are usually followed closely in an inpatient setting, facilitating prompt diagnosis and intervention, and the possible benefits of customary systemic and periocular antibiotic therapy in the prophylaxis of endophthalmitis have already been discussed.

The issue of antibiotic prophylaxis for IOFB injuries merits special consideration. Brinton et al[2] documented a 10.7% incidence of endophthalmitis in the presence of an IOFB. In addition, studies have noted a high incidence of *B. cereus* infections associated with IOFBs.[2,12] This organism typically produces symptoms within 24 hours following injury and rapidly progresses to total loss of vision in the next 24 hours. In view of these findings, a compelling argument may be made for prophylaxis by intravitreal injection in all cases of IOFB and that this prophylaxis be effective against *B. cereus*. The selection of agents for this purpose is unresolved at present. For postoperative cases, the use of intravitreal vancomycin (for gram-positive organisms) and aminoglycoside (for gram-negative organisms) has been widely accepted, but the need for effective coverage of *Bacillus* has led some authors to suggest the use of intravitreal clindamycin for traumatic cases. The most effective regimen for *Bacillus* has been reported to be clindamycin and gentamicin; these agents display a synergistic effect against *B. cereus*.[13] Clindamycin also has a good spectrum against other gram-positive bacteria. However, Pflugfelder et al[20] observed that all recent isolates of *Bacillus* were sensitive to vancomycin; some sensitivity of *Bacillus* to aminoglycoside alone has also been reported.[13] At the present time, clindamycin in combination with aminoglycoside is recommended as the regimen of choice for *Bacillus* species, but vancomycin and aminoglycoside may emerge as equally effective. The latter regimen would have the obvious advantage of being identical with the initial regimen for treating postoperative bacterial endophthalmitis, but this appealing uniformity must await additional careful study. A summary of intravitreal prophylaxis regimens for IOFB is given in the box on p. 245.

TRAUMATIC FUNGAL ENDOPHTHALMITIS

Antibiotic regimens are altered if fungi are observed in a fresh smear of vitreous or aqueous, or if a positive fungal culture is obtained. The use of Calcofluor white and other stains has been mentioned; the detection of fungal elements on the smear at the time of specimen collection is advantageous and may permit initial therapy for fungal endophthalmitis. In more typical cases, the initial smears are not definitive, and presumptive antibacterial therapy is offered as outlined in the box on p. 245. In such cases, therapy for fungi is secondary and is initiated promptly if a positive fungal culture is obtained. This information is usually available one or more days after the culture procedure. Specific details of antifungal therapy are outlined in the box on p. 246.

VITRECTOMY

The initial therapy for suspected endophthalmitis (after appropriate vitreous and aqueous samples have been obtained) includes intravitreal antibiotics, with vitrectomy and perhaps intravitreal steroids considered as adjunctive therapy. The issues involved in the selection of prophylactic antibiotics are also applicable to the initial management of suspected endophthalmitis because treatment must be initiated at the time of vitreous and aqueous sampling, before receiving culture results.

The role of vitrectomy, now considered a useful adjunct in the treatment of endophthalmitis, has been investigated in both clinical and experimental studies. Assessing the results of clinical studies is difficult because of their retrospective character and the acknowledged bias for performing vitrectomy in more advanced cases. Driebe et al[31] reported a 94% success rate (recovery of 20/400 or better visual acuity) with intraocular antibiotics only, compared to a 50% success rate with intraocular antibiotics and vitrectomy. However, they acknowledged that vitrectomy was reserved for cases that were more advanced initially or responded poorly to initial antibiotic treatment. Puliafito et al[11] found better visual results when vitrectomy was performed within the first 24 hours than when performed later; experience with intraocular antibiotics alone as a form of management was not available in this study. Forster, Abbott, and Gelender[32] found virtually equivalent results in patients treated with antibiotics alone and those treated with antibiotics and vitrectomy. Peyman, Carroll, and Raichand[28] recommended vitrectomy if the eye was worse at 24 to 48 hours after intravitreal antibiotic therapy. Pflugfelder et al[14] favored vitrectomy in association with intravitreal antibiotic therapy for fungal cases.

Experimental studies by Cottingham and Forster[33] showed that endophthalmitis with less virulent organisms such as *S. epidermidis* was effectively treated with intravitreal antibiotics alone, but that more virulent organisms were not successfully treated by intravitreal antibiotics alone unless the drugs were given during the first 24 hours. In another experimental model of *S. aureus* endophthalmitis in aphakic eyes, Talley et al[34] observed that the combination of vitrectomy and intravitreal antibiotics was decidedly superior to intravitreal antibiotics alone. Although clinical experience has also shown that infection with a less virulent organism such as *S. epidermidis* can be successfully treated with intravenous antibiotics alone,[35] this information is of limited practical value because the type of organism is not initially known and delay in treating most pathogens is associated with a poor prognosis.

The advantages of vitrectomy include the opportunity to obtain an adequate vitreous sample for culture, clear the ocular media, remove intraocular inflammatory and bacterial toxic products, reduce the number of organisms present in the eye, and possibly permit earlier intravitreal drug administration and better intraocular drug diffusion. Disadvantages include the possibility of a delay in treatment, more rapid clearing of intraocular antibiotics, retinal breaks, and other known complications of vitrectomy.

Nelson, Marcus, and Bovino[36] noted a 21% incidence of retinal detachment in cases treated with intravitreal antibiotics and vitrectomy, compared to a 9% incidence in eyes treated without vitrectomy. Certainly vitrectomy increases the risk of retinal detachment, but it must be emphasized that the introduction of needles into the eye for cultures and intravitreal injections and perhaps endophthalmitis itself are also risk factors for detachment. Successful salvage of any eye with active bacterial endophthalmitis and a coexisting retinal detachment has not been reported. Thus, the presence of a retinal detachment in an eye with active endophthalmitis, whether iatrogenic or otherwise, is disastrous and invariably associated with loss of all useful vision. The treatment of such eyes presents extraordinary difficulties, such as the use of intravitreal antibiotics in the presence of intravitreal air, gas, or silicone oil tamponade, and the employment of scleral buckling materials in eyes with an infected surgical field. Recently, Parke[37] developed an approach in which an air/fluid exchange is performed immediately after intravitreal injection of standard doses of antibiotic. He reasons that the minimal remaining meniscus of fluid in the subsequently air-filled eye will have a nontoxic concentration of drug. These innovative observations suggest a possible opportunity for these otherwise desperate eyes and deserve further evaluation.

Vitrectomy continues to play a prominent role in the treatment of ocular trauma and endophthalmitis, and additional investigation will provide further refinement of its indications and technique.

CORTICOSTEROIDS

Corticosteroids have been increasingly used via the systemic, topical, subconjunctival, and intravitreal routes. Systemic, topical, and subconjunctival steroids have long been noted to be effective in reducing ocular inflammation in endophthalmitis. Prophylaxis with steroids, however, should probably be avoided since signs of early endophthalmitis may be masked and hence delay diagnosis and treatment. In cases with significant anterior segment inflammation following penetrating trauma, topical corticosteroids in moderate doses (e.g., prednisolone acetate 1% 4 times daily) may be cautiously added.

Intravitreal steroid therapy with dexamethasone[21] has been used in endophthalmitis cases since 1974, but a randomized clinical trial has not been performed. At present, a single intravitreal steroid injection may be considered as part of initial therapy for cases with severe inflammation, but the exact indications and safety of intravitreal steroids require further investigation. As a general rule, steroids are omitted in early management of traumatic fungal endophthalmitis but may be used later, in the setting of an improving clinical course, if required.

SUBSEQUENT MANAGEMENT

Topical and intravenous antibiotic therapy is typically continued for 5 to 7 days, but the exact importance and duration of this therapy remain under scrutiny. Clinical status is closely monitored, and subconjunctival injections are not repeated in cases of clinical stabilization or improvement but may be repeated daily in cases of clinical deterioration.

Repeat cultures of the vitreous and aqueous are essential in cases that display clinical deterioration despite initial therapy and also in cases involving fungi. The repeat cultures may be performed about 48 to 72 hours after initial therapy.

The surgeon must weigh factors of safety and clinical indications when considering repeat intravitreal antibiotic injections. Large overdoses of certain drugs—for example, gentamicin—can destroy the retina completely and irreversibly.[38] Single doses of vancomycin and gentamicin, as well as other drugs, are well tolerated, but there appears to be a threshold beyond which retinal damage occurs. Oum, D'Amico, and Wong[39] evaluated the toxicity in rabbit eyes of repeated intraocular combination therapy with vancomycin and gentamicin and with vancomycin and amikacin. Using dosages typical for endophthalmitis therapy, histologic evidence of retinal toxicity was observed in eyes receiving two sets of intravitreal injections (separated by 48 hours), and more advanced histologic and ophthalmoscopic retinal toxicity was noted after a third set of injections (separated by another 48 hours). Amikacin-containing therapy produced less severe changes than gentamicin, which was consistent with previous studies.[40] These results appear to militate against repeated injections in the subsequent management of endophthalmitis. Although intravitreal drug clearance may be increased by inflammation and vitrectomy, it appears that a short duration or momentary peak level is sufficient to cause absorption in the outer layers of the retina and retinal pigment epithelium adequate to cause toxicity, even in the face of enhanced clearance from the vitreous cavity.[41] It therefore seems preferable to avoid repeat intravitreal injections except in cases displaying a positive repeat culture or smear.

PROGNOSIS

The prognosis in traumatic endophthalmitis, although improved over the past 15 years, is still dismal, and it remains the most dreaded complication of penetrating trauma. Success is defined by many authors as retaining 20/400 or better visual acuity. A review of all reported cases of endophthalmitis from 1948 to 1974 revealed a 66% rate of enucleation or no light perception,[42] but these findings did not differentiate traumatic from other clinical settings. Still, traumatic endophthalmitis has a significantly worse prognosis in most series compared with that following intraocular surgery. Visual success for all cases after 1980 was 42% to 73% but only 17% to 50% for the traumatic subgroup.[2] Some recent series show more cause for optimism; Brinton et al[2] reported 42% of eyes retaining visual acuity of 20/200 or better and 26% 20/30 or better. Affeldt et al[10] noted that only 22% of their cases regained visual acuity of 20/400 or better, but *Bacillus* species were involved in 8 of their 27 eyes; 4 of their 5 fungal cases did well. Puliafito et al[11] reported that 5 out of 6 of their traumatic eyes lost all visual acuity. Nobe et al[9] compared the visual outcomes after treatment for traumatic and postoperative endophthalmitis. In cases treated with vitrectomy and intraocular antibiotics, 43% of the traumatic cases did well as opposed to 53% of the postoperative cases. In cases treated without vitrectomy and intraocular antibiotics, 38% in each category did well. Combining their different treatment modalities, 46% of the posttraumatic cases and 41% of the postoperative cases were treated successfully.

There are several important prognostic indicators for endophthalmitis in general. Favorable outcomes are associated with negative cultures or cultures with less virulent organisms, prompt versus delayed therapy, good initial visual acuity, a red reflex at presentation, absence of retinal detachment, and absence of nonsurgical trauma. These prognostic variables have been consistent throughout the literature. Three of these factors impact on traumatic endophthalmitis: a delay in diagnosis, a more virulent spectrum of organisms, and the extent of the associated injury.

The problem of delayed diagnosis is even more important in traumatic endophthalmitis than in the postoperative situation because of the virulent spectrum of the organisms involved.

With *Bacillus* species, a delay of even a few hours may mean the difference between a successful outcome and loss of the eye. Visual results in fungal cases are seemingly superior,[2,10,19] but the issue is confounded by the extent of injury since most reported fungal cases had trauma limited in a corneal laceration.

The extent and nature of the injury are also significant. Brinton et al[2] found that 72% of posttraumatic cases did well if retinal detachment was absent. Affeldt et al[10] noted that 5 of 8 infections following corneal laceration were successfully treated as compared to only 1 of 13 cases associated with posterior segment injury that retained useful vision. IOFBs pose a special hazard because they appear to be associated with an increased rate of endophthalmitis and tend to be associated with organisms that carry the worst prognosis. Often, of course, the extent of the injury limits the best potential posttreatment visual acuity, and for this reason it is difficult to compare series of traumatic endophthalmitis treatment solely in terms of visual results. The association of a retinal detachment and an endophthalmitis caused by any organism is catastrophic; these eyes have an extremely grave prognosis.

References

1. Parrish CM and O'Day DM: Traumatic endophthalmitis, Int Ophthalmol Clin 27:112-119, 1987.
2. Brinton GS et al: Posttraumatic endophthalmitis, Arch Ophthalmol 102:547-550, 1984.
3. Forster RK: Endophthalmitis. In Duane TD, editor: Clinical ophthalmology, vol 4, Philadelphia, 1987, JB Lippincott.
4. D'Amico DJ and Noorily SW: Postoperative bacterial endophthalmitis. In Blumenkranz M and Culbertson W, editors: Infectious diseases of the retina and choroid, New York, Alan R Liss (in press).
5. Mandelbaum S and Forster RK: Postoperative endophthalmitis, Int Ophthalmol Clin 27:95-106, 1987.
6. Pettit TH et al: Fungal endophthalmitis following intraocular lens implantation: a surgical epidemic, Arch Ophthalmol 98:1025-1039, 1980.
7. Stern WH et al: Epidemic postsurgical *Candida parapsilosis* endophthalmitis: clinical findings and management of 15 consecutive cases, Ophthalmology 92:1701-1709, 1985.
8. Mandelbaum S and Forster RK: Endophthalmitis associated with filtering blebs, Int Ophthalmol Clin 27:107-111, 1987.
9. Nobe JR et al: Post-traumatic and postoperative endophthalmitis: a comparison of visual outcome, Br J Ophthalmol 71:614-617, 1987.
10. Affeldt JC et al: Microbial endophthalmitis resulting from ocular trauma, Ophthalmology 94:407-413, 1987.
11. Puliafito CA et al: Infectious endophthalmitis: review of 36 cases, Ophthalmology 89:921-929, 1982.
12. Schemmer GB and Driebe WT Jr: Posttraumatic *Bacillus cereus* endophthalmitis, Arch Ophthalmol 105:342-344, 1987.
13. O'Day DM et al: The problem of *Bacillus* species infection with special emphasis on the virulence of *Bacillus cereus*, Ophthalmology 88:833-838, 1981.
14. Pflugfelder SC et al: Exogenous fungal endophthalmitis, Ophthalmology 95:19-30, 1988.
15. Packer AJ, Weingeist TA, and Abrams GW: Retinal periphlebitis as an early sign of bacterial endophthalmitis, Am J Ophthalmol 96:66-71, 1983.
16. Al-Hemidan A, Bryne-Rhodes KA, and Tabbara KF: *Bacillus cereus* panophthalmitis associated with intraocular gas bubble, Br J Ophthalmol 73:25-28, 1989.
17. Smith MA et al: Treatment of experimental methicillin-resistant *Staphylococcus epidermidis* endophthalmitis with intravitreal vancomycin, Ophthalmology 93:1328-1335, 1986.
18. Talamo JH, D'Amico DJ, and Kenyon KR: Intravitreal amikacin in the treatment of bacterial endophthalmitis, Arch Ophthalmol 104:1483-1485, 1986.
19. Rowsey JJ et al: Endophthalmitis: current approaches, Ophthalmology 89:1055-1066, 1982.
20. Pflugfelder SC et al: Intravitreal vancomycin: retinal toxicity, clearance, and interaction with gentamicin, Arch Ophthalmol 105:831-837, 1987.
21. Peyman GA and Herbst R: Bacterial endophthalmitis: treatment with intraocular injection of gentamicin and dexamethasone, Arch Ophthalmol 91:416-418, 1974.
22. Pavan PR and Brinser JH: Exogenous bacterial endophthalmitis treated without systemic antibiotics, Am J Ophthalmol 104:121-126, 1987.
23. Forster RK: Etiology and diagnosis of bacterial postoperative endophthalmitis, Ophthalmology 85:320-326, 1978.
24. Joondeph BC et al: A new culture method for infectious endophthalmitis, Arch Ophthalmol 107:1334-1337, 1989.
25. Wilson FM: Causes and prevention of endophthalmitis, Int Ophthalmol Clin 27:67-73, 1987.
26. Beatty RF et al: Anaerobic endophthalmitis caused by *Propionibacterium acnes*, Am J Ophthalmol 101:114-116, 1986.
27. Friedman E, Peyman GA, and May DR: Endophthalmitis caused by *Propionibacterium acnes*, Can J Ophthalmol 13:50-52, 1978.

28. Peyman GA, Carroll CP, and Raichand M: Prevention and management of traumatic endophthalmitis, Ophthalmology 87:320-324, 1980.
29. Wong KW et al: The intraocular penetration of rifampin after oral administration, Graefes Arch Clin Exp Ophthalmol 1989 (in press).
30. Schwalbe RS, Stapleton JT, and Gilligan PH: Emergence of vancomycin resistance in coagulase-negative staphylococci, N Engl J Med 316:927-931, 1987.
31. Driebe WT et al: Pseudophakic endophthalmitis: diagnosis and management, Ophthalmology 93:442-448, 1986.
32. Forster RK, Abbott RL, and Gelender H: Management of infectious endophthalmitis, Ophthalmology 87:313-319, 1980.
33. Cottingham AJ and Forster RK: Vitrectomy in endophthalmitis, Arch Ophthalmol 94:2078-2081, 1976.
34. Talley AR et al: The role of vitrectomy in the treatment of postoperative bacterial endophthalmitis: an experimental study, Arch Ophthalmol 105:1699-1702, 1987.
35. O'Day DM et al: *Staphylococcus epidermidis:* visual outcome following noninvasive therapy, Ophthalmology 89:354-360, 1982.
36. Nelson PT, Marcus DA, and Bovino JA: Retinal detachment following endophthalmitis, Ophthalmology 92:1112-1117, 1985.
37. Parke DW: Unpublished observations, presented at the Vail Vitreoretinal Seminar, Vail, Colorado, March 1989.
38. McDonald HR et al: Retinal toxicity secondary to intraocular gentamicin injection, Ophthalmology 93:871-877, 1986.
39. Oum BS, D'Amico DJ, and Wong KW: Intravitreal antibiotic therapy with vancomycin and aminoglycoside: an experimental study of combination and repetitive injections, Arch Ophthalmol 107:1055-1060, 1989.
40. D'Amico DJ et al: Comparative toxicity of intravitreal aminoglycoside antibiotics, Am J Ophthalmol 100:264-275, 1985.
41. Talamo JH et al: The influence of aphakia and vitrectomy on experimental retinal toxicity of aminoglycoside antibiotics, Am J Ophthalmol 100:840-847, 1985.
42. Abel R Jr, Binder PS, and Bellows R: Postoperative bacterial endophthalmitis, Ann Ophthalmol 8:731-744, 1976.

CHAPTER 24

Sympathetic ophthalmia

DOUGLAS HOLMES
DAVID WILSON

Incidence
Clinical features
Histologic features
Role of the penetrating wound
Etiology
Differential diagnosis
Treatment and prognosis
References

Sympathetic ophthalmia is characterized by granulomatous inflammation of the uvea following accidental or surgical penetrating injury to the globe. The inflammation appears in the injured (exciting) eye at a variable time after the injury and usually affects the contralateral (sympathizing) eye soon afterward. It is a unique disease process in that injury to one eye affects the normal, uninjured eye, resulting in severe bilateral visual disability. The specific pathogenesis is uncertain, but experimental evidence suggests an autoimmune, delayed hypersensitivity reaction to retinal tissue antigens. Sympathetic ophthalmia may present a difficult diagnostic challenge owing to the variability of signs and symptoms.

INCIDENCE

Sympathetic ophthalmia is rare.[1] The older medical literature places the incidence after penetrating wounds at approximately 2%. However, it is generally accepted that sympathetic ophthalmia currently occurs in approximately 2 of 1000 eyes after accidental penetrating injuries and approximately 1 of 10,000 eyes after routine surgical procedures.[2] Recent advances in the surgical management of these wounds probably account for this decreased incidence.[3]

Sympathetic ophthalmia is more common in males than females, a reflection of the epidemiology of eye injuries. If only cases following surgery are considered, the incidence of sympathetic ophthalmia is identical in males and females. Sympathetic ophthalmia appears to have a higher incidence in the early decades of life, corresponding to a higher incidence of accidental trauma, and also in the later decades, when surgical trauma is more common.[4] Race and geographic distribution are seemingly not factors that affect the incidence of sympathetic ophthalmia.

In several large series, trauma with scleral perforation accounted for approximately 55% of the cases of sympathetic ophthalmia and surgical wounds for approximately 45%.[5-8] Although virtually all types of intraocular surgery have been reported preceding sympathetic ophthalmia, most frequent are routine cataract and glaucoma filtering procedures. However, sympathetic ophthalmia has also been noted following phacoemulsification, paracentesis, retinal detachment surgery,[9] vitrectomy,[5] and evisceration.[10] In addition, nonsurgical procedures involving subconjunctival scleral ruptures,[11] perforated corneal ulcers, and epibulbar extension of malignant melanoma have been reported to cause sympathetic ophthalmia.[2] The common factor in most cases appears to be incarceration of uveal tissue in the healing wounds.

Sympathetic ophthalmia is a potential risk with essentially every type of surgical intraocular procedure. No particular procedure appears to carry a greater risk of developing the disease. The issue becomes unclear, however, when multiple surgical procedures are performed on a single eye; each procedure may carry additional risk for the development of sympathetic ophthalmia.[12]

CLINICAL FEATURES

The time interval between injury to the exciting eye and the onset of inflammation in the sympathizing eye varies and has been reported to be as early as 5 days and as late as several decades.[6] Generally, however, sympathetic ophthalmia has rarely been reported within the initial 2 weeks. Approximately 65% of cases occur between 2 weeks and 2 months, 80% before 3 months, and 90% before 1 year.[1,6] The initial signs and symptoms are also quite variable. The first clinical evidence is usually a mild anterior uveitis in the sympathizing eye, associated with nonimproving or increasing inflammation in the exciting eye. In the sympathizing eye the patient typically complains of pain, photophobia, and decreased visual acuity, associated with transient episodes of accommodative spasm, visual fatigue, and increased tearing. The exciting eye, which has usually not fully recovered from the original injury, is most often irritated and hyperemic and may exhibit increased pain or tenderness and decreased visual acuity.

Examination generally demonstrates features of uveitis, such as ciliary injection, globe tenderness, and cell and flare in the anterior chamber and vitreous cavity. Even though the earliest signs of sympathetic ophthalmia may be a relatively mild nongranulomatous anterior uveitis with minimal vitritis, most cases detected clinically exhibit a more moderate to severe anterior and posterior uveitis associated with keratic precipitates. These findings may be less prominent, however, especially if topical or oral corticosteroids were used in the primary treatment of the exciting eye.[1] In chronic cases, the advanced sequelae of uveitis can occur, such as posterior synechiae, glaucoma, cataract formation, rubeosis, iritis, and occlusion and seclusion of the pupil. Posterior segment involvement with sympathetic ophthalmia may include papillitis and localized choroidal inflammation. Dalen-Fuchs nodules—small, hypopigmented nodules at the level of the retinal pigment epithelium (RPE)—are frequently evident in the periphery (Fig. 24-1). Exudative retinal detachments may also be present. Although most cases typically involve an anterior and posterior uveitis, approximately 5% have posterior involvement only.[13] In the latter form, the inflammation is confined primarily to the optic nerve, choroid, and ciliary body, but the initiating injury, the time between the injury and onset of sympathetic ophthalmia, and the histopathologic characteristics do not differ. Although there is some disagreement in the older literature, the prognosis and therapy of the posterior form do not differ from those of the classic anterior form.[13]

No clinical diagnostic tests can reliably confirm the diagnosis of sympathetic ophthalmia. The diagnosis is based initially on the clinical characteristics and history and ultimately on histopathologic verification. Many diagnostic tests advocated in the past have been found to be unreliable.

Although not diagnostic, two types of abnormal fluorescein angiographic findings may be helpful in the differential diagnosis of sympathetic ophthalmia. The most frequent pattern is multiple fine spots of hyperfluorescence that enlarge in later frames of the angiogram as a result of dye leakage. These leakage sites correspond to the clinically apparent Dalen-Fuchs nodules.[14,15] In cases with exudative retinal detachments, there may be large areas of pooled fluorescence, similar to those observed in Vogt-Koyanagi-Harada syndrome. The second pattern is characterized by lesions that block fluorescence during the early phase and stain during the late phases. The appearance is similar to that seen in acute posterior multifocal placoid pigment epitheliopathy.[16] These seemingly conflicting fluorescence patterns in the two types of angiographic presentations may simply represent different time points in the evolutionary development of Dalen-Fuchs nodules.[17]

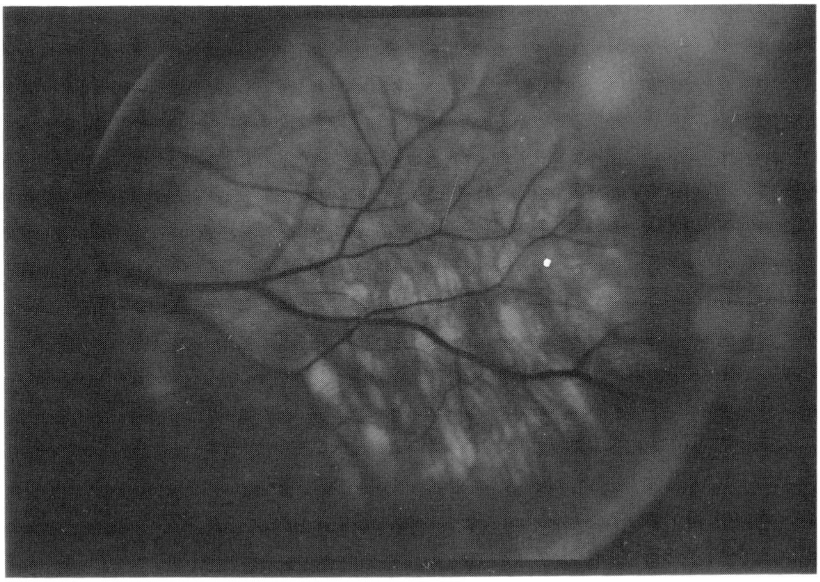

Fig. 24-1. Fundus photograph of Dalen-Fuchs nodules—small hypopigmented nodules at the level of the retinal pigment epithelium (RPE).

HISTOLOGIC FEATURES

Histopathologically, inflammatory changes are similar in both the exciting and sympathizing eyes except for features specifically associated with the original trauma.[18] Classically, the uveal tract is thickened by a diffuse lymphocytic infiltrate containing epithelioid cells and giant cells that have phagocytosed pigment. Eosinophils may be present, especially in early cases, and tend to congregate beneath Bruch's membrane.[19] Plasma cells are absent. In most cases the choriocapillaris and retina are not involved in the inflammatory response, but the inflammation often extends into the scleral emissaria[18] and may involve the optic nerve head. Retinal findings, if any, are usually limited to chronic perivascular inflammation. Debate exists as to whether the Dalen-Fuchs nodules are composed of transformed RPE cells or histiocytes that gain access to this location through breaks in Bruch's membrane (Fig. 24-2). Immunohistochemical studies indicate that Dalen-Fuchs nodules consist of a mixture of monocyte-derived cells and hyperplastic RPE cells.[20,21] Immunohistochemical studies have shown that the choroidal infiltrate seen in sympathetic ophthalmia consists predominantly of T lymphocytes with only 5% B lymphocytes,[21] supporting the theory of a T cell–mediated delayed hypersensitivity reaction.

Atypical histologic patterns have been described that include infiltration of the choriocapillaris and retina with resulting chorioretinal adhesion and scarring, similar to that described in Vogt-Koyanagi-Harada syndrome. Frequently patients with sympathetic ophthalmia show histologic findings of phaco-anaphylactic uveitis with breaks in the lens capsule. This is manifested as granulomataous inflammation surrounding the lens fibers.

ROLE OF THE PENETRATING WOUND

The presence of a penetrating injury to the globe has always been part of the classical description of sympathetic ophthalmia, but only rare cases have been reported after a nonpenetrating injury; one was a recent case following cyclocryotherapy for neovascular glaucoma with no history of prior trauma or surgery.[22] Nonetheless, an ocular penetration should always be suspected. In numerous reports, malignant melanoma associated with sympathetic ophthalmia has ultimately been shown by serial sections to be associated with occult penetrating injury.[6]

ETIOLOGY

The etiology of sympathetic ophthalmia remains unclear, but all of the currently favored hypotheses involve autoimmunity. One hypothesis

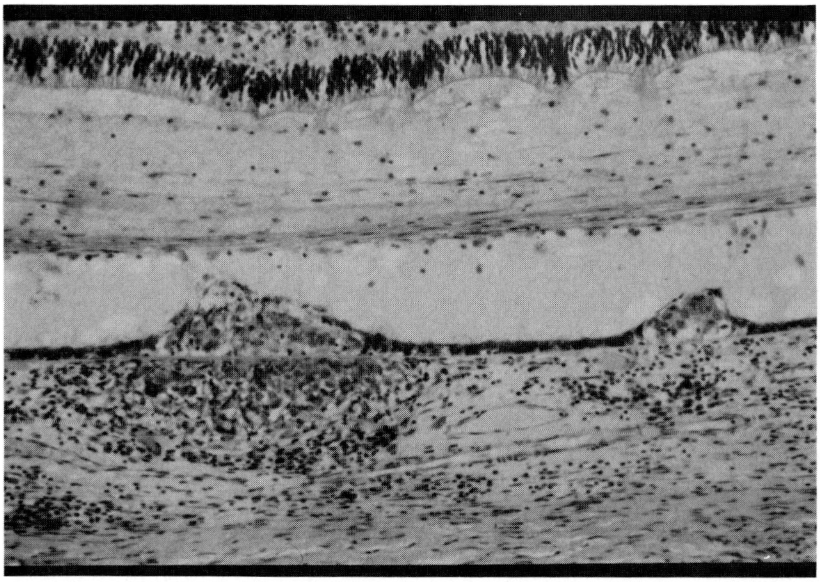

Fig. 24-2. Light photomicrograph of Dalen-Fuchs nodules. Two nodules are present and probably consist of a mixture of monocyte-derived cells and hyperplastic RPE cells. The retina is detached *(above)* and there is extensive subretinal fibrous proliferation.

holds that an infectious agent such as a virus initiates the process by causing direct cell damage or initiating antigenic change in tissue proteins of the exposed intraocular tissues.[6] The presence of a viral or similarly infective agent has not been substantiated by ultrastructural studies, but the possibility of an infectious agent cannot be ruled out.

Autoimmune disease has long been considered a possible factor in the etiology of sympathetic ophthalmia, and most investigators agree that the underlying immune pathogenesis is a delayed hypersensitivity reaction to ocular antigens. Recent immunologic studies on sympathetic ophthalmia and experimental allergic uveitis have provided new insight into the role of uveal-retinal antigens in the development of sympathetic ophthalmia. Debate continues concerning the specific uveal-retinal antigen involved, and various ocular antigens have been considered, including uveal melanin, uveal melanocytes, retinal pigment epithelium, and a retinal soluble protein called S-antigen.[23] Uveal melanin in its pure state has not been shown to be antigenic in biochemical and immunologic studies. Similarly, uveal tissue free of retinal contaminants and devoid of RPE has not produced a picture similar to that of sympathetic uveitis in experimental settings. Experimental studies have implicated S-antigen, a soluble antigen derived from the photoreceptor outer segments. The increased incidence of HLA-A11 antigen in patients with sympathetic ophthalmia suggests the possibility of a genetic predisposition to developing the disorder.[24]

DIFFERENTIAL DIAGNOSIS

Similarities to other ocular diseases can make sympathetic ophthalmia difficult to distinguish by clinical, fluorescein angiographic, or even histopathologic criteria. Causes of bilateral granulomatous uveitis should also be considered, including sarcoidosis, pars planitis, ankylosing spondylitis, Reiter's syndrome, and Behcet's disease. Careful evaluation of the patient's history and appropriate laboratory testing may exclude these possibilities. The infrequent cases in which bilateral penetrating ocular injuries occur can pose a more difficult diagnostic situation because the occurrence of prolonged or recurrent inflammation of one eye may not be attributable solely to the initial injury but rather to sympathetic ophthalmia.

There are many similarities between sympathetic ophthalmia and Vogt-Koyanagi-Harada syndrome, including the fluorescein angiographic pattern and clinical and pathologic findings. Vogt-Koyanagi-Harada syndrome is an idiopathic, bilateral, granulomatous panuveitis that occurs without a history of penetrating injury. This multisystem disease affects the eye, skin, and central nervous system, is more common in darkly pigmented individuals, and is associated with poliosis, vitiligo, alopecia, auditory defects, and signs and symptoms of meningeal irritation. Vitiligo, poliosis, and alopecia have also been noted to occur rarely in cases of sympathetic ophthalmia. Histologically, Vogt-Koyanagi-Harada syndrome characteristically involves the choriocapillaris and the retina, producing significant chorioretinal scarring, which is not typical of classic sympathetic ophthalmia, but such scarring has been reported as a chronic finding in 25% of patients with sympathetic ophthalmia.[7] The clinical distinction of these two disease processes can be difficult, but a diagnosis of sympathetic ophthalmia can usually be made based on a history of penetrating trauma.

Another entity that should be considered in the differential diagnosis is phacoanaphylactic uveitis. The frequency of phacoanaphylaxis associated with sympathetic ophthalmia has been estimated at 23% to 45%.[1,6] Phacoanaphylactic uveitis is characterized by zonal granulomatous inflammation involving the lens; it is usually unilateral, and removal of the remaining lens material usually results in improvement of the uveitis.

TREATMENT AND PROGNOSIS

Before the development of current treatment modalities, the natural history of sympathetic ophthalmia was quite variable. Most cases were complicated by recurrent episodes of acute inflammation with intervals of resolution that could last months to years. Approximately 50% of patients with untreated sympathetic ophthalmia were left with useful vision.[7] In other instances the inflammation would become chronic and ultimately lead to blindness and phthisis. With the development of corticosteroid therapy, a more predictable and favorable outcome has been attained, with approximately 65% of patients obtaining a final visual acuity of 20/60 or better.[7]

Generally, an initial dose of 100 to 160 mg of oral prednisone (or its equivalent) is given daily for the first week and then tapered based on the clinical improvement. Maintenance doses are frequently required to prevent recurrence and may ultimately lead to the well-known complications of long-term systemic steroid administration. Topical and periocular steroids are used as needed. Cases may enter a quiescent period in which steroids may be completely discontinued. Several cases of successful intraocular surgery, including cataract extraction, have been reported during such periods.[25]

In patients unresponsive to steroid treatment and in whom the use of steroids is contraindicated or results in unacceptable systemic complications, the use of immunosuppressive agents should be considered. A variety of cytotoxic agents have been used, including methotrexate, cyclophosphamide, 2-mercaptopurine, azathioprine, and chlorambucil.[26,27] These agents, when used for treating uveitis from a variety of causes, have been found effective in suppressing inflammation and in some cases result in clinical remission. Cytotoxic drugs may be given in association with corticosteroids and may reduce the corticosteroid dose needed to control the uveitis. Because the side effects of these agents include leukopenia, thrombocytopenia, anemia, GI distress, alopecia, and hepatorenal toxicity, patients must be carefully monitored for evidence of bone marrow suppression and renal or hepatic toxicity.

More recently, cyclosporin A has been used investigatively with some effectiveness in treating sympathetic ophthalmia.[28] The mode of action of cyclosporin A is different from that of other, more conventional forms of immunosuppression. Because cyclosporin A inhibits T cell function, it would seem theoretically to be of possible use in this presumed T cell–mediated disease.

Even though corticosteroids have favorably altered the natural history of the disorder, the most effective management of sympathetic ophthalmia is prevention. Immediate closure of all penetrating injuries is imperative. In cases where substantial ocular and orbital trauma has occurred, a ruptured globe should be suspected. Ultrasonography may be helpful, but in questionable cases surgical exploration of each quadrant and inspection underneath each rectus muscle are necessary to exclude the possibility of rupture. If a rupture is present, prolapsed uveal tissue should be reinserted or excised and the sclera closed as far posteriorly as possible.[29]

Enucleation of the injured eye within 2 weeks of the injury is generally considered to protect against the development of sympathetic ophthalmia in the noninjured eye.[30] Enucleation of an injured eye that is blind and painful is seldom controversial. In eyes whose visual status is in question, ultrasonography and bright-flash electroretinogram may be helpful. An injured eye that retains useful vision should not be enucleated. In fact, the injured eye can ultimately be the better-seeing eye in some cases.[8] The issue of enucleating an exciting eye after the onset of symptoms of sympathetic ophthalmia in the sympathizing eye remains quite controversial. Some investigators suggest that enucleation of the exciting eye may favorably affect the course of the sympathetic eye.[6] Other investigators believe that enucleation of the exciting eye provides no therapeutic benefit in terms of visual acuity or clinical course.[8]

References

1. Blodi FC: Sympathetic uveitis. In Freeman HM, editor: Ocular trauma, New York, 1979, Appleton-Century-Crofts, 417-427.
2. Liddy BSL and Stuart J: Sympathetic ophthalmia in Canada, Can J Ophthalmol 7:157-159, 1972.
3. Duke-Elder S and Perkins ES: Diseases of the uveal tract. In Duke-Elder S, editor: System of ophthalmology, vol 9, London, 1966, Kimpton.
4. Marak GE: Recent advances in sympathetic ophthalmia, Surv Ophthalmol 24:141-156, 1979.
5. Gass JDM: Sympathetic ophthalmia following vitrectomy, Am J Ophthalmol 92:552-558, 1982.
6. Lubin JR, Albert DM, and Weinstein M: Sixty-five years of sympathetic ophthalmia: a clinicopathologic review of 105 cases, Am J Ophthalmol 87:109-121, 1980.
7. Makley TA and Azar A: Sympathetic ophthalmia: a long-term follow-up, Arch Ophthalmol 96:257-262, 1978.
8. Winter FC: Sympathetic uveitis: a clinical and pathologic study of the visual result, Am J Ophthalmol 39:340-347 ,1955.
9. Wang WJ: Clinical and histopathological report of sympathetic ophthalmia after retinal detachment surgery, Br J Ophthalmol 67:150-152, 1983.
10. Green WR et al: Sympathetic uveitis following evisceration, Trans Am Acad Ophthalmol Otolaryngol 76:625-644, 1972.
11. Baghdassarian SA, Crawford JB, and Fine LM: Sympathetic ophthalmia following occult indirect scleral rupture, Surv Ophthalmol 14:327-329, 1970.
12. Puliafito CA et al: Sympathetic uveitis, Ophthalmology 87:355-358, 1980.
13. McPherson SD and Dalton HT: Posterior form sympathetic ophthalmia, Trans Am Ophthalmol Soc 73:251-263, 1975.
14. Dreyer WB et al: Sympathetic ophthalmia, Am J Ophthalmol 92:816-823, 1981.
15. Sharp DC et al: Sympathetic ophthalmia: histopathologic and fluorescein angiographic correlation, Arch Ophthalmol 102:232-235, 1984.
16. Lewis ML, Gass JDM, and Spencer WH: Sympathetic uveitis after trauma and vitrectomy, Arch Ophthalmol 96:263-267, 1978.
17. Reynard M, Riffenburgh RS, and Minckler DS: Morphological variation of Dalen-Fuchs nodules in sympathetic ophthalmia, Br J Ophthalmol 69:197-201, 1985.
18. Easom HA and Zimmerman LE: Sympathetic ophthalmia and bilateral phacoanaphylaxis: a clinicopathologic correlation of the sympathogenic and sympathizing eyes, Arch Ophthalmol 72:9-15, 1964.
19. Spencer WH: Autoimmune diseases. In Spencer WH, editor: Ophthalmic pathology: an atlas and textbook, vol. 3, Philadelphia, 1986, WB Saunders, 1913-1956.
20. Chan CC et al: Sympathetic ophthalmia: immunopathological findings, Ophthalmology 93:690-695, 1986.
21. Jakobiec FA et al: Human sympathetic ophthalmia: an analysis of the inflammatory infiltrate by hybridoma–monoclonal antibodies, immunochemistry, and correlative electron microscopy, Ophthalmology 90:76-95, 1983.
22. Sabates R: Choroiditis compatible with the histopathologic diagnosis of sympathetic ophthalmia following cyclocryotherapy of neovascular glaucoma, Ophthalmic Surg 19:176-182, 1988.
23. Rao NA and Wong VG: Aetiology of sympathetic ophthalmitis, Trans Ophthalmol Soc UK 101:357-360, 1981.
24. Reynard M et al: Histocompatibility antigens in sympathetic ophthalmia, Am J Ophthalmol 95:216-221, 1983.
25. Raynard M and Minckler DS: Cataract extraction in the sympathizing eye, Arch Ophthalmol 101:1701-1703, 1983.
26. Andrasch RH, Pirofsky B, and Burns RP: Immunosuppressive therapy for severe chronic uveitis, Arch Ophthalmol 96:247-251, 1978.
27. Godfrey WA et al: The use of chlorambucil in intractable idiopathic uveitis, Am J Ophthalmol 78:415-428, 1974.
28. Nussenblatt RB, Palestine AG, and Chan CC: Cyclosporin A therapy in the treatment of intraocular inflammatory disease resistant to systemic corticosteroids and cytotoxic agents, Am J Ophthalmol 96:275-282, 1983.
29. Charles NC: Sympathetic ophthalmia, Adv Ophthalmic Plast Reconstr Surg 7:239-245, 1988.
30. Reynard M, Riffenburgh RS, and Maes EF: Effect of corticosteroids treatment and enucleation on the visual prognosis of sympathetic ophthalmia, Am J Ophthalmol 96:290-294, 1983.

PART 4

Orbital and adnexal trauma

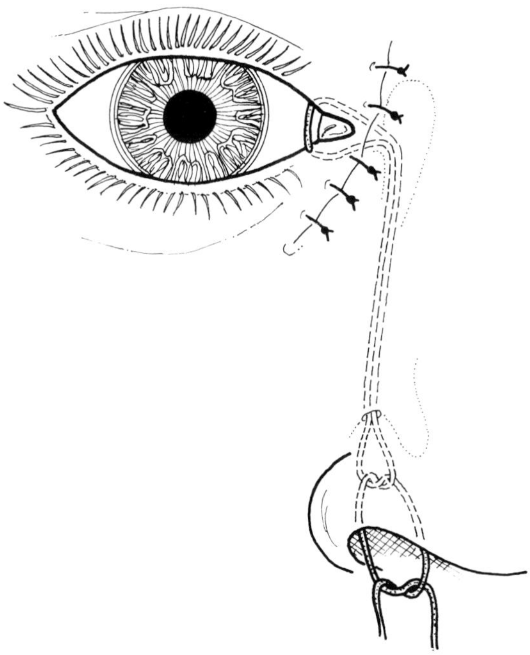

CHAPTER 25

Anatomy of the orbit and ocular adnexa

GEORGE O. STASIOR
BRADLEY N. LEMKE

- Soft tissue anatomy
  - Facial soft tissues
    - Sensory innervation
    - Arterial supply
    - Venous supply
    - Lymphatic supply
    - Muscles of facial expression
    - Facial motor nerves
  - Eyebrow and eyelids
    - Eyebrow
    - Eyelid topography
    - Orbicularis oculi
    - Lateral retinaculum
    - Orbital septum
    - Orbital fat
    - Anterior and posterior lamella
    - Eyelid margin
    - Lacrimal excretory system
- Osteology
  - Orbital dimensions
  - Orbital rim
  - Orbital walls
  - Paraorbital sinuses
- Orbit
  - Periorbita
  - Lacrimal gland
  - Orbital fascia
  - Orbital vessels
  - Orbital nerves
  - Extraocular muscles
  - Orbital imaging
- References

An understanding of orbital and ocular adnexal anatomy is essential to managing trauma to these areas. Familiarity with orbital anatomy will both facilitate recognition of structural injury and guide surgical repair.

SOFT TISSUE ANATOMY

Facial Soft Tissues

Examination of the patient with ocular or adnexal trauma begins with examination of the soft tissues of the face. The extent of the trauma to these tissues depends on the severity, type, and location of the injury and the degree of functional and cosmetic disruption. Careful attention must be paid to degree of symmetry. Asymmetry is often a clue to functional abnormality or deeper bony disruption. Important structures in the facial soft tissues include sensory and motor cutaneous nerves, superficial and deep arteries and veins, lymphatics of the head and neck, and muscles of facial expression.

Sensory Innervation

Cranial nerve V, the trigeminal nerve, comprises three major divisions, which are responsible for sensory input from the three major derma-

All figures for this chapter have been borrowed with permission from Lemke BN: Anatomy of the ocular adnexa and orbit. In Smith BC and others, editors: Ophthalmic plastic and reconstructive surgery, St Louis, 1987, CV Mosby. Medical illustrator: Virginia Hoyt Cantarella.

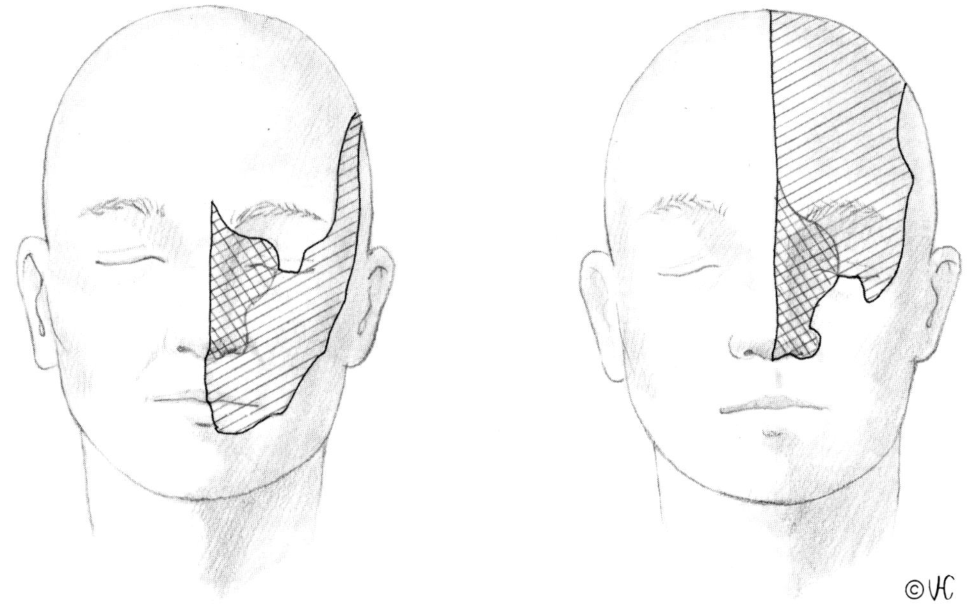

Fig. 25-1. Cutaneous distribution of the fifth cranial nerve, maxillary *(left)* and ophthalmic *(right)* divisions.

tomes of the face. The frontal nerve of the ophthalmic division (V_1) branches into the supratrochlear, infratrochlear, supraorbital, and lacrimal branches of the ophthalmic division and supplies sensory information from the upper lid. Sensation from the nose is supplied by this division through the supratrochlear and infratrochlear nerves and nasal branches. The maxillary division of the trigeminal nerve (V_2) is responsible for sensory information from the lower lid via the infraorbital nerve and the branches of the zygomaticofacial nerve. Disruption of the infraorbital nerve during an orbital floor fracture may result in numbness involving the ipsilateral cheek and maxillary teeth. Together, divisions V_1 and V_2 cover over two thirds of the facial cutaneous distribution (Fig. 25-1). Most of the facial innervation for the mandibular division of the trigeminal nerve (V_3) arises from the facial anastomotic branch of the auriculotemporal nerve and the mental nerve at the chin. The mandibular division also supplies the anterior-superior portion of the external ear.

Arterial Supply

The superficial and deep arteries of the face originate from the external carotid artery. The external carotid courses beneath the digastric and sphenohyaloid muscles, curves over the surface of the submandibular gland, and proceeds to the angle of the eye, terminating as the angular artery (Fig. 25-2). The branches of the facial artery also include the inferolabial, superolabial, lateral nasal, and muscular arteries. The maxillary artery is another large branch of the external carotid artery.

Venous Supply

The deep and superficial veins of the face are a vast and complex network. Beginning at the supratrochlear vein in the middle of the scalp and forehead, they descend to the medial angle of the eye, where they join the supraorbital vein to form the angular vein (Fig. 25-3). Communications of the angular vein course beneath the facial muscles and over the masseter muscles to join branches of the retromandibular vein. Together they form the common facial vein. The superficial temporal vein descends preauricularly to join first the maxillary vein and then the retromandibular vein. There are communications between anterior facial veins and the pterygoid plexus through the deep facial vein. Finally, the facial and posterior auricular veins drain into the external jugular vein.

Lymphatic Supply

The lymphatic drainage system of the face involves vessels from the scalp, eyelids, cheeks, and lips, with regional lymph node drainage areas (Fig. 25-4). Medial lymphatics of the eyelids and conjunctiva follow the anterior facial veins to the submandibular nodes. The lateral group drains the remainder of the lids to the

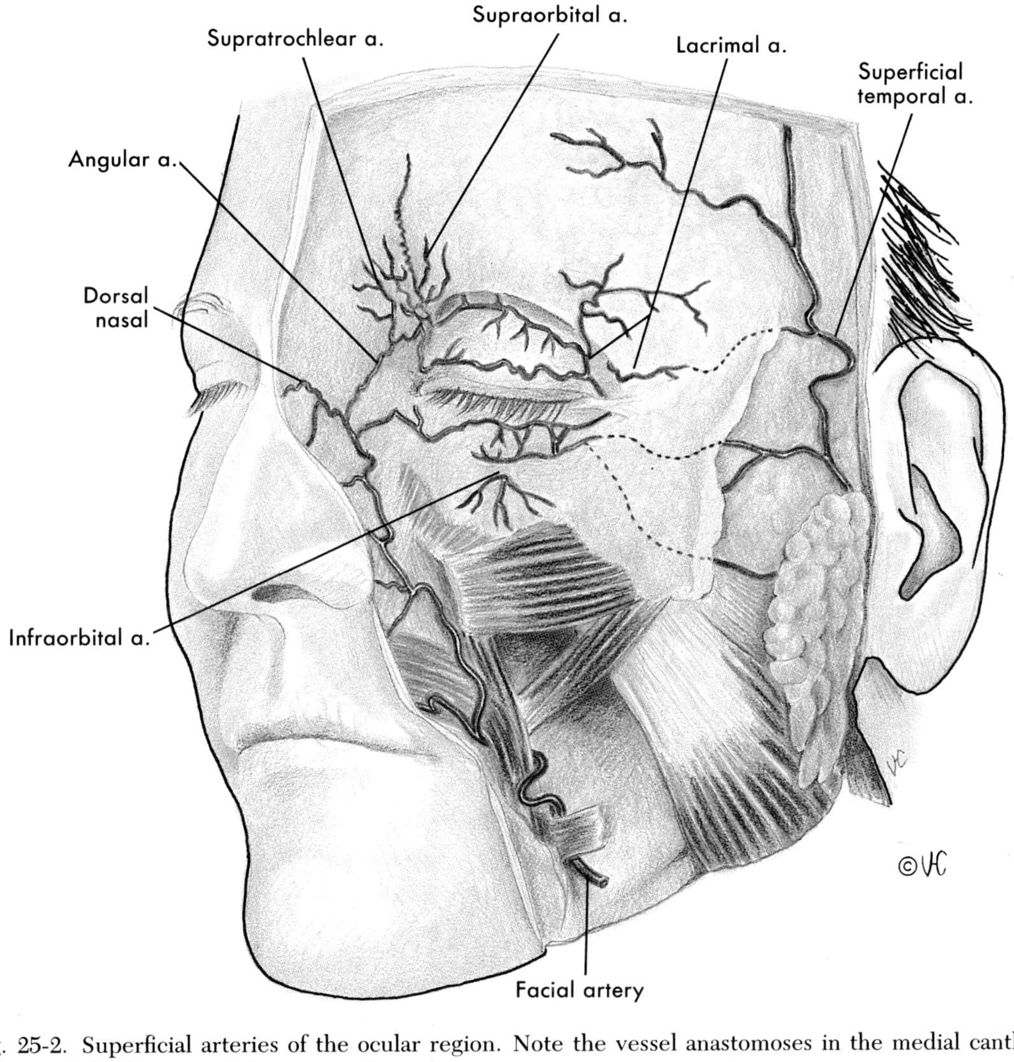

Fig. 25-2. Superficial arteries of the ocular region. Note the vessel anastomoses in the medial canthal region and the location of the marginal arcades.

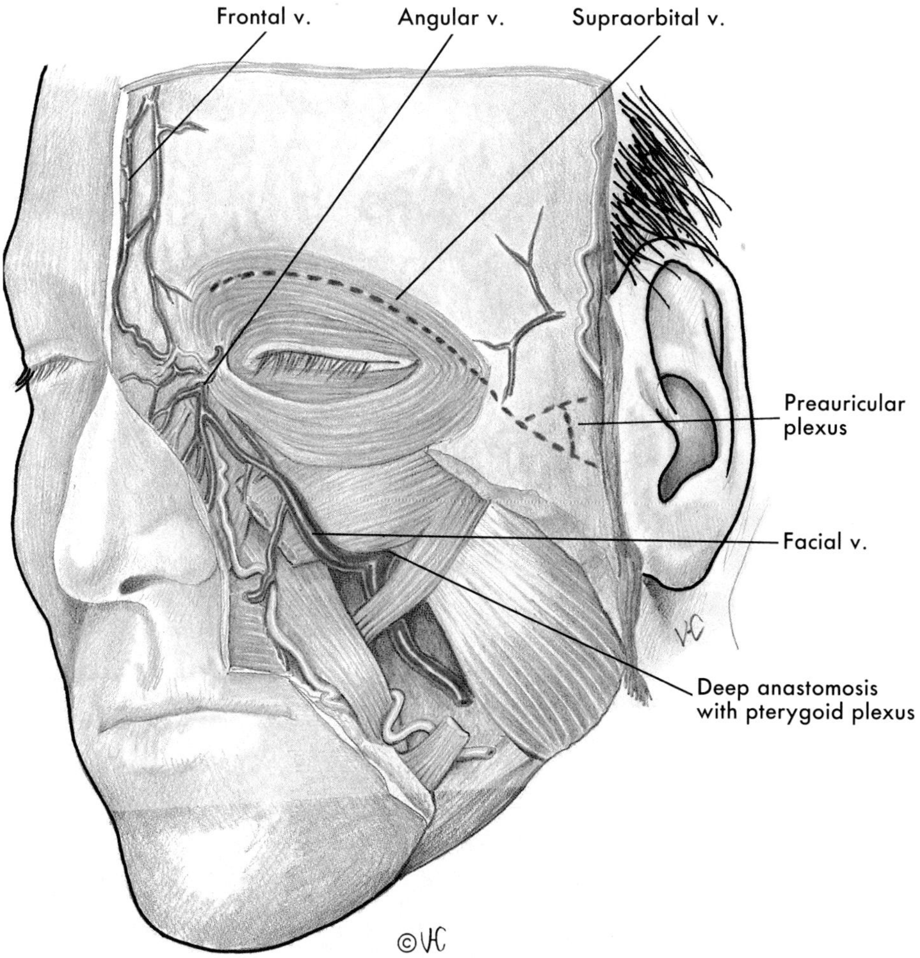

Fig. 25-3. The superficial veins of the ocular region. The angular vein communicates superficially with frontal and facial veins and joins horizontally with the supraorbital vein beneath the orbicularis to become the superior ophthalmic vein after piercing the orbital septum.

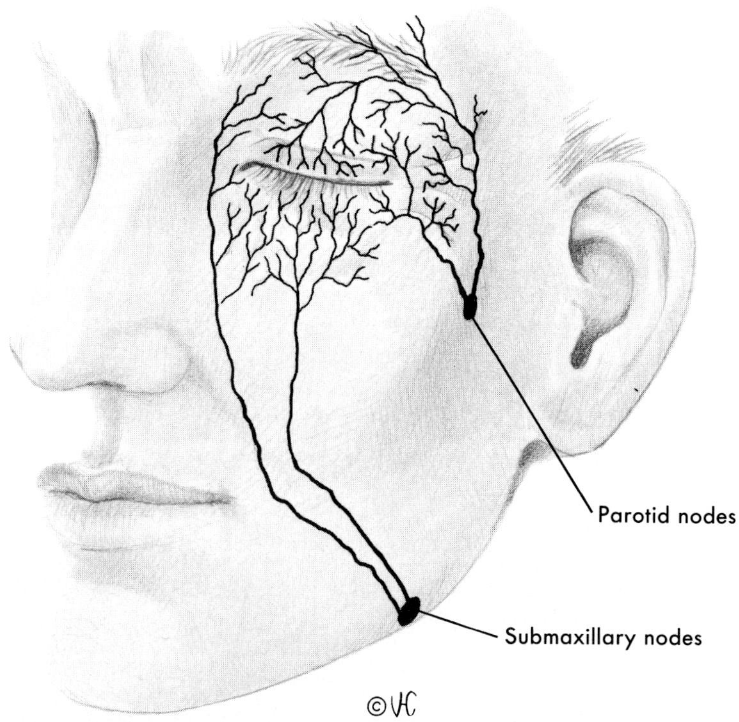

Fig. 25-4. Lymphatic drainage of the eyelids.

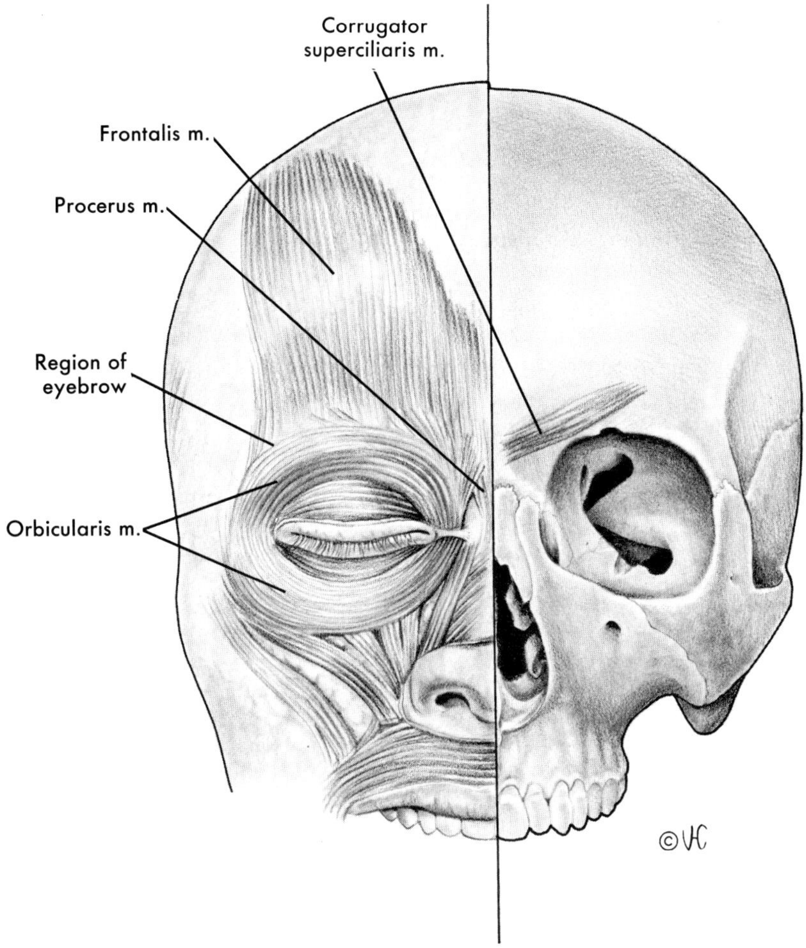

Fig. 25-5. Superficial muscles of facial expression.

superficial parotid lymph nodes in the preauricular area. The cheeks drain to the parotid and submandibular nodes. The side of the nose and the upper and lateral lip drain to the submandibular nodes alone. The medial lower lip drains to the submental nodes. Temporal and infratemporal fossa areas drain into the deep facial and cervical nodes.

It is classically held that there are no lymphatic nodes or vessels in the orbit. Principal drainage accompanies the vessels through the inferior orbital fissure to the internal maxillary or deep cervical nodes. Studies in orbital lymphatic drainage have involved injecting dye into the retrobulbar space.[1] Lymphatic drainage to bilateral deep cervical nodes, with minor concentrations in the ipsilateral superficial cervical mandibular nodes, has been noted.[2]

Muscles of Facial Expression

The muscles of facial expression are cutaneous muscles (Fig. 25-5). They lie on superficial fascia, arising from either bone or fascia and inserting into the skin. They may act separately or in groups.

The muscles that raise the eyebrows and wrinkle the forehead, as in surprise, are the frontalis and the occipitalis. The orbicularis oculi, the protractor muscle of the eyelid, closes the eyelids. The corrugator muscle draws the eyebrows downward and medially in a frowning manner. In the midface the cheek is spanned by the zygomatic major and minor muscles and the levator labii superioris. The zygomaticus minor muscle and the levator labii superioris form the nasolabial fold (see Fig. 25-9). The zygomaticus major muscle draws the angle of the mouth up and back when laughing. Damage to the facial nerve or its branches may produce variable amounts of weakness in the muscles of facial expression.

Facial Motor Nerves

The facial nerve, cranial nerve VII, is a large voluntary motor nerve with a mix of sensory and parasympathetic fibers. It leaves the cranial fossa with the acoustic nerve (VIII) through the internal acoustic meatus. It enters the facial canal, passing laterally and posterior to the medial wall of the tympanic cavity. The facial nerve exits the skull through the stylomastoid foramen and then runs rostrally in the parotid gland. Branches supply the stylohyoid, the posterior belly of the digastric muscle, and all the muscles of expression. The muscles of facial expression are supplied through five designated branches: temporal, zygomatic, buccal, mandibular, and cervical (Fig. 25-6). Taste in the anterior two thirds of the tongue is supplied by the facial nerve via the chorda tympani. Loss of taste in this region indicates an injury to the chorda tympani nerve or to the facial nerve in the posterior facial canal.

Eyebrow and Eyelids

The eyebrow and eyelids represent a functional cosmetic structure for protecting the eye. Integrity of their function is essential.

Eyebrow

The eyebrow is an area of the superficial muscle plane where the frontalis and the orbicularis interdigitate.[3] Eyebrows have a characteristic distribution of hair that is important for facial expression and cosmesis. The eyebrows overlie

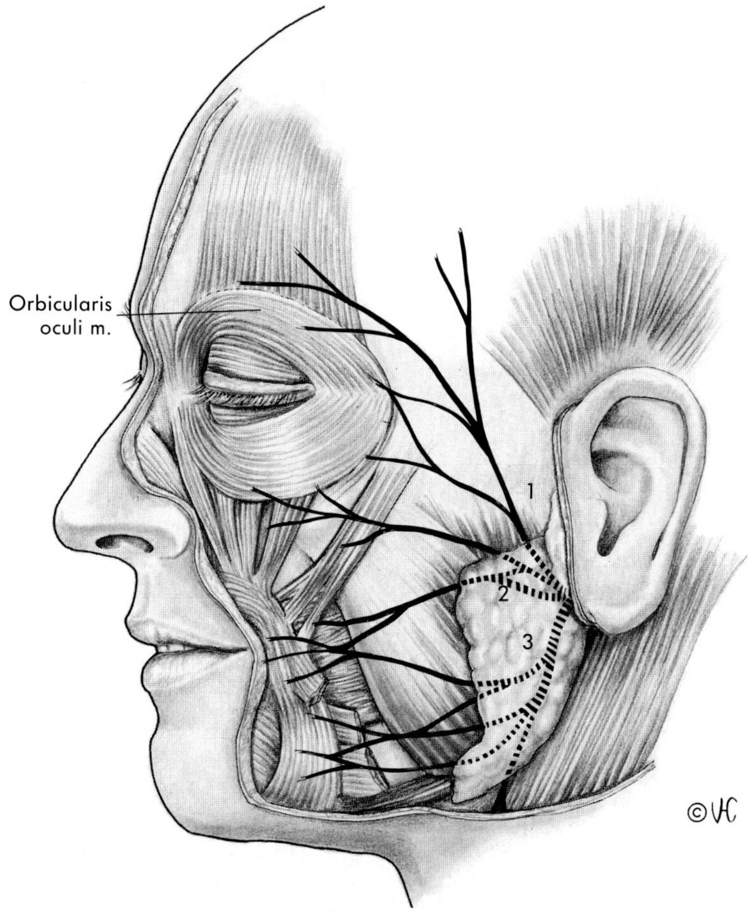

Fig. 25-6. Superficial seventh cranial nerve. *1*, Temporal, *2*, zygomatic, and *3*, cervical facial with three divisions: buccal, mandibular, and cervical.

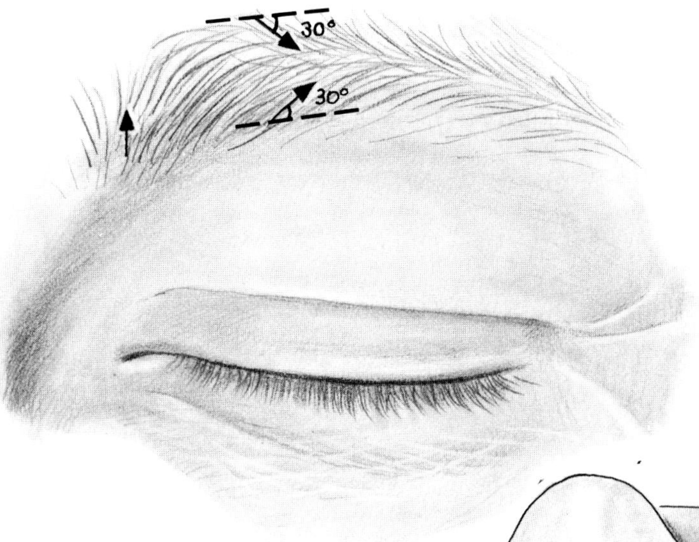

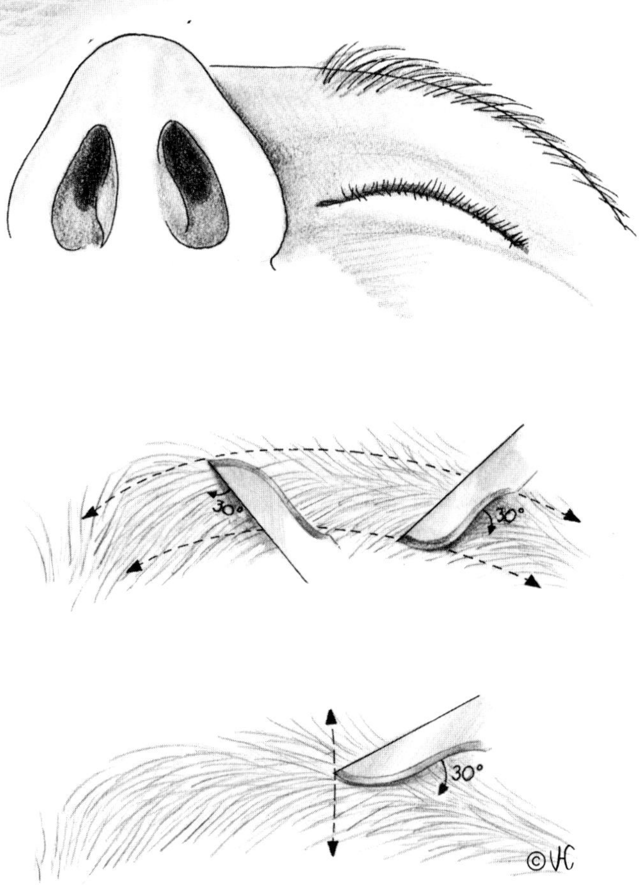

Fig. 25-7. Hair direction in adult eyebrow. Hair angulation is about 30° downward from vertical in the upper eyebrow and 30° upward in the lower eyebrow, with an abrupt reversal at the center of the brow. This reversal does not occur at the medial end of the eyebrow where the hair sweeps upward uninterrupted from below. Hair also angles laterally, at least 30° from vertical. Horizontal and vertical eyebrow hair angulations coincident to about 30° serve as useful "rule of thumb" for surgeon making incisions in this area.

the frontal sinuses nasally and the frontal bone centrally and extend temporally to the zygomatical-frontal suture.

Eyebrow skin is thick and full of sebaceous and sweat glands. There are large hair follicles between the inserting muscle fibers. The direction of hair in the adult eyebrow is angulated differently in the upper and lower eyebrow[4] (Fig. 25-7). Between the medial extension of the eyebrows, the intersupraciliary region is known as the glabella.

The frontalis muscle contracts to elevate the eyebrow. Depression of the eyebrow is caused by contraction of the orbicularis oculi corrugator and procerus muscles. Contraction of the corrugator superciliaris muscle alone (Fig. 25-5) de-

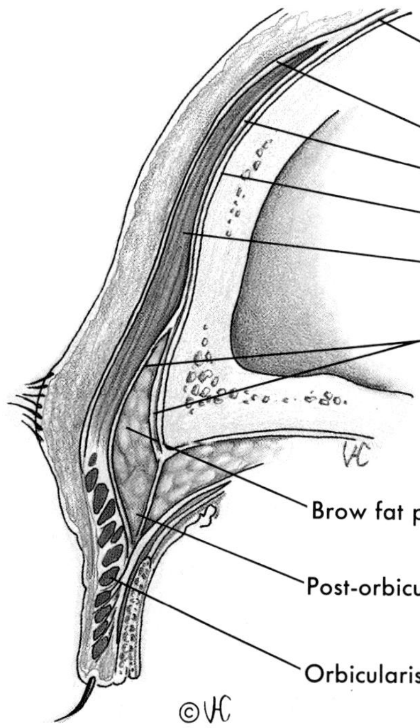

Fig. 25-8. Relationship of galea aponeurotica, frontalis muscle, and brow fat pad.

presses the medial eyebrow and pulls the eyebrows together. The procerus muscle overlies the glabella and is continuous with the frontalis. The frontalis muscle is surrounded by the galea, which splits to form a superficial and a deep layer.[5] The galea aponeurotica is connected to the occipitalis, auricular, and frontalis muscles. The deep galea is the posterior muscle sheath for the frontalis and orbicularis and divides to encompass the fat pad of the eyebrow (Fig. 25-8). The posterior investment of the eyebrow fat pad is a fibrous layer that continues inferiorly into the orbit as the superior orbital septum. The lateral one third of the brow is frequently involved in eyebrow ptosis because of the lack of firm attachment to the frontal bone in this region and the scarcity of frontalis muscle laterally.

Eyelid Topography

The eyelids have a characteristic symmetrical superficial anatomy (Fig. 25-9). This may be disrupted by trauma, and comparison with the undisturbed anatomy of the other side may be the key to finding superficial symmetrical landmarks. Vertically, the palpebral fissure measures approximately 12 mm in an adult. The highest point of the lower eyelid is slightly temporal. The distance between the medial and lateral commissures of the eyelid is approximately 30 mm. The distance from the medial canthus to the midline of the nose should be approximately 15 mm. Trauma to the medial canthal area may result in medial tendon laceration, leading to unilateral telecanthus (lateral displacement of the medial canthus).[6] Damage to the lacrimal outflow system should also be suspected in this setting.

The upper eyelid crease, which is approximately 8 to 10 mm above the eyelid margin, is formed by the superficial attachment of the levator aponeurosis into the subcutaneous tissue. This fusion occurs below the orbital septum. In Occidentals, the cutaneous insertion is higher than in Orientals, in whom the superior orbital septum inserts in the aponeurosis at a lower level, a few millimeters from the eyelid margin. The superior sulcus is the area between the upper eyelid crease and the superior orbital margin. Herniated orbital fat can be seen as a bulge in this area, and orbital volume loss causes deepening of the sulcus.

The lower eyelid crease, when present, is 4 to 5 mm below the margin, sloping inferiorly and temporally. A prominent malar fold accentuates the rise of the cheek and is contiguous

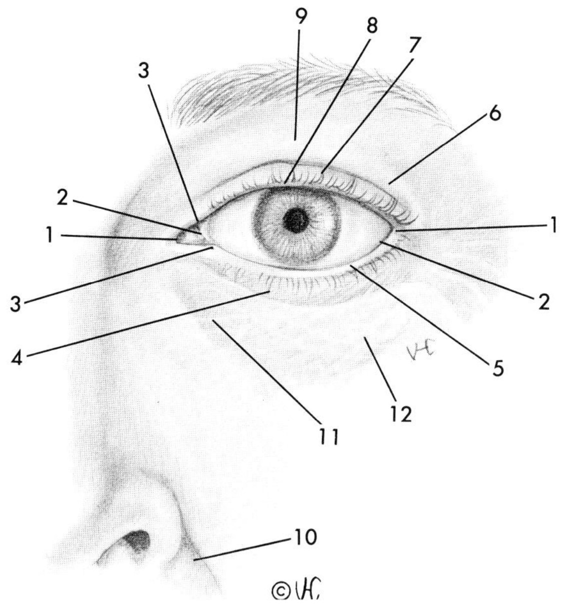

Fig. 25-9. Topographic eyelid anatomy. *1*, Commissures, *2*, canthal angles, medial and lateral, *3*, puncta, *4*, inferior lid crease, *5*, lowest point of curve, *6*, superior eyelid skin fold, *7*, superior orbital sulcus, *8*, highest point of curve, *9*, superior orbital sulcus, *10*, nasolabial fold, *11*, nasojugular fold, *12*, malar fold.

medially with the nasojugular fold (Fig. 25-9). Beneath this fold run the angular vessels.

The skin of the medial upper eyelid is some of the thinnest in the body. The skin in the preseptal portion of the eyelid is loose in texture and has fine attachments to the subcutaneous tissues. The pretarsal skin, however, is attached directly to the underlying orbicularis muscle by connective tissue devoid of fat. There is an abrupt transition from eyelid skin to the thick skin of the eyebrow and malar region. With edema, fluid swells the eyelid tissues with a specific border at these junctions. This thin skin and the fine connective tissue connections allow distensibility of the eyelids following trauma.

Orbicularis Oculi

The orbicularis oculi muscle is divided into three sections: orbital, preseptal, and pretarsal (Fig. 25-10). This superficial muscle inserts deep within the orbital rim medially and laterally. Superiorly, the orbital portion extends into the region of the eyebrow. Laterally, the orbital portion lies anterior to the temporalis muscle and

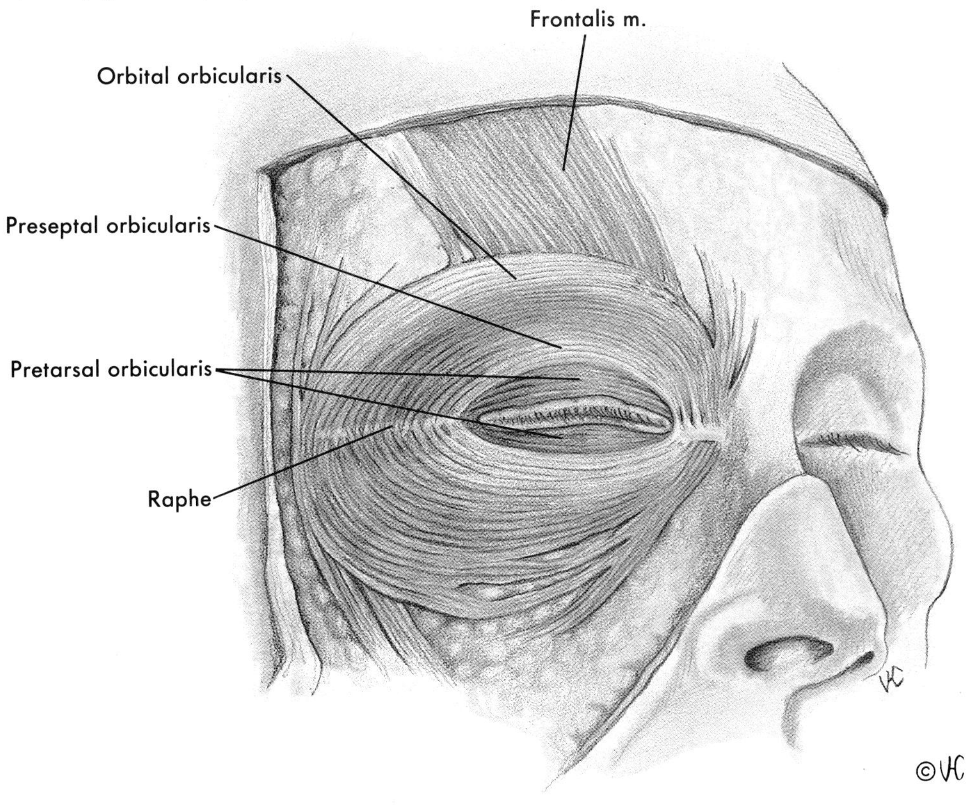

Fig. 25-10. Superficial orbicularis oculi muscle.

extends into the cheek. Fibers also extend into the medial canthal tendon.

The preseptal and pretarsal orbicularis combine to form the palpebral portion of the orbicularis muscle. The pretarsal orbicularis is tightly inherent to the tarsus. The preseptal orbicularis inserts directly into the skin of the inferior nasal part of the lid, causing vertical wrinkles when the skin is pulled medially. When the eyes are squeezed shut, the preseptal layer overrides the pretarsal layers. The preseptal part of the orbicularis oculi overlies the orbital septum, is similar in the upper and lower lids, and arises from the medial canthal tendons and from deep attachments to the lacrimal crest.

The pretarsal muscle has a superficial head, which forms the anterior limb of the medial canthal tendon, and a deep head, known as Horner's muscle, which attaches to the posterior lacrimal crest. The anterior head lies anterior to the canaliculus, and the posterior head passes deep to insert in the lacrimal sac fascia. Directly beneath the anterior portion of the medial canthal tendon is a lacrimal canaliculus, which may be involved in injuries of this area. Injury to the medial canthal tendon may disrupt Horner's muscle, creating negative pressure in the lacrimal sac with lid closure. Weakening of this lacrimal pump mechanism can cause epiphora, despite a normal punctum position.[7]

Lateral Retinaculum

Eyelid trauma can disrupt the lateral retinaculum. Beneath the orbicularis oculi muscle lie the periosteum of the orbital rim and the lateral canthal tendon. The latter is formed by fusion of the pretarsal orbicularis muscle from the upper and lower eyelids.[8] In this area the tendon is approximately 2 mm wide and 6 to 7 mm long. The tendon splits, sending one leaf anteriorly in close association with the lateral rim periosteum. The posterior leaf inserts at the lateral orbital tubercle of Whitnall, approximately 2 to 4 mm behind the lateral rim[9] (Fig. 25-11). The structures that attach to the lateral orbital tubercle with the lateral canthal tendon include the lateral horn of the levator aponeurosis, the suspensory ligament of Lockwood, the lateral rectus muscle check ligament, and the orbital septum and fascia.[2]

Orbital Septum

The orbital septum is the anatomic boundary between the orbita and the superficial muscle plane of the orbicularis oculi. It originates from the arcus marginalis, a white fibrous band at the bony orbit margin. Medially, the septum interrupts into an anterior leaf along the anterior lacrimal crest and a posterior leaf that covers Horner's muscle and inserts to the posterior lacrimal crest. Because of its posterior nasal detachment, the lacrimal fossa and sac lie outside the confines of the orbit. The orbital septum is firmly attached to the arcus marginalis in the superior, inferior, and lateral quadrants.

In the lower lid the orbital septum fuses with the capsulopalpebral fascia 4 to 5 mm below the lower tarsal border to form a single fascial layer with its insertion at the base of the tarsus.[10] In the upper lid the superior orbital septum cannot reach the superior tarsal plate. The intervening aponeurosis meets the septum 10 mm above the superior eyelid margin, helping to form the upper lid crease. The orbital septum (Fig. 25-12) keeps the orbital fat within the orbit.

Orbital Fat

Classically, orbital fat pad pockets have been described as two pockets in the upper lid, one medial and one central, and three pockets in the lower lid.[11] When the orbital septum of the upper lid is reflected, the preaponeurotic fat is seen to be separated from the nasal fat pad by fascia continuous with the trochlear region (Fig. 25-13). Medial and inferior to this trochlear region is the infratrochlear nerve and the terminal branch of the ophthalmic artery. The preaponeurotic fat pad is seen more centrally. Behind the preaponeurotic fascia lies the levator palpebrae superioris muscle complex. Lateral to the preaponeurotic fat pad is the orbital portion of the lacrimal gland.

Although three distinct fat pockets in the lower lid have not been demonstrated anatomically,[12] it is useful clinically to consider three separate fat areas, with middle and medial pockets herniating forward on each side of the inferior oblique muscle (Fig. 25-13). Anterior to the septum is a loose alveolar tissue known as the suborbicularis oris fascia.[13]

Anterior and Posterior Lamellae

In planning eyelid reconstruction following trauma or surgery, it is convenient to divide the upper eyelid into anterior and posterior lamellae. The anterior lamella consists of skin and the orbicularis muscle with associated vascular structures. The marginal artery is approximately

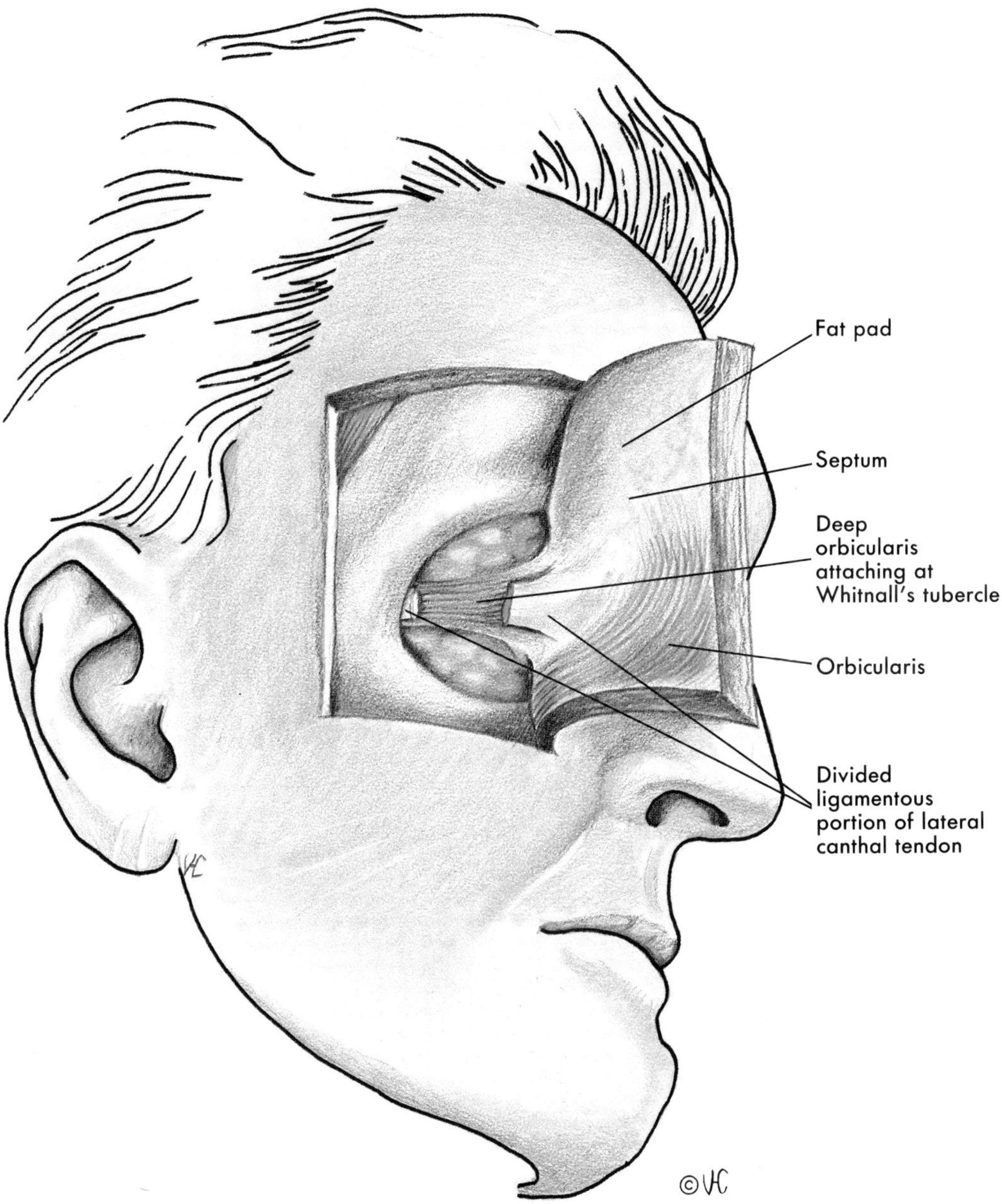

Fig. 25-11. Deep lateral canthal structures. The superficial muscle plan is partly reflected medially. The superficial head of the lateral canthal ligament (tendon) has been divided to show the deep orbicularis (lateral canthal tendon) inserting on Whitnall's tubercle.

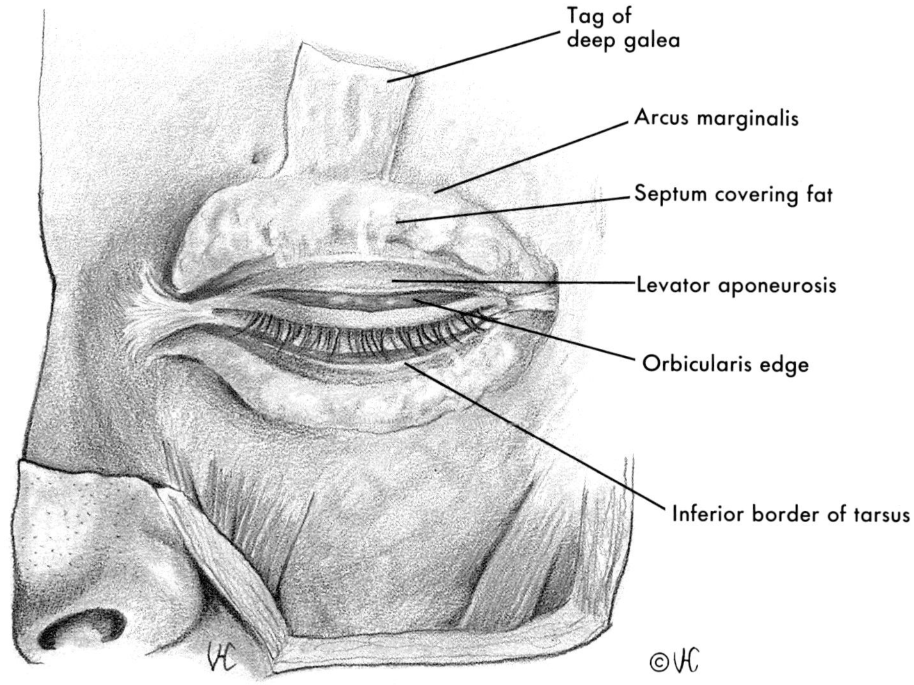

Fig. 25-12. Orbital septum. Superficial and deep orbicularis heads have been removed. A tag of deep galea, which forms the posterior border of the eyebrow fat pad, has been left to show its continuity with the orbital septum. The anterior limit of the septum is the postorbicularis fascia, deep to the orbicularis muscle.

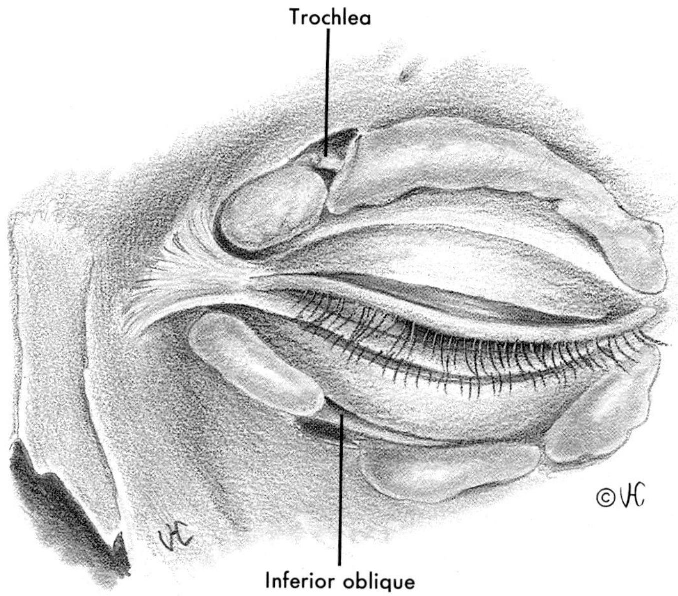

Fig. 25-13. Anterior orbital fat seen after removal of orbital septum. Deep dissection of the orbital fat pad shows the trochlea dividing the fat pad in the upper lid. Fascial attachments from inferior oblique muscle presumably serve to divide the large medial fat pad into two herniations, seen clinically in the lower eyelid.

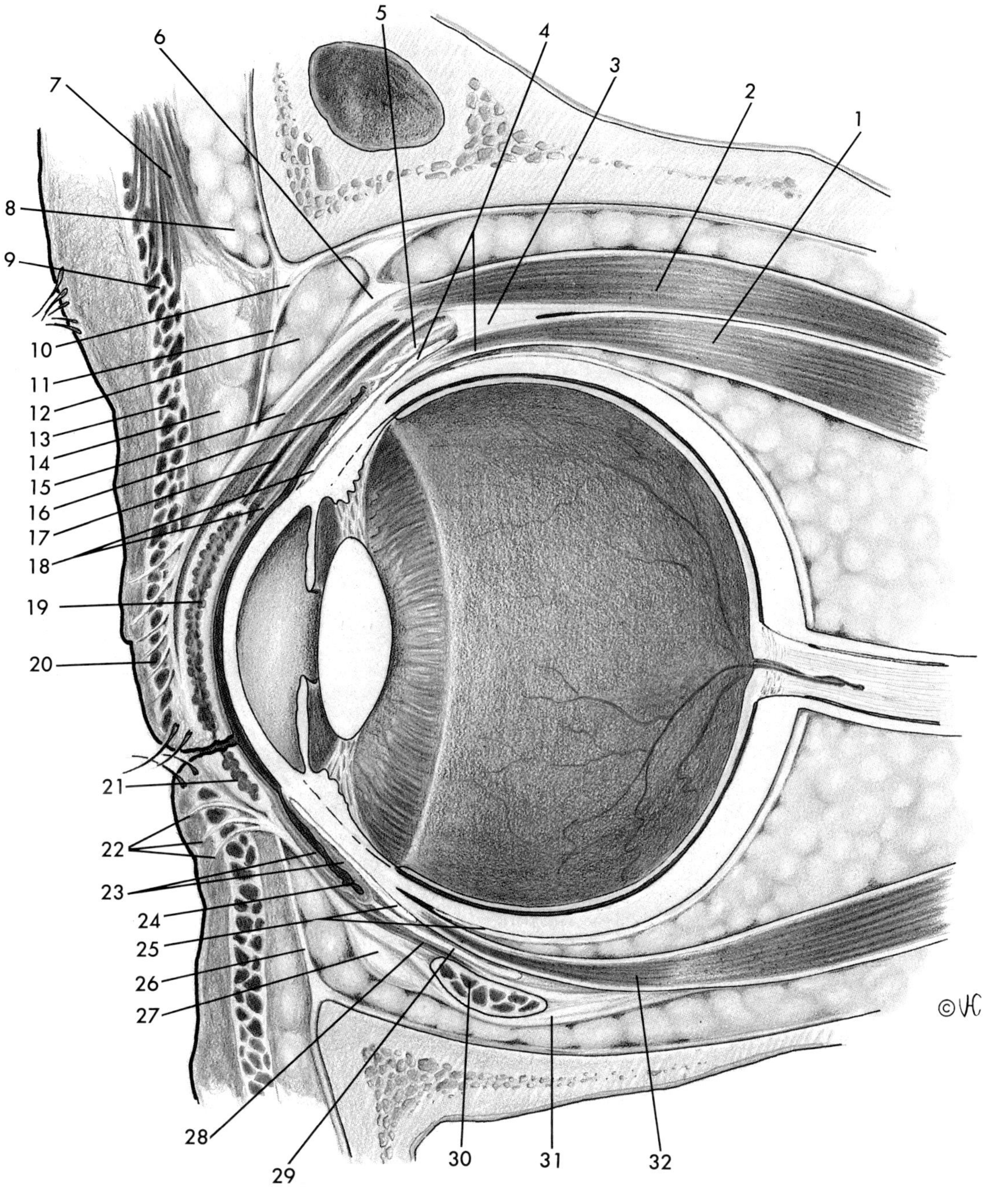

Fig. 25-14. Parasagittal section showing anterior orbital structures. *1,* Superior rectus muscle (SRM), *2,* levator muscle, *3,* conjoining of SRM with levator muscle sheath, *4,* Tenon's capsule, *5,* suspensory ligament of superior fornix, *6,* Whitnall's ligament, *7,* frontalis muscle, *8,* brow fat pad, *9,* orbital orbicularis, *10,* arcus marginalis, *11,* orbital septum, *12,* aponeurotic fat pad, *13,* preseptal orbicularis, *14,* postorbicularis fascia, *15,* levator aponeurosis, *16,* superior conjunctival fornix, *17,* Müller's muscle, *18,* conjunctiva, *19,* superior tarsus, *20,* pretarsal orbicularis, *21,* inferior tarsus, *22,* musculocutaneous retractor insertion, *23,* conjunctiva, *24,* inferior conjunctival fornix, *25,* Tenon's capsule, *26,* inferior septum, *27,* Lockwood's ligament, *28,* inferior tarsal muscle, *29,* suspensory ligament of inferior fornix, *30,* inferior oblique muscle, *31,* capsulopalpebral fascia, *32,* inferior rectus muscle.

3 mm above the lid margin. The posterior lamella consists of the levator aponeurosis, Müller's muscle, tarsus, and conjunctiva (Fig. 25-14). The levator muscle and its aponeurosis make up a complex that is the primary levator of the upper lid. Any horizontal laceration of the upper lid may injure the aponeurosis and should be suspected of having done so until proven otherwise.[14] The aponeurosis courses anteriorly to insert on the lower two thirds of the anterior tarsal plate. The levator muscle arises from the lesser wing of the sphenoid above the annulus of Zinn. Its origin is adjacent to the superior oblique muscle and above the superior rectus muscle (see Fig. 25-21). The levator muscle complex extends for approximately 65 mm through the superior orbit; the rectus muscle is approximately 45 mm long. The levator complex traverses anteriorly in the superior orbit with the supraorbital artery, the frontal nerve, and the trochlear nerve. The levator muscle supplies an origin for Müller's muscle, a nonstriated, sympathetically innervated elevator of the upper lid.

In the upper lid, Müller's muscle inserts into the superior border of the tarsus (Fig. 25-14). In the lower lid, the inferior tarsal muscle (a sympathetically innervated muscle) does not insert directly into the inferior tarsus but is a few millimeters away from its inferior border.[10] Müller's muscle arises 20 to 22 mm above the superior tarsal border. It may be easily separated from the levator muscle as it approaches the tarsus, forming the potential postaponeurotic space. Interruption of sympathetic innervation from the superior cervical ganglion will produce approximately 2 mm of blepharoptosis. The precise anatomic course of innervation for Müller's muscle remains poorly understood.

Müller's muscle and the levator aponeurotic complex are considered the eyelid retractors. In addition to its palpebral insertion, the aponeurosis extends into a broad fiber sheet that inserts behind the medial and lateral commissures of the lids. Laterally, this forms the lateral horn, incompletely dividing the lacrimal glands into two lobes (see Fig. 25-21). The medial horn is "filmy" and passes over the reflection of the superior oblique tendon as it reaches the medial canthal area. The transition between the levator muscle and its aponeurosis occurs at approximately the superior transverse ligament of Whitnall.

Whitnall's superior transverse ligament can be found by tracing 14 to 20 mm posterior from the anterior inferior tarsal border[15] (see Fig. 25-21). Whitnall's ligament is an intermuscular fascial condensation between the levator and the superior rectus muscles. It checks the posterior movement of the levator and provides longitudinal support.[2] Although the ligament does not offer a vertical fulcrum for the levator palpebrae superioris muscle, its damage may lead to upper eyelid dysfunction.

In the lower eyelid, Lockwood's ligament is the analog to Whitnall's ligament. The integrity of this ligament plays a direct role in lower eyelid position and the development of globe ptosis. When managing eyelid trauma, care should be taken to preserve these supportive transverse eyelid ligaments.

The conjunctiva and tarsus, with the eyelid retractors, comprise the posterior lamella of the eyelid. The superior portion of the conjunctiva is about 13 mm from the open eyelid margin and 20 to 25 mm from the closed eyelid margin. The inferior fornix reflection is 10 mm from the lower eyelid margin. The conjunctiva of the superior and inferior fornices is loosely attached to the underlying tissues and can become markedly swollen in trauma. The conjunctival epithelium contains numerous unicellular mucus glands, known as goblet cells. Goblet cells secrete mucin, one of the layers of the tear film responsible for proper wetting of the corneal epithelium. Accessory lacrimal glands located in the conjunctiva's substantia propria, particularly in the fornices,[16] are also important in maintaining a normal tear film. It is thus important to preserve as much viable conjunctival tissue as possible in patients sustaining eyelid trauma. In addition, scarring of the fornices may cause eyelid margin abnormalities and eyelid malposition, including cicatricial entropion.

The tarsus is one of the main elements that give structural integrity to the upper and lower eyelids (Fig. 25-15). The shape of the superior tarsal plate is that of a *D* laid on its side; the lower plate is an elongated band. The upper plate is 10 to 12 mm broad at the center; the lower tarsal plate is 4 to 5 mm wide throughout. The tarsus is thickest at the ciliary border, approximately 1 mm in the center, and tapers off toward the borders. The superior tarsus is covered in front by the terminal fibers of the levator aponeurosis. The inferior plate is covered by the

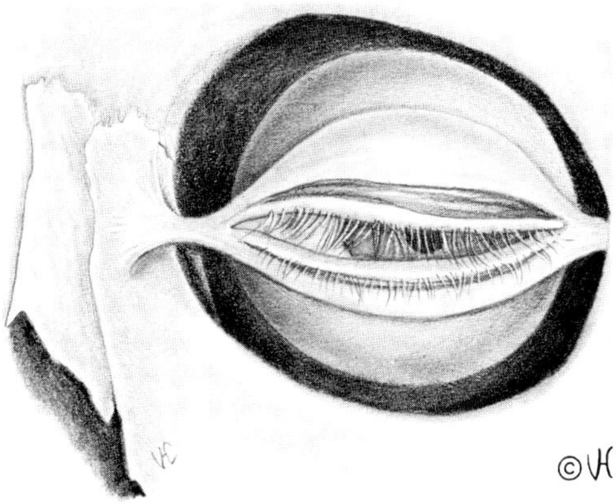

Fig. 25-15. Skeletonized tarsal plates with eyelid margins left intact. Disparity btween upper and lower tarsal dimensions directly reflects the contribution of respective eyelids in covering the globe anteriorly.

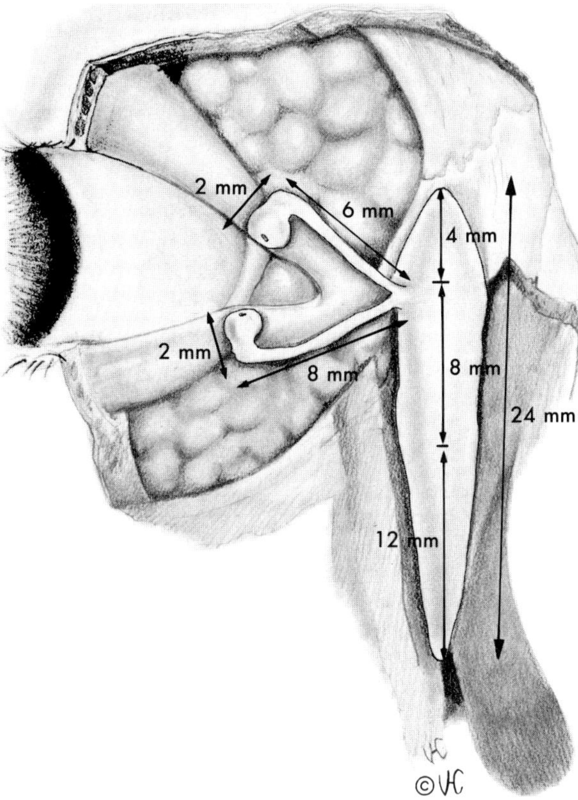

Fig. 25-16. Nasolacrimal excretory system in adults is about 35 mm; in the newborn, about 25 mm.

orbicularis. The plates are molded to the anterior surface of the globe and are adherent to the conjunctiva. Medially and laterally, the tarsal plates form fibrous connections to the orbital rim called ligaments. The lateral canthal ligament attaches at Whitnall's tubercle, in close association with the lateral extension of the levator aponeurosis.[17]

Eyelid Margin

Each tarsal plate contains sebaceous, oil-secreting meibomian glands (Fig. 25-14). The meibomian gland orifices are located anterior to the mucocutaneous junction, and their epithelial lining is keratinized. There are approximately 25 glands in the upper tarsus and approximately 10 in the lower. The central gray line represents the muscle of Riolan near the mucocutaneous junction and is an anatomic landmark of the eyelid margin, helping to identify the anterior and posterior lamellae.[2] The lacrimal puncta divides the eyelid margin into lateral palpebral and medial lacrimal portions (Fig. 25-9). Medially, the lid margin is without lashes and contains the lacrimal canaliculi. The depth of each canaliculus is variable. The canaliculi course posteriorly and medially from the nasal end of the tarsus.

Lacrimal Excretory System

The medial canthal area comprises the canthal tendon, the superficial and deep heads of the pretarsal orbicularis oculi muscle, and the lacrimal excretory system. The deep head of the preseptal ocularis oculis muscle is known as Horner's muscle. The lacrimal excretory system consists of the puncta, the canaliculi, the common canaliculus, the lacrimal sac, and the nasolacrimal duct and is often involved in trauma to this region (Fig. 25-16). The upper and lower puncta open 5 to 7 mm laterally from the medial canthal angle. The lower eyelid punctum is usually 1 to 2 mm more lateral than the upper punctum. The lacrimal papillae is an elevated, pale mound of fibrous tissue around each punctum. If the punctum is apparent on external inspection, there is, by definition, ectropion of the medial eyelid margin. Tears pooling in the medial angle of the eye may not drain correctly in this situation. The vertical length of the canaliculus is 2 mm, and the punctal os is approximately 0.3 mm in diameter. The horizontal length from the canaliculus to the sac is 8 mm.

The common canaliculus usually enters the lacrimal sac approximately 3 to 5 mm from its apex. The lacrimal sac, located in the lacrimal fossa in the medial wall, is sheathed in thick periorbita and surrounding fascia.[1] The lacrimal sac is 15 mm high and extends 3 to 5 mm above the medial canthal tendon. The bony portion of the nasolacrimal duct is 12 mm in length. The duct enters into the inferior meatus 15 mm from the floor of the nose. The approximate length of the nasolacrimal excretory system in the adult is 35 mm and in the newborn 25 mm.[2] The structural integrity of the "lacrimal pump" relies on the function of the superficial and deep pretarsal orbicularis. The anatomic complexity in this region warrants special care and management (see Chapter 30).

OSTEOLOGY

Understanding orbital osteology is extremely important in evaluating the facial trauma patient. The bony orbit and the paraorbital sinuses support, protect, and maximize the function of the eyes. Fractures of the orbit may be extensive and involve injury to the sinuses, the nasolacrimal pathways, and the brain. Carotid-cavernous sinus fistulas and cerebral spinal fluid leaks can be associated with craniofacial trauma (see Chapter 27).

Orbital Dimensions

The orbital cavities are symmetrical on either side of the nose. The orbital volume is approximately 35 cc; its height at the entrance is approximately 35 mm. The orbital width in the adult is 40 mm. Orbital depth, measured to the bone between the optic foramen and the superior orbital fissure, is 45 to 55 mm. The orbital cavities are cone-shaped, tapering posteriorly to the apex of the orbit. The angle between the lateral and medial walls of the orbit on a single side is approximately 45°. The medial walls appear almost parallel (Fig. 25-17).

Orbital Rim

The orbital rim is a rectangular opening at the anterior orbit. The zygomatic bone forms most of the lateral margin and half of the inferior orbital rim. It is important to palpate this bone at its sutures to note possible displacement. The frontal bone encompasses the superior orbital rim and extends laterally and medially.

The medial orbital rim consists of the maxillary process of the frontal bone, the lacrimal bone, and the frontal process of the maxillary bone. Medially, the rim is discontinuous between the anterior and posterior lacrimal crest. In this space lies the lacrimal sac.

The maxillary bone and the zygoma each constitute half of the inferior orbital rim. At the zygomatico-maxillary suture, an elevation is frequently present forming the infraorbital tubercle. Below the suture is the infraorbital foramen, approximately 4 mm in diameter and 7 mm from the inferior orbital rim. In the child, the infraorbital foramen is immediately below the inferior orbital margin.

Laterally, the temporal fossa lies behind the zygomatic bone. The foramen of the zygomatic facial nerve and vessels leaves the lateral orbit through the zygomatic bone. Inside the lateral orbital rim, 10 mm below the zygomatic-frontal suture, is the lateral orbital tubercle of Whitnall. This tubercle of the zygomatic bone is palpable 2 to 4 mm behind the anterior opening of the rim and marks the deep attachment of the lateral retinaculum.

The superior orbital rim is formed by the frontal bone. The newborn rim is sharp but becomes more rounded with development, especially in the male. The medial superior orbital rim is indented at the supraorbital notch, which is formed by the supraorbital nerve and artery.

Orbital Walls

Seven bones contribute to the orbit: frontal, maxilla, zygoma, sphenoid with its greater and lesser wings, palatine, ethmoid, and lacrimal (Fig. 25-18). The superior, inferior, and lateral orbital walls are triangular in shape. The medial orbital wall is rectangular. The superior orbital wall is formed by two bones. The orbital roof is primarily formed anteriorly by the orbital plate of the frontal bone. Posteriorly, the orbital roof at the apex is formed by the lesser wing of the sphenoid bone. The posterior roof is perforated at the optic foramen at an angle of about 45° from the midline, forming the canal of the optic nerve.

The optic foramen measures 6 mm in height and 5 mm in width, and is located in the lesser wing of the sphenoid bone. The optic foramen is the anterior orifice of the optic canal, through which pass the optic nerve and the ophthalmic artery. The artery is located below and lateral to the nerve. The canal is lined by dura. The meninges surrounding the nerve and dura are continuous with the orbital periosteum at the

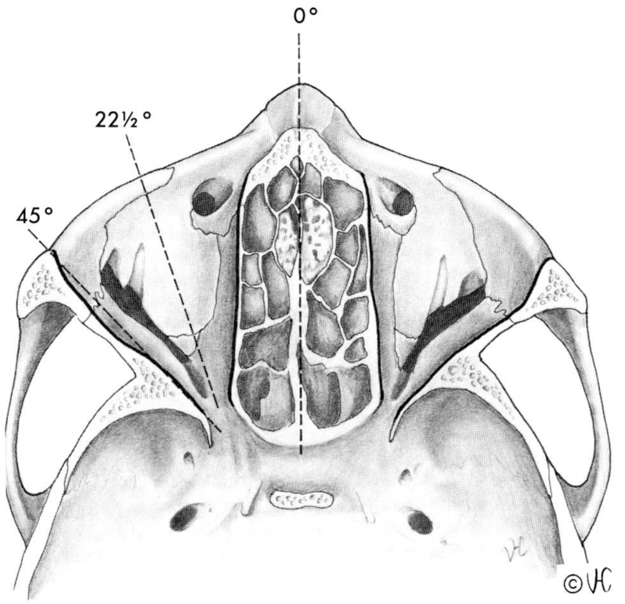

Fig. 25-17. Horizontal section through orbits. The medial walls are nearly parallel, and lateral walls diverge 45°. Thus the orbital axis diverges 22.5° from the midline.

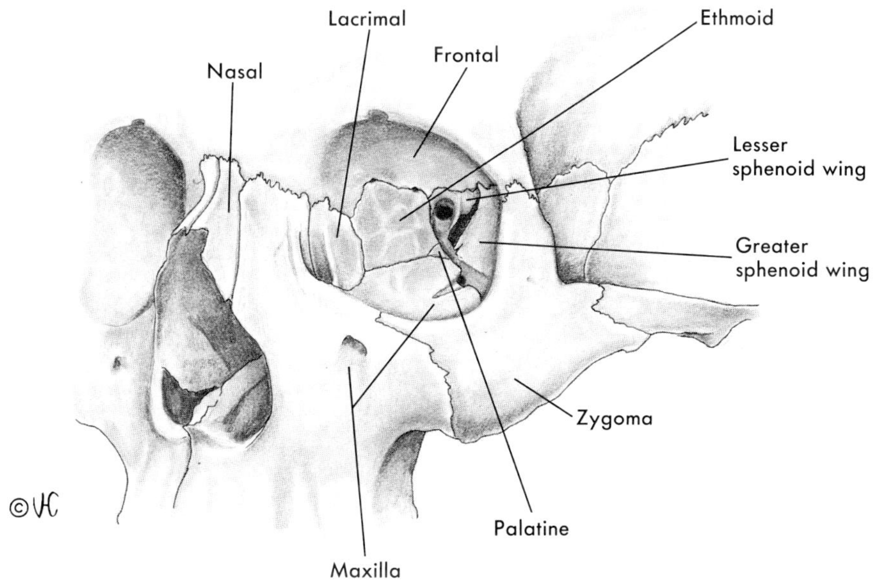

Fig. 25-18. Bones of the orbit.

posterior orbit. Although the posterior globe is only about 18 mm from the optic foramen, the optic nerve's orbital length is about 25 mm. The orbital portion of the optic nerve is 6 to 8 mm longer than the distance from the globe to the orbital apex.[18]

Important landmarks of the orbital roof also include the lacrimal gland fossa seen anterolaterally and the small trochlear fossa anteromedially. The fovea trochlearis in the superior nasal angle of the orbit, 4 mm from the orbital rim, is the point of attachment of the superior oblique tendon.

The lateral orbital wall is formed posteriorly by the greater wing of the sphenoid. In this wing are enclosed the superior and inferior orbital fissures. The anterior lateral orbital wall is formed by the zygomatic process of the frontal bone and the zygomatic bone itself. The zygomatic bone becomes thick anteriorly and is a strong buttress that protects and supports the orbit. Posteriorly, the wall is thinner and separates the orbit from the temporal fossa. The sphenoid portion of the lateral wall is separated from the roof by the superior orbital fissure.

The total length of the superior orbital fissure is 22 mm. It is divided by a tendinous ring of the extraocular muscles called the annulus of Zinn. Through the superior orbital fissure and the annulus, known as the oculomotor foramen, traverse both the upper and lower divisions of cranial nerve III, cranial nerve VI, the nasal ciliary branch of cranial nerve V, the ophthalmic veins, the orbital branch of the middle meningeal artery at times, and the sympathetic nerve fibers. In the superior orbital fissure above the annulus, the trochlear nerve and the frontal and lacrimal branches of cranial nerve V are transmitted (Fig. 25-19). Therefore, in trauma related to the orbital apex and superior fissure, it is important to remember that cranial nerve IV and the frontal and lacrimal branches of the ophthalmic division of cranial nerve V are in the orbit but outside the muscle cone.[9]

The floor of the orbit, the shortest orbital wall, is triangular. It is separated laterally by the inferior orbital fissure and medially by the suture joining it and the ethmoid and lacrimal

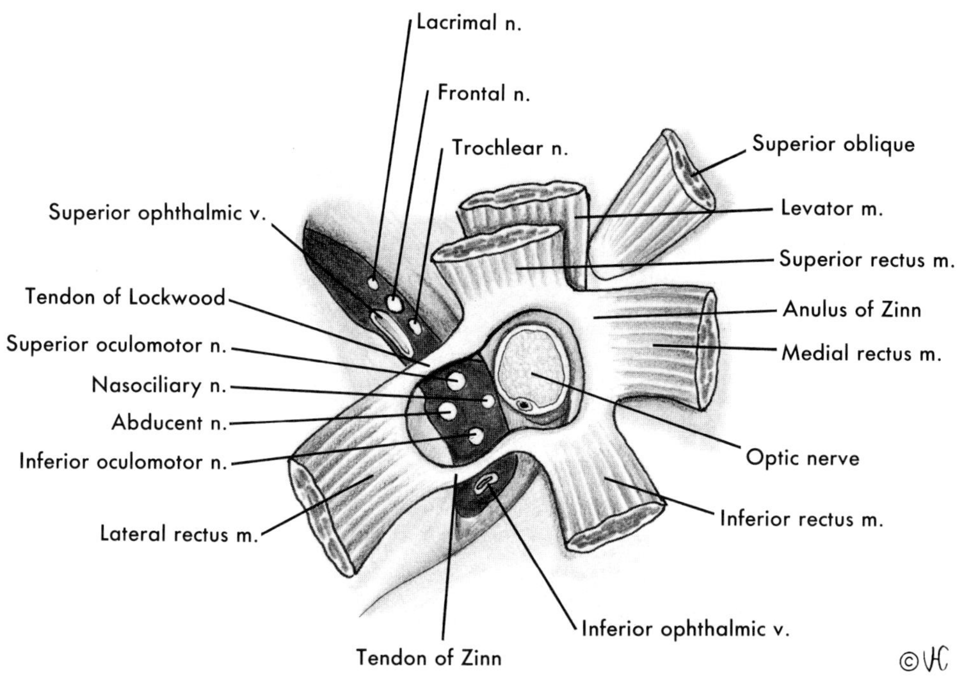

Fig. 25-19. Schematic drawing to show Zinn's annulus spanning the superior orbital fissure. The levator palpebrae superioris and superior oblique muscles arise from the sphenoid lesser wing above and medial to the annulus.

bones. The orbital plate of the maxillary bone constitutes most of the entire floor except for a posterior contribution from the palatine bone and from the zygoma anterolaterally. The inferior orbital fissure, initially narrow, widens anteriorly. It is situated 16 to 18 mm from the orbital rim.[19] The infraorbital groove runs forward from the inferior orbital fissure. Anteriorly, this groove becomes a canal within the maxilla, finally exiting as the infraorbital foramen on the anterior maxillary surface. The nerves of the inferior orbital fissure can best be visualized on coronal sections of the orbital apex.[20]

Through the inferior orbital fissure, anterior to the foramen rotundum, passes the maxillary division of the trigeminal nerve (V_2), its branches, the infraorbital nerve, the branches of the sphenopalatine ganglia, and the branches of the inferior ophthalmic vein that go to the pterygoid plexus. This fissure communicates with both the pterygopalatine and infratemporal fossae. Before the infraorbital nerve exits its foramen, the anterior-superior alveolar nerves branch out medially within the bony floor to descend medially along the inner face and supply sensation to the three anterior teeth and gingiva. Sensory abnormalities of the teeth, therefore, may help focus attention on bony abnormalities of the orbital floor. As a child reaches adulthood, the floor remains strong laterally to the infraorbital nerve but thins medially as a result of maxillary sinus expansion. This thin, unsupported dome of the maxillary sinus is usually where floor fractures, referred to as blowout fractures, occur after blunt orbital trauma.[2]

The medial wall of the orbit is composed of four bones including, from anterior to posterior, the frontal process of the maxillary bone, the lacrimal bone, the orbital plate of the ethmoid bone, known as the lamina papyracea, and the lesser wing of the sphenoid. The anterior and posterior ethmoid foramen can be found at the frontal-ethmoidal suture. This denotes the level of the cribriform plate. The anterior ethmoidal foramen transmits the anterior ethmoidal artery and the nasociliary nerve. The posterior ethmoidal foramen contains the posterior ethmoidal artery. The anterior and posterior ethmoidal foramina are located 20 to 35 mm, respectively, posterior to the anterior lacrimal crest.[2]

Anteriorly, in the medial wall, lies the lacrimal fossa, which is approximately 14 mm in height. The anterior lacrimal crest, which is part of the frontal process of the maxillary bone, is the anterior border; the posterior lacrimal crest of the lacrimal bone is the posterior extension of the fossa. The lacrimal sac rests in this fossa, which gives rise inferiorly to the nasolacrimal canal.

Paraorbital Sinuses

The paranasal sinuses are the maxillary, ethmoid, frontal, and sphenoid sinuses. The maxillary sinuses, the largest sinuses, are situated beneath the orbital floor. The sinus roof declines from the medial wall to the lateral wall at approximately a 30° angle. For this reason, the intermediate Water's view is best used to visualize blow-out fractures that expand into the maxillary sinus (Fig. 25-20).

The ethmoid sinuses arise from the nose below the middle turbinate. The ethmoids are the most exuberantly growing sinuses and may be seen to pneumatize the frontal, ethmoidal, palatine, and lacrimal bones.[2] There are 3 to 15 air cells that expand from the lateral border of the

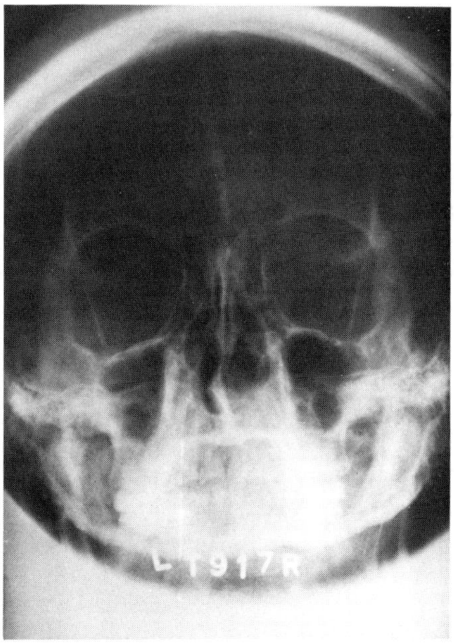

Fig. 25-20. X ray of atraumatic male orbit. Intermediate Water's projection shows intact orbital floors and clear maxillary sinuses.

cribriform plate to the middle and superior turbinates medially.

The frontal sinuses, not well developed until the sixth year of life, expand throughout adolescence. The frontal sinuses attain greater proportion in the male than the female.

The sphenoid sinuses arise from the posterior portion of the nasal route and are divided into two portions, usually unequal. Pneumatization of the sphenoid bone may extend into the greater and lesser wings and even into the pterygoid process. The sphenoid bone requires special attention because many important neurovascular structures of the orbit pass through it.

ORBIT

Periorbita

The periorbita consists of the orbital septum and periosteum. It is a thin, resistant, fibrous membrane that covers the walls of the orbit.[19] The orbital periosteum covers the bony skeleton and constitutes a protective sac for the soft elements of the orbit. This self-contained sac has a superomedial pedicle, which contains the optic nerve, and an inferolateral or sphenoid pedicle, which forms a sheath around the structures that pass through the supraorbital fissure. The periorbital sac generally shapes itself to the form of the orbital walls.[19] The periorbita adheres to the arcus marginalis at the orbital rim. Anteriorly, it inserts into the orbital septum. The periorbita firmly attaches to the suture lines, foramen, fissures, arcus marginalis, and lacrimal crest. The orbital space within the periorbita that is not filled with the globe, muscles, fascia, nerves, or glandular structures is filled with fat. The preaponeurotic fat pad is of some importance because it lies directly beneath the orbital septum superiorly. Inferiorly are the inferior orbital fat pads discussed previously. Inside the muscle cone is the intraconal fat.

The lacrimal gland is located inside the periorbita in the superolateral part of the orbit. It is separated into an orbital and a palpebral part of the lateral "horn" of the aponeurosis (Fig. 25-21). This division is often not discernible on computerized tomography (CT) scan.[20]

Lacrimal Gland

The lacrimal gland, located in the lacrimal fossa, is the main aqueous-producing secretory gland of the orbit. The lacrimal gland is suspended from the periorbita by the loose ligament of Sommering. The lateral levator aponeurosis divides the lacrimal gland into an anterior palpebral third and a posterior orbital two thirds. The levator and the suspensory ligament of Whitnall are important in suspending the lacrimal gland anteriorly in the superior lateral orbit.

Secretory ducts originating in the larger orbital lobe of the lacrimal gland secrete fluid through the palpebral lobe into the superior cul-de-sac. These 12 or so ductules enter the conjunctiva 5 mm above the superolateral tarsal border. Disruption of the palpebral lobe may interrupt the secretory ducts and thus interrupt the aqueous secretion from the orbital lacrimal gland.

The lacrimal nerve supplies innervation to the lacrimal gland. Both sympathetic and parasympathetic fibers play a major role. Disruption of the orbital lobe may interrupt efferent innervation to the palpebral lacrimal gland.

Orbital Fascia

Within the periorbita is a fine, fibrous organization of orbital fascia. The orbital fascia has direct connection with the periorbita, intraocular muscles, and Tenon's capsule. Tenon's capsule, or the fascia bulbi, is a fibrous membrane that extends posteriorly from the anterior aspect of the globe where it fuses with the conjunctiva approximately 2 mm from the corneoscleral limbal junction. The globe is thus loosely attached to the surrounding orbital fascia and is free to move. Tenon's capsule is penetrated by nerves, vessels, and intraocular muscles as they travel anteriorly to reach the globe.[2] There are fascial muscle sheaths that envelop each extraocular muscle. The muscles are connected with the surrounding fascia over the anterior one third of their length. The recti muscles enter Tenon's capsule in front of the equator of the globe. There are attachments between Tenon's capsule and the muscles. The importance of Tenon's capsule is in forming a barrier between the globe and other orbital contents.

Each of the extraocular muscles has a fascial attachment to the adjacent orbital wall, known as check ligaments. Highly developed check ligaments are associated with the medial and lateral recti muscles. The lateral check ligament is very strong and is attached to Whitnall's tubercle. The superior transverse ligament of Whitnall may be considered a check ligament of the levator aponeurosis. Fascial connections to the inferior periorbita, which may also have some

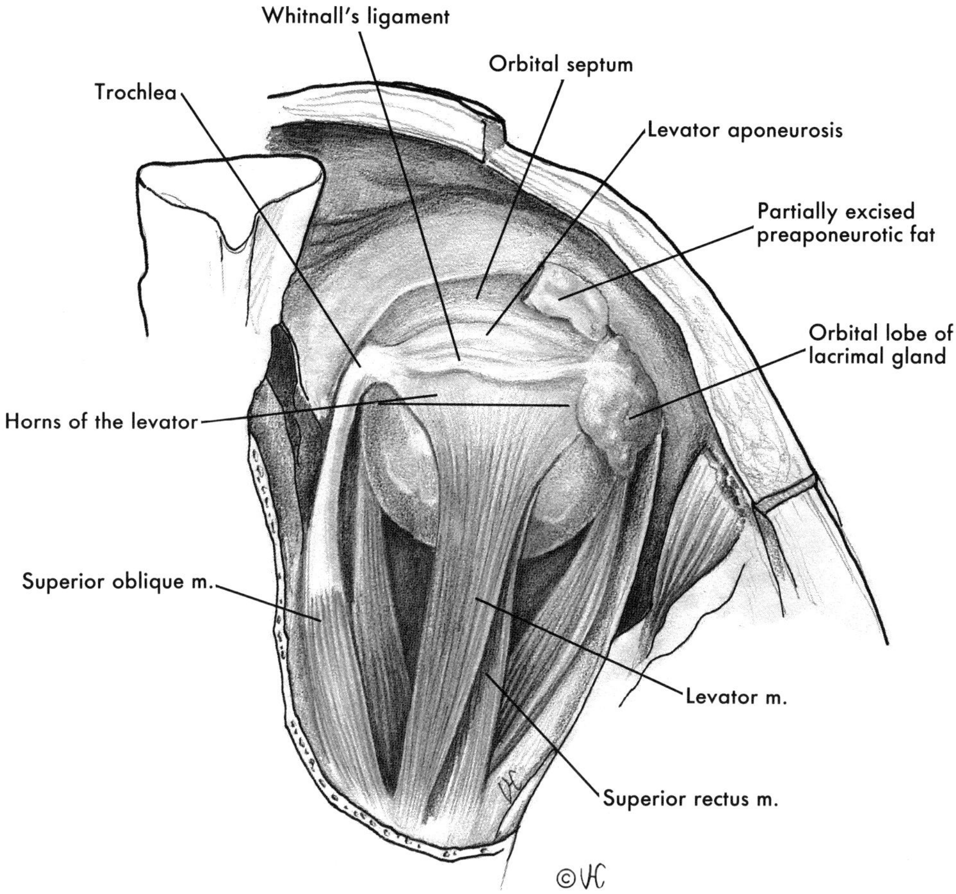

Fig. 25-21. Superior view of the levator palpebrae superioris muscle and its relations. Note superior transverse Whitnall's ligament attached medially to the trochlear fascia and laterally to the fascia investing the lacrimal gland. The levator is bound on its medial side to the superior rectus muscle and is innervated by the same superior oculomotor nerve division.

checking function,[21] exist between the inferior rectus and inferior oblique muscles. Koornneff,[21] who studied the complexity of orbital fascia, documented the interrelationship among all fibrous structures of the orbit. He also demonstrated a fascial hammock support system for veins (i.e., the superior ophthalmic vein) (see Fig. 25-26). The veins are supported by fascia, whereas the arteries are independent.

Orbital Vessels

The orbit is supplied by the ophthalmic artery, with additional blood supply from the infraorbital and middle meningeal branches of the internal maxillary artery. The ophthalmic artery arises from the internal carotid, branching off before the division of the anterior and middle cerebral arteries. The artery leaves the cranial cavity through the optic canal and is embedded in the dural sheath of the nerve as it enters the annulus of Zinn. It winds with the optic nerve posteriorly and then crosses and runs medially between the superior oblique and medial rectus muscles (Fig. 25-22). The ophthalmic artery is tethered to the medial wall by the ethmoid arteries. Anteriorly, it divides into its terminal branches at the eyelid and connects with the tarsal marginal arcades. It passes by the trochlea, with the infratrochlear nerve, and joins with the angular tributary of the fascial artery. The ophthalmic artery is accompanied at various parts of its course by the frontal, lacrimal, nasociliary, and infraorbital nerves[17] (Fig. 25-22).

The central retinal artery branches from the ophthalmic artery and lies beneath the optic nerve 5 to 15 mm posterior to the posterior pole of the eye. The posterior ciliary arteries arise from the ophthalmic artery as it crosses the ophthalmic nerve. These may appear as a single trunk or a group of 6 to 8 vessels, and continue

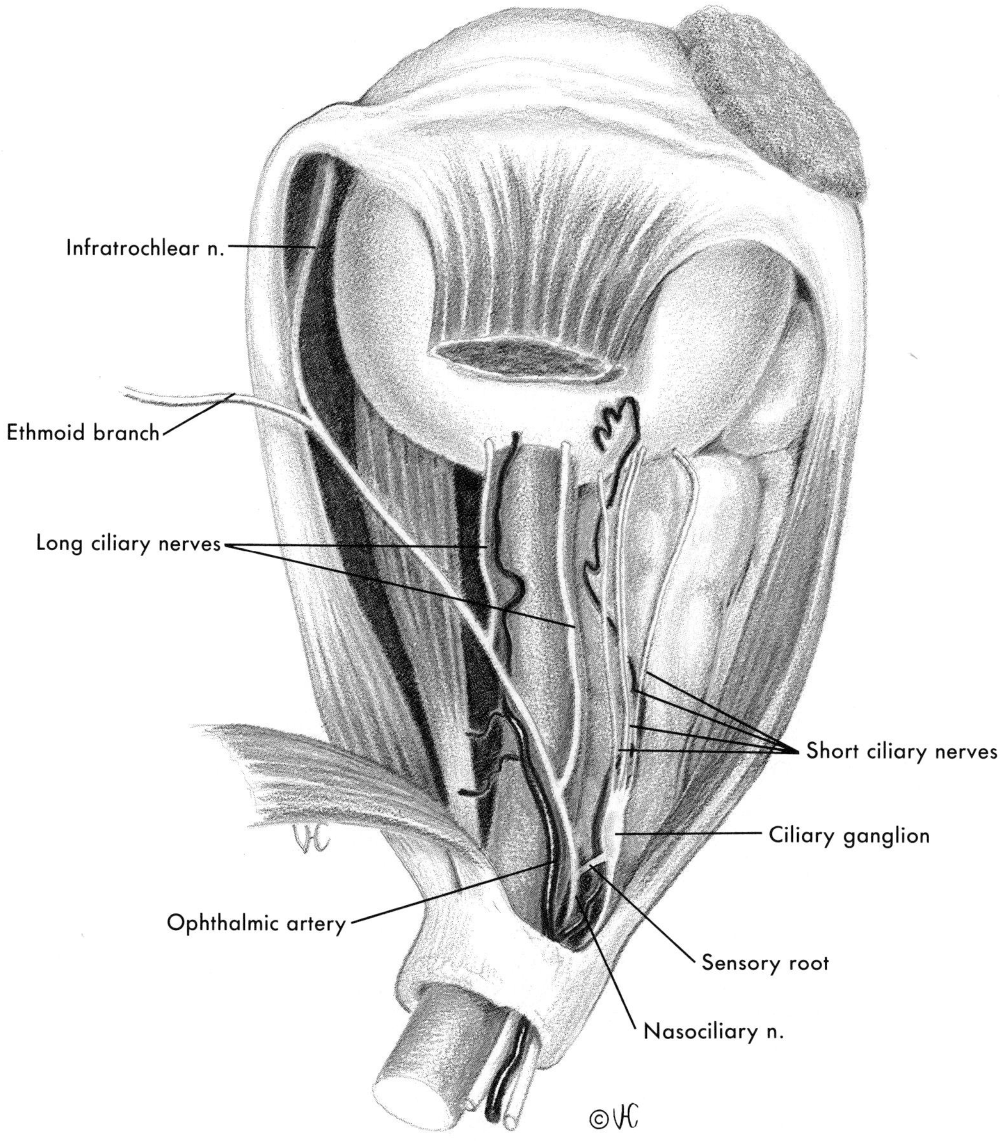

Fig. 25-22. Superior orbital dissection to show intraorbital nasociliary nerve course.

to subdivide into 15 to 20 branches surrounding the optic nerve. Two branches produce the long posterior ciliary arteries that enter the globe on either side of the optic nerve. Their ultimate destination is the ciliary muscle and the iris. The muscular arteries, which usually arise from the two trunks of the ophthalmic artery, supply the muscles of the globe. They pierce the extraocular recti muscle bellies at their midpoints and accompany the tendons. Three of the recti muscles have two arteries; the lateral rectus has only one. These arteries enter the sclera anterior to the tendon insertions and anastomose with the posterior ciliary arteries.

The lacrimal artery arises from the ophthalmic artery on the lateral side of the optic nerve. It accompanies the lacrimal nerve along the upper border of the lateral rectus muscle to reach the gland. It terminates laterally in the marginal arcade and gives off a branch called the recurrent meningeal artery. The supraorbital artery arises from the ophthalmic artery above the optic nerve. It runs forward medially and then superiorly to the levator between it and the roof of the orbit. It is accompanied by its corresponding nerve and exits the orbit through the supraorbital notch. The two ethmoidal arteries leave the ophthalmic artery as it passes along the medial wall of the orbit between the superior oblique and medial rectus muscles.

The palpebral branches of the ophthalmic artery arise from just below the trochlea and enter the eyelid medially to join the superior and inferior tarsal marginal arcades. These arcades anastomose laterally with the palpebral branches of the lacrimal artery and with the supraorbital and infraorbital arteries. The final terminal branch of the ophthalmic artery, the supratrochlear artery, leaves the orbit by piercing the septum to accompany the supratrochlear nerve and anastomose with the supraorbital artery. Connections exist between the external and internal carotid artery systems.

The infraorbital artery, a terminal branch of the internal maxillary artery from the external carotid system, traverses along the floor of the orbit beneath the periosteum. Eventually, it anastomoses with the branches of the facial artery, including the angular artery. Here there is another communication with the terminal branches of the ophthalmic artery, a branch of the internal carotid system. Another communication between the internal and external carotid artery systems is created by the anastomosis between the recurrent meningeal branch of the lacrimal artery and the middle meningeal artery (derived from the external carotid system).

The superior orbital vein is the chief vein of the orbit. It forms behind the medial corner of the upper eyelid by confluence of the angular, supraorbital, and supratrochlear veins to form the superior ophthalmic vein. The supraorbital vein runs below the orbicularis muscle, piercing it medially to communicate at the frontalis muscle with the branches of the superficial temporal vein. The angular vein lies temporal to the angular artery 8 mm from the medial commissure. The superior ophthalmic vein pierces the muscle cone in midorbit. At this point it receives venous drainage from the globe and travels along the lateral border of the superior rectus muscle. It leaves the orbit through the annulus of Zinn. The infraorbital vein, found above the inferior rectus muscle, exits below the annulus of Zinn. It joins the superior orbital vein, bending downward to enter the cavernous sinus or entering the pterygoid plexus above.[17] Venous drainage of the optic nerve by the central retinal vein accompanies the artery through its intraneural course. Ciliary veins accompany the ciliary arteries on their intraorbital routes.

Orbital Nerves

Besides the optic nerve, four other cranial nerves are found in the orbit: oculomotor (cranial nerve III), trochlear (cranial nerve IV), trigeminal (cranial nerve V), and abducens (cranial nerve VI).

The orbital nerves crowd together with the ophthalmic artery as they enter the orbit at its apex. The oculomotor nerve travels through the cavernous sinus and divides into a superior and an inferior branch. It goes through the annulus, separated by the nasociliary nerve. The superior branch travels within the muscle cone and reaches the internal side of the superior rectus 15 mm from the orbital apex. Fibers innervating the levator palpebrae superioris muscle either pass medial to the superior rectus (90%) or pierce through the muscle (10%).[2]

The inferior branch of the oculomotor nerve innervates the medial and inferior rectus muscles, and a large terminal branch to the inferior oblique can be found at the lateral border of the inferior rectus. The oculomotor nerve also carries parasympathetic fibers that synapse in the ciliary ganglion.

The ciliary ganglion is 2 mm in diameter and 10 mm from the orbital apex (Fig. 25-22). It lies between the optic nerve and the lateral rectus. Pupillomotor parasympathetic fibers and sympathetic pupillodilating fibers from the nasal ciliary nerve are found in the ciliary ganglion. Autonomic innervation enters the eye via the short ciliary nerves that pierce the sclera around the optic nerve.

The thin trochlear nerve enters the orbital fissure superotemporally to the annulus of Zinn and medially to the frontal nerve, courses outside the muscle cone, and travels anteromedially to the superior rectus muscle.

The abducens nerve passes through the optic foramen and enters the orbit between the optic nerve and the lateral rectus muscle. It inserts in the inner surface at the posterior third of the lateral rectus muscle.

The ophthalmic and maxillary divisions of the trigeminal nerve enter the orbit and supply sensation to the superior two thirds of the face. The ophthalmic division enters the superior orbital fissure as three branches: the lacrimal, frontal, and nasociliary nerves. The lacrimal nerve, the smallest branch, is situated most laterally. It contains a sympathetic nerve component that is partially responsible for lacrimal gland secretion. It joins the lacrimal artery to pass superotemporally into the posterior aspect of the lacrimal gland. Here it forms superior and inferior branches. The superior branch supplies the gland, conjunctiva, and lateral upper lid. The inferior branch supplies the gland and sends fibers along the zygomaticotemporal nerve. The frontal nerve passes superiorly through the orbit beneath the periorbita, where it divides into a supratrochlear and a larger supraorbital branch. The frontal nerve, large enough to be identified by CT scanning, is located above the levator palpebrae superioris muscle in its anterior orbital route.

The nasociliary nerve is the only branch of the ophthalmic division of the trigeminal nerve that passes through the annulus of Zinn. It gives off sensory roots to the ciliary ganglia (Fig. 25-22). It sends off two long ciliary nerves to the globe, creates the anterior ethmoidal nerve, and terminates as the infratrochlear nerve. The sympathetic nerve supply to the orbit is responsible for pupillary dilation, smooth muscle eyelid function, and vasoconstriction. It is believed that major pupillodilating fibers pass along the nasociliary nerve and then through the posterior ciliaries to the globe.

Extraocular Muscles

Except for the inferior oblique, the average rectus muscle length is about 40 mm, excluding the tendon. Insertions of the rectus muscles attach in a clockwise fashion at the corneal limbus in the spiral of Tillaux (Fig. 25-23). Variations of these insertions are well documented.[22] The orbital nerves for these muscles terminate at approximately the junction of the posterior third of the muscle.

The medial and inferior rectus muscles receive innervation from the inferior division of the oculomotor nerve (cranial nerve III). The superior rectus muscle receives innervation from the superior oculomotor division, as does the levator superioris. The medial rectus muscle remains close to the medial wall unit the anterior third of its course, where it angles medially to insert in the eye. This is the rectus muscle with the greatest mass. Above the muscle lies the terminal branch of the nasociliary nerve and the ophthalmic artery.

The lateral rectus muscle is innervated by the abducens nerve (cranial nerve VI). The lateral rectus muscle is separated from the optic nerve by the ciliary ganglion, the ophthalmic artery, and loose intraconal fat (Fig. 25-22).

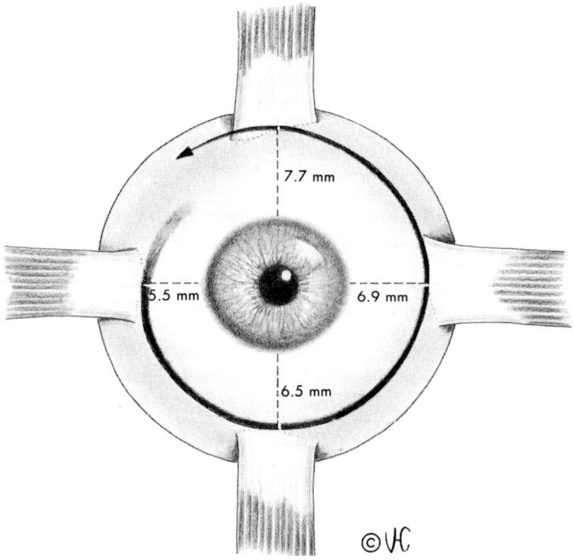

Fig. 25-23. Spiral of Tillaux, left eye.

The inferior oblique muscle travels beneath the inferior rectus muscle. The large inferior oculomotor nerve travels below the optic nerve to the inferior oblique muscle and anteriorly along the lateral border of the inferior rectus.

The superior oblique muscle courses anteriorly and superiorly about 40 mm from its origin until it passes to the trochlea. At the trochlea it makes a 54° angle posteriorly, laterally, and inferiorly to the eye. The tendon begins 10 mm behind the globe. The insertion is thought to be 10 to 11 mm along a posterolateral convex line to the globe, but this insertion is the most variable of the extraocular muscles[23] (Fig. 25-24). The superior oblique is innervated by the trochlear nerve (cranial nerve IV).

Orbital Imaging

When managing orbital trauma, computerized tomography is a valuable diagnostic tool. CT scans can visualize most orbital soft tissues and bony abnormalities. Foreign bodies can be localized accurately by using narrow density windows with three-dimensional imaging.[24] Direct multiplanar high-resolution CT scanning is the modality of choices for studying the vital structures of the orbit (Figs. 25-25 through 25-27).[25] (See Chapter 2.)

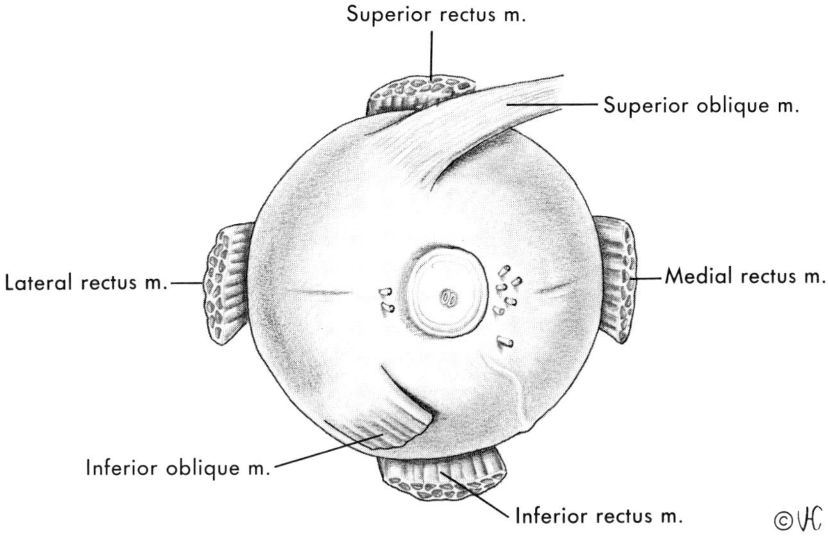

Fig. 25-24. Posterior view of the left globe (rotated slightly externally) to show insertions of the oblique muscles.

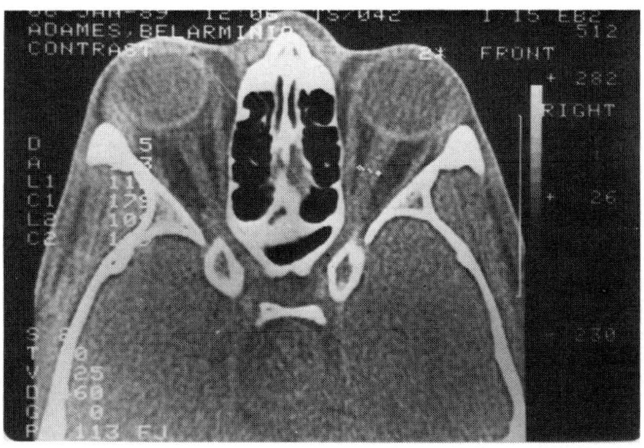

Fig. 25-25. CT scan of atraumatic male orbit with contrast. Axial view of midglobe with medial and lateral recti muscles, ethmoid air cells, and the optic nerve through the orbit and canal.

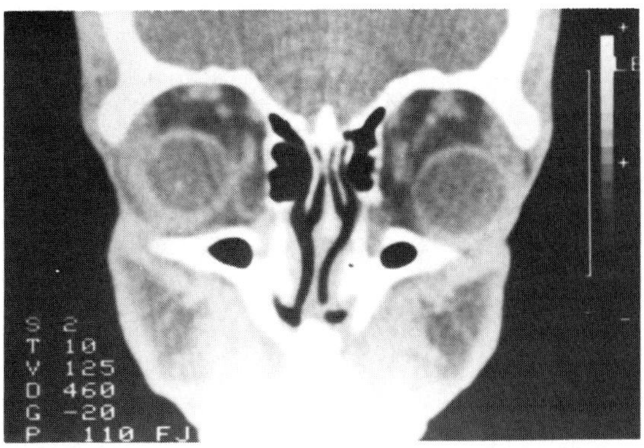

Fig. 25-26. CT scan of atraumatic male orbit with contrast. Coronal view of midglobe with lacrimal gland laterally, superior recti superiorly, and medial recti laterally, with the superior ophthalmic vein suspended between, highlighted here with contrast.

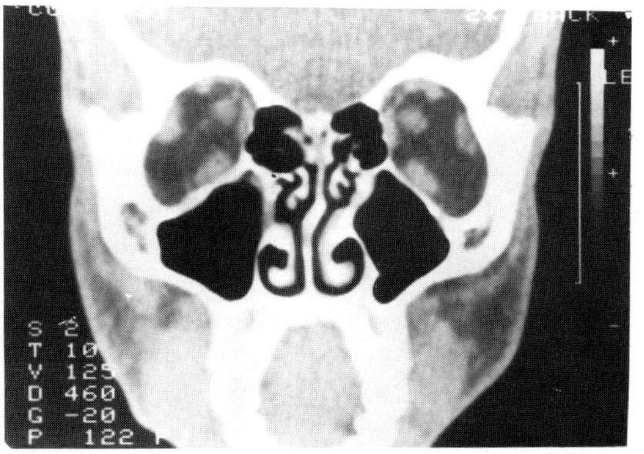

Fig. 25-27. CT scan of atraumatic male orbit with contrast. Coronal view of the posterior orbit. Note the muscle cone and the close relationship between the medial and inferior recti muscles and the lamina papyracea and orbital floor, respectively.

References

1. McGetrick JJ et al: A search for lymphatic drainage of the monkey orbit, Arch Ophthalmol 107:255-260, 1989.
2. Lemke BN: Anatomy of the ocular adnexa and orbit. In Smith BC et al, editors: Ophthalmic plastic and reconstructive surgery, part I, vol 1, St Louis, 1987, The CV Mosby Co, Chap. 1.
3. Lemke BN and Stasior OG: The anatomy of eyebrow ptosis, Arch Ophthalmol 100:981, 1982.
4. Lemke BN and Stasior OG: Eyebrow incision making, Adv Ophthal Plast Reconstr Surg 2:19, 1983.
5. Doxanas MT and Anderson RL: Clinical orbital anatomy, Baltimore, 1984, Williams & Wilkins.
6. Beyer CK, Fabian RL, and Smith B: Naso-orbital fractures, complications and treatment, Ophthalmology 89:458, 1982.
7. Jones LT: Epiphora: its causes and new surgical procedures for its course, Am J Ophthalmol 38:824, 1954.
8. Jones LT and Wobig JL: Surgery of the eyelids and lacrimal systems, Birmingham, 1976, Aesculapius.
9. Zide BM and Jelks GW: Surgical anatomy of the orbit, New York, 1985, Raven Press.
10. Hawes MJ and Dortzbach RK: The microscopic anatomy of the lower eyelid retractors, Arch Ophthalmol 100:1313, 1982.
11. Castanares S: Blepharoplasty for herniated intraorbital fat: anatomical basis for a new approach, Plast Reconstr Surg 8:46, 1951.
12. Hugo NE and Stone E: Anatomy for a blepharoplasty, Plast Reconstr Surg 53:381, 1974.
13. Putterman AM and Urist MJ: Surgical anatomy of the orbital septum, Ann Ophthalmol 6:290, 1974.
14. Garber PF, McDonald D, and Beyer-Machule CK: Management of trauma to the eyelids. In Smith BC et al, editors: Ophthalmic plastic and reconstructive surgery, part V, vol 1, St Louis, 1987, The CV Mosby Co, Chap. 13.
15. Anderson RL and Beard C: The levator aponeurosis: attachments and their clinical significance, Arch Ophthalmol 95:1437-1441, 1977.
16. Newell FW: Ophthalmology: principles and concepts, ed 5, St Louis, 1982, The CV Mosby Co.
17. Whitnall SE: Anatomy of the human orbit and accessory organs of vision, New York, 1979, Robert E Kreiger, (originally published in 1921).
18. Bergin DJ: Anatomy of the eyelids, lacrimal system and orbit. In McCord CD and Tannenbaum M, editors: Oculoplastic surgery, ed 2, New York, 1987, Raven Press.
19. Tessier P et al: Plastic surgery of the orbits and eyelids, Report of the French Society of Ophthalmology, New York, 1977, Masson (Translated by SA Wolfe).
20. Zonnenfeld FW et al: Normal direct multiplanar CT anatomy of the orbit with correlative anatomic cross-sections. In Mafee MF, editor: Imaging in ophthalmology, Part I, Radiologic clinics of North America, vol 25, 3, Philadelphia, May 1987, WB Saunders.
21. Koornneff L: Spatial aspects of orbital musculofibrous tissue in man: a new anatomical and histologic approach, Amsterdam, 1977, Swets & Zeitlinger.
22. Apt L: An anatomic re-evaluation of rectus muscle insertions, Trans Am Ophthalmol Soc 78:365, 1980.
23. Fink WH: A surgical anatomy of the superior oblique muscle, Trans Am Ophthalmol Soc 46:154, 1948.
24. Grove AS and McCord CD: Acute orbital trauma: diagnosis and management. In McCord CD and Tannenbaum M, editors: Oculoplastic surgery, ed 2, New York, 1987, Raven Press.
25. Collin JRO, Beard C, and Wood I: Terminal course of nerve supply to Müller's muscle in the rhesus monkey and its clinical significance, Am J Ophthalmol 87:234, 1979.

CHAPTER 26

Blunt trauma to orbital soft tissues

JEMSHED A. KHAN

Examination
Abrasion, contusion, and crush injury
Edema
Hemorrhage
Emphysema
Ptosis
Ophthalmoplegia
Optic nerve blindness
Therapy
  Ice packs
  Cellulitis/antibiotics
  Intraocular pressure management
  Corticosteroids
Surgery
  Lateral canthotomy
  Peritomy
  Orbital decompression
  Persistent conjunctival prolapse
References

A strong bony perimeter composed of the skull and facial bones affords the orbit's greatest defense against blunt trauma. The orbital bones, however, may be bypassed by relatively small masses such as a fist, table corner, champagne cork, or squash ball. In such instances concussive forces are also absorbed by the globe, eyelids, extraocular muscles, orbital soft tissues, and various fat pads with consequent injury. Soft tissue trauma, moreover, often accompanies orbital fractures[1,2] (see Chapter 27).

EXAMINATION

When confronted with blunt trauma of orbital soft tissue, the ophthalmologist's first priority is evaluation of the globe to determine if emergent medical or surgical intervention is necessary. Attention is then turned to fully documenting the nature and history of the injury. The patient should be specifically questioned regarding symptoms of cerebrospinal fluid (CSF) rhinorrhea, indicating a basilar skull fracture.

The orbital rim, zygomatic arch, forehead, and nasal bridge should be palpated for fractures. The relationship of the globe to the surrounding structures is evaluated for globe ptosis or other displacement. Hertel exophthalmometry readings and neurological examination findings should be recorded, including motility and testing for infraorbital nerve anesthesia and tonic pupil associated with a floor fracture. Ultrasound, X-ray, or computerized tomography (CT) studies should be considered (see Chapter 2). Rhabdomyosarcoma is sometimes misdiagnosed when orbital swelling and proptosis in a child are mistakenly attributed to a previous minor orbital trauma.

ABRASION, CONTUSION, AND CRUSH INJURY

Abrasions result from shearing or denuding of the epidermis and superficial dermis. Abrasions should be irrigated and cleansed of foreign material and necrotic debris to diminish the likelihood of infection and traumatic tattooing. The wound is then appropriately documented by careful drawings or photographs, measured, and explored to rule out injury to deeper structures.

Skin breaks associated with periorbital trauma are responsible for 24% to 35% of cases of periorbital cellulitis,[3-5] and in over 80% of infected cases, staphylococci or streptococci are cultured.[3] Therefore, copious irrigation and early prophylactic topical antibiotic therapy of periorbital skin breaks should be considered. Tetanus prophylaxis may be indicated, especially if the wound is deep or much devitalized tissue is present (see Appendix).

If the abrasion is kept moist with antibiotic ointment and raw dermal surfaces are kept unapposed, the dermis usually reepithelializes without scarring. A moist or nonstick Telfa dressing will avoid denuding the wound during subsequent dressing changes. Partially avulsed or rolled skin edges may be unrolled and sutured back into place, often providing satisfactory coverage. Skin grafting and immobilization in an extended position may be necessary if a large area of the dermis is absent. Injuries penetrating deeper than the dermis require surgical repair.

Contusion injuries result from crushing of subcutaneous muscle and connective tissues with secondary hemorrhage and edema. Ice packs for the first 24 hours and hot packs subsequently help diminish edema and hematoma. Infected, tense, or large hematomas of the eyelid may be incised and drained to diminish the risk of spread of infection, abscess formation, necrosis of overlying skin, and development of excessive scar tissue.

Sufficient blunt force can divide the soft tissues overlying the superior and lateral orbital rims and mimic a sharp laceration.[6] The distinction may be based upon the typical location, stellate versus linear skin disruption, residual strands of tissue bridging the wound, and incomplete penetration of tissues.[6]

EDEMA

Chemosis and edema following periorbital injury result from intravascular leakage into the soft tissues. Because the thin, distensible eyelid skin and the conjunctiva are only loosely adherent to the underlying tissues, edema accumulates to a greater degree in these loose subcutaneous tissues than elsewhere in the body. The lateral spread of edema is limited by the adherent fascia beneath the eyebrows and by the malar and nasojugal folds.[6] Fluid may, however, tunnel subcutaneously across the bridge of the nose resulting in bilateral lid edema following unilateral trauma.[6]

Massive periorbital edema may obscure penetrating injuries, necessitating a careful search for occult lacerations, puncture wounds, and foreign bodies. Edema will also limit the ability to palpate underlying facial bone fractures. When eyelid edema interferes with globe examination, the lids may be gently pried apart under topical anesthesia with the aid of two Desmarres retractors. If the globe still cannot be evaluated, a crude assessment of visual function can be made by shining a bright muscle light through the eyelids to detect light perception. A consensual pupillary response can also be monitored with this technique, providing a rough gauge of optic nerve function. Ultrasonography and CT scanning may be useful adjuncts in evaluation of such cases.

Conjunctival edema may range from minor swelling to dramatic conjunctival prolapse that prevents lid closure. Conjunctival prolapse is often prominent inferiorly, medially, and laterally. A bland topical ointment should be applied to prevent desiccation of chronically exposed conjunctiva. Corticosteroid ointment may hasten resolution of conjunctival swelling. Rarely, persistent conjunctival prolapse of the inferior fornix that fails to improve continually after 1 week becomes organized and may not spontaneously reposition as the edema subsides. Surgical intervention may be necessary (see the section on surgery later).

Orbital edema without significant hemorrhage is usually self-limited. Proptosis, increased resistance of the globe to retropulsion, "tight" orbital tissues, chemosis, and conjunctival vascular congestion are all commonly seen. Orbital edema may result in nonspecific limitations of motility that can be mistaken for muscle entrapment. Forced ductions are usually negative, however, and motility improves dramatically as the edema resolves. Diplopic fields may help quantitate improvements in motility. Orbital edema may temporarily mask an expansion in the bony orbital volume due to blowout fracture. Hertel exophthalmometry readings should be obtained as a baseline for future reference.

Carotid-cavernous fistula may produce immediate or delayed signs and symptoms, including pain, diplopia, florid periorbital swelling, chemosis, proptosis and orbital edema, conjunctival and episcleral vascular congestion, and elevated intraocular pressure.[7] Associated features should be sought, such as orbital pulsation, dilated congested episcleral vessels (corkscrew vessels), ocular or cranial bruit, choroidal thickening, retinal venous congestion, ptosis, and tinnitus, to ensure that such patients are treated appropriately and not mistakenly thought to have suffered marked edema due to direct orbital injury.[7,8] CT scan and ultrasound usually demonstrate a dilated superior ophthalmic vein.[7] Neuroradiological or neurosurgical closure of the fistula may be necessary.

HEMORRHAGE

Hemorrhage is managed conservatively unless there is a threat to vision. Localized visible hemorrhage into the eyelid tissues quickly follows even minor injuries and will eventually migrate beyond the zone of injury. Hemorrhage from skull fractures will often spread diffusely into the eyelid tissues after 24 to 48 hours. Orbital hemorrhage resolves spontaneously over a course of weeks. Eyelid hematomas were discussed in the previous section under contusion injuries.

Patients with a predisposition to bleeding, such as those with hemophilia, vitamin deficiency, alcoholism, platelet abnormality, lymphangioma, scurvy, anticoagulant therapy, or orbital vascular malformation, may suffer severe orbital hemorrhage following otherwise trivial injuries. Eyelid ecchymosis is also seen with metastatic neuroblastoma ("raccoon's eye sign") and amyloidosis.

Blood distribution may range from diffuse to highly confined within the subperiosteal, extraconal, intraconal, Tenon's, or nerve sheath space (Fig. 26-1). Diffuse hemorrhage usually produces axial proptosis, whereas localized hemorrhage produces eccentric proptosis. The site of a fracture causing subperiosteal hematoma may be surmised to lie somewhere opposite the vector of globe displacement.

Visual acuity, pupillary responses, exophthalmometry, tonometry, and fundus evaluation of retinal-vascular perfusion should be recorded. Bleeding time, prothrombin time, partial thromboplastin time, and platelets should be checked and bleeding tendencies reversed. Barring an immediate threat to visual recovery, CT scanning of the orbits is prudent to determine

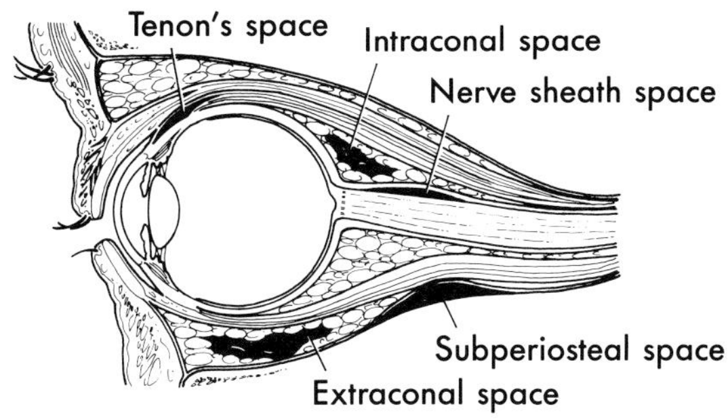

Fig. 26-1. Five potential surgical spaces of the orbit: subperiosteal, extraconal, intraconal, Tenon's, and nerve sheath.

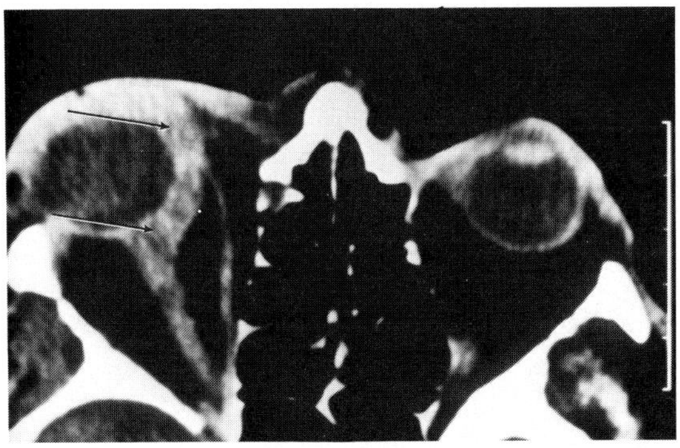

Fig. 26-2. CT scan shows Tenon's space hematoma *(arrows)* that occurred following eye-rubbing in a 65-year-old patient taking coumadin. Clot is impinging on the optic nerve and had reduced vision to finger-counting. Bleeding time was reversed with fresh frozen plasma, and patient noted return of color vision and acuity on the operating table as the clot was evacuated via an anterior peritomy. Final vision was 20/30.

the extent of injury and localize any blood clots (Fig. 26-2).

Orbital hemorrhage may impinge upon the optic nerve, globe, choroidal and retinal circulation, or orbital venous drainage. Aggressive intervention is warranted if there is optic nerve dysfunction, dangerous elevation of intraocular pressure, or retinal or choroidal ischemia. Nonperfusion of the central retinal artery demands immediate measures to establish retinal perfusion.

Rarely, blood may remain loculated as a chronic hematic cyst, also known as a cholesterol granuloma.[9] Subperiosteal hematomas may also become chronic because of a localized disruption of the fibrinolytic system in a manner analogous to chronic subdural hematomas.[10,11]

EMPHYSEMA

Orbital emphysema, although usually self-limited, can cause blindness following orbital fractures. Emphysema is seen radiologically in up to 50% of orbital fractures, especially those involving the floor and ethmoid sinuses.[12]

Emphysema results when a pressure gradient forces air across a disruption of the paranasal sinus mucosa and orbital bone and into the orbital tissues. Emphysema is not necessarily coincident with the initial bone injury but may be manifested hours later in association with coughing, sneezing, blowing of the nose, vomiting, straining, or any other activity that produces a sudden rise in paranasal sinus air pressure.[13] Patients with orbital fractures should avoid such activities.

Orbital emphysema is harmless unless there is a ball, or one-way valve effect that does not allow the air to leave the orbit. In this case the air pressure may build up and constrain blood flow, causing optic nerve or retinal ischemia and blindness—so-called orbital compartment syndrome.[14] Pathogens may also enter the orbit through the fracture site.

Proptosis, subconjunctival air, or subcutaneous crepitus is often present. Plain films and CT scan will reliably demonstrate significant orbital emphysema as an intraorbital air density (Fig. 26-3). Dried wood foreign bodies may occasionally be mistaken for orbital emphysema on CT scan because of their numerous air cells. Pneumocephalus may also occur with orbital fracture.[15] If emphysema is causing visual loss, Marcus-Gunn pupil, central retinal artery occlusion, or compromising intraocular blood flow, emergent decompression is indicated.

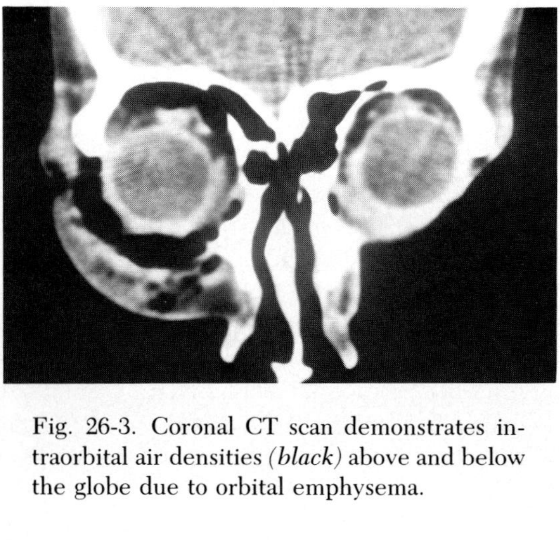

Fig. 26-3. Coronal CT scan demonstrates intraorbital air densities *(black)* above and below the globe due to orbital emphysema.

PTOSIS

Eyelid edema or hemorrhage often results in a transient mechanical ptosis and diminishes the measurable levator function. Levator dihiscence may result from hemorrhage, swelling, or blunt mechanical force—typically a human thumb—without known incision of the lid tissues. Such cases often improve spontaneously over weeks to months.[16] If ptosis persists beyond 3 months without continuous improvement, levator repair is warranted. Paretic ptosis may also accompany blunt trauma, with or without an associated occulomotor or superior rectus nerve paresis.

OPHTHALMOPLEGIA

Limitation of ocular motility following blunt orbital trauma may be due to edema, hemorrhage, emphysema, specific or nonspecific brain or nerve injury, muscle contusion, incarceration of muscle, fat, or orbital tissue connective septae in a fracture,[2] or carotid cavernous fistula. Decompensated phorias may also occur with administration of medications.

Specific nerve palsies may be diagnosed on the basis of typical clinical features and negative forced-duction testing. About 30% to 50% of ocular motor palsies will recover over 6 to 8 months. Temporizing maneuvers such as occluders, prisms, and even botulinum toxin may aid in managing the diplopia until a stable result is obtained. Aggressive management to prevent amblyopia is warranted in high-risk young children.

Thin-section axial and coronal 2-mm CT scanning and forced-duction testing help in diagnosing motility defects due to tissues incarcerated in a fracture. CT scan will also demonstrate emphysema, hematoma, and dilation of the superior ophthalmic vein in carotid-cavernous fistula.

OPTIC NERVE BLINDNESS

Optic nerve blindness can result from direct penetrating injury to the nerve, indirect or remote trauma such as optic canal fractures associated with facial fractures, or blunt forehead trauma without fracture.[17,18] Such patients with remote trauma are usually children or young adults.[17,18] Uniocular decreasing vision, afferent defect, and scotoma with a normal fundus and clear media suggest optic nerve injury. Acuity is sometimes normal, although the patient complains of a "dimness" of vision.

Injury is believed to be due to stretching, tearing, and torsion of the tethered optic nerve during sudden deceleration, as well as to skeletal deformation of the optic canal.[17,18] These forces injure the optic nerve by disruption or compression of nutrient vessels, pressure effects resulting from intranerve sheath hematoma or orbital hematoma, or direct injury to the nerve.[17,18]

Immediate, sudden, and complete optic nerve visual loss at the time of trauma is usually unresponsive to all treatment modalities.[17] Delayed-onset visual loss is initially treated with high-dose corticosteroids (discussed later in the section on steroid therapy). If vision fails to improve, or improves and then relapses during steroid therapy or steroid taper, some authors advocate optic nerve decompression with removal of a portion of the optic canal[17] (see Chapter 35).

Rarely, an intraoptic nerve sheath hematoma may compromise vision. Such clots may be recognized on magnetic resonance imaging (MRI) or CT scan and treated with incision of the optic nerve sheath to decompress the hematoma.

THERAPY

One should not overlook the cosmetic and psychologic impact of periorbital injuries; most patients will demand some type of dressing to protect the injured site from inquisitive stares.

Ice Packs

Topical ice packs applied over a cotton gauze diminish edema, provide minor superficial anesthesia, and provide a purposeful, calming, and repetitive distraction for the patient and family. Ice packs applied as frequently and continuously as possible for up to 1 week will diminish periorbital swelling and help stay the spread of ecchymosis.

Cellulitis/Antibiotics

Infection following blunt adnexal injuries is most often due to skin disruption with subsequent periorbital cellulitis or infected hematoma. Topical erythromycin, bacitracin, and neomycin-bacitracin-polysporin ointment are effective against the prevalent periorbital wound pathogens staphylococci and streptococci[3] and should be considered for prophylaxis[19,20] when the integrity of the skin has been violated.

If a periorbital cellulitis occurs, cultures should be obtained and hot packs applied. Drainage of any abscess, debridement of necrotic or foreign matter, and topical and systemic antibiotics should be considered. Empirical antibiotic therapy is discussed below. Of course, the final decision regarding antibiotic therapy should be guided by the results of bacterial culture sensitivities.

For preseptal cellulitis clearly related to an infection of a skin lesion (i.e., probably staphylococcus or streptococcus), Jackson and Baker[4,5] recommend nafcillin (150 mg/kg/day divided every 6 hours; usual adult dose[21] 1 g every 4 hours IM or IV) or another beta-lactam drug given intravenously. Vancomycin (40 mg/kg/day divided every 6 hours, usual adult dose[21] 1 g every 12 hours IV) may be substituted if there is penicillin allergy. Oral antibiotic therapy may be substituted when systemic symptoms disappear and the patient responds clinically. With mild infection, outpatient oral antibiotic therapy may be used, such as cefaclor (40 mg/kg/day divided every 8 hours; usual adult dose[21] 0.25 to 0.5 g every 8 hours po). A second choice would be the combination of amoxicillin and clavulanate potassium (Augmentin) (40 mg/kg/day divided every 8 hours, usual adult dose[21] 0.25 to 0.5 g every 8 hours po).

Dicloxacillin (25 to 40 mg/kg/day divided in 4 doses, usual adult dose[21] 0.125 to 0.5 g every 6 hours IM or po) provides antistaphylococcal activity. If drug allergy is present, erythromycin (40 mg/kg/day divided in 4 doses, usual adult dose[21] 0.5 g every 6 hours po) may be substituted.

True orbital cellulitis is a surprisingly rare complication of nonpenetrating facial trauma, even with coexistent maxillary or zygomatic fractures.[5,22,23] In children under 12 years of age, *Hemophilus* is an important cause of orbital cellulitis secondary to sinusitis and requires antibiotic therapy different from that for preseptal cellulitis.

Intraocular Pressure Management

The urgency with which measures are undertaken to reduce intraocular pressure (IOP) depends upon the degree of imminent risk of irreversible visual loss. Nonperfusion of the central retinal artery demands immediate intervention to prevent irreversible retinal ischemia. Extremely high IOP or moderate IOP elevation with advanced glaucomatous cupping or poor ocular perfusion pressure may result in irreversible damage to the optic nerve head.

Elevated IOP following blunt orbital trauma may be due to elevated orbital pressure (emphysema, hematoma, edema), elevated episcleral venous pressure (carotid cavernous fistula, diminished orbital venous return due to orbital congestion), or intraocular damage (angle closure, hyphema). IOP following blunt globe trauma is typically highest in the first few hours, normal within 24 hours, 3 to 5 mmHg below the IOP in the uninjured eye for 1 week, and normal by 2 weeks.[24]

Modest IOP elevations due to orbital causes are often managed with topical beta-blocker medications. Miotics are avoided if there is a risk of posterior synechia formation. Oral hyperosmotic agents, such as glycerine, or carbonic anhydrase inhibitors, such as acetazolamide (Diamox) or methazolamide (Neptazane), may be added. Rapid lowering of IOP may be achieved with intravenous acetazolamide, mannitol, or oral glycerine or isosorbide. Many IOP-lowering agents have severe potential side effects and specific contraindications. Steroids should be considered if the IOP rise is believed to be due to orbital edema or congestion. Digital massage, anterior chamber paracentesis, and carbogen inhalation may also be useful (see Chapter 10).

Corticosteroids

Corticosteroids will hasten the resolution of orbital edema and return of motility.[25] They may quicken the return of lid function in a young child in whom periorbital swelling may be causing an occlusion amblyopia. Some ophthalmologists routinely use corticosteroids to aid in determining whether limited ocular motility following trauma is due to entrapment or edema. Corticosteroids may also be useful in helping to prevent sympathetic ophthalmia when uveal tissue has extruded into the orbit, in lowering an IOP rise due to orbital congestion, and in decreasing preoperative or perioperative orbital swelling.

For optic nerve blindness, Anderson, Panje, and Gross[17] recommend an initial dose of 0.75 mg/kg dexamethasone sodium phosphate and then 0.33 mg/kg every 6 hours for 24 hours. (Such high corticosteroid dosages are not indicated in the routine management of other aspects of orbital trauma.) Corticosteroids are then decreased to 1 mg/kg/day of pexamethasone for 24 to 48 hours. If there is no improvement by 48 hours, steroids are rapidly tapered and discontinued. If a response occurs, doses are gradually decreased for 5 to 7 days (see Chapter 35).

SURGERY

Lateral Canthotomy

The most common urgent situation requiring lateral canthotomy is orbital hematoma or hemorrhage with elevated IOP, nonperfusion of the central retinal artery, central visual loss, afferent pupillary defect, and macular cherry-red spot. The orbit is tense, and periorbital subcutaneous hemorrhage is present.

A rapid lateral canthotomy may be performed by following the steps outlined in Figs. 26-4 through 26-6. This usually results in an immediate release of orbital pressure and allows the eyeball to assume a less constrained proptotic position. The fundus is reexamined to determine whether perfusion has been reestablished.

Peritomy

Conjunctival peritomy is useful in relieving tense, sight-threatening, subconjunctival or Tenon's space hematoma. Topical anesthetics or lidocaine injection usually provides adequate anesthesia. Direct incision with sharp-tipped Westcott scissors over a subconjunctival clot may allow adequate anterior escape of hematoma and lower orbital pressure. Tenon's space hematoma may require a more formal limbal peritomy and subtenon's dissection to decompress the clot.

Orbital Decompression

Orbital decompression may be necessary when there is vision loss due to orbital edema, hematoma, congestion, or emphysema that is unresponsive to medical management. Decompression of a subperiosteal orbital hematoma 11 days after visual loss has resulted in return of vision.[26] A determination must be made regarding which orbital compartment is involved—subtenon's, intraconal, extraconal, subperiosteal, nerve sheath, or diffuse (Fig. 26-1). CT scan or ultrasound may be helpful in this determination. An appropriate surgical course can then be planned to drain and decom-

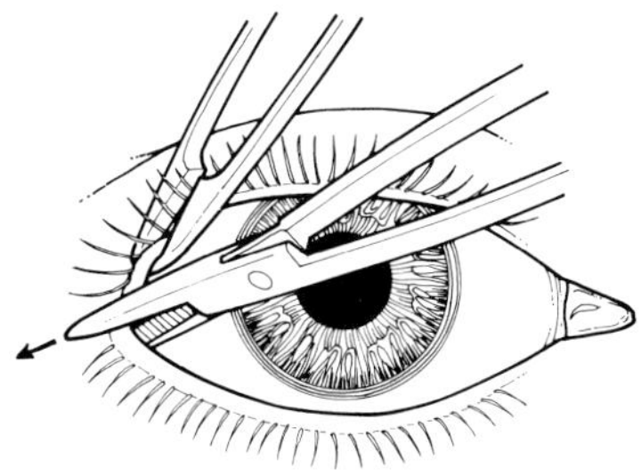

Fig. 26-4. Technique of lateral canthotomy. The lateral canthus is anesthetized with lidocaine and grasped with toothed forceps. A hemostat is angled inferiorly and slightly laterally at the lateral canthus, with the lateral lower eyelid margin passing between the open jaws. The hemostat is advanced with open jaws to the base of the fornix and then closed, crushing the most lateral lower eyelid tissues between the jaws.

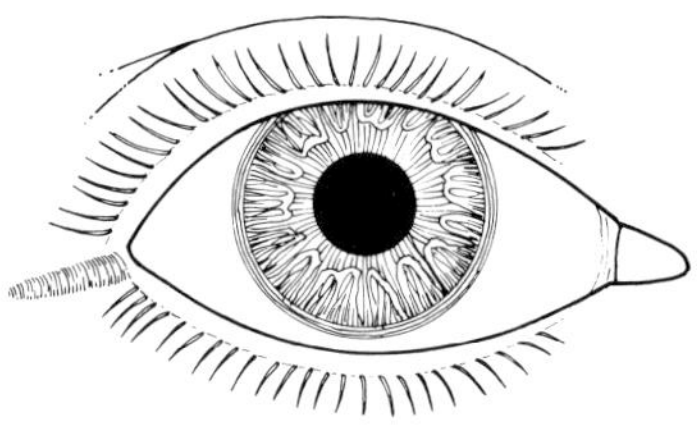

Fig. 26-5. The hemostat leaves a crush mark along the lateral lower eyelid.

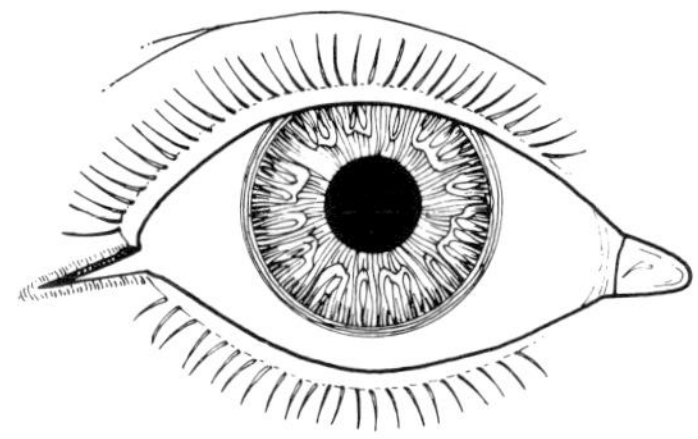

Fig. 26-6. Scissors have been used to divide the lateral lower eyelid from the inferior lateral canthal tendon along the crush mark, which helps ensure hemostasis. The lateral canthus is repaired at a later date by reattaching the tarsal plate and lateral canthal tendons and reestablishing continuity of the lid margin and skin.

press the involved compartment. Entering the traumatized orbit is not an easy procedure and may require special expertise in orbital surgery. Diffuse orbital hemorrhage unresponsive to lateral canthotomy may require decompression of the bony orbit.

Persistent Conjunctival Prolapse

Persistent conjunctival prolapse that fails to improve beyond 1 week's duration may become organized and may not spontaneously reposition as the edema subsides. In such cases, three double-armed 5-0 chromic gut sutures may be passed through the prolapsing inferior conjunctiva, inferior to the tarsal plate and exiting anteriorly and inferiorly onto the upper cheek. Each double-armed suture is then tied down tightly and left to dissolve spontaneously.

References

1. Giovinazzo VJ: The ocular sequelae of blunt trauma, Adv Ophthalmic Plast Reconstr Surg 6:107-114, 1987.
2. Fujino T and Makino K: Entrapment mechanism and ocular injury in orbital blowout fracture, Plast Reconstr Surg 65:571-576, 1980.
3. Israele V and Nelson JD: Periorbital and orbital cellulitis, Pediatr Infect Dis J 6:404-410, 1987.
4. Jackson K and Baker S: Periorbital cellulitis, Head Neck Surg 9:227-234, 1987.
5. Jackson K and Baker S: Clinical implications of orbital cellulitis, Laryngoscope 96:568-574, 1986.
6. Duke-Elder S and MacFaul PA: Mechanical injuries. In Duke-Elder S, editor: System of ophthalmology, vol XIV, part 1, St Louis, 1972, The CV Mosby Co.
7. Keltner JL et al: Dural and carotid cavernous sinus fistulas: diagnosis, management, and complications, Ophthalmology 94:1585-1600, 1987.

8. Katzen LB, Katzen BT, and Katzen MJ: Treatment of carotid-cavernous fistulas with detachable balloon catheter occlusion, Adv Ophthalmic Plast Reconstr Surg 7:157-165, 1987.
9. Bergin DJ et al: Chronic hematic cyst of the orbit, Ophthalmic Plast Reconstr Surg 4:31-36, 1988.
10. Giangiacomo J et al: Sequential cranial computed tomography in infants with retinal hemorrhages, Ophthalmology 95:295-299, 1988.
11. Itoh KT et al: Role of local hyperfibrinolysis in the etiology of chronic subdural hematoma, J Neurosurg 45:26-31, 1976.
12. Lloyd GA: Orbital emphysema, Radiology 39:933-938, 1966.
13. Jordan DR et al: Orbital emphysema: a potentially blinding complication following orbital fractures, Ann Emerg Med 17:853-855, 1988.
14. Linberg JV: Orbital compartment syndromes following trauma, Adv Ophthalmic Plast Reconstr Surg 6:51-62, 1987.
15. Waring GO III and Flanagan JC: Pneumocephalus: a sign of intracranial involvement in orbital fracture, Arch Ophthalmol 93:847-850, 1975.
16. Silkiss RZ and Baylis HI: Management of traumatic ptosis, Adv Ophthalmic Plast Reconstr Surg 7:149-155, 1987.
17. Anderson RL, Panje WR, and Gross CE: Optic nerve blindness following blunt forehead trauma, Ophthalmology 89:445-455, 1982.
18. Purvin V: Evidence of orbital deformation in indirect optic nerve injury; weight lifter's optic neuropathy, J Clin Neuroophthalmol 8:9-11, 1988.
19. Halasz NA: Wound infection and topical antibiotics: the surgeon's dilemma, Arch Surg 112:1240-1244, 1977.
20. Leyden JJ and Sulzberger MB: Topical antibiotics and minor skin trauma, Am Fam Physician 23:121-125, 1981.
21. Sanford JP: Antibiotic dosage and side effects. In Sanford JP, editor: Guide to antimicrobial therapy 1988, Bethesda, Md., 1988, Antimicrobial Therapy.
22. Chole RA and Yee J: Antibiotic prophylaxis for facial fractures: a randomized clinical trial, Arch Otolaryngol Head Neck Surg 113:1055-1057, 1987.
23. Goldfarb MS, Hoffman DS, and Rosenberg S: Orbital cellulitis and orbital fractures, Ann Ophthalmol 19:97-99, 1987.
24. Tonjum AM: Intraocular pressure disturbances early after ocular contusion, Acta Ophthalmol 46:874-885, 1968.
25. Char DH: Thyroid eye disease, Baltimore, 1985, Williams & Wilkins.
26. Kersten RC and Rice CD: Subperiosteal orbital hematoma: visual recovery following delayed drainage, Ophthalmic Surg 18:423-427, 1987.

CHAPTER 27

Orbital fractures

ROBERT A. WEISS
CLINTON D. McCORD, JR.
ROBERT M. ELLSWORTH

Examination
- Globe displacement
- Palpation of the orbital rim
- Intercanthal distance
- Nasolacrimal drainage system
- Infraorbital nerve sensation
- Orbital emphysema
- Ocular motility
- Forced-duction testing
- Pupillary reactivity
- Photography

Radiographic evaluation
- Plain films
- Axial hypocycloidal tomography
- Specialized plain film applications
- Computerized tomography

Classification of orbital fractures
- LeFort fractures
- Orbital roof fractures
- Nasoorbital and medial wall fractures
- Orbital floor and tripod fractures

Management of orbital fractures
- Indications for surgery
- Timing of surgical repair
- Repair of orbital floor fracture

References

Orbital fractures are frequently associated with acute ocular and adnexal injuries, including those involving the eyelids, canthi, and lacrimal apparatus.[1-5] Temporal considerations are important for the appropriate workup and treatment of fractures to the orbit. Immediate signs of orbital injury include mechanical restriction of eye movements, enophthalmos, orbital bony deformity, and damage to the orbital and ocular neurovasculature or to the globe itself. Delayed or long-term manifestations include bony remodeling, secondary abscess formation, external fistulization from a retained foreign body, persistent subperiosteal or bony blood cysts, and carotid-cavernous sinus fistulas, arteriovenous malformations, and aneurysms.

EXAMINATION

Globe Displacement

After assessing the integrity of the globe and the status of the optic nerve in a patient with orbital injury, the examiner should step back from the patient and evaluate the symmetry of globe position. The globe may be ptotic or inferiorly displaced or axially malpositioned compared with the opposite eye in patients with orbital fractures.

Posttraumatic exophthalmos is usually a transient event related to hemorrhage and edema of the orbital soft tissues. Exceptions include rare instances of major orbital roof defects with orbital herniation of the anterior cranial contents, and space-occupying hematic bone cysts. In contrast, enophthalmos is almost always a chronic condition due to one or more mechanisms. Orbital fractures, which most commonly occur in the floor or medial wall, cause an expansion of the orbital volume into the adjacent maxillary or ethmoid sinuses. The loss of orbital support or herniation of orbital contents through fracture sites or the development of cicatricial changes in the orbital soft tissues with fibrosis and possibly atrophy may also contribute to the development of posttraumatic enophthalmos.

Although significant asymmetry of the globe position is readily apparent, it should be documented and quantitated for future comparison and for identification of subtle asymmetries. The gross relative axial position of the globes can easily be ascertained by establishing the examiner's position at a central vantage point such as the top of the patient's head and, while holding the patient's eyelids open, looking down at the corneal apices. The presence of axial displacement (exophthalmos or enophthalmos) is usually readily apparent. This anterior/posterior deviation can be accurately quantitated by use of a Hertel or Leudde exophthalmometer if the lateral orbital rims are intact and normally positioned. These devices align a millimeter scale in the axial plane of the globe for measuring the distance from the lateral orbital rims to the corneal apices in the meridian of the canthal angles. The relative anterior/posterior position of the globes can be quantitated accurately in cases where the lateral orbital rims are not intact by use of a Mutch exophthalmometer. This device, while resting on the bones adjacent to the superior and inferior orbital rims, has a central calibrated projection whose foot plate touches the center of the closed upper eyelid overlying the corneal apex. The position of the globes relative to the superior and inferior orbital rims, and each other, can thereby be measured objectively.

Globe malposition may not develop, even in the presence of major fractures, if the globe's normal suspensory ligamentous sling remains intact (see Chapter 25). However, if the supporting elements of the globe, such as Lockwood's ligament and the orbital floor, are disrupted, the globe may develop inferior displacement and become hypophthalmic or ptotic (Fig. 27-1). Orbital floor or large rim fractures can result in unilateral hypophthalmos; extensive maxillary fractures tend to cause bilateral globe ptosis. The degree of hypophthalmos may be measured clinically by aligning a straightedge over the bridge of the nose and across the medial canthal tendons and measuring the relative vertical position of the globes using the centers of the pupils as reference points.

Palpation of the Orbital Rim

Palpation of the orbital rim is a quick, important technique for evaluating the integrity of the bony orbit. Fracture of the orbital rim involves much more forceful trauma than do medial wall and floor fractures. Palpation of the orbital rim readily cues the examiner to the presence of subtle rim fractures, especially if the deformity is masked by associated soft-tissue swelling.

Orbital rim fractures often localize at bony suture lines. For example, inferior rim fractures frequently develop at the zygomaticomaxillary suture. These fractures are often characterized as the classically described "step-deformity," in which a definite malunion or misalignment of the fractured bones is readily palpable. Similarly, lateral orbital rim fractures frequently involve the frontozygomatic suture. Crushing zygomatic complex, trimalar, or tripod fractures involve both the lateral and inferior orbital rims in addition to the zygomatic arch. These fractures are discussed later in the sections on classification and management of orbital fractures.

Tactile evaluation of the superior and nasal aspects of the orbital rim is also useful in detecting the presence of an orbital fracture (Fig. 27-2). Diagnosis of superior rim fractures is particularly important because they are often associated with orbital roof fractures as well. In these cases, potential intracranial injury becomes the clinician's priority, especially since these injuries may be life threatening.[6] Tactile evaluation of the medial rim is often unnecessary since these fractures are typically readily apparent. Clinical suspicion of medial rim fractures is usually aroused by a history of direct nasal or medial rim trauma. Multiple fractures of the nasoethmoidal complex are often present as well.[7,8]

A

B

C

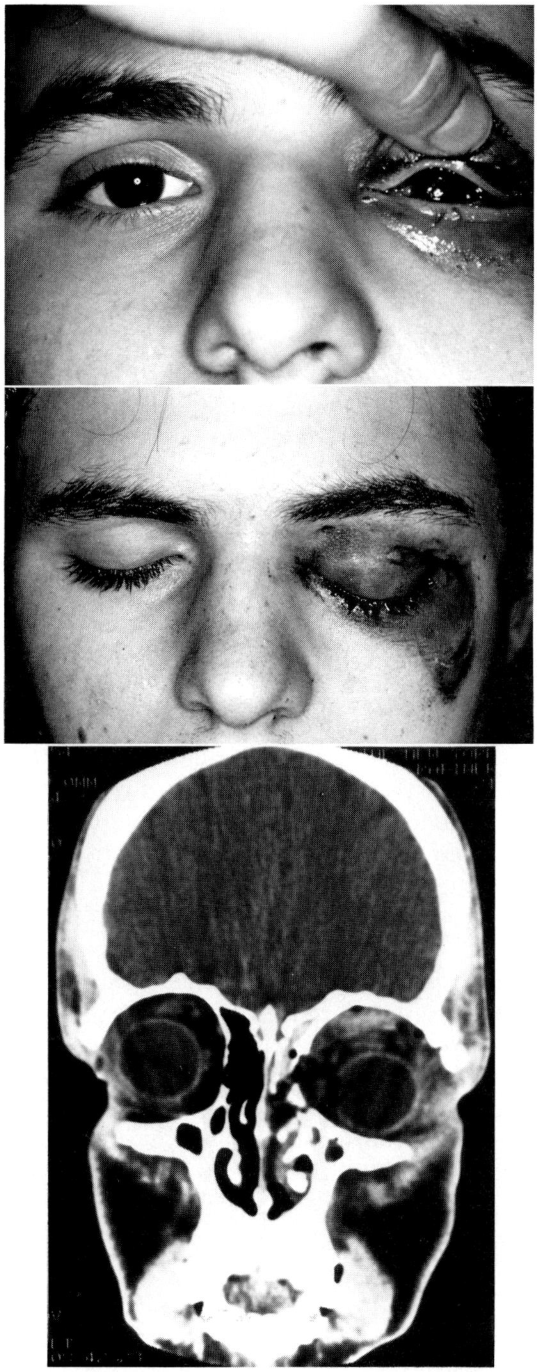

Fig. 27-1. **A**, **B**, Clinical photographs, and **C**, coronal computerized tomography (CT) scan of a patient with multiple orbital and sinus fractures that have resulted in inferior displacement of the globe. The globe ptosis can be appreciated in the clinical photographs even with the eyelid closed.

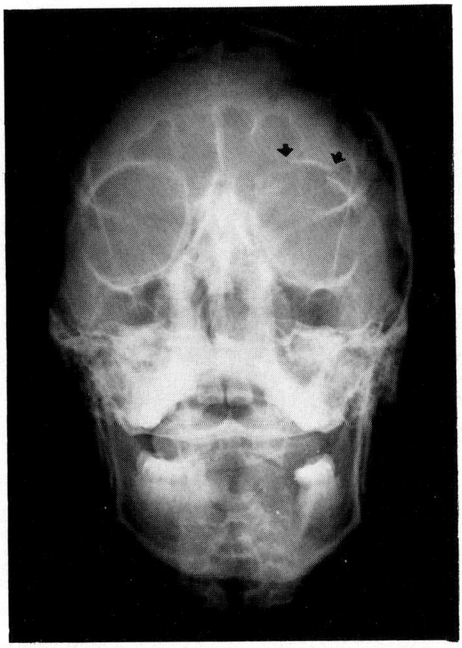

Fig. 27-2. Waters view plain film radiograph of a patient with a superolateral orbital rim fracture. This fracture may be readily diagnosed on clinical examination since the areas of orbital rim discontinuity *(arrows)* are easily palpable.

Intercanthal Distance

Expansion of the distance between the medial canthal angles of each eye is termed telecanthus. This change in intercanthal distance is sometimes seen with midfacial fractures in which there is disruption of the normal nasal bone anatomy and in cases involving soft-tissue injury with severing or disinsertion of the medial canthal tendon. Disruption of the medial canthal area anatomy is often manifested by a rounding of the normal sharp canthal angle, as well as enlargement of the intercanthal distance. Such changes are readily apparent to the examiner in unilateral cases but less so in bilateral cases. For these patients the examiner can assess and document the expanded intercanthal distance by comparing a straightedge measurement of the interpupillary distance with the intercanthal angle distance. A ratio of these measures of less than 2:1 in a setting of orbital or midfacial trauma is usually indicative of telecanthus. Posttraumatic telecanthus often requires transnasal wiring for optimal reconstruction of the canthal angle.

Nasolacrimal Drainage System

The lacrimal drainage system is frequently disrupted in patients with orbital or nasoorbital trauma because of its close proximity to the medial canthal structures. A 20% incidence of nasolacrimal duct laceration has been estimated in patients with nasoethmoidal fractures.[5]

Epiphora is not meaningful in the setting of acute orbital, nasoorbital, or midfacial trauma unless frank soft-tissue injury is evident in the lacrimal sac area or drainage pathway. Evaluation and repair of the system is typically deferred until soft-tissue swelling has subsided, except for the immediate repair of lacerations of the canalicular system (see Chapter 30). In general, when a patient has posttraumatic telecanthus and loss of adequate lacrimal system function, the surgeon should repair the lacrimal system before the telecanthus. The exception to this rule is the patient who requires a Jones' tube, since a normal medial canthal angle is necessary for this tube to function properly.[9]

Infraorbital Nerve Sensation

Since the floor of the orbit serves as the roof of the canal that carries the infraorbital nerve, it is not unusual to find decreased sensation along the distribution of this nerve and its three branches in patients with orbital floor fractures. This division of the trigeminal nerve is completely sensory in nature, transmitting sensation from the skin and conjunctiva of the lower eyelid, the skin and subcutaneous tissues of the side of the nose, and the skin and mucous membrane of the upper lip, gingiva, and labial glands. In general, fracture of the orbital floor is always suspected when diminished sensation along the distribution of this nerve is evident, although perineural edema and hemorrhage may affect the infraorbital nerve in the absence of a true fracture of the floor.

Orbital Emphysema

Palpable air in the periorbital tissues, known as orbital emphysema, is a clear clinical sign of an orbital fracture since this phenomenon occurs only when a communication exists between the orbital tissues and the periorbital sinuses. Orbital emphysema is frequently encountered with medial orbital fractures as a result of communication with the ethmoid sinuses. The presence of air in the periorbital soft tissues is clinically evident with gentle direct palpation of the area and in radiographic studies.

Ocular Motility

Ocular motility should be evaluated in all cardinal fields of gaze. Posttraumatic limitation of movement is not an unusual phenomenon, and the presence of such limitation is not pathognomonic of entrapment or mechanical restriction of one or more of the extraocular muscles. Posttraumatic limitation of ocular motility or lid elevation can result from a number of circumstances, including direct injury to the muscles or their innervation, mechanical restriction due to orbital bony fractures, and central nervous system causes including increased intracranial pressure. The last cause frequently occurs in association with unilateral or bilateral sixth cranial nerve palsies.

The indications for surgical intervention in cases of motility limitations are the presence of true mechanical restriction or significant enophthalmos, as opposed to neuromuscular limitations of motility or "prophylaxis" against the development of enophthalmos. Therefore, it is important to establish the cause of any motility limitations. Horizontal and vertical limitations usually develop as a result of hemorrhage, edema, and associated neuromuscular causes. Patients with this type of diffuse motility limitation commonly improve spontaneously as the edema and hemorrhage resolve. The same is true of any patient with purely horizontal limitations, especially of abduction, which may be associated with increased intracranial pressure.

In contrast, patients with relatively purely vertical limitations are most likely to have true entrapment. Entrapment, which refers to capture or tethering of the inferior rectus muscle, its adventitial tissues,[10,11] or, in some cases, the inferior oblique muscle in an orbital floor fracture, must be distinguished from self-limited causes of mechanical restrictions, such as edema and hemorrhage, which do not usually require surgical intervention. Although pure limitation of upgaze with no limitation of downgaze is frequently neuromuscular in origin, limitations of both upgaze and downgaze are typically associated with true mechanical restriction. An entrapped inferior rectus muscle, for example, will be tethered with attempted movement of the globe in either direction in the vertical plane. The distinction between true entrapment and neuromuscular limitation of motility can be made in some cases by forced-duction testing.

Compared with larger fractures, small orbital floor fractures are more likely to cause entrapment from a trap-door effect with incarceration of prolapsed tissues, and less likely to cause enophthalmos due to expansion of orbital volume. The opposite association is true for larger fractures.

Forced-Duction Testing

Limitation of vertical ocular motility following orbital trauma, without evidence of significant horizontal limitation or innervational disturbance, is often the result of mechanical restriction. Entrapment of the inferior rectus and possibly the inferior oblique muscles and their adventitial attachments are the usual cause of true mechanical restriction associated with orbital floor or blowout fractures.

The forced-duction, or traction, test is helpful in determining whether mechanical restriction is the actual cause of limited eye movements. Local anesthesia and vasoconstriction of the superficial vasculature of the globe are obtained by placing a 4% cocaine-saturated pledget over the inferior surface of the globe or in the inferior cul-de-sac. A toothed forceps is used to grasp either the inferior rectus muscle insertion or the inferior perilimbal conjunctiva-Tenon's tissue between the inferior limbus at 6 o'clock and the inferior rectus muscle insertion. The globe is then passively moved in the vertical meridian while having the patient attempt to gaze in the same direction. Inability to move the globe up and down readily in the vertical plane suggests either actual entrapment or secondary adhesions that mechanically restrict globe movement. Limitation of forced duction can also occur with significant orbital edema, edema or hematoma of the extraocular muscles or their sheaths, and atraumatic restrictive myopathies, as may be found in patients with thyroid orbitopathy.

Pupillary Reactivity

Pupillary reactivity, an integral aspect of any ophthalmic examination, is especially important after trauma, since it quickly, effectively, and noninvasively gives the examiner essential information about globe status and optic nerve function. Lack of reactivity to direct light, irregularity of pupillary shape, or pupillary malposition may indicate traumatic damage to the iris sphincter muscle. A normal-appearing iris that is relatively nonreactive may indicate the presence of a traumatic iridoplegia from damage to parasympathetic fibers, as may occur with orbital apex, ciliary ganglion, or third nerve injury. The presence of a relative afferent pupillary defect directs the examiner to assess the status of the optic nerve, chiasm, and, less frequently, the optic tract and its posterior pathway as far as the pregeniculate area.

Photography

The importance of photographic documentation should not be underestimated. Full-face photographs in addition to close-up or slit-lamp photos are important for medicolegal documentation and occasionally for insurance review (see Chapter 37). In addition, photographs are extremely important to demonstrate the starting point to the patient, whose memory of the initial appearance may have been softened by time, and as a guide in the operating room to assist in maximizing symmetries and contours. Photographs of the patient in an upright position are preferred to demonstrate the appearance with the full normal effect of gravity.

RADIOGRAPHIC EVALUATION

A number of advanced diagnostic imaging techniques have proven extremely useful in ophthalmology; however, conventional radiography remains the diagnostic imaging method of choice for the initial evaluation of orbital fractures. Especially important is simple plain film roentgenography and its contrast-related applications (dacryocystography, orbital venography, and angiography) and computerized tomography (CT). Other important techniques such as ultrasonography and magnetic resonance imaging (MRI) are less useful for the initial evaluation of the orbital trauma patient (see Chapter 2).

Plain Films

Plain films are particularly useful in assessing blunt trauma involving bony injury.[12] Although soft-tissue swelling and large areas of hemorrhage may be evident in plain film radiographs, bony fractures are very well demonstrated as is intraorbital or intracranial air.

The Waters, Caldwell, and lateral projections are the standard plain film radiographic views used for routine imaging of the traumatized orbit. The *Waters* projection is an oblique coronal view that is particularly useful for evaluating orbital floor and blowout fractures[13] (Fig. 27-3). It is also useful for evaluating the neighboring maxillary and frontal sinuses and the orbital roof and lacrimal fossa. The Waters projection may demonstrate a dislocated bony fragment or inferiorly displaced orbital soft tissues. The radiographic appearance of this inferiorly displaced tissue is often referred to as the teardrop sign since the prolapsed tissue often assumes this shape (Fig. 27-4). Accompanying hemorrhage appearing as an air-fluid level or complete opacification of the maxillary sinus is highly suggestive of an orbital floor fracture.

The *Caldwell* projection is a plain film radiograph inclined in the posteroanterior plane. This view is useful in assessing the medial orbital wall, lateral and superior orbital rims, superior orbital fissure, and ethmoidal and frontal sinuses (Fig. 27-5). Fractures of the medial wall and ethmoid sinuses are particularly difficult to assess accurately in these films because the bones that make up these structures are extremely thin and detail is obscured by overlying shadows. Fracture is suggested when the ethmoid sinuses appear clouded, which results from hemorrhage accompanying the traumatic fracture.[14]

The orbital roof, lateral orbital margin, and zygoma, in addition to the frontal, sphenoid, and maxillary sinuses (including the posterior wall), can all be evaluated by use of plain film radio-

A

B

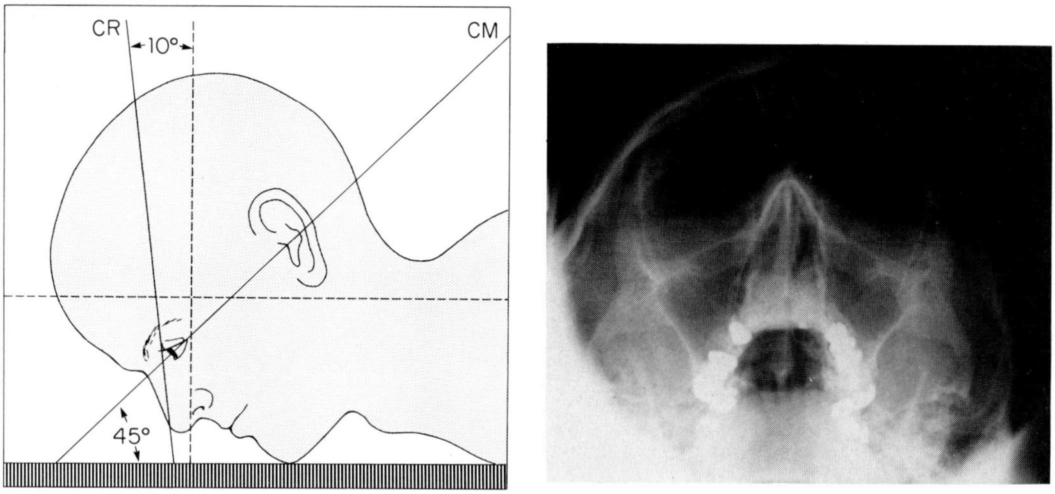

Fig. 27-3. **A,** Waters projection. *CR*, central ray; *CM*, canthomeatal line. **B,** Normal Waters projection (oblique coronal view) plain film radiograph, used in evaluating orbital floor and blowout fractures. The orbital roof, petrous pyramids, lacrimal fossa, ethmoid air cells, and neighboring maxillary and frontal sinuses are clearly shown. (Reprinted, with permission, from Weiss RA et al: Advanced diagnostic imaging techniques in ophthalmology, Adv Ophthalmic Plast Reconstr Surg 6:207-63, 1987.)

A

B

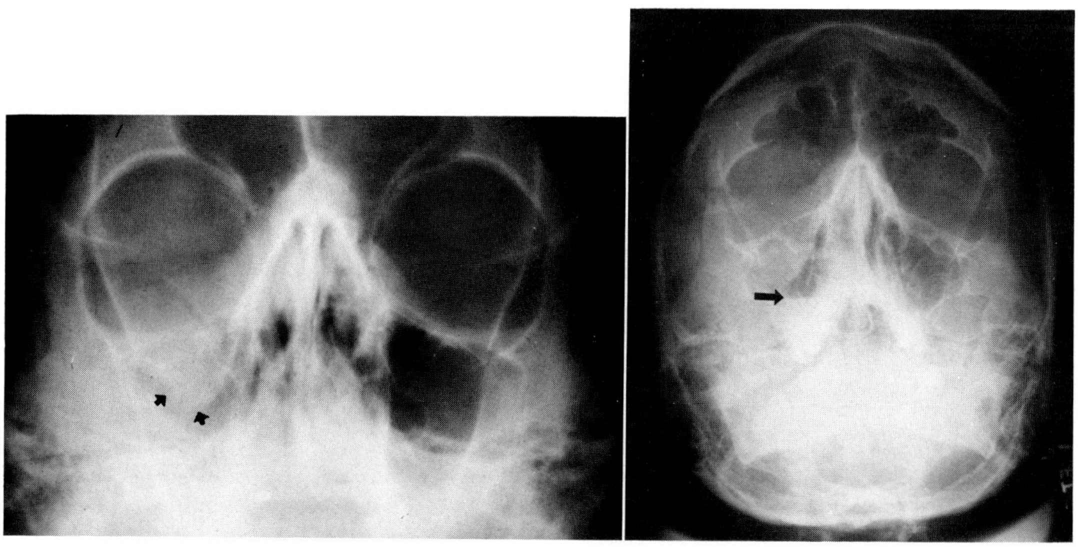

Fig. 27-4. Waters view plain film radiographs of two cases involving large floor fractures in the right orbit with opacification of the right maxillary sinus. **A,** The bony orbital floor is depressed and a well-defined soft-tissue mass extends below the floor of the orbit into the sinus. This mass, the teardrop sign, represents herniation of orbital fat *(arrows)*. **B,** Maxillary sinus air-fluid level *(arrow)*. Edema of the eyelids and soft tissues is also apparent. (Reprinted, with permission, from Weiss RA et al: Advanced diagnostic imaging techniques in ophthalmology, Adv Ophthalmic Plast Reconstr Surg 6:207-63, 1987.)

A

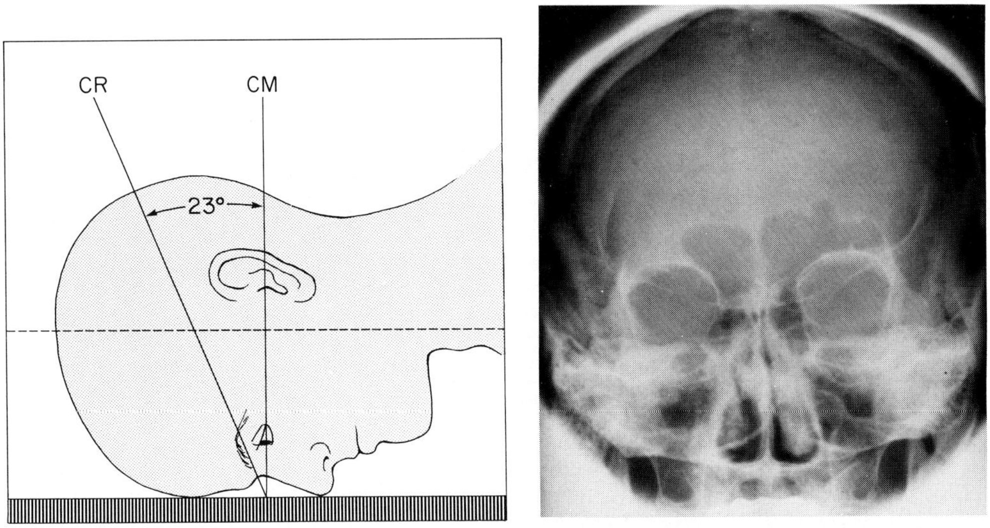

B

Fig. 27-5. **A,** Caldwell projection. *CR,* central ray; *CM,* canthomeatal line. **B,** Caldwell projection (inclined in posteroanterior plane) plain film radiograph, useful in evaluating medial orbital wall, superior and lateral orbital rims, superior orbital fissure, and ethmoid and frontal sinuses. (Reprinted, with permission, from Weiss RA et al: Advanced diagnostic imaging techniques in ophthalmology, Adv Ophthalmic Plast Reconstr Surg 6:207-63, 1987.)

A

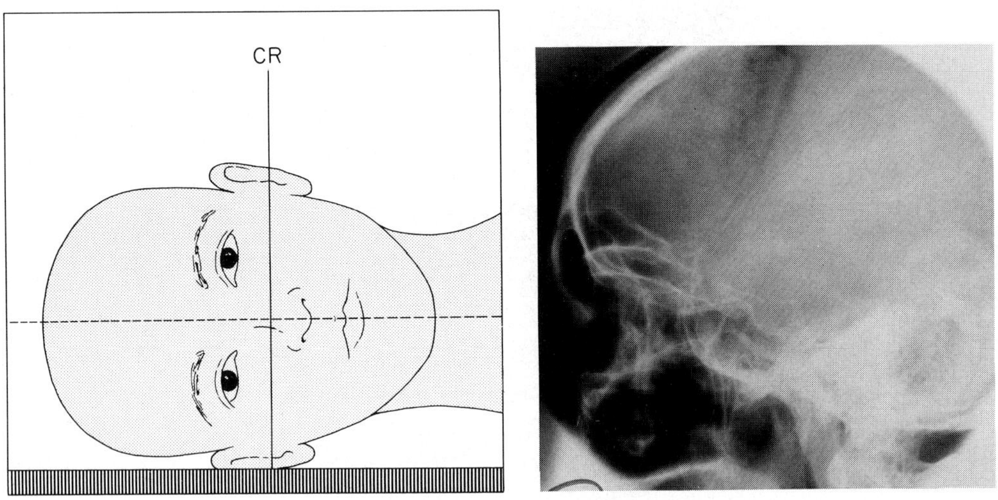

B

Fig. 27-6. **A,** Lateral projection. *CR,* central ray. **B,** Normal lateral projection plain film radiograph, useful in evaluating orbital roof, lateral orbital margin, zygoma, maxillary and frontal sinuses, and sella turcica. (Reprinted, with permission, from Weiss RA et al: Advanced diagnostic imaging techniques in ophthalmology, Adv Ophthalmic Plast Reconstr Surg 6:207-63, 1987.)

graphs in the *lateral* projection (Fig. 27-6). This projection is also important in assessing the status of the pterygoid plates in the evaluation of LeFort fractures. Furthermore, lateral views can demonstrate opacification of the mastoid air cells, fractures of the calvarium, and abnormalities of the sella turcica.

Plain film evaluation of the orbital apex in orbitofacial trauma patients can best be achieved by the use of Caldwell, Rhese, and cranial base views. *Rhese* views are oblique projections that demonstrate the optic foramina (Fig. 27-7). *Cranial base*, or *submentovertex*, views are useful for assessing the integrity of the lateral orbital

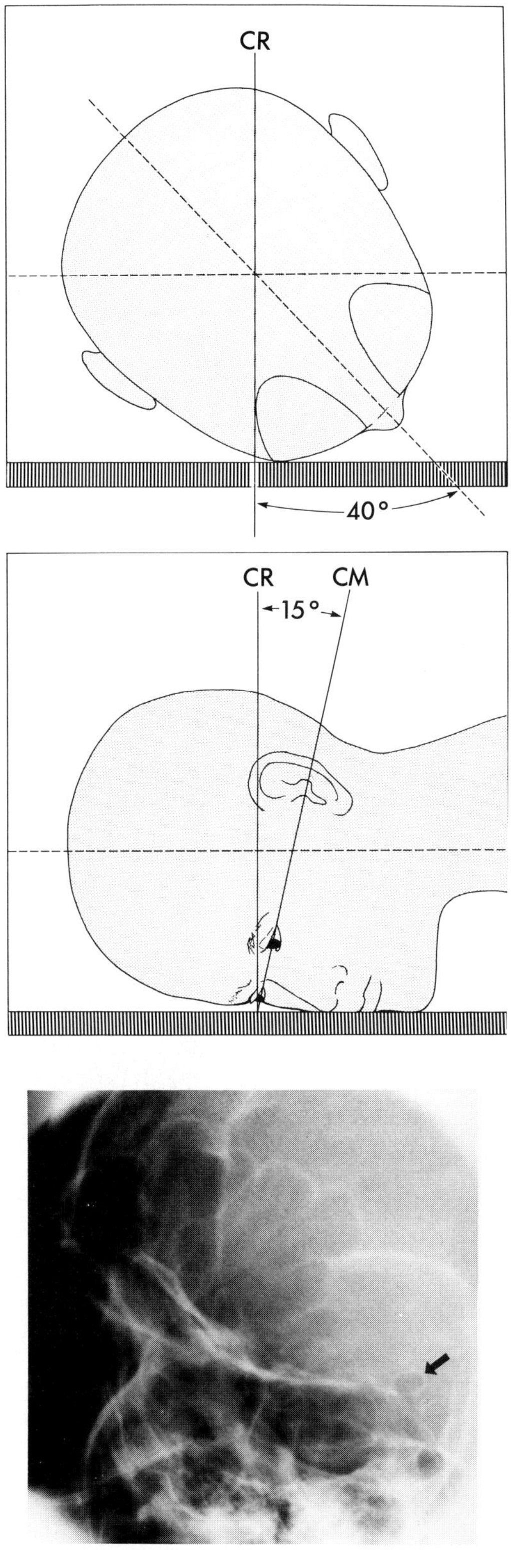

A

B

Fig. 27-7. **A,** Rhese projection. *CR,* central ray; *CM,* canthomeatal line. **B,** Normal Rhese (oblique) projection plain film radiograph, useful in evaluating optic foramina *(arrow)*. (Reprinted, with permission, from Weiss RA et al: Advanced diagnostic imaging techniques in ophthalmology, Adv Ophthalmic Plast Reconstr Surg 6:207-63, 1987.)

A

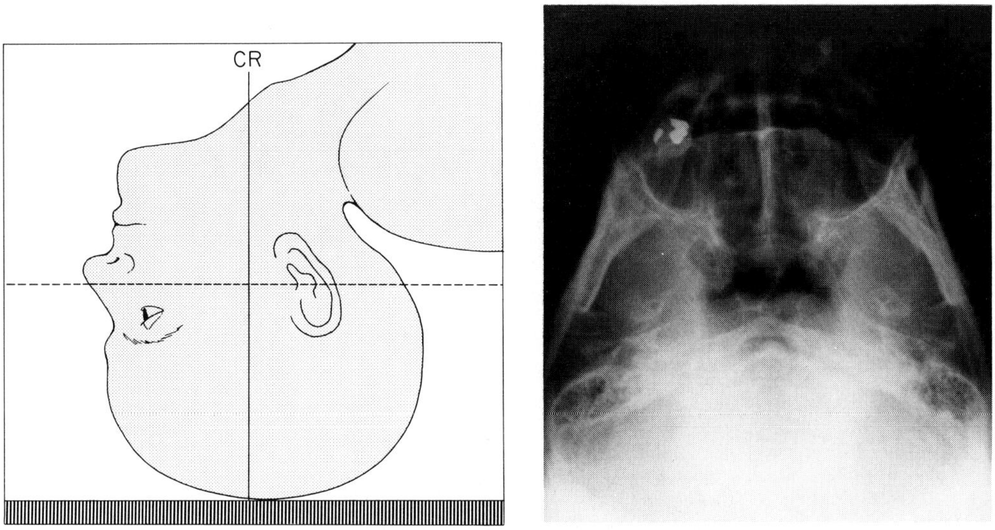

B

Fig. 27-8. **A,** Cranial base, or submentovertex, projection. *CR,* central ray. **B,** Normal cranial base projection plain film radiograph, useful for assessing integrity of lateral walls, zygomatic arches, and ethmoid, maxillary, sphenoid, and frontal sinuses. (Reprinted, with permission, from Weiss RA et al: Advanced diagnostic imaging techniques in ophthalmology, Adv Ophthalmic Plast Reconstr Surg 6:207-63, 1987.)

walls and zygomatic arches, in addition to the periorbital sinuses (Fig. 27-8).[14] Unfortunately, positioning requirements may preclude the use of these projections, especially the cranial base view, in orbital trauma patients who may have associated cranial or cervical injuries.[15]

Specialized Plain Film Applications

The superb quality of soft-tissue detail and the noninvasive means of vascular imaging afforded by CT scanning and MRI has, for the most part, eliminated the need for axial hypocycloidal tomography, dacryocystography, orbital venography, and angiography. Nevertheless, these important applications of plain film radiography still have their place in specific instances of ophthalmic trauma. For instance, dacryocystography performed by injecting oil-based, iodinated, low-viscosity contrast materials into the eyelid puncta is useful in the evaluation of lacrimal drainage system anomalies (Fig. 27-9).

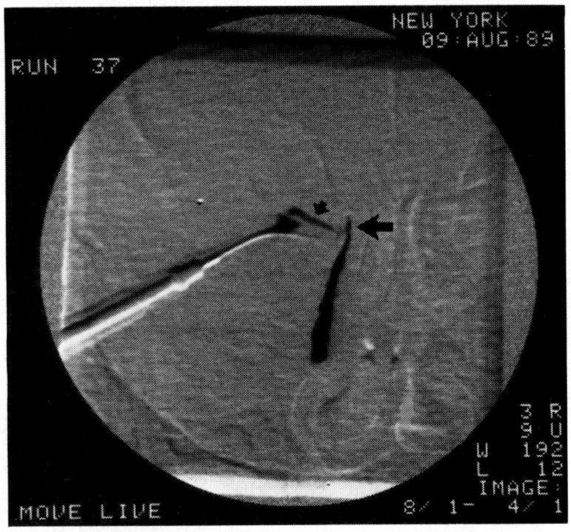

Fig. 27-9. Digital subtraction dacryocystogram in a patient with a functional partial obstruction of the nasolacrimal drainage outflow system. The dacryocystogram demonstrates reflux of radioopaque material into the superior canaliculus *(small arrow)* and possible narrowing of the fundus of the lacrimal sac *(large arrow).*

Orbital venography, a similar but less useful technique since the advent of CT scanning, enables the examiner to evaluate variances and assess the patency of the ophthalmic veins by injecting contrast material through superficial veins. The primary use of this technique is to evaluate the status of the superior ophthalmic vein in cases of possible orbital venous thrombosis or cavernous sinus thrombosis, as may occur in association with orbital fractures (Fig. 27-10). Because CT scanning clearly demonstrates the caliber of the superior ophthalmic vein, in addition to clearly resolving orbital varices, it has essentially replaced venography.

The final plain film application that continues to have specific indications in the assessment of the orbit is angiography. Angiography performed by arterial or digital venous (DIVA) techniques is indicated when vascular lesions such as dural arteriovenous malformations, cavernous sinus fistulas, and aneurysms are suspected (Fig. 27-11). In addition, angiography may be essential in planning the safe surgical removal of a retained penetrating orbital foreign body (Fig. 27-12).

Computerized Tomography

CT is extremely useful for the initial assessment of orbital trauma because it allows simultaneous evaluation of the globes, orbital and facial bony structures and soft tissues, and intracranial contents.[16,17] Standard CT studies are obtained in the axial or horizontal plane, perpendicular to the orbital walls. This permits the examiner to visualize the medial, lateral, and posterior walls of the orbit. Coronal sections are useful in assessing the integrity of the orbital floor and in-

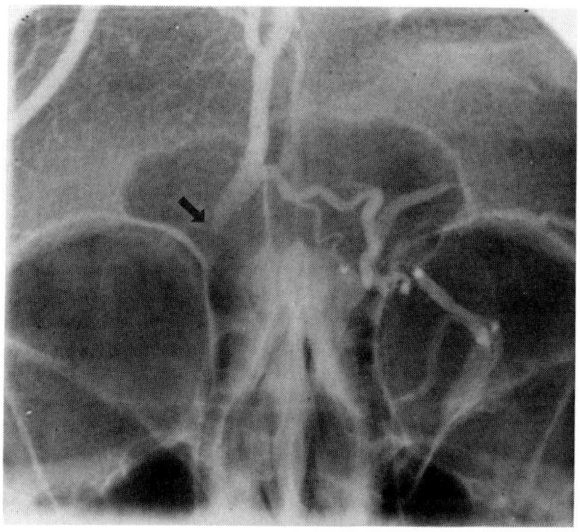

Fig. 27-10. Orbital venogram performed after injection of contrast material through a butterfly needle placed in a forehead vein. The venogram shows unilateral filling of the left superior ophthalmic vein. The occluded right superior ophthalmic vein does not fill *(arrow)*. (Reprinted, with permission, from Weiss RA et al: Advanced diagnostic imaging techniques in ophthalmology, Adv Ophthalmic Plast Reconstr Surg 6:207-63, 1987.)

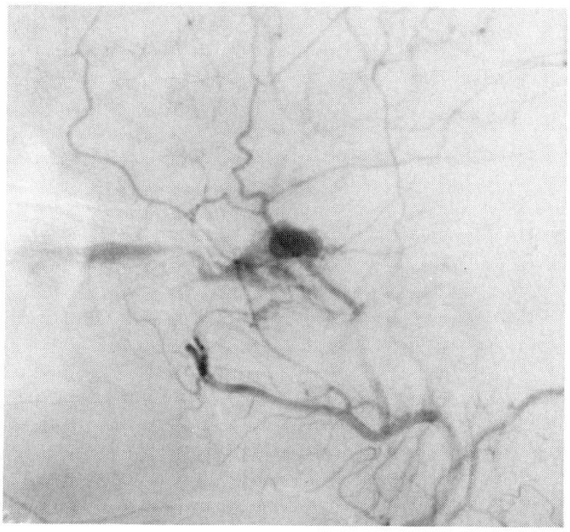

Fig. 27-11. Angiogram of a dural arteriovenous fistula. The external carotid artery shows feeding of the dural fistula through the internal maxillary artery by way of the foramen rotundum, with retrograde filling of the cavernous sinus region and dilatation of the superior ophthalmic vein. (Reprinted, with permission, from Weiss RA et al: Advanced diagnostic imaging techniques in ophthalmology, Adv Ophthalmic Plast Reconstr Surg 6:207-63, 1987.)

A 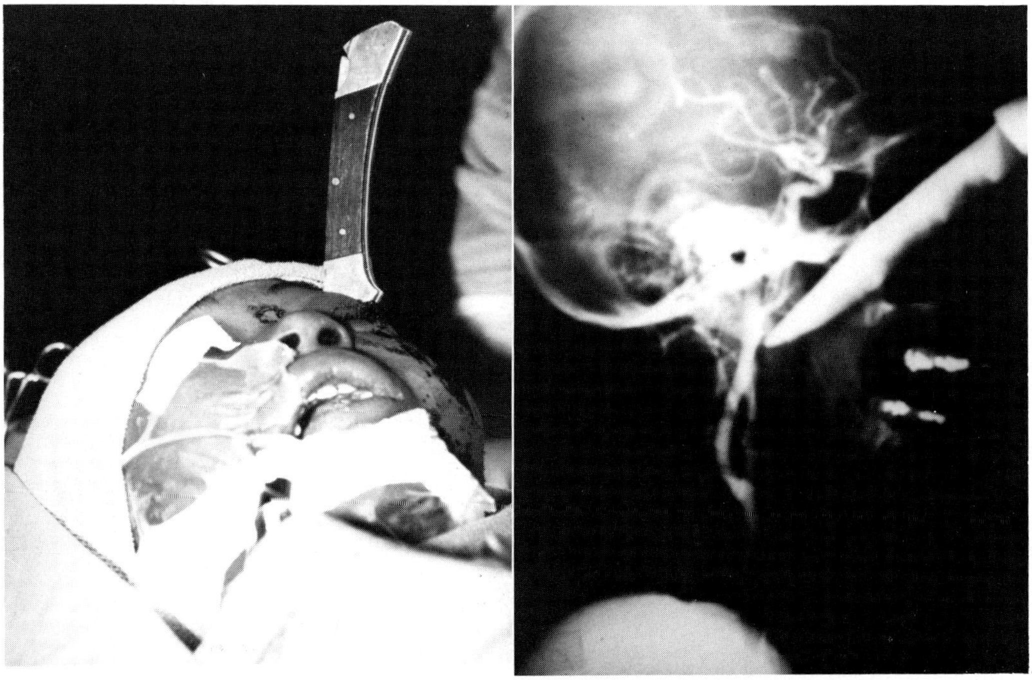 B

Fig. 27-12. **A,** Clinical photograph, and **B,** lateral plain film projection of a carotid angiogram in a patient with a knife foreign body in the orbit. The angiogram shows the close proximity of the knife's tip to the internal carotid artery. (Reprinted, with permission, from Weiss RA et al: Advanced diagnostic imaging techniques in ophthalmology, Adv Ophthalmic Plast Reconstr Surg 6:207-63, 1987.)

ferior rectus muscle. They are also helpful in imaging the extraocular muscles, sinuses, anterior fossa, and oropharyngeal and nasal cavities.

The possibility of optic nerve injury with orbital apex fractures in the absence of clinical signs and symptoms of optic nerve compression makes accurate CT evaluation of these fractures particularly important. Traumatic optic nerve compression typically occurs acutely as a result of hemorrhage, displaced bony fragments, or inflammation; however, such injury may also occur as a result of callus formation as the fracture heals.[16]

In addition, CT scans clearly demonstrate abnormalities associated with bony fractures such as opacification, air-fluid levels, or soft-tissue incarceration in the maxillary or ethmoid sinuses. They may also show subperiosteal hematomas, which, although rare, may develop after only minor trauma. Subperiosteal hematomas in the orbit are most commonly found in the orbital roof of young people since the attachments between the bone and periosteum are relatively weak at younger ages. Because high attenuation and blood density are so sharply defined by CT scanning, the extent, as well as the presence, of a subperiosteal collection of blood is well demonstrated.[18] CT also allows retained air to be identified in periorbital, intraocular (perforation or endophthalmitis with a gas-producing organism), retroorbital, and intracranial locations.[19]

Although ultrasonography is particularly helpful in evaluating and localizing intraocular foreign bodies, it is very limited in evaluating foreign bodies in the orbit.[21,22] In contrast, CT has demonstrated some use in localizing foreign bodies, especially with the use of bone review algorithms. Experimental techniques have been used to demonstrate the minimum detectable quantities of various metals, glass, and wood. Intraocular metals including steel and copper were detectable with fragments as small as 0.06 mm^3. Different types of glass were detectable at sizes smaller than 2 mm^3 although wooden pine splinters were not detectable in trials of 2.4 mm^3.[20] Other studies have shown similar or slightly less impressive results.[22,23] The minimum detectable sizes of the various materials depend on their size, density, attenuation coefficients, and, in some cases, orientation with

A 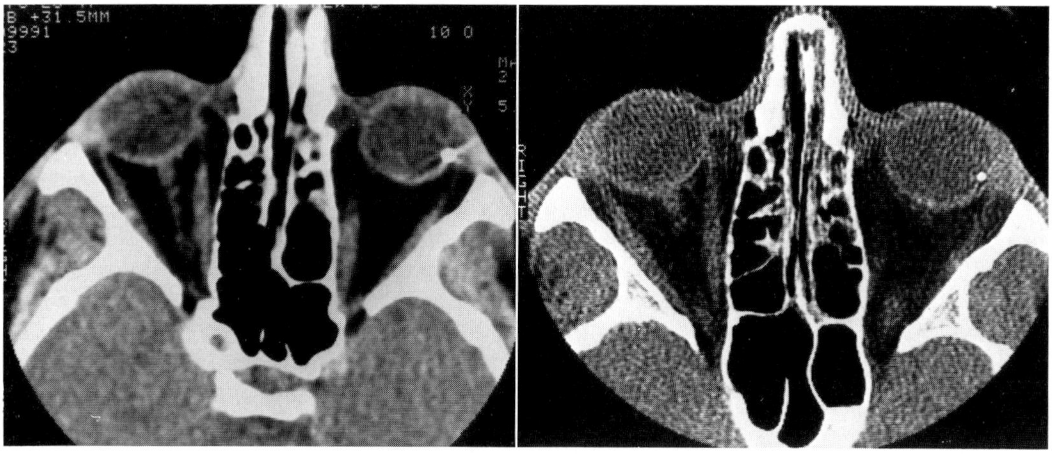 B

Fig. 27-13. Axial CT scan of a patient with an intraocular foreign body. **A,** Soft-tissue window shows a metallic fragment in a lateral aspect of the left globe. Whether the foreign body is intrascleral, intravitreal, or extrascleral cannot be ascertained because of a beam-hardening artifact. **B,** A bone review algorithm (bone window) shows the metallic density to be intravitreal. (Reprinted, with permission, from Weiss RA et al: Advanced diagnostic imaging techniques in ophthalmology, Adv Ophthalmic Plast Reconstr Surg 6:207-63, 1987.)

respect to the radiation beam.[20,23] Accurate localization of intraocular and intraorbital foreign bodies has been demonstrated at even smaller sizes, and in some cases the specific composition of certain nonmetallic foreign bodies can be determined by the use of advanced software techniques.[24]

Different tissues vary in their radiodensity, which enhances the yield of CT studies. For example, retroocular fat is clearly delineated and distinguished from extraocular muscles and the optic nerve by the inherent contrast between them. Fat is imaged as low density or black, whereas muscle and optic nerve are imaged as high density or relatively white. Contrast variation in generated images can also be achieved by the use of soft-tissue windows or bone review algorithms in which the examiner can enhance soft-tissue detail or subtle bony abnormalities on the computer screen (Fig. 27-13). Exogenous contrast agents can also be used; they are particularly helpful in evaluating acute orbital trauma and diagnosing vascular lesions such as varices. A complete discussion of radiography in orbital trauma is presented in Chapter 2.

CLASSIFICATION OF ORBITAL FRACTURES

LeFort Fractures

Orbital fractures are usually classified based on their extent and involvement with periorbital structures. An important group of orbital fractures that extend beyond the orbit are known as midfacial fractures. These fractures are frequently assymmetric and complex. They are generally categorized by the LeFort classification, which divides midfacial fractures into three groups. The LeFort I fracture, also known as Geurin's fracture, is a relatively inferior transverse fracture within the body of the maxilla in the region above the teeth without true involvement of the orbit. The LeFort II fracture is a pyramidally shaped maxillary fracture extending to the medial floors and walls of the orbit. This fracture typically involves the nasal and lacrimal bones in addition to the maxillary bones. The LeFort III fracture is a complex, extensive, midfacial fracture also known as craniofacial dysjunction or "free-floating" maxilla since the midface is essentially detached from the skull and is suspended in place by soft tissues alone. This fracture extends through the ramus of the mandible, in addition to the lateral walls, floors, and medial walls of the orbit.

Depending upon the extent of the injuries, the trauma patient with a midfacial LeFort fracture may be best served by a multispeciality approach. The patient's condition may require arch bars for stabilization in conjunction with dental occlusion alignment, open reduction with internal fixation using bone plates, interosseous wire fixation, and possibly autologous bone grafts or alloplastic supporting materials. Skull fractures and intracranial injuries that require neurosurgical intervention can be associated with severe LeFort fractures.[25]

Orbital Roof Fractures

Orbital roof fractures may represent a threat to life by direct CNS injury, an intracranial foreign body, or the presence of a dural tear with cerebrospinal fluid leakage.[6] The last complication is usually transient since these leaks are often self-sealing. Pneumocephalus and a brain abscess or infectious meningitis may develop in association with an orbital roof fracture.[26] Therefore, extensive CNS evaluation and possible neurosurgical management is required in the presence of an orbital roof fracture.[27-30]

Fracture and involvement of the nasofrontal duct or frontal sinus can also accompany an orbital roof fracture. Large defects, which on rare occasion can be associated with herniation of anterior cranial contents, may require repair using primary pericranium or bone grafts or both. Alloplastic graft materials should be avoided since nonautogenous materials carry a greater risk of infection, especially in these cases, since the grafts are in contact with the frontal sinus. In general, calvarial bone is preferred in all cases that require grafting of autogenous tissue. Some authors recommend considering obliteration of the frontal sinus at the time of primary surgical repair to avoid the risk of delayed development of a frontal sinus mucocele.[31,32]

Bony fragments from orbital roof fractures can cause mechanical restriction of the superior muscle complex, but this situation is most unusual. Dysfunction of the superior rectus or levator muscle much more commonly results from edema, hemorrhage, or neurogenic etiologies. Therefore, if direct bony displacement is not the apparent cause of superior rectus or levator muscle dysfunction, a period of 6 months or longer is typically allowed to pass before attention is directed toward surgical repair of these muscles because they often regain or improve function spontaneously.

Nasoorbital and Medial Wall Fractures

Fracture of the lamina papyracea that serves as the lateral wall of the ethmoid sinus is relatively common in nasoorbital and medial wall fractures because this bone is so thin. Ethmoidal wall fractures frequently develop by transmission of hydraulic forces when an individual receives blunt trauma or a blow to the globe or anterior orbit.[13] In a large number of these cases, signs and symptoms are limited to epistaxis or orbital emphysema. Since these findings generally have no long-term importance and leave no permanent sequelae, the appropriate treatment is to instruct the patient to avoid nose-blowing until symptoms have resolved.

In some cases, nasoorbital fractures may contribute to the development of posttraumatic enophthalmos, which results from orbital volume expansion if the periorbita is violated and orbital tissues and fat prolapse into the ethmoid air cells. In addition to the lateral wall of the ethmoid sinus, nasoorbital or medial wall injury may involve fracture of the frontal process of the maxilla and the lacrimal bone. These fractures are usually the result of direct trauma to the nose or medial orbital rim but may also occur in association with an indirect or blowout fracture.

A problem that can occur in association with these fractures is direct or secondary injury to the medial canthal tendon with subsequent functional or cosmetic problems such as medial lid or canthal angle malposition, punctal eversion, and telecanthus. In addition, disruption of the lacrimal sac and drainage system can occur with development of dacryostenosis or a sac mucocele.[8] Associated nasal fractures must be addressed as well.

On occasion, medial fractures may interfere with normal globe motility by tethering the medial rectus muscle. The presence of mechanical restriction of the eye may warrant surgical exploration to prevent or minimize permanent limitation of motility from fibrosis and scarring.

Orbital Floor and Tripod Fractures

Orbital floor fractures are often classified as direct or indirect. Direct fractures result from trauma to the inferior orbital rim of enough force to directly fracture the relatively thick bones that make up the rim. The fracture usually occurs along the proximal aspect of the zygoma or at its articulation with the medial or maxillary portion of the inferior rim. Forceful or crushing trauma may result in multifocal zygomatic fractures, often involving the zygomatic arch or its posterior articulation in addition to its lateral and inferior orbital rim articulation (the frontozygomatic and zygomaticomaxillary sutures, re-

A 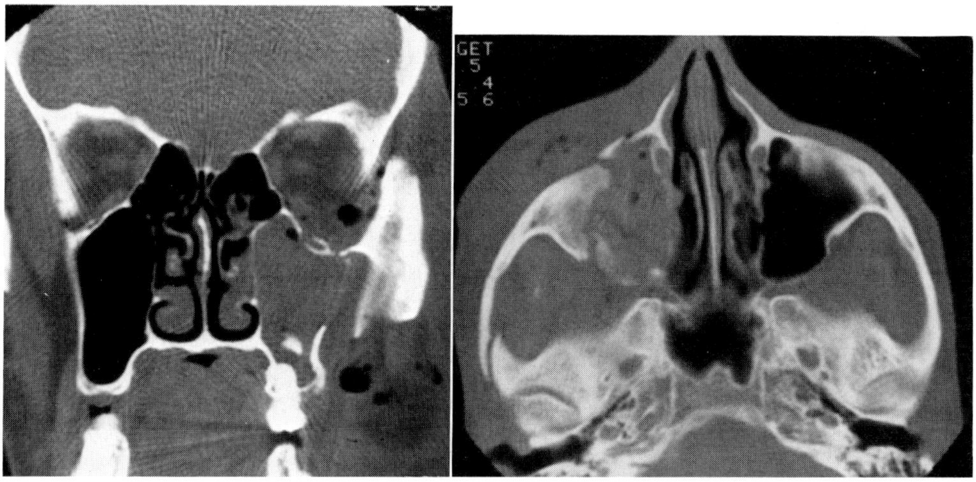 B

Fig. 27-14. Bone review algorithms of a tripod fracture in the coronal and axial planes. **A,** Coronal scan shows fractures of the orbital floor, lateral orbital wall, and lateral maxillary wall, with a bone fragment in the maxillary sinus. **B,** Axial scan shows fractures through the zygoma and anterior and posterior maxillary sinus walls. (Reprinted, with permission, from Weiss RA et al: Advanced diagnostic imaging techniques in ophthalmology, Adv Ophthalmic Plast Reconstr Surg 6:207-63, 1987.)

spectively). This three-part zygomatic fracture is referred to as a tripod fracture (Fig. 27-14). When nondisplaced, these fractures often require no reduction or fixation. However, displaced, depressed, or rotated tripod fractures result in loss of the normal prominence of the cheek and may limit the normal excursion of the mandible. Fractures causing cosmetic or functional sequelae should be repaired primarily by simple open or closed reduction or by open reduction and internal fixation, as indicated.[25,33] An oral surgeon should be involved when mandibular excursion or dental occlusion is affected by the injury.

Direct inferior rim fractures and tripod fractures rarely affect ocular motility, and late enophthalmos or globe ptosis does not usually occur. In contrast, all these ocular sequelae may develop following indirect or "blowout" fractures. Blowout fractures involve fractures of the orbital floor with an intact inferior orbital rim. These fractures typically develop as a result of blunt trauma with a nonpenetrating object such as a fist or ball, which results in a sudden increase in intraorbital pressure.[25,34] The orbit is acutely decompressed by "blowing out" the thin bones of the orbital floor, with or without prolapse and incarceration of orbital soft tissues. Transmission of the hydraulic forces from the orbit can involve fracture of the lamina papyracea, which serves as the medial orbital wall, and the thin orbital floor, which is also the roof of the maxillary sinus.[13]

There is often both indirect and direct clinical evidence suggesting the presence of a blowout fracture. The indirect evidence may include orbital emphysema, infraorbital paresthesia, and restriction of globe motility in the vertical meridian (see previous discussion on examination). Direct, overt signs of a blowout fracture include globe ptosis and acute enophthalmos from expansion of the bony orbit (Figs. 27-1 and 27-15).

Smaller orbital floor fractures are more likely to cause entrapment. This is due to a ball-valve effect in which the bony fragment is acutely displaced as the hydraulic force is transmitted to the maxillary sinus and then instantly replaced, entrapping incarcerated tissue when the acute pressure rise ceases. In contrast, larger orbital floor fractures are more likely to cause enophthalmos as a result of expansion of orbital volume.

The best diagnostic imaging techniques for confirming the presence of a blowout fracture are simple plain film radiography and CT. The most important plain film radiograph for evaluating a blowout fracture is the Waters view. CT provides more information than does its plain film counterpart, especially in terms of soft-tissue detail. For evaluation of the orbital floor, finely cut (1.5 to 2 mm), direct, coronal views are most helpful.

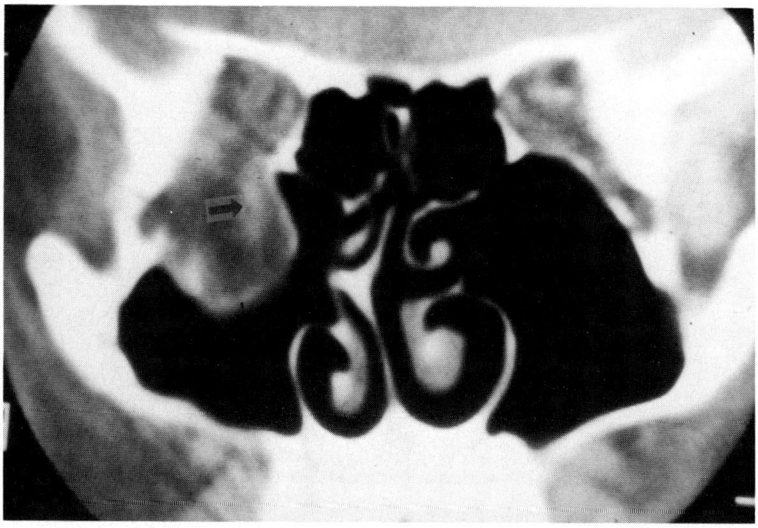

Fig. 27-15. Coronal CT scan through the midorbit of a patient with a blowout fracture. The floor fracture is displaced laterally and medially. Significant herniation of orbital fat into the maxillary sinus is apparent, with muscle herniating downward into the defect *(arrow)*. (Reprinted, with permission, from Weiss RA et al: Advanced diagnostic imaging techniques in ophthalmology, Adv Ophthalmic Plast Reconstr Surg 6:207-63, 1987.)

MANAGEMENT OF ORBITAL FRACTURES

Indications for Surgery

There is controversy regarding the indications for and timing of surgical repair of orbital fractures. Indications for surgical intervention and repair of a blowout fracture include diplopia accompaning motility limitation, positive forced-duction testing, gross enophthalmos, radiographic evidence of a blowout fracture, and the suggestion of subtle or asymptomatic findings such as tissue incarceration in the maxillary sinus. Minor clinical symptoms such as infraorbital paresthesia (which may result from edema and hemorrhage without the presence of an accompanying fracture) have been considered additional indications for surgical intervention.[7,13,35-43]

Simple radiographic presence of a blowout fracture is not an indication for surgical repair. Rather, the three standard indications for surgical intervention are enophthalmos, motility disturbance due to entrapment, and hypoophthalmos. The latter two account for the majority of surgical repairs.[41]

A most important aspect of posttraumatic enophthalmos is often cosmetic and not functional in nature. With surprising frequency patients are dissatisfied with their appearance because of axial asymmetry of globe position following blowout fractures (Fig. 27-16). This consideration should be taken into account as appropriate for each patient.

Timing of Surgical Repair

The timing of surgical intervention depends on the presence of associated injuries, the degree of impairment, and the patient's age, general health, and preference. Blowout fracture surgery should not be approached in a cavalier manner since numerous postsurgical complications have been reported, including infraorbital paresthesia, implant extrusion, diplopia and delayed extraocular muscle restriction, and blindness.[34,44]

Surgical intervention, when appropriate, is technically easier in terms of scarring and fibrosis and may have a better functional result if performed within the first 10 days after injury. It is often better to wait a few days after the traumatic event to allow for some resolution of soft tissue swelling and hemorrhage before considering surgical intervention. This is true even when true entrapment is evident clinically or verified by forced-duction testing, because of the greater technical ease of repair and the possibility of more accurate estimation of secondary or delayed enophthalmos development. This

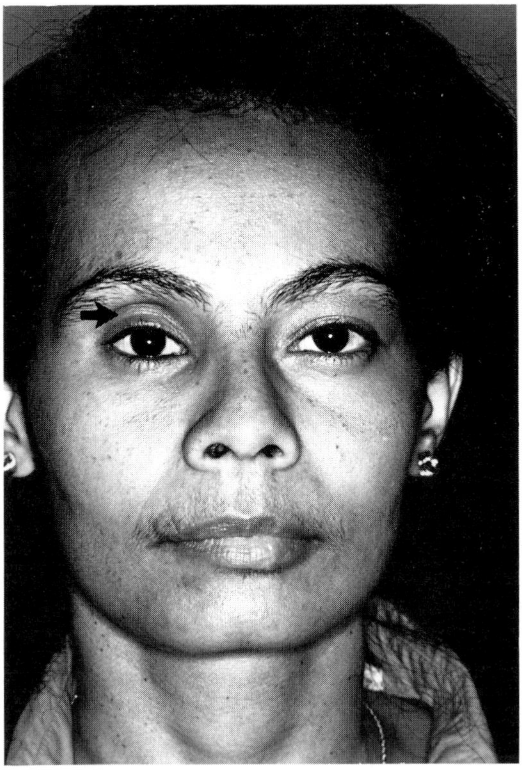

Fig. 27-16. Clinical photograph of a patient with significant posttraumatic enophthalmos. Note the asymmetry in her appearance as a result of the secondary superior sulcus deformity *(arrow)*.

knowledge enables the surgeon to more accurately gauge the size of the orbital implant needed and its shape, if contoured, and to appropriately correct globe ptosis and avoid hyperophthalmos. A short course of systemic corticosteroids may be helpful in distinguishing neuromuscular edema or related motility disturbance from true entrapment. The use of systemic steroids appears to speed the resolution of diplopia when present, unmask enophthalmos more quickly, and reduce patient discomfort and disability.[45] Systemic steroids, however, carry the potential risk of sinus-orbital infections, particularly in cases with hemorrhage and stagnant fluid in the sinuses. Therefore, such patients should be watched closely.

Globe ptosis and progressive or late enophthalmos may undergo delayed repair with generally successful results. In fact, if acute surgical intervention is not appropriate for any reason and delayed repair is ultimately warranted, it may be preferable to wait more than 6 weeks after injury. At this time inflammation of the orbital tissues is usually resolved and accurate assessment of globe ptosis or enophthalmos can be made to guide the surgeon's judgment and surgical approach.

Repair of Orbital Floor Fracture

A number of surgical approaches to gain exposure of the orbital floor have been described, including translid–inferior orbital rim, subciliary, Caldwell-Luc (gingival sulcus), and inferior fornix or transconjunctival/cul-de-sac incisions. An inferior forniceal-lower limb lateral canthotomy approach[9,46] gives excellent exposure. After the patient is placed under general anesthesia, the lateral canthal region and the length of the inferior orbital floor is infiltrated with 1%or 2% lidocaine (Xylocaine) with 1:100,000 epinephrine and hyaluronidase (Wydase). An adequate interval is allowed to elapse for the optimal hemostatic effect of epinephrine to occur.

A lateral subciliary incision line is delineated extending adjacent to the point of the lateral canthal angle, after which the incision is angled 45° downward in a natural smile line for 3 to 4

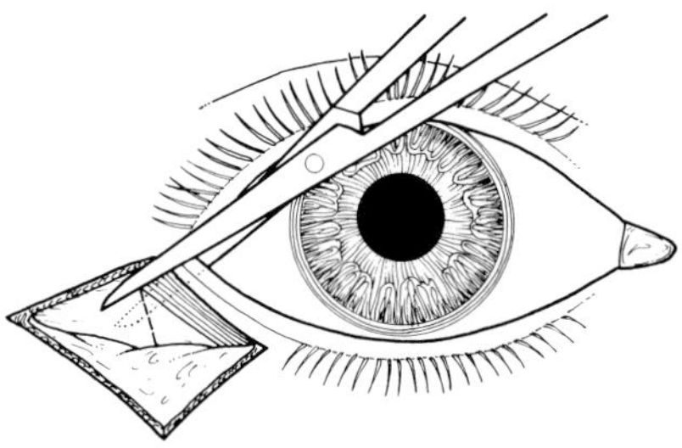

Fig. 27-17. Surgical approach for disinsertion of the lower limb of the lateral canthal tendon and lateral septal attachments of the lower lid *(dashed line)*.

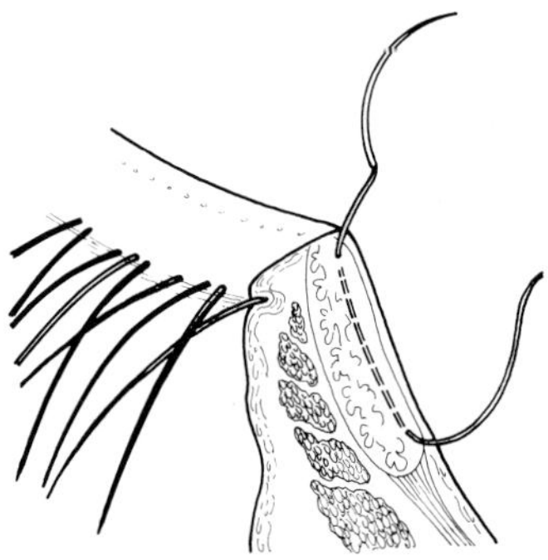

Fig. 27-18. Proper placement of the lateral tarsal suture used to retract the lid during the procedure and reattach it to the lateral orbital rim at the end of the procedure. The suture is passed through the most posterior aspect of the tarsus from its lower to upper border such that the suture exits immediately deep to the lid margin.

mm. This line is incised and a skin-muscle flap raised. The lower limb of the lateral canthal tendon is detached with a sharp iris or Stevens scissors, and the incision is continued inferiorly along the orbital rim to detach the lateral septal attachments (Fig. 27-17). The lid can be freely retracted at this point since the canthal tendon and the lateral septal attachments have been disinserted. The cut edge of the lid margin is then cleaned by full-thickness excision of a minimal amount of tissue (usually less than 1 mm) such that a smooth edge of tarsus can be appreciated. A permanent suture (e.g., 4-0 Prolene or Polydek) with a strong semicircular needle (PS-5 or ME-1) is passed through the most posterior aspect of the tarsus from its lower to upper border such that the suture exits just deep to the lid margin. This suture is used to retract the lid for exposure during the fracture repair and to reattach it to the lateral orbital rim at the end of the procedure (Fig. 27-18).

Two 4-0 silk ligatures are placed under the horizontal rectus muscles for traction; the lid is then retracted, exposing the inferior fornix. The conjunctiva and lower lid retractors are incised with a scalpel, scissors, or needle-tip bovie, and the incision is carried deep to the periosteum overlying the orbital rim. Care must be exercised to remain just within the inferior orbital rim to avoid buttonholing the lower lid or traumatizing the infraorbital nerve. Some surgeons find the use of a malleable retractor placed at the outer edge of the infraorbital rim or against the globe useful to direct the incision and protect the globe and lower lid. The periosteal incision is extended medially and laterally, and the periosteum is elevated using a periosteal elevator (Fig. 27-19). A malleable retractor is used to elevate the orbital contents superiorly and enhance exposure of the fracture site. This gives excellent exposure of the fracture and any incarcerated tissue. Entrapped tissues are bluntly freed with care taken to avoid trauma to the infraorbital neurovascular tissues (Fig. 27-20). Autologous or alloplastic implant material is then placed over the fracture site. The type and amount of material used depends on the surgeon's preference and the size of the fracture.

Many surgeons feel that autologous material is the implant of choice to lessen the risk of infection and prevent obstructive sinus disease. Autologous material may be harvested with relative ease from iliac bone, rib, or calvarium. The last may be preferred because variable graft sizes can be harvested with ease and patients appear

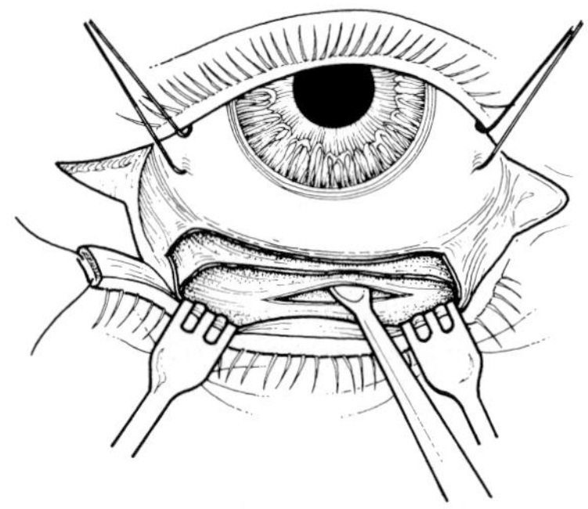

Fig. 27-19. Use of a periosteal elevator to expose the fracture site after incising the conjunctiva, capsulopalpebral fascia, and periosteum.

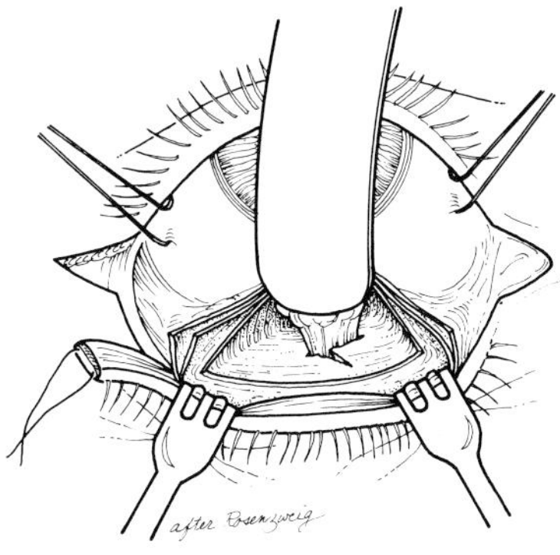

Fig. 27-20. Use of a malleable retractor to retract the periorbita and orbital contents upward. This gives excellent exposure of the fracture site and any incarcerated tissue. This exposure facilitates dissection of entrapped tissues and placement of orbital implant material.

to have less postoperative discomfort. In addition, it appears that there may be slightly less resorption of grafted bone harvested from the calvarium. Autologous bone grafts, however, demonstrate variable and unpredictable resorption and may cause scarring that complicates secondary surgery should delayed enophthalmos or superior sulcus deformity develop. In cases of severe sinus disruption or destruction of a significant portion of the orbital floor, as may occur following shotgun injuries, autologous bone is the implant of choice.

When using alloplastic material, the use of Howmedica Bone Cement is useful because it allows the surgeon to mold, adjust, and customize the implant. If globe ptosis is present, the implant is typically left smooth, following the normal contour of the orbital floor. If the globe is not ptotic, a central groove is cut using a Stryker or Hull burr, paralleling the course of the inferior rectus muscle such that the implant has a gull wing shape, filling volume medially and laterally while avoiding displacement of the globe superiorly. Other alloplastic material can be used such as Cranioplast, RTV silicone, Supramid, silastic, Teflon, and titanium mesh.

The globe may be pulled forward passively using the previously placed 4-0 silk traction sutures while positioning the floor implant. The conjunctiva is closed with a 6-0 plain suture. The lower lid retractors and deep tissues need not be sutured, which may help avoid postoperative lid retraction. The 4-0 Prolene or Polydek suture, previously placed in the lateral tarsal cut edge and used for traction up to this point, is then used to reattach the lateral canthal tendon and lateral lower lid septum. This approach may be used for delayed repair or for orbital augmentation to correct late enophthalmos and superior sulcus deformities. Other approaches, such as the use of dermis-fat grafts to correct superior sulcus deformities, are also acceptable. For these cases, the dermis-fat graft is harvested from the flank area and sutured via a lid crease incision to the arcus marginalis.

References

1. Greenwald HS, Keeney AH, and Shannon GM: A review of 128 patients with orbital fractures, Am J Ophthalmol 78:655-664, 1974.
2. Miller GR and Tenzel RR: Ocular complications of mid-facial fractures, Plast Reconstr Surg 39:37-42, 1967.
3. Smith B, Varr DR, and Langham EJ: Complications of orbital fractures, NY State J Med 71:2407-2411, 1971.
4. Petro J et al: Ocular injuries associated with periorbital fractures, J Trauma 19:730-733, 1979.
5. Cruse CW, Blevins PH, and Luce EA: Naso-ethmoid-orbital fractures, J Trauma 20:551-556, 1980.
6. McLachlan DL, Flanagan JC, and Shannon GM: Complications of orbital roof fractures, Ophthalmology 89:1274-1278, 1982.
7. Converse JM and Smith B: Naso-orbital fractures, Trans Am Acad Ophthalmol Otolaryngol 67:622-634, 1963.
8. Beyer CK, Fabian RL, and Smith B: Naso-orbital fractures: complications and treatment, Ophthalmology 89:456-463, 1982.
9. Shore JW and McCord CD Jr: Delayed repair of orbital and adnexal deformities following trauma. In Stewart WB, editor: Ophthalmic plastic and reconstructive surgery, San Francisco, 1984, American Academy of Ophthalmology, 400-412.
10. Koornneff L: Orbital septa: anatomy and function, Ophthalmology 86:876-880, 1979.
11. Koornneff L: Spatial aspects of orbital musculo-fibrous tissue in man, Amsterdam, 1977, Swets & Zeitlinger.
12. Moseley IF and Sanders MD, editors: Computerized tomography in neuro-ophthalmology, Philadelphia, 1982, WB Saunders, pp. 11-14.
13. Smith B and Regan WF: Blow-out fracture of the orbit, Am J Ophthalmol 44:733-739, 1957.
14. Ballinger PW: Merrill's atlas of radiographic positions and radiologic procedures, ed 5, St Louis, 1982, The CV Mosby Co, 404-418.

15. Unger JM: Orbital apex fractures: the contribution of computed tomography, Radiology 150:713-717, 1984.
16. Sevel D et al: Value of computed tomography for the diagnosis of a ruptured eye, J Comput Assist Tomogr 7:870, 1983.
17. Healy JF: Computed tomography of orbital trauma, CT 6:1-10, 1984.
18. Seigel RS et al: Subperiosteal hematomas of the orbit: angiographic and computed tomographic diagnosis, Radiology 143:711-875, 1982.
19. Bristow JH, Kassar B, and Sevel D: Gas gangrene panophthalmitis treated with hyperbaric oxygen, Br J Ophthalmol 55:139-142, 1971.
20. Tate E and Cuppes H: Detection of orbital foreign bodies with computed tomography: current limits, AJNR 2:363-365, 1981.
21. Niirnanen M. Perforating eye injuries. a comparative epidemiological, prognostic and socioeconomic study of patients treated 1930-39 and 1950-59, Acta Ophthalmol 56 (suppl 135):1-87, 1978.
22. Totsuka K and Takao M: CT scanner and the reliable limit of detection of intraocular foreign bodies, Nippon Ganka Gakkai Zasshi (Acta Soc Ophthalmol Jpn) 82:368-374, 1978.
23. Kadir S, Aronow S, and David KR: The use of computerized tomography in the detection of intra-orbital foreign bodies, Comput Tomogr 1:151-156, 1977.
24. Zinreich SJ et al: Computed tomographic three-dimensional localization and compositional evaluation of intraocular foreign bodies, Arch Ophthalmol 104:1477-1482, 1986.
25. Converse JM: Fractures of the zygoma. In Converse JM, editor: Kazanjian and Converse's surgical treatment of facial injuries, ed 3, vol 1, Baltimore, 1974, Williams & Wilkins, 287-306.
26. Waring GO III and Flanagan JC: Pneumocephalus: a sign of intracranial involvement in orbital fracture, Arch Ophthalmol 98:847-850, 1975,
27. Leech PJ and Paterson A: Conservative and operative management for cerebrospinal fluid rhinorrhea after closed head trauma, Lancet 1:1013-1016, 1973.
28. Jamieson KC and Yelland JDN: Surgical repair of the anterior fossa because of rhinorrhea aerocele or meningitis, J Neurosurg 39:328-331, 1973.
29. Maxwell JS and Goldware SI: Use of tissue adhesive in the surgical treatment of cerebrospinal fluid leaks: experiences with isobutyl 2-cyanoacrylate in 12 cases, J Neurosurg 39:332-336, 1973.
30. McCabe BF: The osteo-mucoperiosteal flap in repair of cerebrospinal fluid rhinorrhea, Laryngoscope 86:537-539, 1976.
31. Gross CW, Teague PF, and Nakamura T: Reconstruction following severe nasofrontal injuries, Otolaryngol Clin North Am 5:653-671, 1972.
32. Montgomery WW: Surgery of the frontal sinuses, Otolaryngol Clin North Am 4:97-102, 1971.
33. Nunery WR: Lateral canthal approach to repair of trimalar fractures of the zygoma, Ophthalmic Plast Reconstr Surg 1:175-83, 1985.
34. Converse JM: On the treatment of blow-out fractures of the orbit, Plast Reconstr Surg 62:100-4, 1978.
35. Converse JM and Smith B: Blowout fracture of the floor and orbit, Trans Am Acad Ophthalmol Otolaryngol 64:676-688, 1960.
36. Emery JM and Van Noorden GK. Orbital floor fracture: long-term follow-up of cases with and without surgical repair, Trans Am Acad Ophthalmol Otolaryngol 75:802-812, 1971.
37. Jones SEP and Evans JNG: Blowout fractures of the orbit: investigation into their anatomical basis, J Laryngol 81:109, 1967.
38. Metz HS, Scott WE, and Madson E: Saccadic velocity and active force studies in blowout fracture of the orbit, Am J Ophthalmol 78:655-670, 1974.
39. Putterman AM, Stevens T, and Urist M: Nonsurgical management of blowout fractures of the orbital floor, Am J Ophthalmol 77:233-239, 1974.
40. Fujino T and Makino K: Entrapment mechanism and ocular injury in orbital blowout fracture, Plast Reconstr Surg 65:571-76, 1980.
41. Wilkins RB and Havins WE: Current treatment of blowout fractures, Ophthalmology 89:464-472, 1982.
42. Smith B et al: Volkmann's contracture of the extraocular muscles following blowout fracture, Plast Reconstr Surg 74:200-209, 1984.
43. Pfeiffer RL: Traumatic enophthalmos, Adv Ophthalmic Plast Reconstr Surg 6:301-312, 1987.
44. Nicholson DH and Guzak SV: Visual loss complicating repair of orbital fractures, Arch Ophthalmol 86:369-375, 1971.
45. Millman AL et al: Steroids and orbital blowout fractures: a new systematic concept in medical management and surgical decision-making, Adv Ophthalmic Plast Reconstr Surg 6:291-300, 1987.
46. McCord CD Jr and Moses JL: Exposure of the inferior orbit with fornix incision and lateral canthotomy, Ophthalmic Surg 10 (6):53-63, 1979.

CHAPTER 28

Eyelid burns

ARTHUR TYRONE GLOVER

Epidemiology
Classification
Examination
Early management
Tarsorrhaphy
Intermediate management
Skin grafting
Tarsoconjunctival advancement flap
Late reconstruction
References

EPIDEMIOLOGY

Annually, over 2 million people in the United States suffer burn injuries; 95% of the burns do not cover more than 10% to 15% of the body surface.[1] Severe burn injuries frequently involve the face,[2-5] and the incidence of eyelid involvement is 20% to 30%.[2,5,6] The cornea and conjunctiva are usually spared because of the blink reflex, Bell's phenomenon, rapid reflex movement of the head, and reflex shielding of the eyes with the arms and hands. Most acute corneal or globe burn injuries are superficial and heal well. Loss of an eye from the initial burn injury occurs in less than 4% of cases.[7]

Flame, flash, and chemical burns account for most oculopalpebral burns. Asch et al[8] report a 7.5% incidence of ocular complications in 1400 burn patients. The cause of the injuries was most often flame (53.8%), but chemical agents (25.9%) and explosion (16.3%) were also major contributors. Ectropion was the most common complication. Primary corneal coagulation occurred in only 1% of patients.

Linhart[5] reported 110 cases of ocular involvement in 552 severe burn cases. In a study by Burns and Chylack,[9] flame and flash burns accounted for 85% of their 40 admissions over an 11-year period; scald and chemical, for 2.5% each.

Residential fires are the most common cause of burn death. Most of these fires are preventable, considering that each year in the United States fires caused by cigarettes kill more than 2300 people and burn more than 5000 others.[1] The elderly and the very young are at highest risk since their lack of physical agility makes them less likely to escape.

Chemical injuries are more likely to occur in an agricultural, military, or industrial setting. Monzingo et al[10] reviewed the clinical records of 4212 consecutive patients admitted to the U.S. Army Institute of Surgical Research from 1969 through 1985 and found 5 globe injuries, 3 from penetrating trauma and only 2 from direct contact of a chemical with the eye. The actual incidence of chemical ocular burns is much higher than the statistics cited here because many chemical burn victims are managed as outpatients. The management of the chemically burned eye is discussed in Chapter 7.

Electrical burns are often more serious than

they appear at first inspection. In passing through the body, the current may destroy muscles, nerves, and blood vessels. Every part of the eye may be involved in such injuries, but the most common sequela seems to be cataract formation.[11] Ignition of clothing by electrical sparks or arcing may result in flame burns.

CLASSIFICATION

Clinical assessment of the depth of the burn wound is important in planning for care and predicting functional and cosmetic results. First- and second-degree burns are known collectively as partial-thickness injuries and third-degree burns as full-thickness injuries.

First-degree burns involve only the epidermis. They are characterized by mild swelling, erythema, skin warmth, and pain.[12] Healing generally takes place in 5 to 10 days without compromising eyelid function since tissue damage is quite superficial. A first-degree burn may result from prolonged exposure to sunlight, brief contact with a hot liquid, or a gas explosion.

Second-degree burns, a more severe injury, are characterized by erythema, bulla formation, considerable edema, and pain.[12] Most of these burns heal uneventfully within 7 to 14 days without compromising lid function. However, deep second-degree burns often result in cicatricial eyelid deformities and readily become full-thickness injuries if infection occurs.

Third-degree, or full-thickness, burns represent the most severe injuries. The burned lids may have a dark, leathery appearance or appear translucent or waxy white.[12] Unlike partial-thickness injuries, these burns are not very painful because the terminal nerve endings have been destroyed.

Full-thickness injuries heal with considerable scarring and disfigurement. The thick, black, rigid eschar separates in 2 to 3 weeks. The granulation tissue that forms develops myofibroblasts, leading to severe contracture and eyelid deformity (Fig. 28-1).

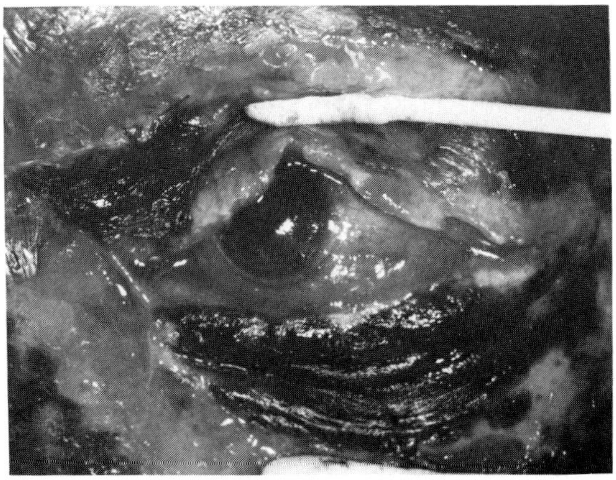

Fig. 28-1. Third-degree eyelid burn with marked lid margin (tarsal) deformity.

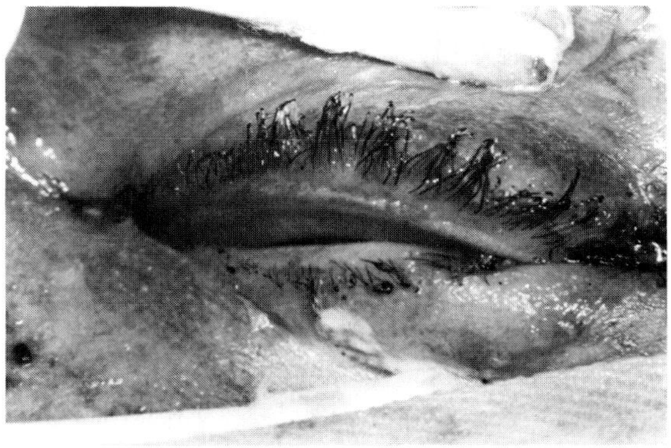

Fig. 28-2. Marked early postburn eyelid edema. Examination of the globe, although often difficult in this situation, must be performed to ensure corneal integrity.

EXAMINATION

The critical condition of most severe burn victims often precludes a prompt eye examination; life-threatening problems such as hemodynamic and pulmonic instability take priority. To prevent visual disability, however, the ocular examination should proceed as soon as possible. Examination of the eye within 8 hours of injury is desirable because the later onset of eyelid edema will make exposure of the globe and fornices more difficult (Fig. 28-2). As with other ocular injuries, some initial estimate of visual acuity should be made. The instillation of a topical anesthetic (proparacaine) often facilitates examination of the eye by relieving blepharospasm. The use of a lid speculum or Desmarres retractor may be necessary to permit inspection of the fornices. Orbicularis function, levator function, and Bell's phenomenon (Fig. 28-3) are evaluated; orbicularis and levator function almost always remain intact even in full-thickness lid burns. The extent and depth of eyelid burns are then determined, often an extremely difficult task. Potential skin donor sites are sought.

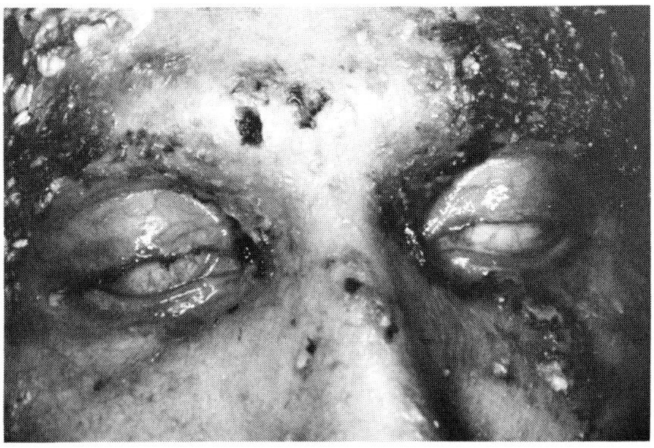

Fig. 28-3. Bilateral cicatricial lower lid ectropion. Bell's phenomenon protects the corneas. Both lower lids were grafted 1 week after these photographs were taken.

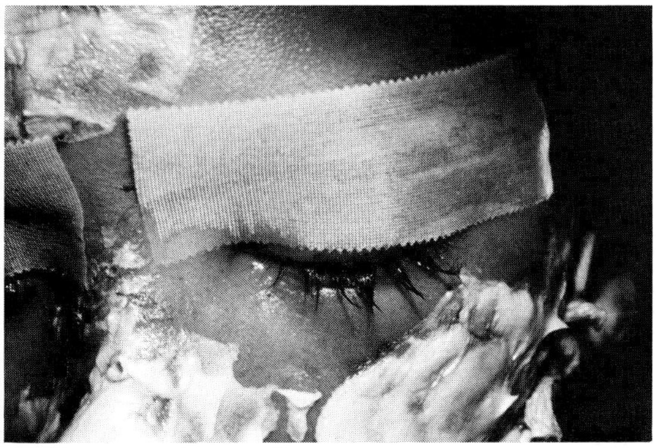

Fig. 28-4. Horizontal application of tape narrows the palpebral fissure in this obtunded patient with flash corneal burns and second-degree periorbital facial burns.

The postauricular and supraclavicular areas provide the best texture and color match, and shrinkage is less than with split-thickness grafts taken from the limbs or other sites. If one of the upper eyelids is not involved, it also serves as a potential skin donor site, but in most cases a large enough graft cannot be obtained. If none of these areas is available, the inner surface of the arm or thigh can be used.

EARLY MANAGEMENT

The guiding principle in the management of eyelid burns is to maintain protection of the cornea. First-degree burns generally require only symptomatic treatment. However, frequent, careful eye examinations are necessary in managing second- and third-degree thermal burns. Loss of vision because of corneal exposure and ulceration may be associated with cicatricial eyelid deformities.

The application of frequent moist dressings to the burned eyelids helps to achieve sloughing of eschar and necrotic debris.[13] Lid hygiene should be carried out to remove hard crusts that form on the lid margins. Repeated impingement of the eyelid against the edge of eschar in the supraorbital and eyebrow areas can result in eyelid perforation.[14] Exposure keratopathy, corneal ulceration, and even perforation may occur when there is inadequate lid closure, ectropion, or poor blink reflex.

The mainstay of medical treatment is the frequent instillation of artificial tears and ointment. As exposure of the cornea progresses, topical lubricants alone may be insufficient to maintain corneal hydration. A moisture chamber can be constructed using Saran Wrap, OpSite, or a Guibor Expo Bubble. Horizontal lid taping (Fig. 28-4) narrows the vertical palpebral fissure and slows tear film evaporation. This technique is useful in managing obtunded patients and those with minimal lid burns and mild corneal exposure. Bandage soft contact lenses are not recommended because they are difficult to maintain in place and may dry in patients with cicatricial ectropion and lagophthalmos.[6] In addition, corneal infections are more likely to occur in dry eyes treated with a continuously worn soft contact lens.[15] Prophylactic topical antibiotics may be used in eyes with corneal burns, abrasions, or extensive exposure keratopathy. Polysporin (polymyxin B-bacitracin) ophthalmic ointment provides good coverage against both *Pseudomonas* and *Staphylococcus*. Topical antibiotics, however, should be used with caution since prolonged use may result in overgrowth of resistant organisms, including fungi. For eyes with extensive surface defects, topical 0.25% scopolamine or 5% homatropine 2 to 3 times per day prevents posterior synechiae formation and relieves ciliary spasm.

TARSORRHAPHY

When exposure keratopathy progresses despite aggressive medical management or when contracture and lid eversion are noted early after injury, the use of a properly placed intermarginal suture or tarsorrhaphy may protect the eye and prevent the development of severe contracture.[3,6,16] These procedures should be done by the end of the second week following the burn injury[17] but should not be performed in serious burn injuries that extend to the lid margin. The placement of a lid adhesion more than 2 weeks postburn is discouraged since rapid contracture of the lids may cause the sutures to erode through, leaving the lids deformed.[16] In cases of relentless cicatricial lid retraction or ectropion, the tarsorrhaphy should be separated and early skin grafting performed. Some surgeons recommend abandoning the use of tarsorrhaphies because of the possibility of severe, permanent eyelid margin deformity.[2,7,18-20] Instead, they use early excision and grafting of the eyelid and repeat grafting when needed. Tarsorrhaphies, however, are generally very effective early in the treatment. With proper case selection, timing, and monitoring they will not cause significant additional damage to the eyelid.

Placement of an intermarginal suture (Fig. 28-5) or tarsorrhaphy (Fig. 28-6) begins with an estimation of the amount of ocular surface coverage required. While observing the cornea, the surgeon pinches the upper and lower lids together laterally between the thumb and index finger. The quality of Bell's phenomenon is judged with the patient's eyelids closed. The lid is then marked to delineate the extent of the planned tarsorrhaphy, and the lids are infiltrated with 1% xylocaine with 1:100,000 epinephrine. A corneal protector is inserted. Both needles of a double-armed 4-0 polypropylene (Prolene) or nylon suture are passed through a silicone or rubber bolster. The needles are then passed through the skin and muscle 4 to 5 mm from the lower lid margin, exit through the lid margin at the gray line, pass through the gray line of the upper lid, and emerge 4 to 5 mm above the lid margin, where they are tied over a rubber or silicone bolster. The corneal protector is removed before tying the sutures. A similar mattress suture can be placed nasally to ensure complete coverage of the cornea. Both sutures should be removed within 14 days.

To achieve more permanent adhesion, small strips from the lid margin posterior to the lashes are removed. This incision should include a small amount of tarsus. A 5-0 nylon or Prolene suture is passed through the skin and muscle of the upper eyelid several millimeters above the lid margin. The needle should emerge from the shaved tarsal margin. While advancing toward the lateral canthus, the suture should be passed alternately from the superior to the inferior tarsus in a serpentine manner and exit through the skin. Tightening the two suture ends brings the lids together, and friction keeps the sutures from moving freely through the tissues. Both suture ends are passed through silicone pegs and knotted. The suture should be removed in 3 to 4 weeks. After the tarsorrhaphy is no longer needed, the adhesion may be divided with little or no defect of the eyelids.[21]

INTERMEDIATE MANAGEMENT

Skin Grafting (Figs. 28-7 and 28-8)

In cases of severe eyelid burns, it is probably best to proceed with early skin grafting. Early application of a skin graft to close the defect can minimize eyelid retraction and ectropion. Contracture with lid retraction and ectropion are likely to lead to exposure keratopathy with consequent corneal ulceration and perforation. Intrinsic contracture (resulting from loss of eyelid tissue) and extrinsic contracture (resulting from pull of tissues in brow and forehead) may coexist. Correction of extrinsic contracture should precede correction of intrinsic contracture.[9,22]

Early eschar removal can be achieved by an aggressive approach, using frequent changes of moist dressing (4 to 5 times daily).[7,13] After the necrotic eschar has sloughed, grafting can be done to minimize contracture, usually by the end of the third week. Either a full-thickness or thick split-thickness graft can be used, depending on the available tissue. Whenever possible, a full-thickness postauricular or supraclavicular graft should be used since they provide superior cosmesis and contract less than do split-thickness grafts.

The surgery can be done under local or general anesthesia; the choice is often dictated by the patient's overall condition. A corneal protector is inserted, and the lids are gently debrided of all necrotic tissue and superficial granulation tissue with a No. 15 Bard-Parker blade. Hemostasis is obtained with a bipolar cautery. A suitable donor site is selected and the skin graft harvested. For a split-thickness graft, the dermatome thickness should be set at 0.014 to 0.016 in. for the lower lid and 0.018 to 0.020 in. for the upper lid. The graft is then placed in the

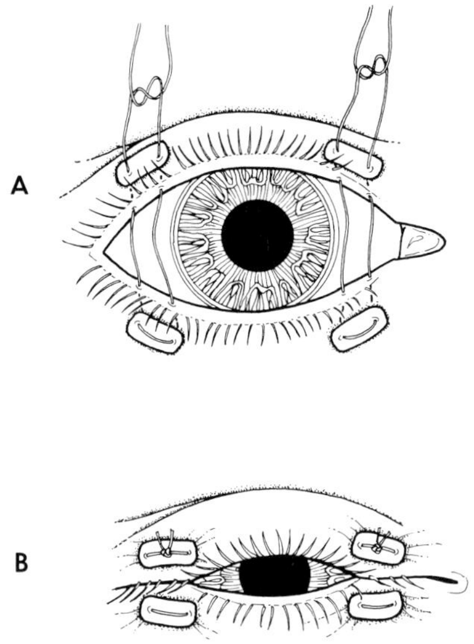

Fig. 28-5. Intermarginal suture. **A,** Horizontal mattress sutures pass from margin of lower lid to margin of upper lid. Silicone or rubber pegs prevent sutures from pulling through soft tisuses of the eyelid. **B,** Horizontal mattress sutures are pulled up and tied securely. Suture ends can be left long and tied in a large bow to permit periodic inspection of the cornea.

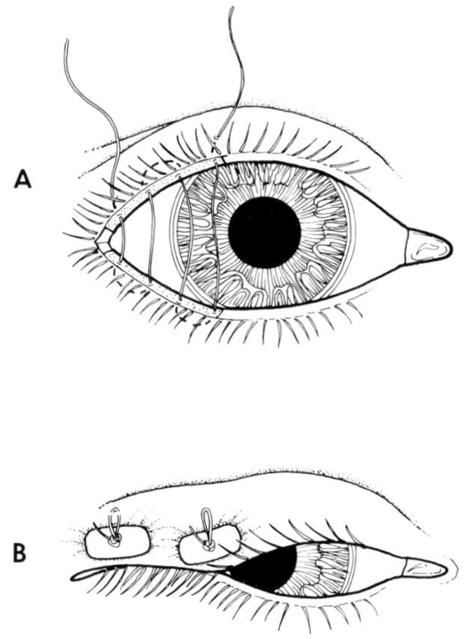

Fig. 28-6. Tarsorrhaphy. **A,** Continuous 5-0 nylon or Prolene suture passed alternately between upper and lower lid tarsus. **B,** Suture ends are drawn tight, approximating the shaved tarsal margins, and knotted on the skin surface of the upper lid.

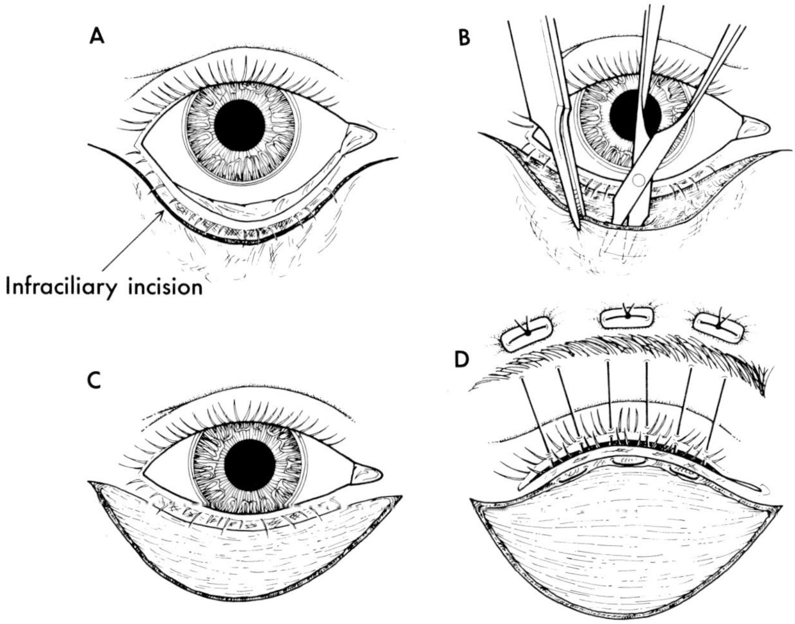

Fig. 28-7. Skin graft with lysis of adhesions. **A,** Infraciliary incision extends beyond medial and lateral canthi. **B,** Lower lid is placed on stretch, and lower lid adhesions are lysed. **C,** Lower lid is mobilized to a point above the pupil, and **D,** horizontal mattress sutures are passed from lower to upper lid margin and anchored through the brow.

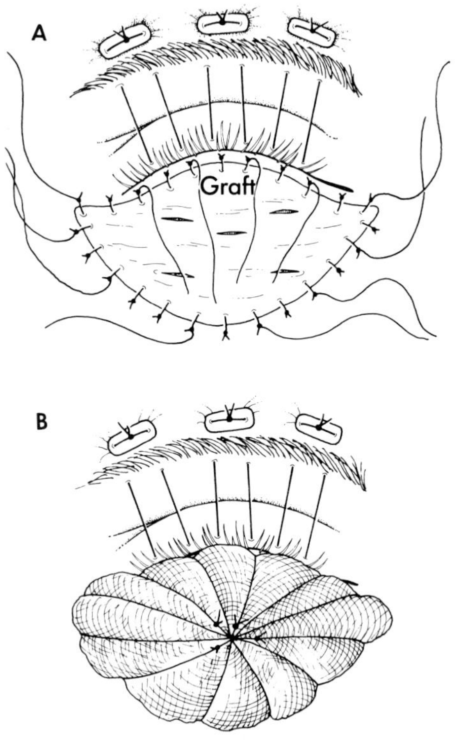

Fig. 28-8. **A,** Skin graft sutured into recipient bed and small incisions made for drainage. **B,** Bolster sutured over graft to act as a stent.

recipient bed and sutured into place with interrupted 5-0 nylon sutures. Alternate suture ends are left long. The corneal protector is removed. Small incisions are made full-thickness through the graft for drainage. A bolus of cotton soaked in glycerin and/or Telfa is applied using the tie-over sutures. The lid is placed on stretch using several 4-0 Prolene mattress sutures (described later). To achieve maximal stretch, one eyelid of each eye should be done at a time. The grafts should also proceed one eye at a time so that patients can maintain visual contact with their surroundings.[17] The bolster and the traction sutures are removed in 5 to 7 days. During this time the graft should be kept moist with saline or antibiotic solution.

When cicatrization is progressive, skin grafting should be combined with release of the contracture. The involved lids are injected with 1% xylocaine with 1:100,000 epinephrine to promote hemostasis. A corneal protector is inserted to protect the globe. For a lower lid, the proposed incision is marked 2 to 3 mm below the lid margin; for an upper lid, the incision is made 8 to 9 mm above the lid margin. The incision should extend beyond the medial and lateral

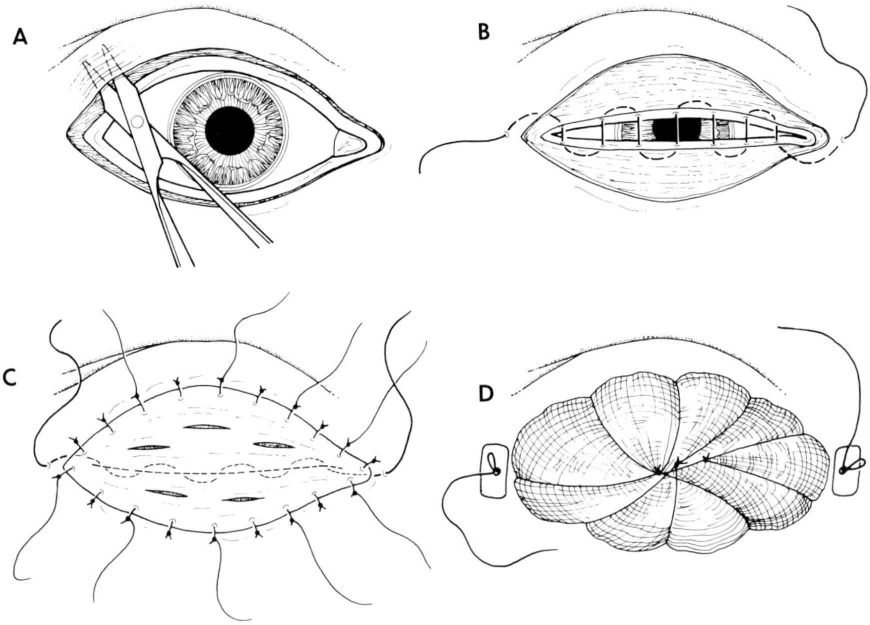

Fig. 28-9. Tarsoconjunctival flap. **A,** Incision made 2 mm from lid margin for 360°; anterior lamellae (skin and obicularis) recessed along with lysis of adhesions. **B,** Tarsoconjunctival flaps advanced to midline and coapted with continuous intratarsal 5-0 nylon suture; suture ends brought out through skin at medial and lateral canthi. **C,** Skin graft sutured over tarsoconjunctival flaps and bolster secured with tie-over sutures. **D,** Bolster sutured over graft to act as a stent.

canthal angles to allow for maximal mobilization of the lid. The skin incision proceeds with a scalpel and is carried down through the subcutaneous tissue and orbicularis. The orbicularis is preserved if possible, but if involved, it should be excised along with overlying scar bands. The dissection should proceed inferiorly until all cicatricial bands are released. This can best be ascertained by placing the lid on stretch and palpating the recipient bed with the fingertip. One should be able to easily mobilize the lower lid margin above the pupil. This overcorrection is desirable, especially when split-thickness grafts are used. There will be some shrinkage of the graft postoperatively, and some later contracture is inevitable. Hemostasis is achieved with the bipolar cautery. The corneal protector is removed. The lid is then secured to the brow with 4-0 Prolene mattress sutures passed from the depths of the recipient bed, through the upper and lower lid margins, through the eyebrow, and tied over silicone or rubber pegs. A pattern of the defect is made by tracing its margins on an overlying sheet of Adaptic gauze. The pattern is transferred to the donor site, and a full-thickness or an oversized, thick, split-thickness graft is harvested and sutured into the recipient bed with interrupted 5-0 nylon or Prolene sutures. Alternate suture ends are left long. Small holes are cut in the graft for drainage, and a stent is applied as described previously.

Tarsoconjunctival Advancement Flap (Fig. 28-9)

When the lid margins are partially or completely destroyed, a tarsoconjunctival advancement flap may be useful. A skin incision is made several millimeters from the deformed lid margin completely around the palpebral fissure. The skin is dissected free of underlying orbicularis until all cicatricial bands are released inferiorly and superiorly. Tarsoconjunctival flaps are fashioned for the full width of both lids, advanced, and approximated with a continuous, pullout intratarsal 5-0 nylon suture (similarly to tarsorrhaphy). To prevent eye irritation, this suture must be buried. The suture ends are brought out through the skin at the medial and lateral canthal angles and knotted over silicone pegs. A thick split-thickness skin graft is sutured over the entire defect, and a tie-over dressing is applied. The continuous 5-0 nylon suture can be removed in 3 to 4 weeks, or it can be retained longer to serve as a guide when the newly formed upper and lower eyelids are separated in 6 weeks to 2 months.[23]

If there is full-thickness loss of tarsus, coverage of the globe can be accomplished by approximating conjunctival flaps advanced from the superior and inferior fornices.[17,19] A skin graft is used to reconstruct the anterior lamella. Marrone[16] has described a potentially useful reconstruction for full-thickness loss of an upper lid and portion of a lower lid by advancing the levator muscle and covering it with a full-thickness skin graft.

LATE RECONSTRUCTION

Unless the integrity of the cornea is threatened by an eyelid burn, definitive reconstructive procedures should be delayed. This waiting period is necessary to allow for complete resolution of inflammation and for scar maturation. Because hypertrophic scars become paler in color, softer in texture, and smaller in size with the passage of time,[23] a premature attempt at reconstruction often results in a wasted operation and the need for further surgery.

Late reconstruction efforts are directed at repair of forward medial canthal displacement, palpebral fissure stenosis, punctal and canalicular obstruction, and eyebrow deformities.[3,4,9,22]

References

1. Warden GD: Epidemiology and prevention. In Boswick JA Jr, editor: The art and science of burn care, Rockville, Md, 1987, Aspen Publishers.
2. Frank DH, Wachtel T, and Frank HA: The early treatment and reconstruction of eyelid burns, J Trauma 23:874-877, 1983.
3. Garber PF, Macdonald D, and Beyer-Machule CK: Management of trauma to the eyelids. In Smith BC et al, editors: Ophthalmic plastic and reconstructive surgery, vol 1, St Louis, 1987, The CV Mosby Co, 437-469.
4. Huang TT, Blackwell ST, and Lewis SR: Burn injuries of the eylids, Clin Plast Surg 5:571-581, 1978.
5. Linhart RW: Burns of the eyes and eyelids, Ann Ophthalmol 10:999-1001, 1978.
6. Guy RJ et al: Three-years' experience in a regional burn center with burns of the eyes and eyelids, Ophthalmic Surg 13:383-386, 1982.
7. Boswick JA: Burns of the head and neck, Surg Clin North Am 53:97-100, 1973.
8. Asch MJ et al: Ocular complications associated with burns: review of a five-year experience including 104 patients, J Trauma 11:857-861, 1971.
9. Burns CL and Chylack LT: Thermal burns: the management of thermal burns of the lids and globes, Ann Ophthalmol 11:1358-1368, 1979.
10. Monzingo DW et al: Chemical burns, J Trauma 28:642-647, 1988.
11. Johnson EV, Kline LB, and Skalka HW: Electrical cataracts: a case report and review of the literature, Ophthalmic Surg 18:283-285, 1987.
12. Weiner SL and Barret J: Trauma management for civilian and military physicians, Philadelphia, 1986, WB Saunders, 53-76.
13. Artz CP, Moncrief JA, and Pruitt BA: Burns: a team approach, Philadelphia, 1979, WB Saunders, 314-317.
14. Beatty RF and Smith RE: Eschar-induced eyelid perforation, Am J Ophthalmol 103:336-338, 1987.
15. Rosen JE and Brown SI: Other uses of soft contact lenses. In Duane TT, editor: Clinical ophthalmology, vol 1, Philadelphia, 1988, JB Lippincott, Chap 56, 1-5.
16. Marrone AC: Thermal eyelid burns. In Hornblass A and Hanio CT, editors: Oculoplastic, orbital and reconstructive surgery, vol 1, Eyelids, Baltimore, 1988, Williams & Wilkins, 433-447.
17. Hartford CE: Methods of reducing burn scar deformity. In Stark RB, editor, Plastic surgery of the head and neck, vol 1. New York, 1987, Churchill Livingstone, 282-285.
18. Falvey MP and Brody GS: Secondary correction of the burned eyelid deformity, Plast Reconstr Surg 62:564-570, 1978.
19. Peterson HD: Eyelids. In Boswick JA Jr, editor: The art and science of burn care, Rockville, Md, 1987, Aspen Publishers, 339-345.
20. Tsur H: Eyelid burns: a general plastic surgeon's approach. In Hornblass A and Hanio CT, editors: Oculoplastic, orbital and reconstructive surgery, vol 1, Eyelids, Baltimore, 1988, Williams & Wilkins, 448-454.
21. Grove AS: Marginal tarsorrhaphy: a technique to minimize premature eyelid separation, Ophthalmic Surg 8:56-59, 1977.
22. Converse JM: Burn deformities of the face and neck, Surg Clin North Am 47:323-354, 1967.
23. Converse JM and Smith B: Repair of severe burn ectropion of the eyelids, Plast Reconstr Surg 23:21-26, 1959.

SURGICAL PRIORITIES

Nonophthalmic intervention*

Neurosurgical
Ear, nose, throat, head, and neck
Cardiothoracic
Gastrointestinal and genitourinary
Vascular
Orthopedic

Ophthalmic intervention

Examination under anesthesia (if required)
Exploration and repair of globe injuries
Optic nerve decompression
Orbital fracture repair
Removal of intraorbital foreign body
Repair of lacrimal outflow system trauma
Eyelid laceration repair

*May precede or follow ophthalmic intervention, depending on relative severity of injuries.

Regardless of the interval from wounding to repair, the wound should be carefully assessed immediately before closure. If the wound appears grossly contaminated or infected, surgical repair should be delayed and a therapeutic regimen of wound hygiene and antibiotic therapy initiated. The wound may then be closed on a delayed primary basis or be allowed to heal secondarily.[18]

Anesthesia

Repair of eyelid lacerations may be accomplished under either general or local anesthesia. In the presence of documented nonophthalmic injuries or of uncertainty concerning the extent of trauma, general anesthesia is preferred. It is often difficult, for example, to adequately examine the eye of a child sustaining eyelid trauma, and examination under anesthesia may be the only way to exclude the possibility of penetrating ocular injury with certainty. Silicone intubation of lacerated canaliculi and the nasolacrimal duct may be easier and more comfortable for both patient and physician when general anesthesia is used. Other circumstances in which general anesthesia may be appropriate are as follows:

Potential Indications for General Anesthesia

Uncertainty concerning extent of injuries
Associated neurosurgical trauma
Associated ear, nose, throat, head, and neck trauma
Associated bony orbital trauma
Lacrimal outflow system injury necessitating transnasal silicone intubation
Extensive trauma
Uncooperative patient

Less extensive eyelid lacerations without associated injuries may be amenable to repair under local anesthesia. A 1:1 mixture of 2% lidocaine (Xylocaine) with 1:200,000 epinephrine and 0.75% bupivacaine (Marcaine) is generally used. To minimize patient discomfort, the mixture may be injected directly into the wound bed through a 30-gauge needle before wound cleansing. Care is taken to inject sufficient anesthetic to obtain adequate anesthesia without producing undue distortion of eyelid anatomy. Alternatively, satisfactory regional anesthesia may be achieved through the use of appropriate sensory nerve blocks (see Chapter 4).[19]

Suture Materials

Sutures may be classified as monofilament (nylon, polypropylene) or multifilament (silk, plain gut, chromic gut) and as absorbable or nonabsorbable. Absorbable sutures lose their tensile strength within 60 days; nonabsorbable sutures retain significant tensile strength beyond 60 days.[20] Table 29-2 lists the important biomechanical characteristics of absorbable sutures used in oculoplastic surgery.[21] Suture absorption and related changes in tensile strength may be influenced by local factors, including the presence of inflammation or infection in the wound bed.

Nonabsorbable sutures are derived from natural (silk, cotton) or synthetic (nylon, Dacron, polypropylene, Polydek) sources. Silk and nylon are perhaps the most commonly used nonabsorbable materials in eyelid surgery. Silk is more accurately considered slowly absorbable, losing 100% of its tensile strength by 2 years after surgery. Nylon retains approximately 75% of its tensile strength during this interval.[22]

The suture materials may be obtained on a variety of stainless steel needles (Fig. 29-3).[23] Conventional cutting and spatulated (side-cutting) needles are most useful in oculoplastic surgery.

Suture Technique

Meticulous closure of eyelid wounds may be facilitated by the use of one or a combination of the following basic suture techniques.[24]

Table 29-2. Biomechanical characteristics of absorbable sutures

Suture material	Construction	Time for 50% tensile loss (days)	Time for total absorption (days)
Fast absorbing plain gut	Multifilament	2-3	21-42
Plain gut	Multifilament	7-10	50-70
Chromic gut	Multifilament	10-14	60-90
Polyglactin 910	Braid	14	56-70
Polydioxanone	Monofilament	28	180

Modified from Reference 20.

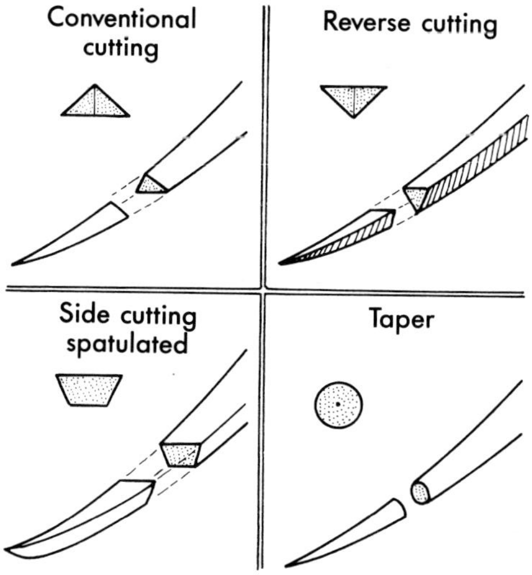

Fig. 29-3. Profile and cross-sectional view of needle shapes used in soft tissue surgery.

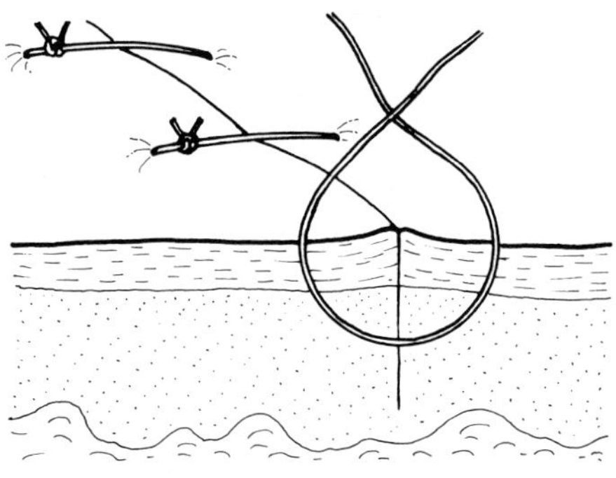

Fig. 29-4. Simple interrupted suture.

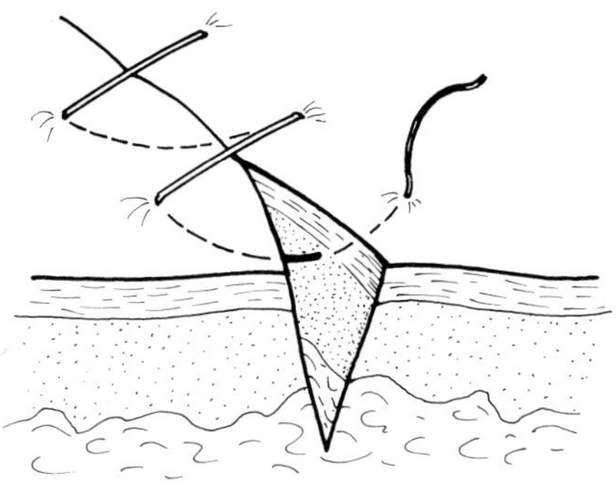

Fig. 29-5. Running percutaneous suture.

Interrupted sutures (Fig. 29-4) are useful in approximating the skin edges and wounds where there is minimal tension. Mild eversion of the skin edge produced by properly placed interrupted sutures helps to achieve a minimally conspicuous scar.

Running sutures (Fig. 29-5) may be used in closing relatively long wounds in areas of mild skin tension.

Buried subcutaneous sutures (Fig. 29-6) serve to eliminate dead space and relieve tension on the wound edges. Burying the knot in

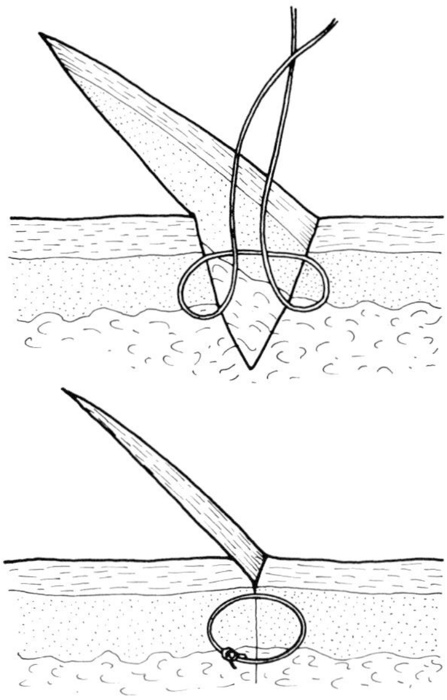

Fig. 29-6. Buried subcutaneous suture.

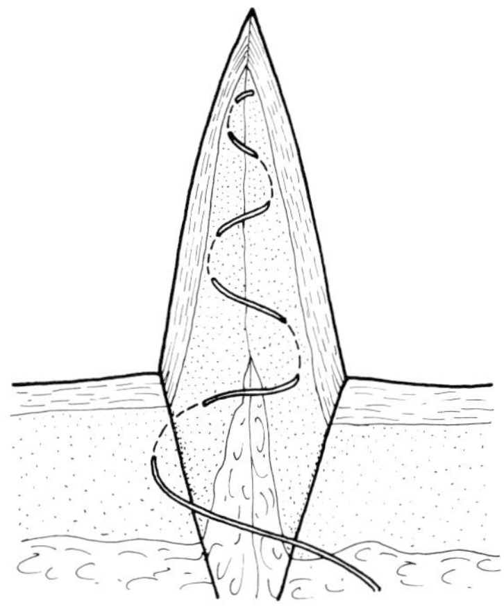

Fig. 29-7. Running subcuticular suture.

this wound closure avoids the problems of knot migration to the wound surface, where it may be seen or palpated by the patient, and subsequent knot extrusion. Buried subcutaneous sutures may be supplemented by percutaneous interrupted or running sutures to achieve eversion of the wound edges. Alternatively, subcutaneous sutures may be used in conjunction with surgical tape closure to approximate the skin edges precisely. This approach is particularly helpful in patients at risk for keloid formation with the placement of transcutaneous sutures or in patients who will be unavailable or uncooperative for suture removal.[10]

Running subcuticular sutures (Fig. 29-7) are often used in areas of thick dermis, such as the forehead and extremities. A pullout subcuticular suture of 6-0 polypropylene may be useful in closing cutaneous wounds in patients uncooperative for extensive suture removal.

Horizontal mattress sutures (Fig. 29-8) may be useful in subcutaneous closure, particularly in larger wounds. A half-buried horizontal mattress suture may be especially helpful in closure of wounds in which the wound edges are of different thicknesses, closure of stellate lacerations, and anchoring of the tip of a triangular flap as in Y-V plasty.

Vertical mattress sutures (Fig. 29-9) provide

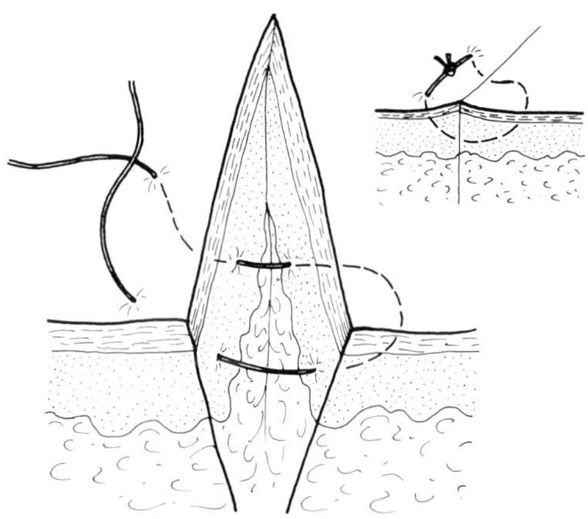

Fig. 29-8. Half-buried horizontal mattess suture.

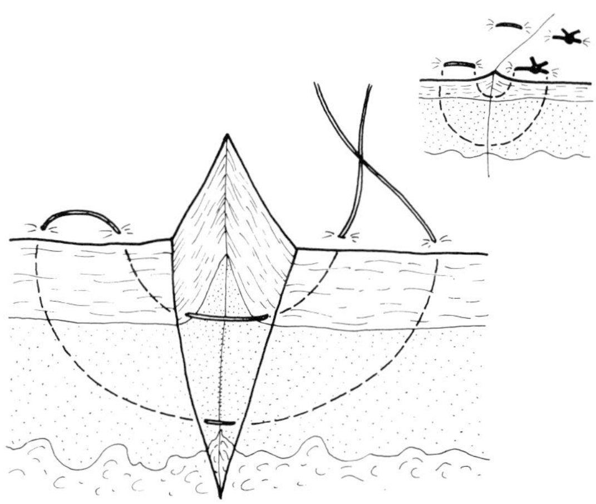

Fig. 29-9. Vertical mattress suture.

superficial and deep support of the wound and aid in achieving eversion of the wound edges. They are often used to close wounds in the lateral canthal area, cheek, brow, and temporal region. Vertical mattress sutures may also be useful in closing full-thickness defects involving the eyelid margin.[25]

Wound Hygiene

The area around the wound may be cleansed with a commercially available povidone-iodine solution or with soap followed by alcohol. Instillation of the preparatory solution into the wound, however, may cause additional tissue inflammation and necrosis and should be avoided.[18] Foreign material is removed from the wound, and grossly necrotic tissue is carefully debrided. If the presence of a ruptured globe has been excluded, a protective scleral contact lens is inserted, and the periorbital wounds are irrigated with normal saline. A 25-ml syringe and 17-gauge plastic cannula (available as part of a disposable intravenous catheter set) are useful in generating sufficient pressure during irrigation to dislodge retained foreign material and bacteria from wound tissues with a concomitant reduction in wound infection rates.[26]

SURGICAL REPAIR OF EYELID LACERATIONS: SPECIFIC CONSIDERATIONS

Partial-Thickness Lacerations

Partial-thickness lacerations involving the anterior lamella (skin and orbicularis muscle) may be associated with disruption of deeper eyelid tissues, including the orbital septum, preaponeurotic and nasal fat pads, and levator aponeurosis or capsulopalpebral fascia. It is thus important to explore the depths of the wound carefully to deal with injuries to these tissues in a stepwise fashion working from the posterior to anterior tissues. The defects in the eyelid retractor layers are repaired with interrupted or horizontal mattress sutures of 6-0 polyglactin 910. Visible orbital fat may be repositioned carefully if apparently viable or excised if grossly necrotic or contaminated. Meticulous hemostasis is achieved with wet-field bipolar cautery. Defects in the orbital septum are best left open to prevent cicatrix formation with subsequent development of lagophthalmos or eyelid retraction. The orbicularis muscle may be closed with buried interrupted sutures of 6-0 polyglactin 910. If there is significant residual tension on the wound edges, buried subcutaneous sutures of the same material may then be placed to achieve better approximation of the dermal edges. The maximal tensile strength of the wound is not achieved until 2 to 4 weeks following wound repair. Therefore, the judicious placement of subcutaneous sutures may prevent widening of the subcutaneous scar and wound dehiscence that might otherwise occur following the customary removal of skin sutures 7 to 10 days after surgery. In the cooperative adult patient, the skin edges are then closed with running or interrupted sutures of a nonabsorbable material. Synthetic monofilament sutures may produce less potentiation of postoperative infection,[27,28] and 6-0 nylon or polypropylene is preferred for skin closure in most patients. For closure of uncontaminated cutaneous wounds and in patients unlikely to be cooperative for suture removal, 6-0 mild chromic gut or, alternatively, a 6-0 pullout subcuticular suture and surgical tape closure may be used. The latter technique may be associated with a higher incidence and greater severity of postoperative infection and should not be used in patients at high risk for this complication.[10]

Beveled anterior lamella wounds may be managed by careful "freshening" of the wound edges followed by layered closure as described previously (see Fig. 29-2).

Partial-thickness lacerations involving the tarsus, conjunctiva, and Müller's muscle are encountered less frequently than anterior lamella injuries. Lacerations involving the posterior aspect of the lid margin in isolation should generally be closed with a single interrupted suture of 6-0 silk or polyglactin 910 to evert the tarsal edges and prevent the development of a posterior eyelid notch. The ends of the suture are left long and are sutured or taped to the skin surface to prevent corneal irritation.

Small extramarginal lacerations involving the tarsus or conjunctiva may be allowed to heal spontaneously. Larger lacerations involving the conjunctiva and eyelid retractor layer may be closed with buried running or interrupted sutures of 6-0 polyglactin 910.

Full-Thickness Lacerations

Reconstruction of full-thickness injuries is begun with repair of the eyelid margin, starting with the placement of a vertical mattress suture of 6-0 silk through the lid margin and tarsus using

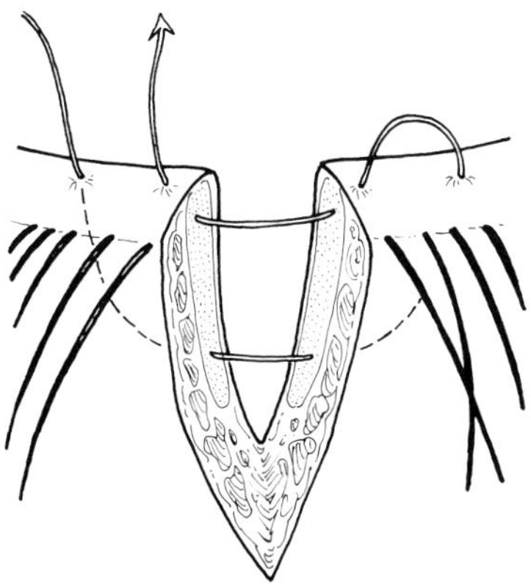

Fig. 29-10. Placement of vertical mattress suture through tarsus in eyelid margin repair.

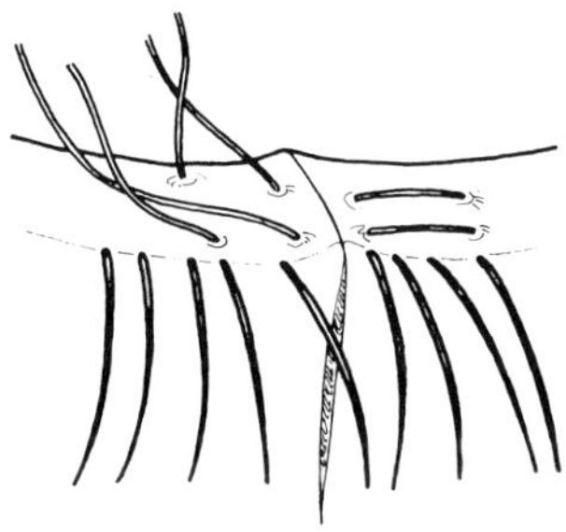

Fig. 29-11. Placement of second vertical mattress suture through lid margin posterior to ciliary line in eyelid margin repair.

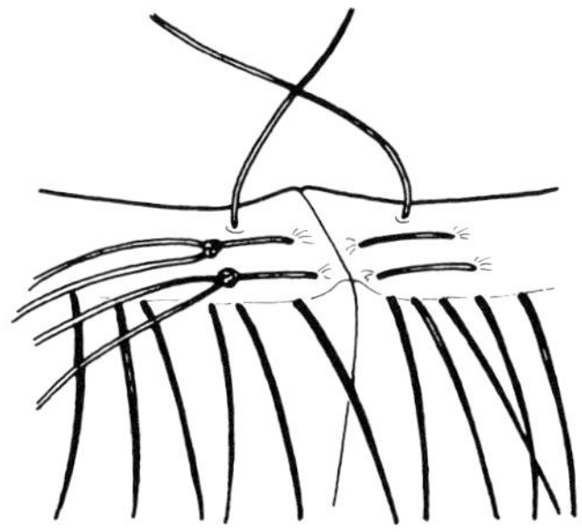

Fig. 29-12. When tied, vertical mattress sutures through eyelid margin result in mild eversion of the wound edges. An additional simple interrupted suture is placed in the posterior lid margin.

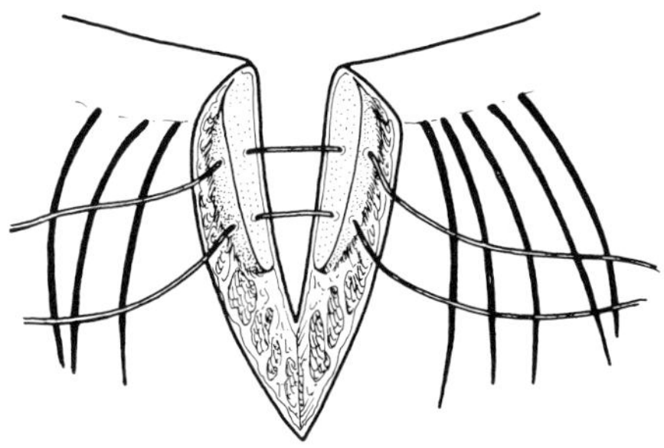

Fig. 29-13. Placement of partial-thickness tarsal sutures.

the gray line as a landmark, and followed by placement of a vertical mattress suture of 6-0 silk or polyglactin 910 through the lid margin and orbicularis muscle just posterior to the ciliary line (Figs. 29-10 and 29-11). Each suture is placed and tied temporarily, and approximation of the lid margin is assessed to ensure that satisfactory closure is obtained. To prevent the development of an eyelid notch with wound healing, eyelid margin edges should demonstrate an everted appearance at this point (Fig. 29-12). Vertical mattress sutures through the eyelid margin are helpful in producing this desired eversion of the wound edges while obviating the use of eyelid margin traction sutures customary in other closure techniques.[25] The tarsal and orbicularis vertical mattress sutures are generally supplemented by a single interrupted suture of 6-0 silk or polyglactin 910 placed to further approximate the posterior lid margin (Fig. 29-12).

Following placement and assessment of the marginal sutures, the sutures are untied, and large associated partial-thickness lacerations of the conjunctiva and lower lid retractors, if any, are repaired, as described previously, while readily accessible. Attention is then turned to tarsal closure. Multiple sutures of 6-0 polyglactin 910 are placed at the anterior half of the tarsal plate with care taken to avoid conjunctival penetration (Fig. 29-13). Use of the spatulated needle during suture placement is helpful in this regard. The marginal sutures are then carefully tightened and tied, with the assistant approximating the wound edges with forceps. The ends of the marginal sutures are left long and are tied anteriorly under the skin sutures at the end of the procedure to prevent corneal irritation. The tarsal sutures are then tied. Additional defects involving the levator aponeurosis and lower eyelid retractors may then be repaired, and the orbicularis muscle and skin are closed, as described in the discussion on partial-thickness laceration repair.

Eyelid marginal sutures are generally removed approximately 2 to 3 weeks following surgical repair. During this period, ophthalmic antibiotic ointment is administered 3 times a day, and the patient is advised to wear a protective shield over the injured eyelids at bedtime.

Special Considerations

Lateral Canthal Tendon Reconstruction

Lacerations involving the lateral one third of the upper or lower eyelid may transect the superior or inferior crus of the lateral canthal tendon (Color Plate 29-1, *A* and *B*), respectively. The lateral canthal tendon anchors the lateral canthus to the periosteum posterior to the lateral orbital rim and plays an important role in maintaining normal eyelid position and function. The lateral canthal tendon may be reconstructed with the placement of a double-armed horizontal mattress suture of a nonabsorbable material (such as 4-0 Tevdek) through the lateral border of the tarsal plate in a half-thickness fashion. Each suture arm is then passed through the periorbita internal to the lateral orbital rim, with care taken to place each suture approximately 2 mm posterior to the orbital rim to ensure satisfactory posterior curvature of the eyelid (Fig. 29-14).

Lacrimal Gland Resuspension

Injuries involving the lateral portion of the upper lid may result in ptosis or prolapse of the lacrimal gland. The lacrimal gland may be returned to its fossa beneath the superolateral orbital rim by placement of a horizontal mattress suture of 5-0 polyglycolic acid through the periosteum in this region and through the capsule surrounding the lacrimal gland. When the suture is tied, the lacrimal gland will be resuspended and in its normal anatomic position (Fig. 29-15).

Avulsive Injuries

Partial-thickness eyelid lacerations associated with tissue loss may necessitate the use of local flaps or skin grafts to achieve adequate wound closure (Color Plate 29-2, *A* and *B*). Similarly, various sophisticated techniques incorporating the use of semicircular advancement flaps, lid-sharing procedures, and free tarsoconjunctival and skin grafts may be required in managing patients sustaining full-thickness loss of eyelid tissue.

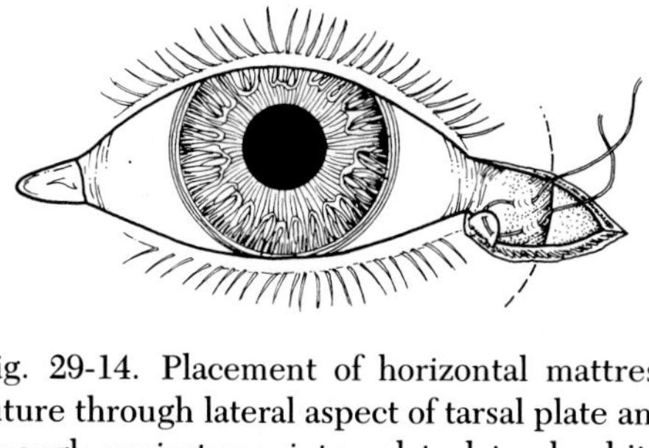

Fig. 29-14. Placement of horizontal mattress suture through lateral aspect of tarsal plate and through periosteum internal to lateral orbital rim.

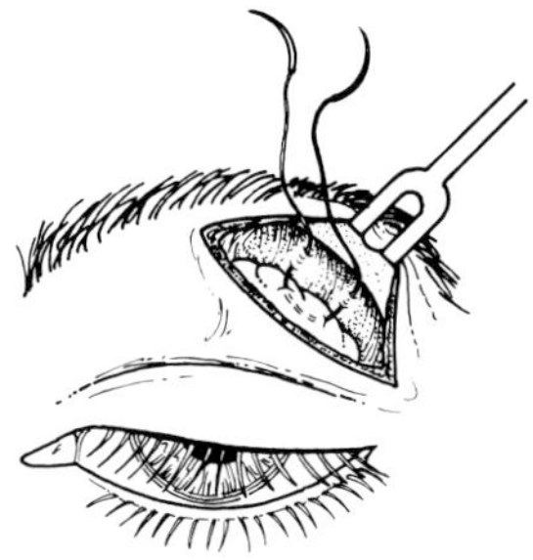

Fig. 29-15. Placement of horizontal mattress suture through capsule of prolapsed lacrimal gland and through periosteum of lacrimal gland fossa.

Medial Canthal Injuries

Trauma to the medial canthal area may result in disruption of the medial canthal tendon and lacrimal drainage system. The management of these injuries is discussed in Chapter 30.

References

1. Gillman PJ: Studies on the repair of cutaneous wounds, Med Proc Suppl 2:121-186, 1956.
2. Peacock EE and van Winkel W: Wound repair, ed 2, Philadelphia, 1976, WB Saunders, 1-21.
3. Wilkins RB and Kulwin DR: Wound healing, Ophthalmology 86:507-510, 1979.
4. Peacock EE and van Winkel W: Wound repair, ed 2, Philadelphia, 1976, WB Saunders, 61.
5. Fox SA: Repair of nasocanthal malignancies by combined laissez-faire and chemosurgery techniques, Trans Am Acad Ophthalmol Otolarynogol 79:654-657, 1975.
6. Irvin TT: Wound healing: principles and practice, New York, 1981, Chapman & Hill, 34-63.
7. Trunkey DD: Priorities in trauma management. In Najarian JS and Delaney JP, editors: Trauma and critical care surgery, Chicago, 1987, Year Book Medical, 29.
8. Committee on Trauma of the American College of Surgeons, Prophylaxis against tetanus in wound management, Bull Am Coll Surg 69:22-23, 1984.
9. Immunization Practice Advisory Committee, General guidelines on immunization, MMWR 32:1-17, 1983.

10. Edlich RF et al: Principles of emergency wound mangement, Ann Emerg Med 17:1284-1304, 1988.
11. Chodak GW and Plaut ME: Use of systemic antibiotics for prophylaxis in surgery, Arch Surg 112:326-334, 1977.
12. Kaplan EL et al: Prevention of bacterial endocarditis, Circulation 56:139A-143A, 1977.
13. Cardany CR et al: The crush injury: a high risk wound, JACEP 5:965-970, 1976.
14. Dellinger EP: Antibiotics in trauma. In Najarian JS and Delaney JP, editors: Trauma and critical care surgery, Chicago, 1987, Year Book Medical, 108-110.
15. Burke JF: The effective period of preventive antibiotic action in experimental incisions and dermal lesions, Surgery 50:161-167, 1961.
16. Halasz NA: Wound infections and topical antibiotics, Arch Surg 12:1240-1244, 1977.
17. Schultz R: Facial injuries, Chicago, 1977, Year Book Medical, 91.
18. Robson MC and Zachary LS: Repair of traumatic cutaneous injuries involving the skin and soft tissue. In Georgiade NG et al, editors: Essentials of plastic, maxillofacial, and reconstructive surgery, Baltimore, 1987, Williams & Wilkins, 117-122.
19. Snow JC: Anesthesia in otolaryngology and ophthalmology, New York, 1982, Appleton-Century-Crofts, 142-145.
20. Edlich RF et al: Physical and chemical configuration of sutures in the development of surgical infection, Ann Surg 177:679-687, 1973.
21. Guido R, Ethicon Inc: Personal communication, 1990.
22. Postlethwait RW: Long-term comparative study of absorbable sutures, Ann Surg 171:892-897, 1971.
23. Wound closure manual, Somerville, N.J., 1985, Ethicon, Inc., 43.
24. Woog J et al: Flap techniques in oculoplastic surgery, American Academy of Ophthalmology Instructional Course, 1987.
25. Divine R and Anderson R: Techniques in eyelid wound closure, Ophthalmic Surg 13:283-287, 1982.
26. Stevenson TR et al: Cleansing the traumatic wound by high pressure irrigation, JACEP 5:17-21, 1976.
27. Peacock EE and van Winkle W: Wound repair, ed 2, Philadelphia, 1976, WB Saunders, 21.
28. Sharp WV et al: Suture resistance to infection, Surgery 91:61-63, 1982.

CHAPTER 30

Lacrimal system trauma

W. JACKSON ILIFF

Evaluation
Anesthesia
Instrumentation
Surgery
Complications
References

Lacrimal system injuries frequently accompany lid and facial injuries. Canalicular lacerations in particular may be subtle and therefore must be suspected so that a careful search for canalicular disruption and appropriate repair will be carried out. Injuries to the canalicular system may occur with blunt injuries or sharp lacerations. Falls, motor vehicle accidents, and blows with blunt objects may apply shearing or tearing forces to the lid, causing an avulsion in the medial canthal area. The lid tends to tear at its weakest point, which is the attachment of the medial canthal tendon to the tarsus lying just nasal to the punctum (Fig. 30-1 and Color Plate 30-1). Occasionally the tear will occur more medially, producing a laceration of the canaliculus, which is more difficult both to identify and to repair because it occurs near the common canaliculus.

Sharp lacerations such as those produced by stab wounds and glass or metal fragment injuries in motor vehicle accidents may occur at any portion of the canalicular system or lacrimal sac area (Figs. 30-2 and 30-3 and Color Plate 30-2). Concurrent injuries to both canaliculi are more common with such sharp injuries. Dog bites are, moreover, a major source of lid and canalicular lacerations, particularly in children. They produce lacerations (Color Plate 30-2) that may have components of both sharp and avulsive injuries. Bite injuries are discussed in greater detail in Chapter 32. Because the lacrimal sac is somewhat protected by the lacrimal fossa, it is less commonly involved in such trauma, but the lacrimal sac and the nasolacrimal duct may be disrupted if nasoethmoid fractures occur. The medial canthal tendon is, of course, also disrupted in many of these injuries. In all these cases, the goal of surgical repair is to restore the normal anatomic architecture and physiologic function of the lacrimal system as well as to minimize cosmetic deficit.

EVALUATION

In examining the patient with damage to the lacrimal system, a careful history must be taken to determine the likelihood of retained foreign bodies (for example, tree branches, twigs, gravel, or other contaminants) and an assiduous search must be made, both before and during surgery, for unsuspected foreign bodies. The

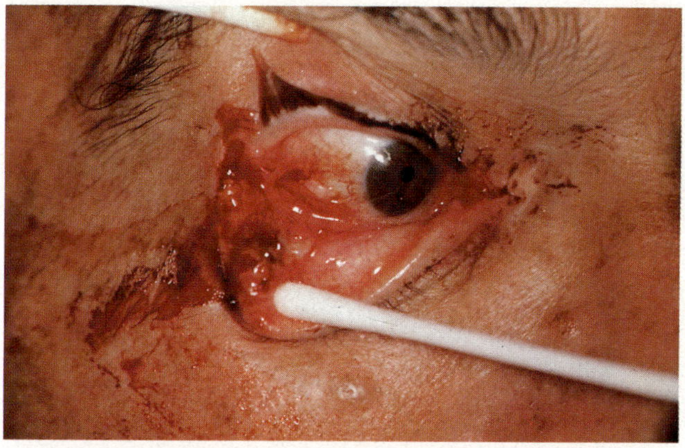

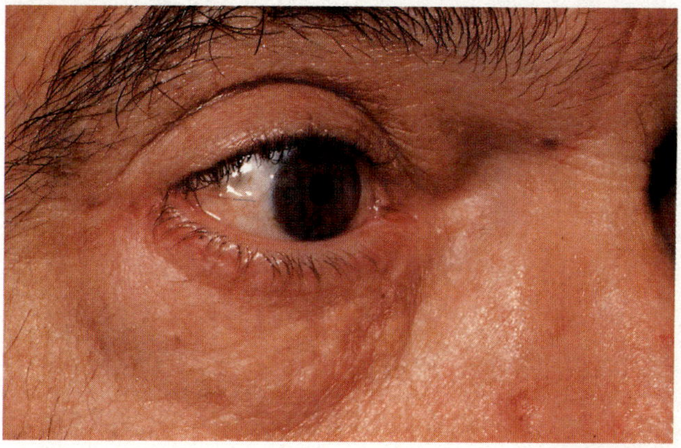

Color Plate 29-1. Right lateral canthal and lower eyelid laceration with disruption of inferior crus of lateral canthal tendon. **A**, Before, and **B**, after repair.

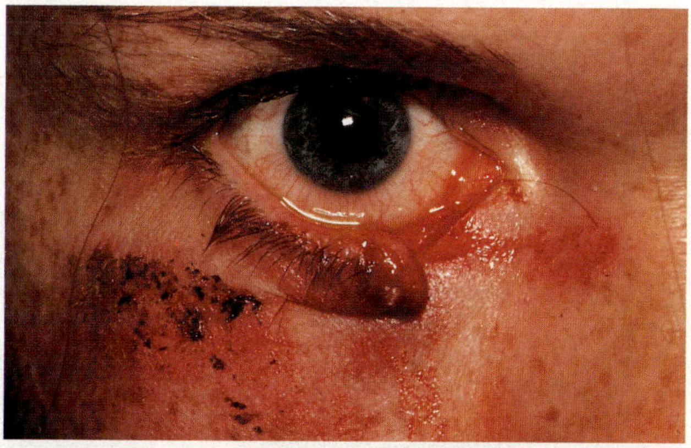

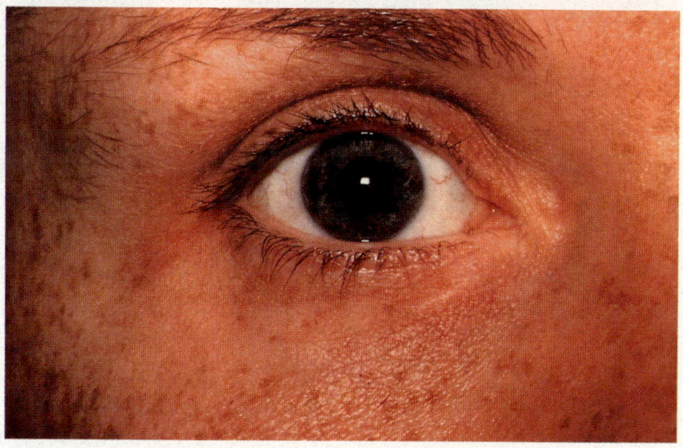

Color Plate 29-2. Partial avulsion of right lower eyelid secondary to dogbite injury. **A**, Before and **B**, after surgical repair.

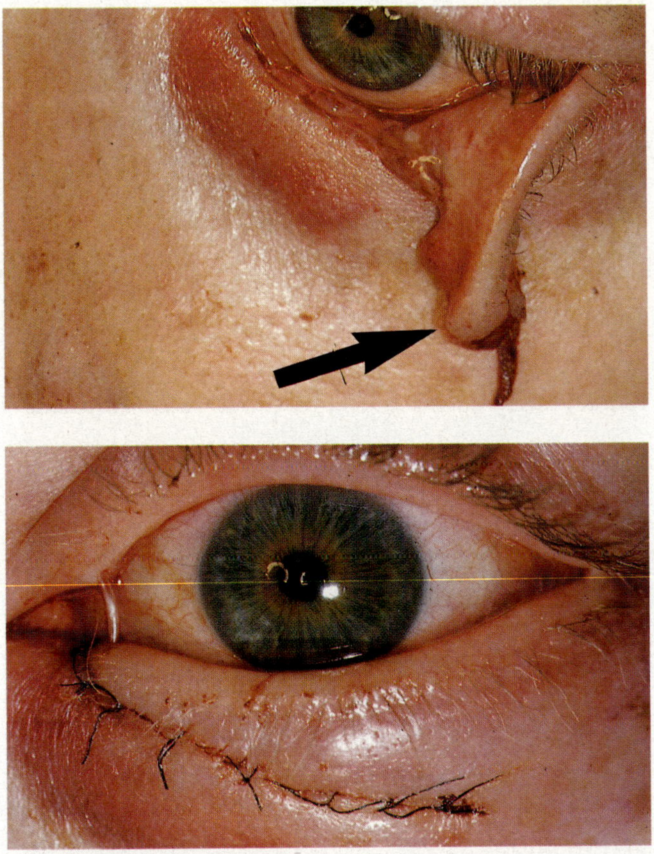

Color Plate 30-1. **A,** Lower lid laceration caused by hooking the lid on a door latch. Note location of punctum *(arrow)*. **B,** Operative photograph with tubes in place and laceration sutured. Tubes were removed at 3 months with normal lacrimal function postoperatively.

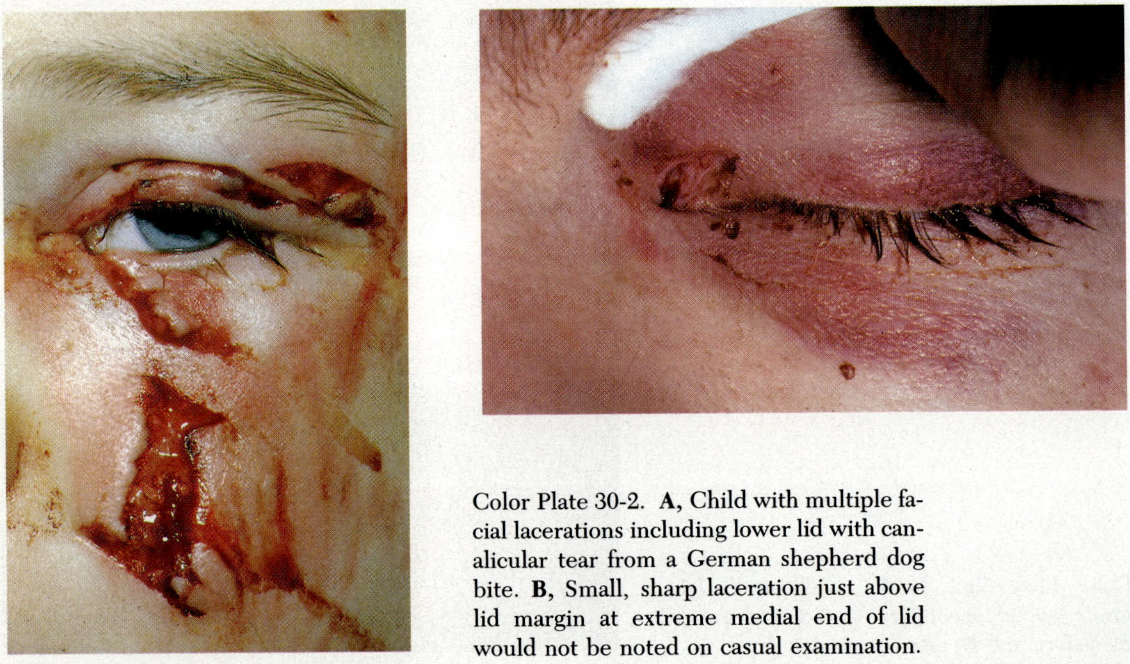

Color Plate 30-2. **A,** Child with multiple facial lacerations including lower lid with canalicular tear from a German shepherd dog bite. **B,** Small, sharp laceration just above lid margin at extreme medial end of lid would not be noted on casual examination.

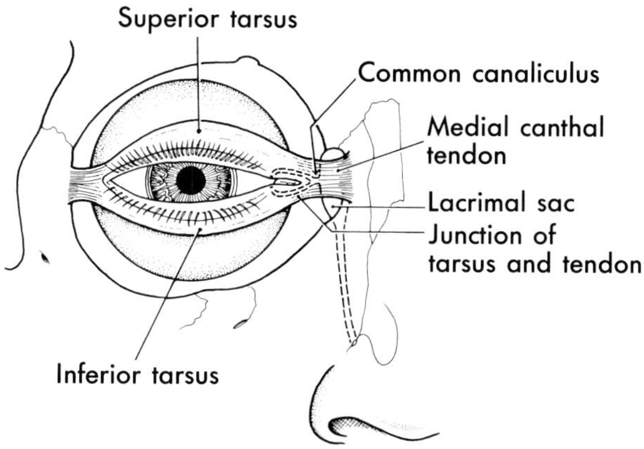

Fig. 30-1. Schematic of anatomy of lids and lacrimal tract. Note the site of junction of the tarsus and medial canthal tendon with respect to the punctum.

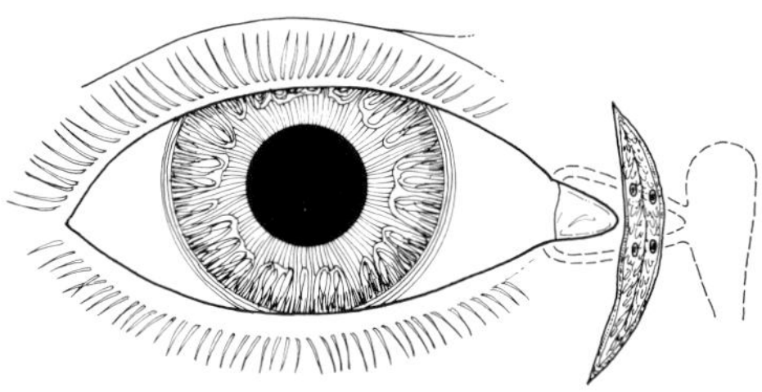

Fig. 30-2. Sharp medial canthal lacerations often cut both canaliculi or the common canaliculus and the medial canthal tendon (see Fig. 30-3).

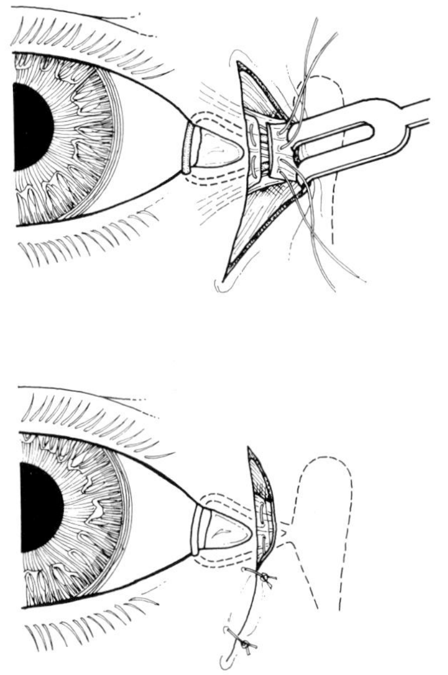

Fig. 30-3. After intubation of the canaliculi, the tendon is repaired with mattress sutures of nonabsorbable material such as Prolene or Mersilene.

slit-lamp and operating microscope are of great benefit in determining whether the canalicular system has been traumatized and in facilitating subsequent repair. Perhaps the most difficult part in the early stages of canalicular repair is identification of the medial cut end of the canaliculus. Generally, a laceration in the midportion of the canaliculus or near the punctum is identified relatively easily. However, when the laceration occurs near the common canaliculus and deeper in the medial canthus, the cut end may be more difficult to find, especially since the canaliculus may retract slightly. The operating microscope is especially helpful in this effort. Irrigation of methylene blue, fluorescein-tinged water, or air through the opposite system may be a useful adjunct in identification of the cut end.[1] Some reports suggest the use of sodium hyaluronate (Healon).[2,3]

In some settings, careful nasal examination with speculum, appropriate decongestion of the nasal mucosa, and a good light source may be helpful in identifying nasal trauma and avoiding problems with the subsequent repair. Facial fractures must be considered and appropriate radiologic studies obtained. Computed tomography is often very helpful in evaluating nasoethmoidal and orbital fractures. If the ophthalmologist performs the initial evaluation of a patient with midfacial trauma, otolaryngological or plastic surgical consultation may be appropriate. If the condition of the patient allows, early primary repair of all these injuries produces the best final result.

Although not generally appropriate for acute lacerations, standard diagnostic techniques may be used in the late evaluation of canalicular injuries to evaluate the lacrimal secretory and excretory systems. These include Schirmer's test, basic secretor tests, Jones 1 and Jones 2 dye tests, and the dye disappearance test, in conjunction with careful probing and irrigation of the lacrimal system.[4-6]

ANESTHESIA

Anesthesia requirements vary, but general anesthesia is usually preferred. It is mandatory with children and is preferred with many adults having other than the simplest of lid lacerations in the lateral to midportion of the canalicular system. The experience of the surgeon in intubating the nasolacrimal system under local anesthesia is also important since this involves adequate anesthesia of the lacrimal sac, nasolacrimal duct, and nose. Although often seemingly straightforward, the repair of canalicular lacerations occasionally becomes quite time-consuming, making general anesthesia more desirable.

INSTRUMENTATION

Appropriate lacrimal system repair requires some special instrumentation, including a full-range of punctum dilators, canalicular probes, and intubation materials. Though it has generally fallen in disfavor, the Worst pigtail probe may also be used and is still popular with some surgeons. Rarely is a dacryocystorhinostomy necessary as part of a primary repair, but some bone instruments may be required, particularly if transnasal wiring or repair of nasoethmoid fractures will be required. Most of this equipment will be available in an ophthalmologic or general operating room.

There is general agreement that silastic tubing is the best lacrimal system intubation material since it is soft and readily placed and produces no tissue reaction. Polyethylene tubing is too stiff and tends to produce erosion of the punctum and lacrimal system. Several varieties of silastic tubing exist, the preferred being small-diameter tubing of the Quickert-Dryden type.[7] Intubation sets are commercially available in prepackaged sterile units in a number of modifications including the Guibor design[8] (Concept) with stainless wires swaged onto the silastic tubing. The stainless wires have variable malleability, with a greater degree at the tips and less at the shank. They are somewhat stiffer than the malleable silver wires originally described by Quickert and Dryden[7] and the Jackson intubation set (Storz).

The Crawford[9] intubation set includes somewhat smaller stainless probes with a small knob on the end and a special hook that is used to retrieve the wire from beneath the inferior turbinate. Concept also markets an intubation set that uses a slightly different system, a fine stainless wire introduced inside the silastic tubing with a reinforcing cuff at its upper end. The tip has a rounded silastic end that may be slightly less traumatic on passage through the lacrimal system. The stainless guide wire is removed after the tip has passed into the nose, and the silastic tubing is pulled through in the usual fashion. The Quickert- and Guibor-type probes are retrieved from the nose using a grooved director placed under the inferior turbinate.[7,10]

One drawback of the silastic intubation sets is the necessity of manipulating and intubating the uninjured canaliculus in the case of a single canalicular laceration. At least two monocanalicular intubation sets and several other methods have been described.[10,13-16] These include the Gavaris set (cited by Beyer[10]) which is, in essence, a single-armed Quickert-Dryden type of intubation probe with silastic tubing. To one end of the silastic tubing, a small button has been affixed that provides a small flat plate that can be secured at the punctum. This allows a single-armed intubation with other aspects of the repair being quite similar to the double-armed intubation. A shorter monocanalicular intubation set (EV monocanalicular stent #0085, Eagle Vision, Memphis, Tenn.) has a silicone tube with a punctum plug (Freeman punctum plug, Eagle Vision) attached to one end.[15] This allows simple intubation of the injured canaliculus only, and the tube is held in place by the punctum plug. If these materials are not available, a regular silastic intubation set may be used in a single-armed fashion by looping the tubing externally between the external naries and the medial canthus.[17] In a young child, however, this may be difficult to maintain. In a less desirable repair, the end of the silastic may be sutured or otherwise fixated to the skin or in the conjunctival cul-de-sac. Since silastic tubes should be left in place for several months or more, these fixation methods are not as reliable.

Other stents that have been used include the Veirs rod,[11] which is a malleable stainless rod with a swaged 4-0 black silk suture attached. This rod may be placed in the lacerated canalicular system and the canaliculus sutured over the top of it using the rod as a stent. The lid is then closed normally. The suture material extends out through the punctum and is sutured to the anterior surface of the lid. Veirs rods have one disadvantage, that they occasionally detach from the silk suture and require surgical retrieval from the canalicular system or the lacrimal sac. They are somewhat rigid and may cause erosion as well. Moreover, there may be some surgical difficulty in repairing the lid over the long rigid stent. The Veirs rod is not appropriate for lacerations near the punctum or the common canaliculus.

The Johnson rod[12] and its modifications[10] are malleable silver rods with a loop on one end that can be bent to conform to the canalicular system. It extends out through the punctum, where it is sutured on the anterior surface of the lid.

Suture materials of large diameter, including Mersilene, nylon, polypropylene, and others, have been intubated through the lacrimal system using a pigtail probe or other threading mechanisms. Though these materials may be useful in some situations, silastic is considered the preferred material for repair.

In the past, many surgeons did not recommend repairing an upper canaliculus with an isolated injury. One factor was the paucity of techniques available and the relatively poor results with any canalicular repair before the development of silastic intubation. Moreover, it was thought that the upper canaliculus carried considerably less than half the total volume of tears drained into the lacrimal sac. Because recent radionucleide flow studies[18] have demonstrated virtually equal flow in the upper and lower canalicular systems, it is currently felt that repair of all canalicular lacerations should be attempted to avoid epiphora.[10,18]

SURGERY

Surgical repair of the lid and lacrimal system has two basic phases: intubation of the canaliculus and lacrimal system as necessary, and repair of the lid laceration. As with all such repairs, the surgery is preceded by careful examination of the wound, inspection for foreign bodies, and copious irrigation to remove contaminants.

In intubation of the lacrimal system, an intact punctum may need careful dilation to allow passage of the lacrimal probes. Exceedingly tight puncta may require a one-snip procedure[13] to allow intubation. The probe is passed through the punctum and out through the wound in the lid unless the canaliculus is only partially severed, in which case it may be passed directly into the medial cut edge of the canaliculus and then to the lacrimal sac (Fig. 30-4). Identification of the medial cut end of the lacrimal sac is then undertaken using good magnification and lighting, with ancillary help from irrigation through the opposing system. When rotating the lacrimal probes superiorly to pass them down through the nasolacrimal duct, care must be taken, particularly with lower lid lacerations to avoid placing excessive tension on the occasionally very narrow portion of lid remaining temporally, thus causing further canalicular trauma or lacerating the punctum. The probe is then passed through the nasolacrimal duct and retrieved from the nose by a grooved director, Crawford hook (Fig. 30-4), or other means. The opposing canaliculus is then intubated. After placement, the tubes can be knotted together

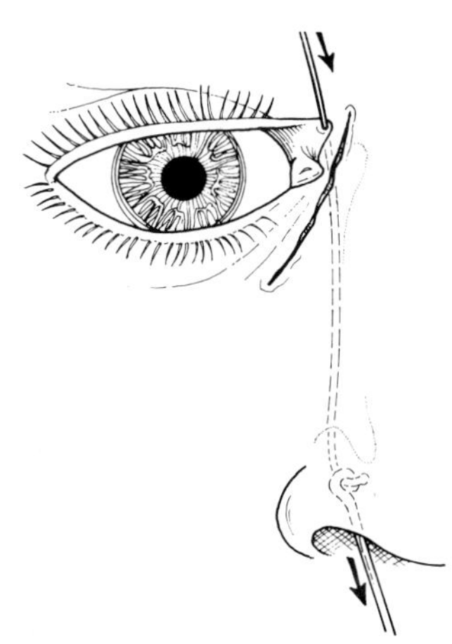

Fig. 30-4. The lacrimal system is intubated before suturing with any of the available silicone tubing sets. The Crawford intubation set uses a hook to extract the probe from under the turbinate and may be easier in some cases than the Quickert-Dryden system using a grooved director.

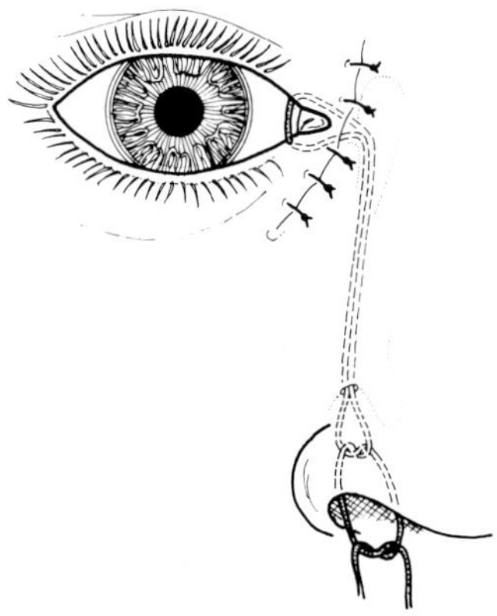

Fig. 30-5. After intubation, the tubes are knotted together.

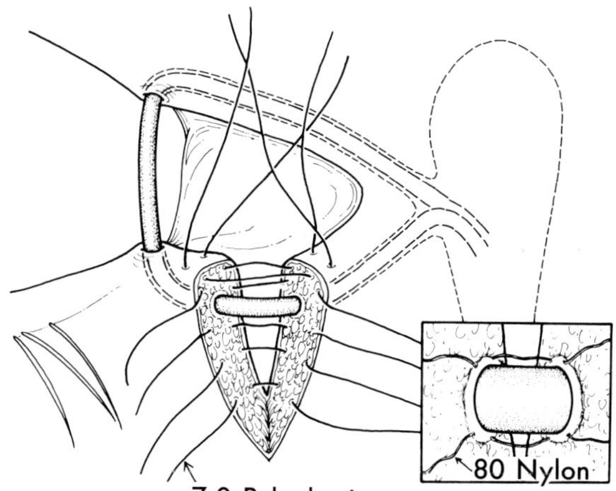

Fig. 30-7. A stay suture placed laterally in the tarsus and running medially to exit the skin and tied over a button or bolster is necessary to prevent tension on the wound.

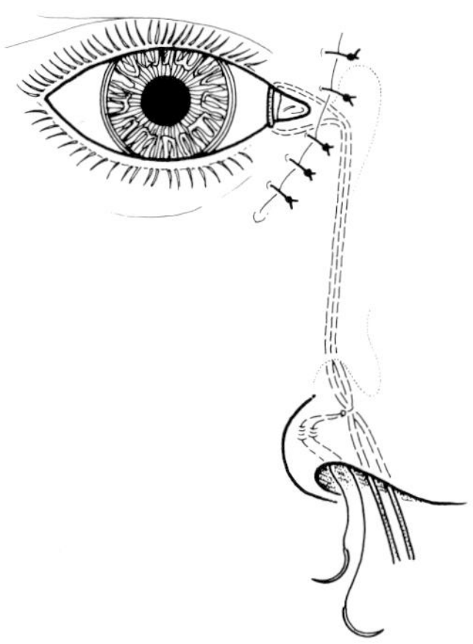

Fig. 30-6. The tubes may be tied with a suture (nylon), which is then sutured to the lateral wall of the nose for fixation.

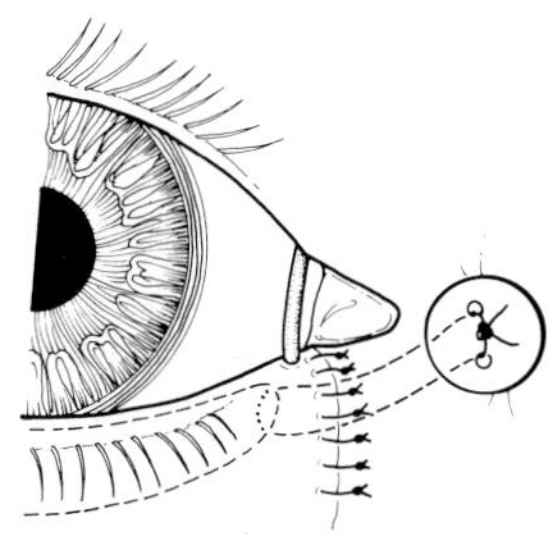

Fig. 30-8. Fine nylon or absorbable sutures placed with microscopic control in the canaliculus will aid reapproximation.

(Fig. 30-5), tied over a silicone sponge, or tied together with a silk or nylon suture, which is then sutured to the lateral wall of the nose (Fig. 30-6). If monocanalicular intubation is being performed, the silastic is fixated to prevent its being pulled out of position during the remainder of the repair.

With the stent in place and under the operating microscope, sutures of fine nylon or polypropylene can be used to reapproximate the ends of the canaliculus (Fig. 30-7). Additional sutures of a fine (7-0 or 8-0) absorbable material such as chromic collagen or Vicryl are then used to close the tissues anterior and posterior to the canaliculus.

If the laceration is near the puncture, the medial canthal tendon is not easily identified, and no distinct ends are generally available for repair. However, more medial lacerations, particularly if they are medial to the medial canthal commissure, will require direct repair of the medial canthal tendon (Figs. 30-2 and 30-3). Often it is difficult to repair the deep heads of the tendon because of adjacent structures and limited access, but unless there is significant tension, repair of the anterior limbs alone will be sufficient.

Injuries directly at the punctum are difficult to repair since there is little tissue available for suturing around the punctum without placing sutures directly through the canaliculus. Either bicanalicular intubation or the Gavaris monocanalicular tube may be useful for such repairs (the Eagle Vision punctum plug-fixated stent probably would not be appropriate). Careful suturing with magnification should allow reconstruction of the punctum. If the area is too badly damaged, the development of an auxiliary punctum or opening into the canaliculus may be attempted,[19] as for excision of tumors in the area of the punctum.

Bicanalicular trauma is approached in the same fashion but of course requires intubation of both systems. There is no question that an attempt at repairing both systems should be undertaken when both are damaged, since repairs are not always successful. Late repairs are very difficult, and ultimate placement of a Jones tube is often necessary.

The surgical repair of the lid follows standard plastic surgical techniques (see Chapter 29). If there has been any suggestion of loss of lid tissue, it may be necessary to relax the lid by performing lateral cantholysis. Although techniques similar to those used in repair of central lid lacerations or lid excisions can be used, with careful suturing of the lid margin and tying of sutures anteriorly to prevent corneal abrasion, the location of canalicular repairs generally does not require these techniques. However, if there is a possibility that the suture ends will irritate the globe, they should be fixated externally to the skin. Canalicular lacerations heal quite well if there is no tension on the wound. A medial supporting stay suture may also be helpful to relieve tension on the wound (Fig. 30-8).

Lacerations caused by avulsion of the lid deep in the medial canthus are difficult to repair because of the small space in which to work. It is often not possible to suture the canaliculus directly. Therefore, careful approximation of the tissues is necessary to prevent rotation and avoid the likelihood of scarring, which might later distort the repair. Direct reapposition of the medial canthal tendon may be possible in these circumstances. It is performed with relatively large (4-0 or 5-0) nonabsorbable sutures. Mattress sutures are placed as necessary to reapproximate the ends of the tendon (Fig. 30-3).

Lacrimal sac trauma is relatively unusual, with the exception of nasoethmoid fractures[20] and severe penetrating injuries to the medial canthal area. Identification of the lacrimal sac may be difficult, but if it can be primarily repaired, it is reasonable to do so. Since nasolacrimal duct obstruction often occurs after any form of lacrimal sac injury, surgical or traumatic, silastic intubation should be performed as a primary procedure if possible. Dacryocystorhinostomy and conjunctivodacryocystorhinostomy are generally not necessary as part of the primary repair and should be delayed for later evaluation and determination of need. However, late obstruction of the lacrimal system, through failed or inadequate primary repair, may require either dacryocystorhinostomy or Jones tube placement.

COMPLICATIONS

A number of complications may occur following repair of the canalicular and lacrimal drainage system. Several may be due to poor surgical technique, but some injuries are so severe that even the most meticulous repair may be doomed to failure. The primary complication is inability to attain both anatomic and physiologic patency. This may be caused by failure to use a stent, early removal of the stent, excessive scarring caused by the initial injury, or distortion by improper apposition of the canaliculus and surrounding lid structures.

Punctal erosion may be caused by pressure from tight silastic tubing. This might be avoided by careful fixation of the tubes in the nose, by monocanalicular intubation, or by the use of loops of silastic material through the canalicular system[10] rather than down into the nasolacrimal duct.

Displacement of silastic tubing can be troublesome. Suture fixation of the tubes in the nose will prevent displacement. However, the sutures occasionally erode, leaving the tubes free. A slight displacement can often be corrected by pushing the tubing back into the sac, having the patient blow the nose forcefully, or occasionally by visualizing the tubes in the nose and manually repositioning them. However, tubes pulled up into the sac require surgical repositioning (or removal). Several methods for repositioning have been described[21-23] and may be useful if removal is not reasonable.

Lid notches occasionally occur, particularly if there is loss of tissue or extensive distortion that might make identification of structures difficult. However, careful surgical reapproximation of the lid margin, paying close attention to all landmarks, will generally prevent notching. Lacrimal pump problems from distortion of the lateral portions of the lid or ectropion of the lower lid may result from widespread injury in the periorbital area but can often be prevented by good surgical technique. Late obstructions and scarring will require revision and possible conjunctivodacryocystorhinostomy.

REFERENCES

1. Morrison FD: An aid to repair of lacerated tear ducts, Arch Ophthalmol 72:341-342, 1964.
2. Lerner HA and Boynton JR: Sodium hyaluronate (Healon) as an adjunct to lacrimal surgery, Am J Ophthalmol 99:365, 1985.
3. Seiff SR and Ahn JC: Locating cut medial canaliculi by direct injection of sodium hyaluronate into the lacrimal sac, Ophthalmic Surg 20:176-178, 1989.
4. Jones LT and Wobig JL: Surgery of eyelids and lacrimal system, Birmingham, 1976, Aesculapius, 141-151.
5. Jones LT: The cure of epiphora due to canalicular disorders, trauma and surgical failures on the lacrimal passages, Trans Am Acad Ophthalmol Otolaryngol 66:506-524, 1962.
6. Reeh MJ, Beyer CK, and Shannon GM: Practical ophthalmic plastic and reconstructive surgery, Philadelphia, 1976, Lea & Febiger, 141-145.
7. Quickert MH and Dryden RM: Probes for intubation of lacrimal drainage system, Trans Am Acad Ophthalmol Otolaryngol 74:431-433, 1970.
8. Guibor P: Canaliculus intubation set, Trans Am Acad Ophthalmol Otolaryngol 79:419-420, 1975.
9. Crawford JS: Intubation of obstruction in the lacrimal system, Can J Ophthalmol 12:289-292, 1977.
10. Beyer CK: Lid trauma. In Heilmann K and Paton D, editors: Atlas of ophthalmic surgery, vol 1, New York, 1985, Thieme-Stratton, 1.64-1.71.
11. Veirs ER: Malleable rods for immediate repair of traumatically severed lacrimal canaliculus, Trans Am Acad Ophthalmol Otolaryngol 66:263-264, 1962.
12. Johnson CC: A canaliculus wire, Am J Ophthalmol 78:854-855, 1974.
13. Fox SA: Ophthalmic plastic surgery, ed 5, New York, 1976, Grune & Stratton, 582-590.
14. Gonnering RS: Simplified monocanalicular silicone intubation, Arch Ophthalmol 105:1024, 1987.
15. Long JA: A method of monocanalicular intubation, Ophthalmic Surg 19:204-205, 1988.
16. Romaro PE: Single silicone intubation for repair of single canaliculus laceration, Ann Ophthalmol 18:112-113, 1986.
17. Braverman DE and Brown RE Jr: Externalized silicone tube in single canalicular intubation, Am J Ophthalmol 103:335-336, 1987.
18. White WL et al: Relative canalicular tear flow as assessed by dacryoscintigraphy, Ophthalmology 96:167-169, 1989.
19. McCord CO: Canalicular resection and reconstruction by canaliculostomy, Ophthalmic Surg 11:440-445.
20. Beyer CK, Fabian RL, and Smith B: Naso-orbital fractures, complications, and treatment, Ophthalmology 89:456-463, 1982.
21. Anderson RL and Edwards JJ: Indications, complications and results with silicone stents, Trans Am Acad Ophthalmol Otolaryngol 86:1474-1487, 1979.
22. Crawford JS and Pashby RC: Lacrimal system disorders, Int Ophthalmol Clin 24(1):39-53, 1984.
23. Gonnering RS: Gentle, technically simple repositioning of displaced lacrimal tubing, Ophthalmic Surg 16:307-308, 1985.

CHAPTER 31

Intraorbital foreign bodies

CHRISTOPHER T. WESTFALL
JOHN W. SHORE

Fundamentals of management
Imaging modalities
Initial management
Surgical treatment
Late effects of retained intraorbital foreign bodies
References

The presence of an intraorbital foreign body suggests the potential for significant injury. At risk are not only the orbital contents, but also the surrounding structures including the sinuses, central nervous system, and great vessels of the head and neck. The proper management of such patients hinges on three basic principles. First and foremost is a comprehensive understanding of the anatomy of the orbit. Second is a complete history and physical examination. Finally, each trauma patient must be approached with a high index of suspicion for the presence of an intraorbital foreign body.

FUNDAMENTALS OF MANAGEMENT

The path and final location of a foreign body determine the degree of injury to the highly specialized structures situated within the orbit. The orbit is a small, closed space, and the structures within it are delicate and easily injured by laceration, contusion, or compression against the surrounding bones. Secondary hemorrhage within the closed orbital space may further compromise the viability of intraorbital tissues. Finally, foreign material carried into the closed space sets the stage for acute infection or chronic inflammation.

In the examiner's review of the anatomy of the orbit, particular attention should be paid to the orientation of the structures within the superior orbital fissure, inferior orbital fissure, and optic canal—the locations of the most severe damage from an intraorbital foreign body (see Chapter 25). The pyramidal shape of the orbit directs penetrating foreign bodies toward the orbital apex,[1] and the foramina provide direct communication to the brain. Therefore, missiles and other foreign bodies that enter the orbit may easily gain access to the cranial vault.[2] The thin medial orbital wall, floor, and roof are also particularly susceptible to penetration by foreign bodies.

A detailed history is necessary for the proper evaluation of a potential intraorbital foreign body. The patient, however, may be unable or unwilling to give an accurate history. For instance, a patient struck by a metal fragment while passing a construction site may not be aware of the origin of the ocular problem. A child struck by a pellet from a friend's air rifle (Fig. 31-1) may not be willing to report the nature of the injury. Constant vigilance and probing questioning are indicated to learn the possible mechanism and time of injury, force and nature of the penetrating object, direction of the entering for-

A 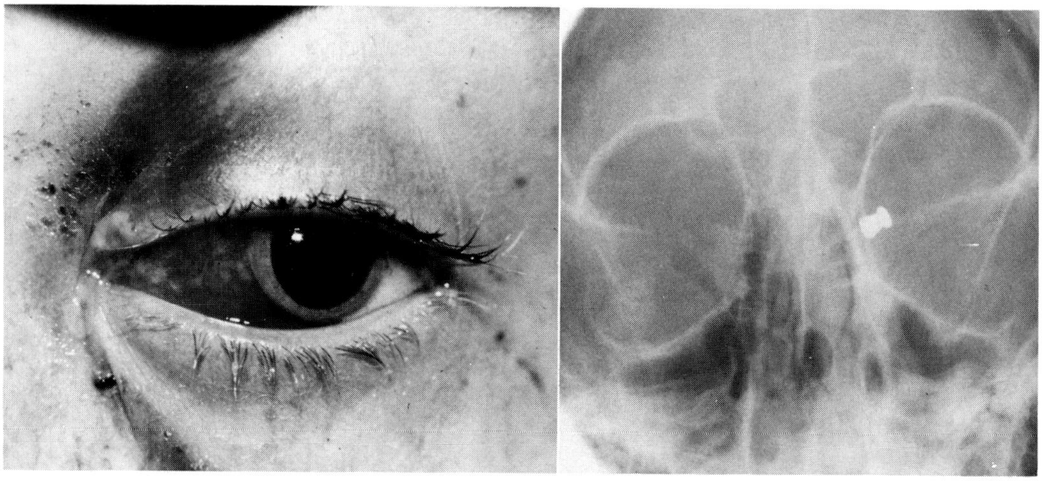 B

Fig. 31-1. **A,** An 11-year-old boy arriving in the emergency room said he had been hit in the eye with a rock. **B,** Plain X-ray films of the orbit indicated otherwise. The child later admitted that a friend had shot him with a pellet gun.

A 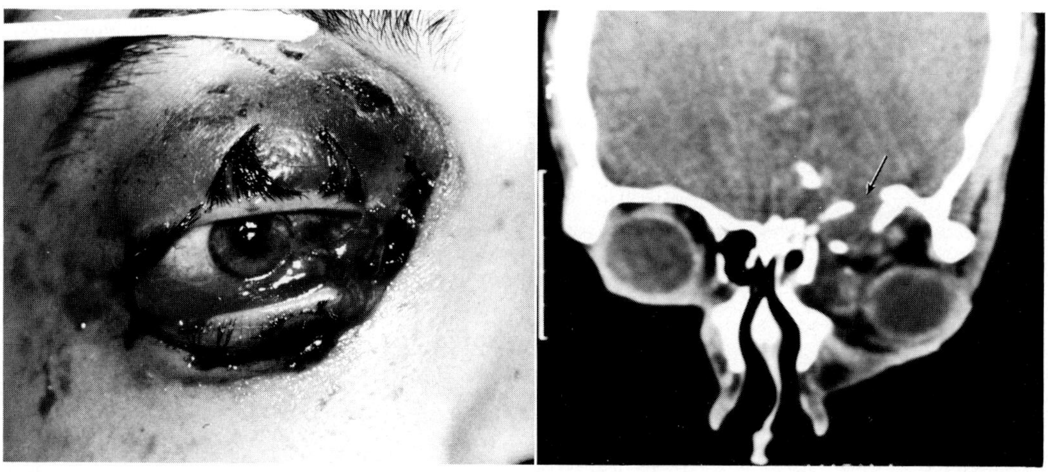 B

Fig. 31-2. **A,** A young man fell from a roof and landed on a rhododendron bush with resultant puncture wound to the orbit. A deep penetrating orbital injury was suspected. **B,** Computerized tomography scan demonstrated an orbital roof fracture *(arrow)*. During neurologic exploration a dural tear along the base of the frontal lake was found. With prompt diagnosis and appropriate neurosurgical intervention, recovery was uneventful.

eign body, and whether it exited or was retrieved from the orbit. It is of paramount importance to determine whether a portion of the object may still remain within the orbital cavity. This is particularly true when vegetable matter, such as sticks or branches, has entered the orbit; a portion may have broken off and remain buried deep in the orbital soft tissues (Fig. 31-2).

As with the history, the physical examination should be conducted with a high index of suspicion. Intraorbital foreign bodies are easily hidden within orbital soft tissue and may not be observed or suspected on examination. The clinician should search diligently for penetration sites. Drainage from the eye is an ominous sign. If an adequate examination cannot be made because of periorbital swelling or lack of patient cooperation, the use of local anesthetic infiltration or a regional nerve block should be considered (see Chapter 4). This will reduce pain and eliminate reflex blepharospasm, permitting a thorough examination. Special care must be taken not to apply pressure to the globe or orbit. In the prehospital or emergency room setting, it may be best to cut short a foreign body protruding from the orbit to allow transport or examination. However, the portion of the foreign body lodged within the eye or orbit should not be removed until all studies have been completed and the patient is properly positioned, anesthetized, and otherwise prepared for foreign body removal in the operating room. Some protruding orbital foreign bodies may require shielding or support to prevent inadvertent displacement during transport and testing.

IMAGING MODALITIES

Following the patient interview and physical examination, appropriate radiologic testing should be performed. If suspicion is low and the potential foreign body metallic, plain films are adequate. Although occasionally helpful, ultrasound is usually not necessary. Greater levels of concern require computed tomography (CT) imaging.[3,4] CT scan will identify most foreign bodies,[5] but small objects and objects composed of wood[6] or plastic may not be imaged by this modality. Glass may also be difficult to detect. Thus, a normal CT scan does not completely rule out the presence of an intraorbital foreign body.[7] The scan cuts must be 1.5 to 2 mm, and direct coronal views are mandatory. If the patient cannot be positioned in the gantry for direct coronal views, reformatted images will suffice, provided thin (2-mm) slices are obtained on the axial views.[8] An additional advantage of the CT scan is the imaging of contiguous anatomic areas, specifically the brain and sinuses. Findings of interest include blood within the sinus cavities, the presence of orbital fractures, and air within the orbital or intracranial cavity. Arteriography is the other imaging modality that may occasionally be necessary, particularly, when posttraumatic pseudoaneurysm, arteriovenous communication, or direct vascular injury may have occurred. Foreign bodies directed toward the orbital apex, and particularly injuries in which a break in the orbital roof or apex has been identified, should trigger consideration of arteriography (Fig. 31-3).

INITIAL MANAGEMENT

Initial management is directed toward protecting the globe from further injury. The role of nerve block in limiting an orbicularis effect has been emphasized. During transport and examination, the orbit should be covered with a protective shield.

When a penetrating orbital injury has occurred, the patient's tetanus immunization status must be determined. Tetanus toxoid and gamma globulin should be administered according to established guidelines (see Appendix). Broad-spectrum antibiotic coverage should be administered intravenously and the patient prepared for general anesthesia if immediate foreign-body removal is anticipated. As the nature and extent of the injury become clear, other specialists should be consulted for development of a surgical plan. Areas of special interest during this critical phase include the potential for infection, for neurologic, vascular, or airway injury, and for damage from secondary missiles generated by the offending foreign body.

The potential for infection is of particular concern in cases involving vegetable matter.[9] Contrary to popular belief, bullets and the material they carry into wounds are not sterile. The use of antibiotics is probably appropriate for all orbital foreign bodies, although no controlled clinical study has established this controversial point. The potential for infection is one aspect of the decision-making process that will determine whether the foreign body is removed primarily, at a later date, or not at all. The most important factor in preventing subsequent infection and inflammation is total removal of the foreign matter with debridement of devitalized tissue.

Neurologic injury is always a possibility in orbital trauma. Neurologic testing, attention to the patient's mental status, and CT imaging are instrumental in evaluating the nature and extent of injury. An otherwise trivial eye injury may be associated with significant neurologic trauma. These cases tend to involve in-and-out penetrating injuries, where a sharp foreign body momentarily enters the cranial fossa through the thin roof of the orbit or through the superior orbital fissure. These injuries may be easily missed. Important clues include air in the intracranial fossa, and frontal, sphenoid, or ethmoid sinus fracture. Rhinorrhea and increasing chemosis caused by cerebrospinal fluid leaking into the nose and the closed orbital space, respectively, are extremely important physical findings.

Not all foreign bodies must be removed. The

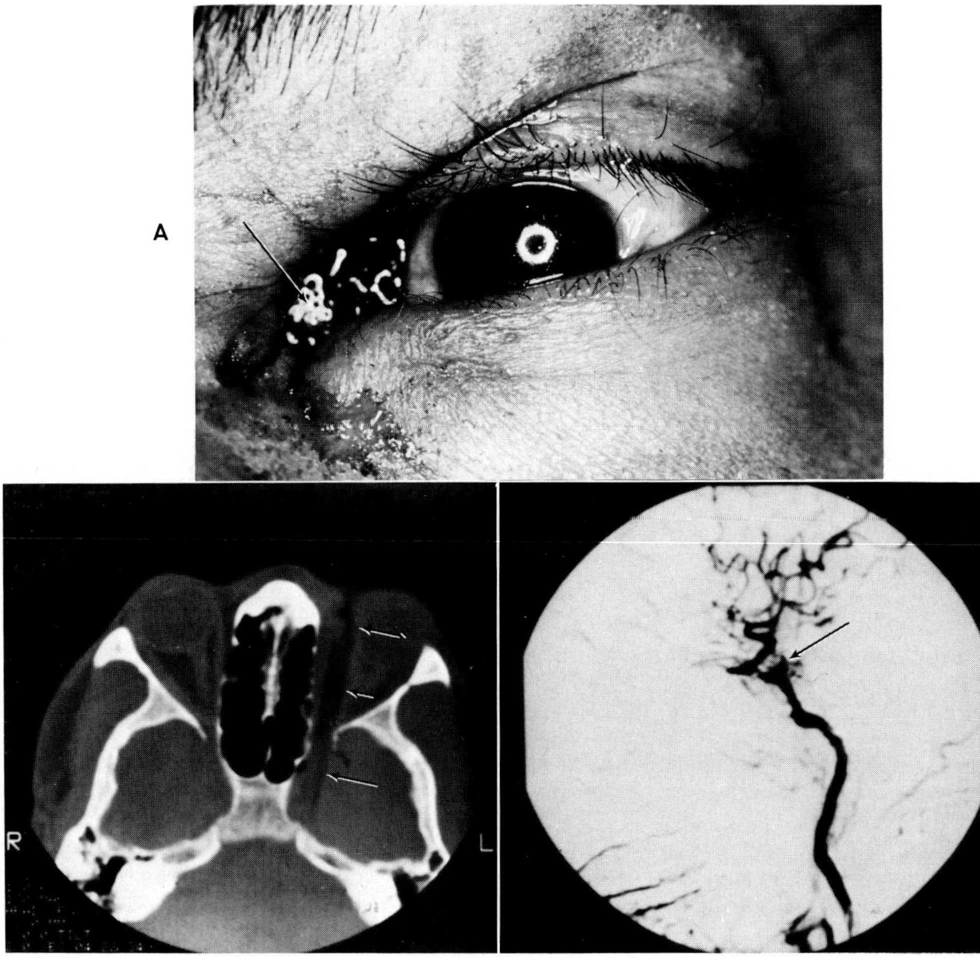

Fig. 31-3. A young man gave a history of having fallen on a stick. **A,** The end of a solid object *(arrow)* was observed in the medial canthal region but was obscured by soft-tissue swelling and chemosis. **B,** A CT scan revealed a fracture of the apex of the orbit with penetration of the cranial vault *(arrows)*. The direction of penetration and location of the foreign body raised concern of cavernous sinus involvement. **C,** This led to an arteriogram that demonstrated a pseudoaneurysm and arteriovenous communication *(arrow)*. Balloon-initiated thrombosis of the cavernous sinus by an interventional radiologist was necessary before the stick could safely be removed by anterior orbitotomy following external ethmoidectomy.

orbit will tolerate most metal fragments without adverse effect. It is only when the foreign body interferes with function or poses other risks, such as infection or chemical toxicity,[10] that removal becomes necessary.[11] It may be judicious to delay removal, particularly in the case of metal fragments, because exploration at the time of injury may produce more harm than benefit. One argument in favor of primary removal is the opportunity to remove secondary foreign bodies such as hair, skin, vegetable matter, bony fragments, or other objects that may have been carried into the orbit.

By the end of the evaluation, the clinician will have decided whether there is an intraocular foreign body and, if so, whether it should be removed. If removal is elected, consultation should be obtained with an ear, nose, and throat surgeon, plastic surgeon, and neurosurgeon as appropriate. The importance of a team approach (in those cases in which the injury extends beyond the orbit) cannot be overemphasized (see algorithm, Fig. 31-4).

SURGICAL TREATMENT

In planning the surgical approach to an intraorbital foreign body, it is important to review the

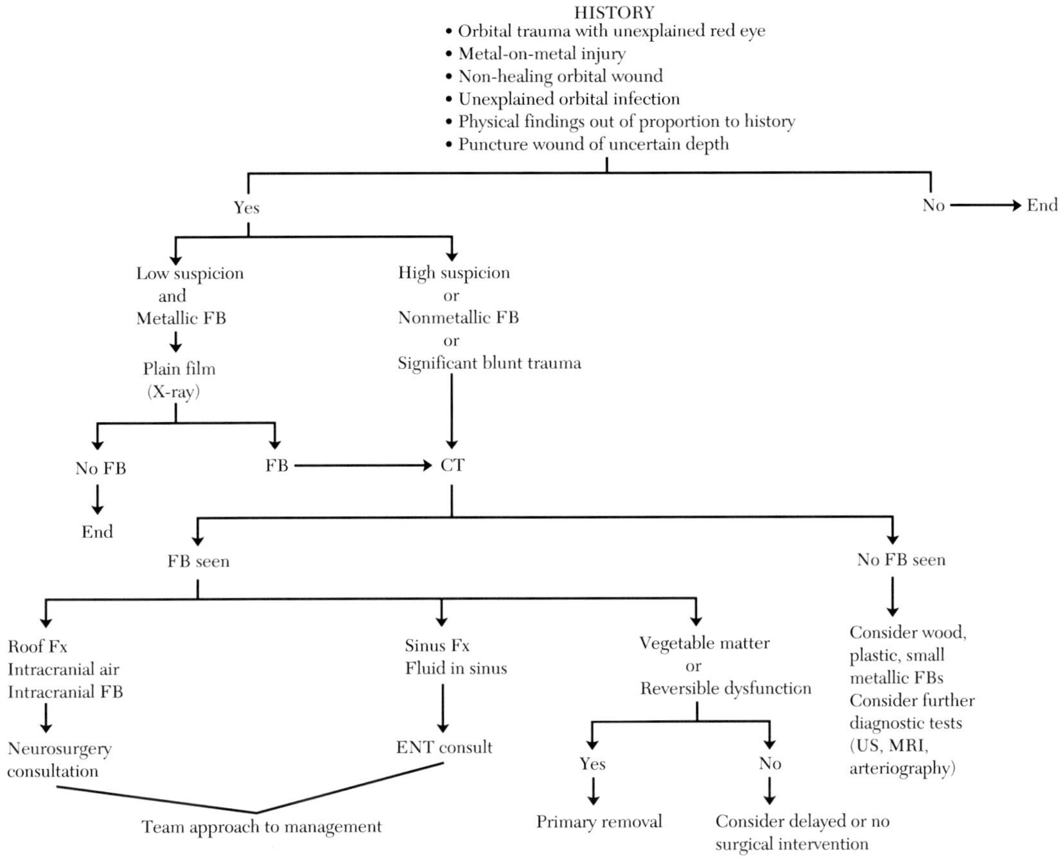

Fig. 31-4. Algorithm for intraorbital foreign body without globe injury.

goals of surgery. Primary consideration should be given to the status of the globe. Exploration of the globe can be accomplished at the time of foreign body removal. If there is evidence of a neurologic or sinus injury, a combined approach must be planned and executed with the appropriate surgical consultants.[12] The incision should provide optimal exposure. Care must be taken to minimize damage to adjacent intraorbital vascular and neurologic structures. Existing lacerations may be incorporated into the surgical incision to enhance the final cosmetic result, but exposure and visualization must not be sacrificed for cosmetic purposes. Vegetable matter, which may fragment easily, is particularly difficult to remove. Once the initial fragment has been retrieved, the surrounding area must be carefully examined for residual material.[13]

The decision as to whether the wound should be closed, left open, or drained will vary with the circumstances. In general, wounds associated with a low risk of infection should be closed. Contaminated wounds, particularly those involving vegetable matter, and wounds in which bleeding into the orbital space is likely may be packed open or a drain inserted deep into the wound.

LATE EFFECTS OF RETAINED INTRAORBITAL FOREIGN BODIES

Infection, nonhealing wounds, mucocele, motility disturbance, and vascular complications are late effects associated with retained intraorbital foreign bodies. In cases of infection in which a foreign body is not recognized, abscess formation with extrusion of the foreign body may have occurred. Any nonhealing orbital wound should be evaluated for the presence of a retained subcutaneous or deep orbital foreign body.[14] A careful history and a high index of suspicion in conjunction with a low threshold for orbital CT imaging are essential in such cases.

Injuries to the sinuses carry the late risk of

mucocele formation. This complication is best prevented rather than treated, and early involvement of an ear, nose, and throat surgeon is appropriate. Obliteration, ablation, or cranialization of the involved sinus are the usual options.

In the absence of orbital fracture, motility disturbances may result from contusion of muscles or nerves. Remarkable improvement may occur within the first 6 months after injury without intervention, and strabismus surgery should be delayed for this period of time.

Injuries to the vessels of the orbit or the intracranial cavity can result in late development of aneurysms and arteriovenous fistulas.[15] Early identification and prevention are the key to management of these patients, and arteriograms should be obtained as indicated. Treatment should involve consultation with an interventional radiologist because obliteration of the vessels with microspheres or balloons may be the optimal approach.

References

1. Simonton JT and Arthurs BP: Penetrating injuries to the orbit, Adv Ophthalmic Plast Reconstr Surg 7:217-227, 1988.
2. Bard LA and Jarrett WH: Intracranial complications of penetrating orbital injuries, Arch Ophthalmol 71:332-343, 1964.
3. Charteris DG: Posterior penetrating injury of the orbit with retained foreign body, Br J Ophthalmol 72:432-433, 1988.
4. Zinreich SJ et al: Computed tomographic three-dimensional localization and compositional evaluation of intraocular and orbital foreign bodies, Arch Ophthalmol 104:1477-1482, 1986.
5. Wilson WB et al: Magnetic resonance imaging of nonmetallic orbital foreign bodies, Am J Ophthalmol 105:612-617, 1988.
6. Weisman RA et al: Computed tomography in penetrating wounds of the orbit with retained foreign bodies, Arch Otolaryngol 109:265-268, 1983.
7. Topilow HW and Ackerman AL: Limitations of computerized tomography in the localization of intraocular foreign bodies, Ophthalmology 91:1086-1091, 1984.
8. Spoor TC: Penetrating orbital injuries, Adv Ophthalmic Plast Reconstr Surg 7:193-216, 1988.
9. Kazarian EL, Stokes NA, and Flynn JT: The orbital puncture wound: intracranial complications of a retained foreign body, J Pediatr Ophthalmol Strabismus 17:247-250, 1980.
10. Sherman S and Levine MR: Gunshot wounds of the orbit, Adv Ophthalmic Plast Reconstr Surg 7:181-192, 1988.
11. Jacobs NA and Morgan LH: On the management of retained airgun pellets: a survey of 11 orbital cases, Br J Ophthalmol 72:97-100, 1988.
12. Doucett T, Harper DW, and Rogers J: Penetrating orbital foreign body with intracranial involvement, Ann Ophthalmol 15:325-327, 1983.
13. Brock L and Tannenbaum HL: Retention of wooden foreign bodies in the orbit, Can J Ophthalmol 15:70-72, 1980.
14. Wang WJ et al: Orbital fistula: causes and treatment of 20 cases, Arch Ophthalmol 101:1721-1723, 1983.
15. Schneider RC and Henderson JW: Penetrating orbital wound with intracranial complications, Arch Ophthalmol 47:81-85, 1952.

CHAPTER 32

Dog bite injuries

RUSSELL S. GONNERING

Epidemiology
History
Examination
Therapy
- Wound decontamination
- Surgical repair
- Adjunct medical therapy
  - Tetanus
  - Rabies
  - Wound infection and antibiotics
- Postoperative care

References

Periorbital and orbital bite injuries represent a distinct subset of trauma cases seen by the ophthalmologist. Patients arrive with a combination of sharp and blunt injury, contaminated with a large inoculum of pathogenic organisms. Successful management depends on accurate assessment of ocular and adnexal injury in an often young and uncooperative patient, recognition of potentially lethal associated injuries and aspects of medical history, prompt wound decontamination and surgical repair, and logical use of intraoperative and postoperative chemotherapeutic agents. Unfortunately, until relatively recently little attention has been given to this area of trauma in the ophthalmic literature. It is one with which all ophthalmologists need facility.

EPIDEMIOLOGY

Mammalian bites, the vast majority of which are dog bites, have reached epidemic numbers in the United States. An estimated 1 to 2 million bites occur each year, most of which are unreported.[1,2] Such injuries account for approximately 1% of all emergency room visits in this country.[3]

Fortunately, most bites are of a minor nature and are treated easily and successfully. However, approximately 44,000 facial bites occur, 16,000 of which are severe. Most involve the so-called "central target area" of lips, cheeks, and nose; orbital and periorbital injuries occur in 4% to 8% of cases.[4,5]

Most severe facial bites occur in children.[4,5] In a recent series in the ophthalmic literature, over half of such bites occurred in children under 5 years of age, and two thirds in children under 10.[6] Males and females are equally victims. Possible explanations for the age distribution have ranged from close facial proximity because of short stature and inexperience with dogs[7,8] to extension of the face/mouth biting behavior dogs use to establish intrapack relationships.[1]

In almost all instances, the dog is either the family pet or otherwise known to the victim.[9,10] Fortunately, since few bites involve strays, the dog's health and rabies vaccination status are usually easy to ascertain. It is absolutely essential, however, that such information be obtained early so that appropriate examination and confinement of the dog can be instituted. In most localities the treating physician is required to report dog bites to the public health department, and the health and rabies information will be needed.

Most dog bites are from large working dogs, with the German shepherd or shepherd-mix accounting for a disproportionate share.[1,8,10,11] Although any dog is capable of biting, the most likely such animal is a young male between 6 and 11 months of age.[12]

In most instances the examiner searching for a specific cause of the attack will be frustrated with the same monotonous history. Invariably, the parent or responsible adult turns his or her back for a moment, hears the commotion, and finds the child bleeding and screaming and the dog cowering in a corner. Although an injured animal or one purposely teased may occasionally bite, most bites seem at first glance to be unprovoked. Daniels[13] has emphasized that dogs usually behave in a logical fashion, however, and almost every bite can be explained as a response to a threat to the dog's sense of territory. Dogs are one of the few animals that do not limit territoriality to conspecifics, viewing humans in much the same way they view other dogs.

Although the circumstances of the bite often seem not to fit a pattern, certain aspects of the timing are constant. The incidence of dog bites peaks in the afternoon and early evening.[2,7,9,10,13] Because of the crepuscular nature of dogs, this is the time of day they are most likely to be on their home ground and prone to displays of territoriality.[13] Most bites occur in the summer and winter as opposed to spring and fall[10,14]; the exact significance of this is unclear.

HISTORY

Most victims of periorbital dog bites come for treatment early, within 4 hours of the injury.[6,10] In addition to the usual items in the medical history, the status of tetanus immunization should be determined so appropriate prophylaxis can be instituted if necessary.

The physician must also ascertain if the patient has undergone prior splenectomy, is otherwise immunocompromised, or is suffering from alcoholism or chronic obstructive pulmonary disease. Such patients are at particular risk for development of fulminant septicemia 24 to 48 hours postbite, caused by overwhelming infection with Dysgonic Fermenter-2 (DF-2), a poorly characterized gram-negative rod.[15-19] Infection with this organism has been reported in an otherwise healthy infant following severe dog bites of the head and neck.[20] This fastidious organism has been found, when appropriate culture techniques are used, to be the most common isolate from the dog's mouth.[21]

The medical history of the dog should be obtained at the time of initial evaluation of the patient. A dog that has not received rabies vaccination must be examined by a veterinarian. In most localities, a 10-day quarantine is mandatory. If there is any question of possible rabies, it is imperative that the public health department be contacted immediately for advice on examination of the dog's brain with immunofluorescent technique at an approved laboratory. The results of this examination can be obtained in 3 hours and appropriate therapy instituted.

EXAMINATION

Although the ophthalmic injury may be the most obvious sequela of the attack, a strong suspicion of associated injury, especially in the young child, must be present. Seemingly innocuous scalp punctures may belie occult intracranial injury[22,23] or facial fracture.[24] Appropriate X-ray examinations may be indicated, particularly in children under the age of 2. Associated abdominal visceral injury may be present,[24] and potentially serious hand injuries may be overlooked in the physician's concentration on the facial deformity.

Dog jaws can exert a force of 200 to 450 psi, enough to penetrate sheet metal.[25] Most dog bites are a combination of jagged lacerations and relatively open puncture wounds with associated crush injury (Figs. 32-1 and 32-2). These are usually the result of a single "nip." Occasional vicious attacks occur that can only be described as an attempted kill, with associated injuries of the neck and throat (Fig. 32-3) and sometimes death.[11]

In a study of 16 periorbital dog bites, Gonnering[6] found no penetrating injuries of the globe and no tissue loss. Disruption of the lacrimal system was present in 14 cases. This is usually the result of laceration/avulsion of the medial aspect of the lid, sometimes with disruption of both the upper and lower canaliculi

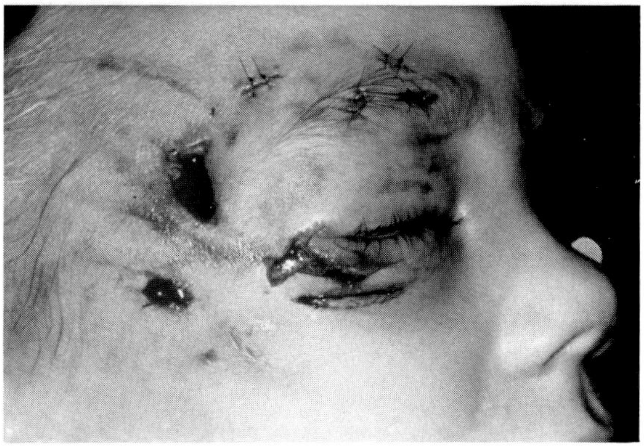

Fig. 32-1. Combination of lacerations and puncture wounds typical of a dog bite. (From Gonnering RS: Orbital and periorbital dog bites. In Bosniak SL and Smith BC, editors: Advances in ophthalmic plastic and reconstructive surgery, vol 7, Orbital trauma, part 2, Elmsford, N.Y., 1987, Pergamon.)

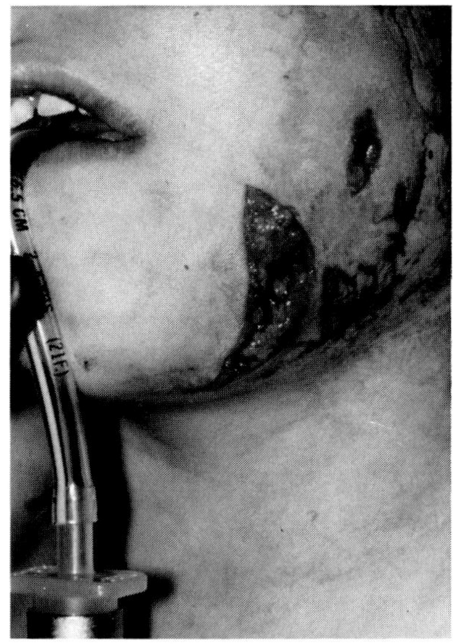

Fig. 32-3. Laceration from dog bite in "central target area."

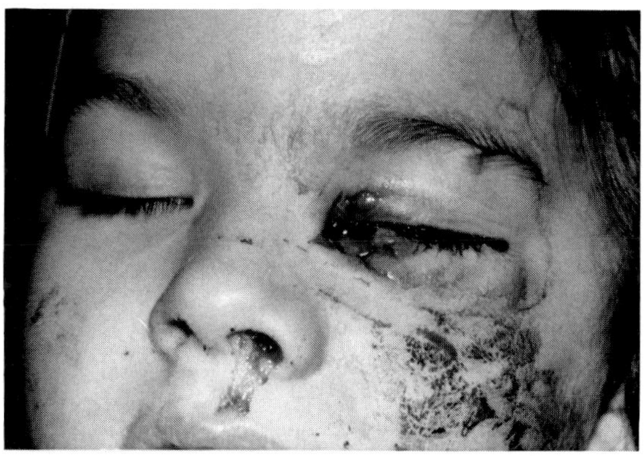

Fig. 32-2. Puncture wound of medial canthus with disruption of inferior and superior lacrimal canaliculi.

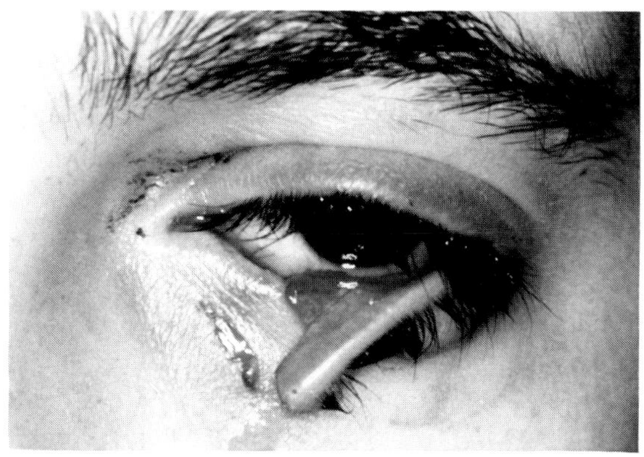

Fig. 32-4. Disruption of inferior canaliculus and medial canthal tendon from dog bite. (From Gonnering RS: Orbital and periorbital dog bites. In Bosniak SL and Smith BC, editors: Advances in ophthalmic plastic and reconstructive surgery, vol 7, Orbital trauma, part 2, Elmsford, N.Y., 1987, Pergamon.)

(Fig. 32-4). As complete an examination as possible should be attempted on initial presentation, but thorough evaluation may be possible only under anesthesia. Lacrimal system injury should be suspected in all cases with medial canthal involvement. Likewise, injury to the upper lid may involve the levator muscle and trochlea (Fig. 32-5).

THERAPY

All periorbital dog bites need prompt, definitive wound decontamination, and most require surgical repair. The upper limit of elapsed time following a bite in which primary repair can be safely undertaken is not known. Goldstein et al[26] found no signs of clinical infection in 34 patients seen within 8 hours of bite, whereas 19 of 27 seen after 12 hours without wound decontamination showed signs of clinical infection. Edlich et al[27] recommended that primary repair be undertaken only in facial wounds less than 6 hours old, but Gonnering[6] found this could be extended to at least 8 hours. Because secondary repair of severe eyelid and lacrimal system injuries often gives less than optimum results and all bites need early wound decontamination, repair should be undertaken in all cases unless signs of frank infection are present.

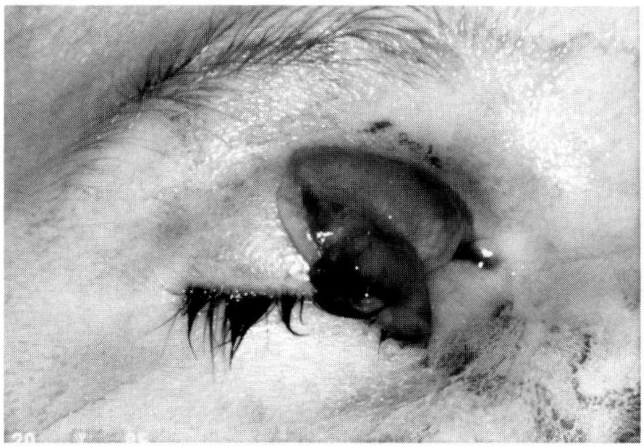

Fig. 32-5. Disruption of levator muscle, superior canaliculus, and medial canthal tendon from dog bite. (From Gonnering RS: Orbital and periorbital dog bites. In Bosniak SL and Smith BC, editors: Advances in ophthalmic plastic and reconstructive surgery, vol 7, Orbital trauma, part 2, Elmsford, N.Y., 1987, Pergamon.)

Wound Decontamination

In most cases, particularly in children, wound decontamination is best done under general anesthesia as part of the surgical repair in the operating room. Following examination of the globe and exclusion of penetrating ocular injury, wound decontamination must be carried out. Dog saliva contains 10^6 organisms/ml,[27] more than enough to cause clinical infection. Thus, all wounds are contaminated, and something must be done to decrease this inoculum of pathogens. Experimental studies have shown that the most effective way of doing this is by forceful hydraulic debridement. Forceful irrigation with at least 200 ml of normal saline using a 35-ml syringe and 19-gauge needle reduced bacteria count by 1.5 log units and decreased experimental wound infection by 90%.[28] During irrigation, the cornea should be protected with a scleral contact lens.

Surgical Repair

The goal of repair is restoration of normal anatomic structure and function. If the lacrimal system is injured, repair should commence with bicanalicular silicone intubation and microsurgical repair, using standard techniques. Anatomic repair of the avulsed medial canthal tendon with permanent suture is vital (see Chapter 30).

Following this, repair of full-thickness lid injuries should be undertaken with standard techniques. Excellent results can be obtained in children using absorbable skin sutures, obviating the trauma and possible need for general anesthesia when permanent sutures are used. In most instances, unlike injuries of the "central target area,"[5] there is no tissue loss, although retraction of the cut orbicularis may mimic such loss.[6] Aggressive surgical debridement of wound edges should not be done on eyelids and, if done at all, should be limited to obviously devitalized muscle and fat.

Once the lid margin is restored, repair of horizontal components of the laceration, which may include levator muscle in the upper lid and retractors in the lower lid, is undertaken. The orbital septum should not be repaired, because tethering of the lid often results. Particularly deep orbital penetration may benefit from placement of a small drain for 24 hours. Finally, layered repair of extramarginal defects with absorbable skin sutures is carried out.

Adjunct Medical Therapy

Tetanus

Tetanus prophylaxis must be considered in all victims of dog bites.[29] In cases without adequate prior vaccination (history of fewer than two immunization doses), use of tetanus immunoglobulin and toxoid should be undertaken (see Appendix).

Rabies

Rabies is extremely rare following dog bites in the United States.[30] Rabies prophylaxis should be instituted only if the dog cannot be found or if questions regarding its health are raised by the examining veterinarian. The preferred prophylaxis is a combination of active and passive immunization.[27,31] On day 0, 20 IU/kg of rabies immunoglobulin is administered, with half infiltrated at the site of the bite and half given intramuscularly. In addition, 1 ml of human diploid cell rabies vaccine is given intramuscularly on days 0, 3, 7, 14, and 28. In immunosuppressed patients, it is important to test the serum for rabies antibodies to ensure adequate immune response. Local and mild systemic reactions to human diploid cell vaccine occur in 25% of patients.[27] Rare, serious systemic reactions to rabies immunoglobulin or human diploid cell vaccine occur. Advice on managing such problems can be obtained from the Centers for Disease Control in Atlanta.

Wound Infection and Antibiotics

The need for prophylactic antibiotics in dog bites is controversial. Numerous studies have attempted to answer basic questions regarding wound microbiology, development of clinical infection, and impact of prophylactic antibiotics.[9,14,26,32-40] Unfortunately, many nonstandardized variables in the studies make comparison extremely difficult.

Reported rates of infection following dog bites in all anatomic locations vary from 50%[41] to less than 0.5%,[40] with the single most important factor being adequate wound decontamination. Zook et al[40] reported an incidence of infection of 1 in 215 in wounds mostly of the head and neck when prophylactic antibiotics were used. The same protocol but without the antibiotics yielded an infection incidence of 2 in 145.[42] They concluded that prophylactic antibiotics were not needed in bites of the head and neck unless the wounds were over 6 hours old. Because of the potentially serious nature of such an infection, however, it seems prudent to employ prophylactic antibiotics in dog bites of the ocular adnexae.[6,10,43]

If prophylactic antibiotics are to be used, the choice must be made when the patient is first seen. Unfortunately, no testing modality is available to point the way toward proper choice. Gram stain is unreliable in predicting possible pathogens.[38] Wound cultures before the development of clinical infection have little predictive value,[8,9,14] and results are not available for at least 24 hours.

Although many possible pathogens can be isolated from dog bite wounds, it is most useful to plan prophylactic treatment to match the isolates found in untreated bites that actually go on to clinical infection. Surprisingly different findings have been reported by different investigators. Brook[32] found most bite infections to be mixed, with *Staphylococcus aureus, Pasteurella multocida,* and anaerobic cocci the most frequent pathogens. In a study of 457 patients with dog bites, Ordog[38] noted multiple pathogenic bacteria in 36.5% of infected patients. *Enterobacteriaceae, Pseudomonas aeruginosa,* and *S. aureus* were found most frequently, with no growth seen in 30% of patients. Significantly, no *P. multocida* were isolated. In contrast, Findling, Pohlmann, and Rose[16] found *P. multocida* present in 48% of infected dog bites and *S. aureus, Staphylococcus epidermidis, Streptococcus* species, and anaerobes also frequent. Aghababian and Conte[44] reported that wounds showing signs of infection within 24 hours of the bite were more likely to contain *P. multocida,* whereas those showing infection after 24 hours contained *S. aureus* or *Streptococcus viridans.*

No single antimicrobial agent is optimal against all of these pathogens. Recommended possible choices include penicillin,[36,43] a penicillinase-resistant penicillin,[38,45] penicillin plus a penicillinase-resistant penicillin,[14,26,32] amoxicillin/clavulanic acid,[26,32,36,37] cephalexin,[6,10,45] cefadroxil,[43] cephradine,[38] and cefuroxime.[37] Alternatives in patients allergic to penicillin include erythromycin,[38,45] tetracycline for adults,[32,43] and intravenous cefazolin.[27,43]

In patients at risk for development of DF-2 septicemia (splenectomy, immunocompromise, alcoholism, and chronic obstructive pulmonary disease to a lesser degree), penicillin must be included in the prophylaxis.

Postoperative Care

Normal postoperative wound care is employed. The bandage can usually be removed after the first postoperative day, with a protective shield worn during sleep. Antibiotic ointment is applied twice a day, and the wound is gently cleansed with warm water and cotton as needed. Young children with prolonged mechanical ptosis must be checked for the development of amblyopia. A wound infection usually requires admission to the hospital for wound culture and appropriate intravenous antibiotics. The presence of a wound infection in a patient at risk for DF-2 septicemia demands urgent treatment of the infection and associated systemic abnormalities. In such patients, examination of the buffy coat by gram stain may provide the diagnosis when blood cultures are equivocal.[17]

With definitive primary repair, secondary reconstructive surgery should not be necessary.[6] As in all periorbital trauma, secondary scar revision should be delayed for at least 6 months unless such delay would compromise visual function.

References

1. Beck AM, Loring H, and Lockwood R: The ecology of dog bite injury in St Louis, Missouri, Public Health Rep 90:262-267, 1975.
2. Harris D, Imperato P, and Oken B: Dog bites: an unrecognized epidemic, Bull NY Acad Med 50:981-1000, 1974.
3. Marcy SM: Infections due to dog and cat bites, Pediatr Infect Dis 1:351-356, 1982.
4. Karlson TA: The incidence of facial injuries from dog bites, JAMA 251:3265-3267, 1984.
5. Palmer J and Rees M: Dog bites of the face: a 15 year review, Br J Plast Surg 36:315-318, 1983.
6. Gonnering RS: Ocular adnexal injury and complications in orbital dog bites, Ophthalmic Plast Reconstr Surg 3:231-235, 1987.
7. Kizer KW: Epidemiologic and clinical aspects of animal bite injuries, J Am Coll Emerg Physicians 8:134-141, 1979.
8. Schultz RC and McMaster WC: The treatment of dog bite injuries, especially those of the face, Plast Reconstr Surg 49:494-500, 1972.
9. Boenning DA, Fleisher GR, and Campos JM: Dog bites in children: epidemiology, microbiology and penicillin prophylactic therapy, Am J Emerg Med 1:17-21, 1983.
10. Gonnering RS: Orbital and periorbital dog bites. In Bosniak SL and Smith BC, editors: Advances in ophthalmic plastic and reconstructive surgery, vol 7, Orbital trauma, Elmsford, N.Y., 1988, Pergamon, 171-180.
11. Pinckney LE and Kennedy LA: Traumatic deaths from dog attacks in the United States, Pediatrics 69:193-196, 1982.
12. Parrish MH et al: Epidemiology of dog bites, Public Health Rep 74:891-903, 1959.
13. Daniels TJ: A study of dog bites on the Navajo reservation, Public Health Rep 101:50-59, 1986.
14. Goldstein EJC, Citron DM, and Finegold SM: Dog bite wounds and infections: a prospective clinical study, Ann Emerg Med 9:508-512, 1980.
15. Butler T et al: Unidentified gram-negative rod infection: a new disease in man, Ann Intern Med 86:1-5, 1977.
16. Findling JW, Pohlmann GP, and Rose HD: Fulminant gram-negative bacillemia (DF-2) following a dog bite in an asplenic woman, Am J Med 68:154-156, 1980.
17. Hicklin H, Verghese A, and Alvarez S: Dysgonic fermenter 2 septicemia, Rev Infect Dis 9:884-890, 1987.
18. Kalb R et al: Cutaneous infection at dog bite wounds associated with fulminant DF-2 septicemia, Am J Med 78:687-690, 1985.
19. Perez RE: Dysgonic fermenter-2 infections, West J Med 148:90-92, 1988.
20. Dankner WM, Davis CE, and Thompson MA: DF-2 bacteremia following a dog bite in a 4-month-old child, Pediatr Infect Dis J 6:695-696, 1987.
21. Bailie WE, Stowe EC, and Schmitt AM: Aerobic bacterial flora of oral and nasal fluids of canines with reference to bacteria associated with bites, J Clin Microbiol 7:223-231, 1978.
22. Klein DM and Cohen ME: *Pasteurella multocida* brain abscess following performing cranial bite, J Pediatr 92:588-592, 1978.
23. Wilberger JE and Pang D: Craniocerebral injuries from dog bites, JAMA 249:2685-2688, 1983.
24. Wiseman NE, Chochinov H, and Fraser V: Major dog attack injuries in children, J Pediatr Surg 18:533-536, 1983.
25. Chambers GH and Payne JF: Treatment of dog-bite wounds, Minn Med 52:427-430, 1969.
26. Goldstein EJC et al: Outpatient therapy of bite wounds: demographic data, bacteriology, and a prospective, randomized trial of amoxicillin clavulanic acid versus penicillin ± dicloxacillin, Int J Dermatol 26:123-127, 1987.
27. Edlich RF et al: Emergency department management of mammalian bites, Emerg Med Clin North Am 4:595-604, 1986.
28. Stevenson TR et al: Cleansing the traumatic wound by high pressure syringe irrigation, J Am Coll Emerg Physicians 5:17-21, 1976.
29. American College of Surgeons Committee on Trauma, Prophylaxis against tetanus in wound management, Bull Am Coll Surg 69:22-23, 1984.
30. Immunization Practices Advisory Committee (ACIP), Rabies prevention—United States, 1984, MMWR 33:393-402, 1984.
31. Flanigan TJ, Rippert ET, and Nieusma GE: Rabies therapy for animal bites in the head and neck region, J Oral Maxillofac Surg 43:704-706, 1985.
32. Brook I: Microbiology of human and animal bite wounds in children, Pediatr Infect Dis J 6:29-32, 1987.
33. Callaham ML: Treatment of common dog bites: infection risk factors, J Am Coll Emerg Physicians 7:83-87, 1978.
34. Callaham M: Prophylactic antibiotics in common dog bite wounds: a controlled study, Ann Emerg Med 9:410-414, 1980.
34. Rosen RA: The use of antibiotics in the initial management of recent dog-bite wounds, J Emerg Med 3:19-23, 1985.
35. Elenbaas R, McNabney WK, and Robinson W: Prophylactic oxacillin in dog bite wounds, Ann Emerg Med 11:248-251, 1982.

36. Feder HM, Shanley JD, and Barbera JA: A review of 59 patients hospitalized with animal bites, Pediatr Infect Dis J 6:24-28, 1987.
37. Goldstein EJC and Citron DM: Comparative activities of cefuroxime, amoxicillin/clavulanic acid, ciprofloxacin, enoxacin and ofloxacin against aerobic and anaerobic bacteria isolated from bite wounds, Antimicrob Agents Chemother 32:1143-1148, 1988.
38. Ordog GJ: The bacteriology of dog bite wounds on initial presentation, Ann Emerg Med 15:1324-1329, 1986.
39. Zook EG et al: Successful treatment protocol for canine fang injuries, J Trauma 20:243-247, 1980.
40. Thompson HJ and Svitek V: Small animal bites: the role of primary closure, J Trauma 13:20-23, 1973.
41. Guy RJ and Zook EG: Successful treatment of acute head and neck dog bite wounds without antibiotics, Ann Plast Surg 17:45-48, 1986.
42. Herman DC, Bartley GB, and Walker RC: The treatment of animal bite injuries of the eye and ocular adnexa, Ophthalmic Plast Reconstr Surg 3:237-241, 1987.
43. Aghababian R and Conte JE: Mammalian bite wounds, Ann Emerg Med 9:79-83, 1980.
44. Callaham M: Controversies in antibiotic choices for bite wounds, Ann Emerg Med 17:1321-1330, 1988.

CHAPTER 33

Enucleation and evisceration

DAVID B. LYON
RICHARD K. DORTZBACH

- Enucleation
  - Indications and advantages
  - Limitations
  - Surgical procedure
    - Patient preparation
    - Anesthesia
    - Technique
    - Additional considerations
  - Complications
    - Hemorrhage
    - Globe perforation
    - Orbit injury
    - Infection
    - Implant migration
    - Blepharoptosis
    - Socket contracture
    - Conjectival cysts
- Evisceration
  - Indications and advantages
  - Limitations
  - Surgical procedure
    - Patient preparation and anesthesia
    - Technique of evisceration with retention of the cornea
    - Technique of evisceration with keratectomy
    - Additional considerations
  - Complications
- References

Despite recent advances in anterior segment and vitreoretinal surgery in severely traumatized eyes, enucleation or evisceration is still necessary in many cases. Enucleation is the surgical removal of the entire globe and a portion of retrobulbar optic nerve. Evisceration is the surgical removal of the intraocular contents and sometimes the cornea, leaving the sclera and optic nerve intact. An orbital implant is usually placed to help replenish orbital volume, and an ocular prosthesis is fabricated when the anophthalmic socket is healed.

The decision to enucleate or eviscerate a traumatized eye may be difficult for both patient and surgeon. The psychological implications of the permanent loss of an eye require compassion from the ophthalmologist when counseling the patient. A thorough discussion of surgical alternatives, their attendant risks, the operative plan, postoperative management, and potential complications must always be undertaken. Persons wearing prosthetic eyes may be available for advice and support. Postoperative photographs of such patients will help allay fears of disfigurement. Literature on adapting to a monocular world is also valuable.[1]

The indications for enucleation and evisceration are often not mutually exclusive or absolute. Advantages and disadvantages of each procedure must be weighed in accordance with the patient's injury and wishes. A second opinion is often beneficial.

Both enucleation and evisceration have the objectives of preserving life, preserving vision in the fellow eye, limiting operative complexity and risk, limiting perioperative morbidity and early and late complications, and achieving optimal cosmesis.[2]

Following removal of an eye, the management of the anophthalmic socket and ocular prosthesis remains a challenge for the ophthalmologist and ocularist. Preventive maintenance and medical and surgical interventions for socket and lid complications are best handled with a team approach.

ENUCLEATION

Indications and Advantages

Traditionally there have been certain absolute indications for enucleation: suspected intraocular malignancies, severely traumatized eyes with large posterior ruptures, and blind painful eyes.[3] However, advances in clinical knowledge, surgical techniques, and alternative therapies have modified these indications. Frequently the choice among enucleation, evisceration, and other therapies is based on the preference of the ophthalmologist and the patient. Decisions should be made on an individual basis with the patient fully informed. Patient age, general health, associated injuries, and availability of services must be taken into account.

Primary enucleation, even in severely traumatized eyes with complete visual loss, is generally not advisable. In most cases, it is better to repair the cornea and anterior scleral defects immediately, with repositioning of prolapsed uvea. Development or persistence of no light perception vision for 3 consecutive days should lead to enucleation secondarily within 7 to 10 days from the time of injury. This allows patients time to realize that the lost vision will not return. Rarely, when primary repair is impossible or other injuries or health problems contraindicate a second anesthesia or operation, primary enucleation is undertaken.

Historically, the risk of sympathetic ophthalmia after severe trauma with uveal prolapse has been a major impetus for enucleation. Enucleation allows more complete removal of uveal tissue, especially along scleral emissaria, than does evisceration. Evisceration performed soon after trauma, however, appears to have a very low risk of sympathetic ophthalmia, although no good statistics are available to substantiate this. Well-documented cases of sympathetic uveitis after evisceration for traumatic visual loss are few, but they have been reported.[4] The patient, therefore, must be informed of this risk. Some authors feel that enucleation of the inciting eye is advantageous in sympathetic ophthalmia if performed within 2 weeks of the onset of symptoms in the sympathizing eye[5,6] (see Chapter 24).

Limitations

Enucleation requires extensive dissection in the orbit and induces multiple changes in orbital anatomy and physiology, including decreased orbital blood flow, as reflected by thermography, fat atrophy and decreased orbital soft tissue volume, disturbance of the levator palpebrae superioris–Whitnalls' ligament complex, disturbance of extraocular muscles, leading to poor prosthesis mobility, prosthesis-induced interference with upper and lower eyelid position, and, in children, retardation of bony orbital growth.[2,7,8] Precise surgery with current enucleation techniques and delicate handling of tissues help to minimize these changes. Many anatomic socket deformities can be camouflaged to give good cosmetic and functional results.

Surgical Procedure

Patient Preparation

Before surgery, informed consent is obtained and the goals of the surgery reviewed. Orbital hemorrhage, infection, and implant extrusion are mentioned as possible complications. An appointment with an ocularist for fitting of the prosthesis may be scheduled for about 1 month postoperatively. The patient is reminded that although the prosthesis is custom-made and will be a good match for the fellow eye, its motility will not be normal. Antiplatelet and anticoagulant medications should be discontinued 10 to 14 days preoperatively.

Anesthesia

Enucleation may be performed under either local or general anesthesia. Local anesthesia supplemented by intravenous narcotics and anxiolytics (e.g., fentanyl and midazolam) is very successful and is particularly desirable for outpatient surgery. A facial nerve block and a 4- to 5-ml retrobulbar injection of a 1:1 mixture of 2% lidocaine with 1:100,000 epinephrine and 0.75% bupivacaine is used, and hyaluronidase (150 units) is added to the mixture.

For psychological reasons, general anesthesia is preferred for young patients and anxious adults. A supplementary retrobulbar anesthetic injection for postoperative pain relief is generally not added in general anesthesia cases.

Technique

Before and after prepping and draping the patient, the surgeon should confirm which eye is

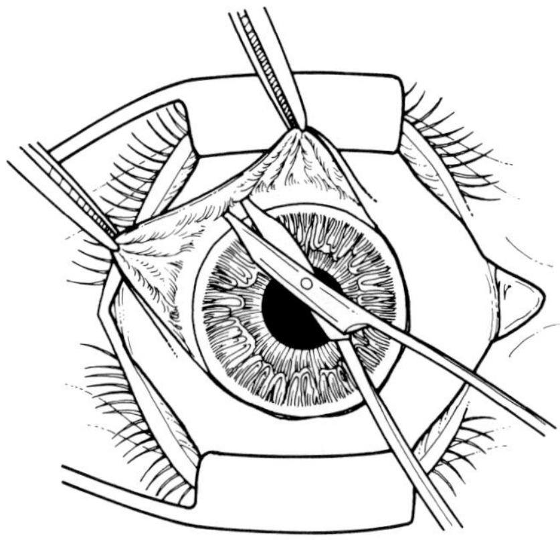

Fig. 33-1. Enucleation technique: peritomy. The conjoined bulbar conjunctiva and anterior Tenon's capsule are dissected as a single layer, taking care to preserve the maximum amount of tissue.

to be enucleated. The patient's chart and operative permit must be rechecked to ensure that the correct eye is being removed. Following trauma, the external appearance of the involved eye is usually abnormal and further identifies the eye to be enucleated. Operating loupe magnification should be used throughout the operation.

A lid speculum or 4-0 silk lid margin traction sutures secured with clamps to the drapes are used. Soll[8,9] recommends placement of 4-0 silk mattress sutures in the superior conjunctival fornix to reduce the chance of levator aponeurosis or muscle damage during dissection.

A 360° limbal peritomy is performed with Westcott scissors, preserving as much conjunctiva and Tenon's capsule as possible (Fig. 33-1). Dissection is continued in the sub-Tenon's space to the rectus muscle insertions. Stevens scissors are then used for blunt dissection beneath Tenon's capsule in the oblique quadrants between the muscle insertions.

The rectus muscles are then sequentially hooked with a muscle hook. Double-armed 6-0 Vicryl sutures are placed just posterior to the insertions of the horizontal recti. Westcott scissors are used to disinsert the recti flush with the sclera except medially, where a small tendinous stump is left on the globe. Dissection of the intermuscular membrane and check ligaments should be avoided, especially around the superior rectus, because this results in unnecessary weakening of orbital tissues and increases

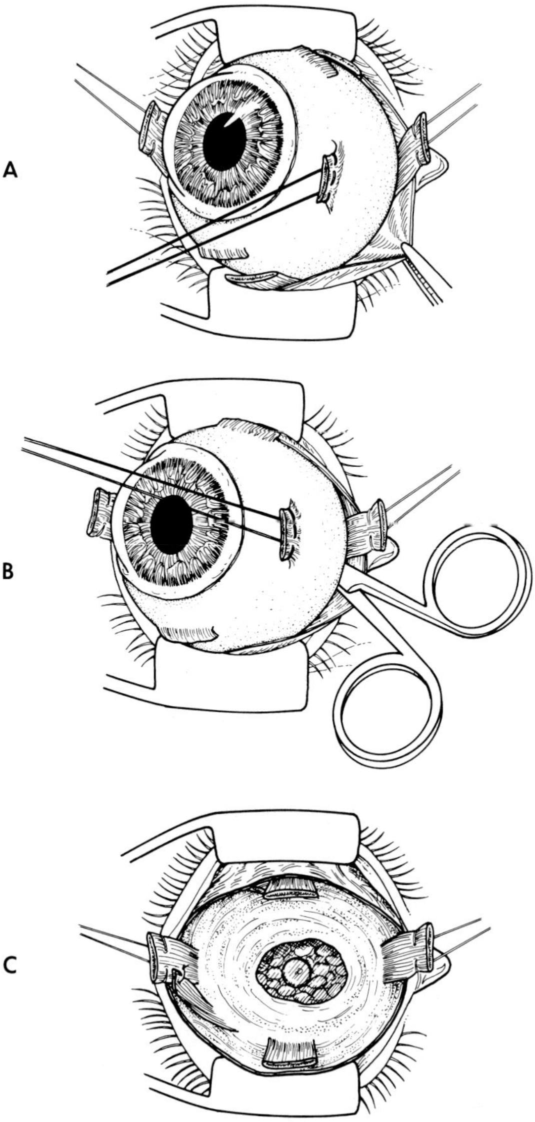

A

B

C

Fig. 33-2. Enucleation technique: removal of globe. **A,** The extraocular muscles are disinserted and a 4-0 silk suture is passed several times through the medial rectus stump on the globe; 6-0 Vicryl sutures are passed through the horizontal rectus muscle tendons prior to disinsertion. The inferior oblique is sutured to the inferior border of the lateral rectus. **B,** Using the medial traction suture, the globe is abducted and proptosed, allowing passage of the enucleation scissors medially to perform the neurectomy. **C,** After the globe has been removed and hemostasis achieved, the opening in posterior Tenon's capsule through which the optic nerve passed is identified. Intraconal orbital fat should be visible through this opening. Note the inferior oblique sewn to the lateral rectus.

the possibility of postoperative ptosis. A 4-0 silk suture is passed several times through the medial rectus stump on the globe, to be used for traction (Fig. 33-2, *A*).

The oblique muscles are hooked next and disinserted under direct visualization by appropriate rotation of the globe: depression and abduction for the superior oblique tendon, elevation and adduction for the inferior oblique. A 6-0 Vicryl suture is used to attach the inferior oblique to the inferior border of the lateral rectus 8 to 10 mm behind its free end, thus allowing the inferior oblique to provide postoperative support for the implant in the socket. This may also be done after globe removal.

The medial traction suture is used to lift and abduct the globe, and enucleation scissors are passed in the sub-Tenon's space medially (Fig. 33-2, *B*). Gentle blunt dissection is usually needed to separate posterior Tenon's from the posterior sclera and emissaria. The scissors are then used to strum the optic nerve, first with the blades closed and then again when open, to confirm the nerve's position. This is done blindly and by feel, to engage the nerve without accompanying posterior sclera, Tenon's capsule, or orbital fat. After ascertaining correct scissors positioning, the surgeon performs a neurectomy well posterior to the globe without excessive posterior compression into the orbital apex. Ideally, a 2- to 4-mm segment of optic nerve is removed with the globe (Fig. 33-3).

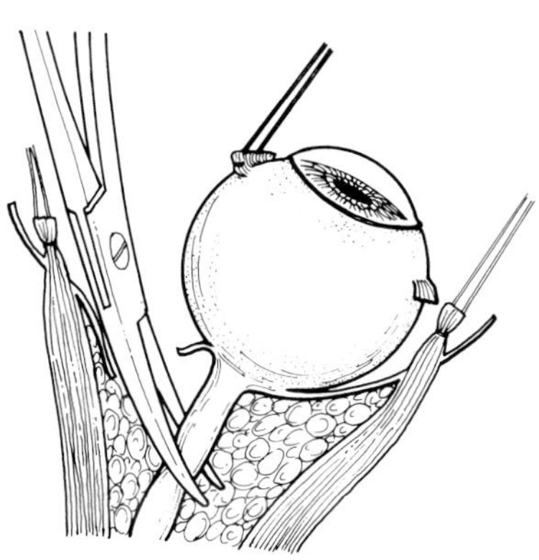

Fig. 33-3. Enucleation technique: neurectomy. Scissor blades are positioned by feel to straddle and then sever the optic nerve, which is held on stretch by traction on the globe. Care is taken to avoid including a large amount of posterior Tenon's capsule and orbital fat between the scissor blades.

After cutting the nerve, the surgeon slowly delivers the detached globe anteriorly and severs any remaining attachments. Tenon's space is then quickly packed with dry 4 × 4-inch gauze sponges, and firm digital pressure is applied for 5 minutes. During this time, the globe is inspected to confirm that it has been completely removed, has no scleral laceration, and has an adequate length of optic nerve. The packing is then slowly removed and hemostasis checked. If bleeding continues, the space is repacked with gauze or gelatin sponges (Gelfoam) soaked in thrombin, and an additional 5 minutes of pressure is applied.

Packing is often ineffective in providing hemostasis if anterior Tenon's is not retracted to allow the packing to fill Tenon's space. Occasionally, identifiable bleeders require cautery to gain hemostasis. With hemostasis achieved, the surgeon inspects the socket to assure the absence of ocular contents. The size of the opening in posterior Tenon's capsule is noted and identified by the presence of intraconal fat posterior to the opening (Fig. 33-2, *C*).

The surgeon is now ready to place the orbital implant. A myriad of implants are available and have been advocated by others, but in most cases noncovered silicone spheres are preferred. Spheres of various sizes are soaked in gentamicin solution before use. The sphere is placed in the muscle cone posterior to posterior Tenon's capsule. The goal is restoration of orbital volume with the largest-diameter implant (usually 20 to 22 mm) that allows closure of posterior Tenon's in front of the implant without undue tension. The rent in posterior Tenon's may have to be enlarged horizontally to allow passage of the implant into the intraconal space (Fig. 33-4, *A*).

After implant placement, attention is directed to meticulous closure in three layers: posterior Tenon's, anterior Tenon's, and conjunctiva (Figs. 33-4, *B* through *D*, and 33-5). The edges of posterior Tenon's are approximated with a horizontal row of simple interrupted 5-0 Vicryl sutures. The double-armed sutures securing the horizontal recti are passed through anterior Tenon's and conjunctiva beyond the medial and lateral extent of the conjunctival opening. Anterior Tenon's, undissected from the conjoined conjunctiva, is closed with multiple interrupted buried sutures of 5-0 Vicryl. A running 5-0 plain catgut suture is used to close the conjunctiva horizontally. The Vicryl sutures from the medial

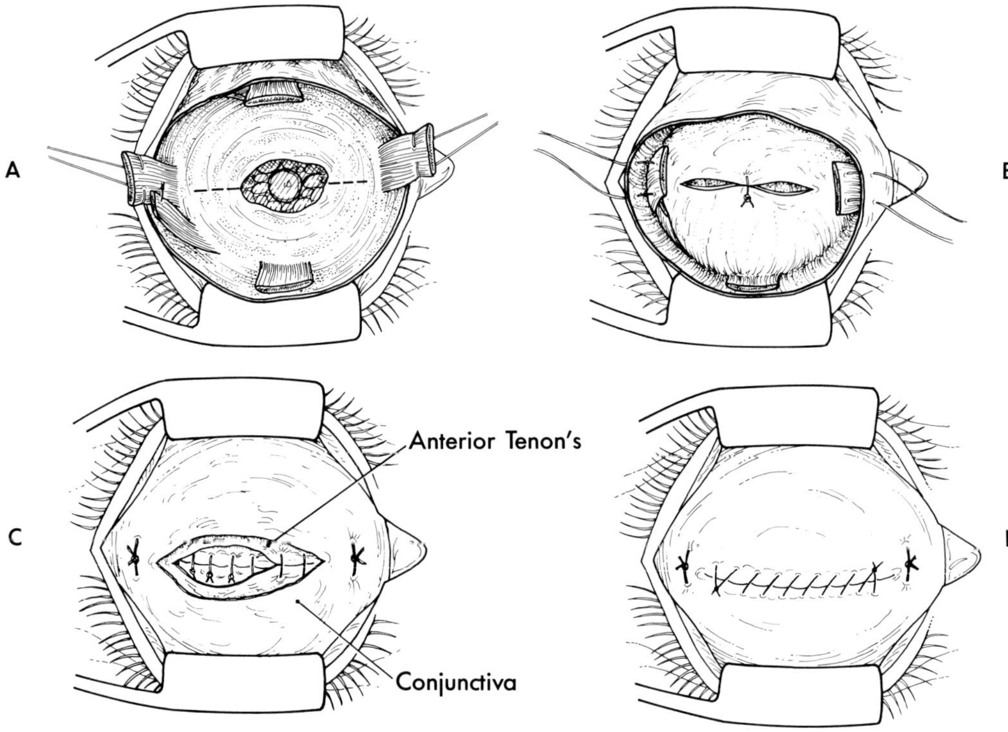

Fig. 33-4. Enucleation technique: orbital implant placement. **A,** The opening in posterior Tenon's may need to be enlarged (dashed line) to allow placement of the orbital implant. **B,** The largest possible sphere that allows closure of posterior Tenon's capsule over it is placed. The double-armed sutures on the horizontal recti are passed through anterior Tenon's capsule and conjunctiva and tied in the medial and lateral fornices. **C,** Anterior Tenon's is closed without dissection away from the conjoined conjunctiva. **D,** The conjunctiva is closed with a running suture.

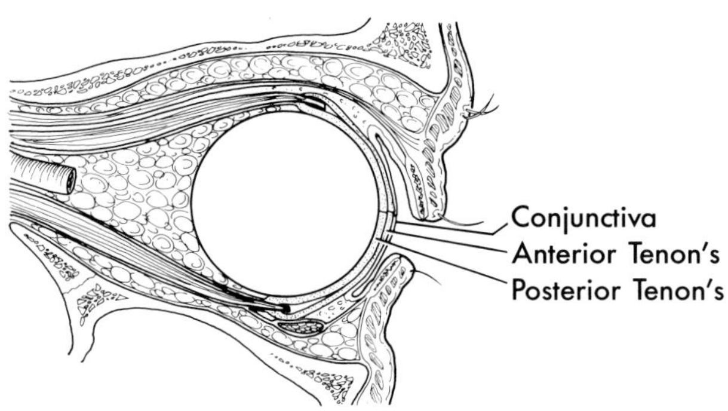

Fig. 33-5. Enucleation technique. A sagittal cut through the orbit shows the implant within the muscle cone with a three-layered closure over it.

and lateral rectus muscles are now tied on the conjunctival surface to secure them to the lateral fornices. No conformer is used. Broad-spectrum antibiotic ointment is instilled in the socket, and a pressure dressing of two eye pads secured with tincture of benzoin and 1-inch tape is applied. Systemic antibiotics are not routinely administered.

After 3 to 4 days the pressure dressing is removed and the socket examined. Topical antibiotic ointment is begun 3 times a day, and a follow-up exam is scheduled 1 month later, just before fitting of the prosthesis.

Additional Considerations

Unique situations may arise in traumatized eyes that need enucleation. In the very rare instance when primary enucleation is done in a severely disrupted globe, partial repair of the globe may be required to reapproximate large pieces of sclera. It is preferable to remove the traumatized scleral shell in one piece, if possible. If not, meticulous exploration of the socket is necessary to extract all uveal and scleral remnants. Copious irrigation with antibiotic solution should be done in contaminated orbits, and intra- and postoperative systemic antibiotics should be prescribed.

In primary enucleation after trauma, an intraconal implant and layered closure are preferred. Extensive defects in posterior Tenon's capsule may require precise repair. Smaller implants may be necessary for adequate closure. Loss of large amounts of conjunctiva or Tenon's fascia may necessitate autogenous or homologous graft materials. Buccal mucosa, dermal fat, autogenous or homologous fascia, and preserved sclera are available materials.

Associated injuries may include orbital fractures and eyelid defects. Ignored large orbital-floor defects result in redistribution of orbital volume. Large fractures identified radiographically may be repaired at the time of enucleation. General principles of ophthalmic plastic surgery should be used in repair and reconstruction of the eyelids (see Chapter 29).

Complications

Intraoperative complications include removal of the wrong eye, orbital hemorrhage, perforation of the globe, and injury to orbital structures. Postoperative complications include infection, migration and extrusion of the implant, blepharoptosis, socket contracture, deep superior sulcus syndrome, and formation of socket cysts.

Removal of the wrong eye is a great tragedy, and the possibility of this error must be continually in the surgeon's mind. The chart and operative consent must be reviewed, and ophthalmoscopy should be performed after draping the patient to ensure removal of the correct eye.

Hemorrhage

Hemorrhage arising from the central retinal vessels usually follows neurectomy. Although crushing the optic nerve with a clamp before cutting it is recommended by some, this additional step induces crush artifact and may damage the posterior globe or Tenon's capsule. Adequate hemostasis is possible with application of firm pressure after placing gauze packing within Tenon's space. Topical thrombin and Gelfoam and electrocautery are sometimes necessary. Development of a tense orbit during closure reflects delayed hemorrhage in spite of adequate hemostasis earlier. Firm digital pressure over the closed lids for 5 to 10 minutes followed by observation for a similar period may be necessary before continuing with the procedure. If signs of hemorrhage persist, the implant is removed, the hematoma evacuated, and the posterior orbit explored to identify and control the source of bleeding.

Globe Perforation

Perforation of the globe most commonly occurs when the posterior sclera is incised during neurectomy. This complication is usually discovered upon inspection of the enucleated specimen. Perforation of the globe is managed by complete removal of extruded or retained contents. Careful blunt dissection within the muscle cone is performed to locate the scleral stump, which may be buried in billowing orbital fat.

Orbit Injury

Overzealous dissection with clamps or enucleation scissors posterior to the globe risks injury to structures in the orbital apex. Damage to the levator muscle or its innervation may result in complete ptosis postoperatively, which may require a frontalis suspension procedure for correction. Increased orbital fat atrophy with associated volume deficit may also be induced.

Infection

The risk of postoperative cellulitis can be reduced by soaking alloplastic implant material in antibiotic solution before use. Meticulous layered closure prevents entry by organisms from the mucosal surface of the socket. If infection does develop, a culture is taken and appropriate topical and systemic antibiotics administered. Implant removal may be necessary.

Before the antibiotic era, enucleation in the presence of infectious endophthalmitis or panophthalmitis was thought to increase the possibility of postoperative meningitis or encephalitis through direct spread along the severed meninges of the optic nerve. The intensive medical and surgical treatment of endophthalmitis today has minimized, if not eliminated, central nervous system infection after enucleation.[10] A single case of postenucleation meningitis has been reported in the more recent literature.[11]

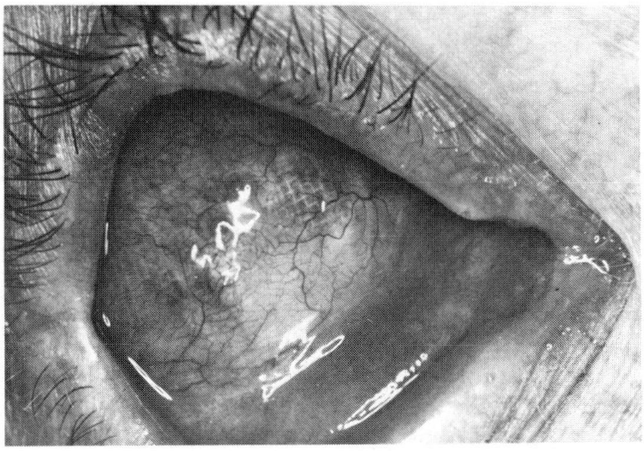

Fig. 33-6. Extruding wire mesh implant. Note that only a thin layer of conjunctiva covers the implant.

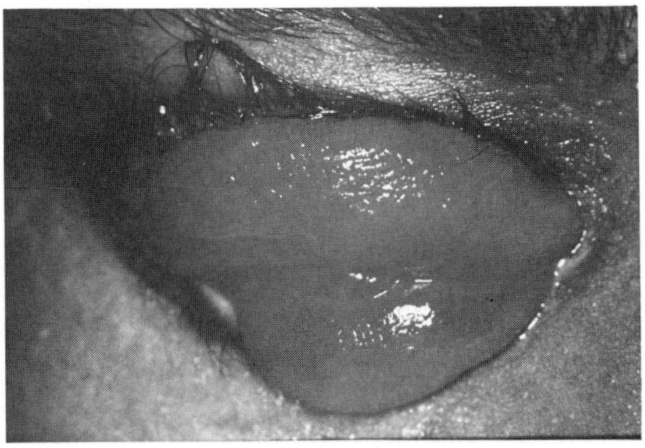

Fig. 33-7. Massive postoperative socket edema with conjunctival prolapse between the lids.

Implant Migration

The goal of enucleation surgery is a well-centered, well-covered, well-supported orbital implant with deep mobile fornices. However, a perfect implant does not exist. Migration and extrusion of orbital implants remain a problem (Fig. 33-6). The choice of implant and the surgical technique should aim to minimize these complications.

A noncovered, light-weight, silicone sphere is generally preferred. Integrated or quasiintegrated (Iowa, Universal) implants have irregularly shaped front surfaces that can erode tissues at friction points with the prosthesis and result in extrusion. Scleral or fascial wrapped spheres are recommended by some authors.[9,12,13] When these are used, Tenon's capsule or rectus muscles can be attached to the scleral coating in various ways. Homologous donor sclera, preserved in 50% ethanol, is available from eye banks. Blood from donors is screened to exclude HIV infection and hepatitis. Nevertheless, there is a remote risk of the transmission of slow-virus infection with the use of homologous sclera. In addition, the anterior tissue barrier to implant extrusion in a cynomolgus monkey model has been shown to be less for a scleral-wrapped sphere than for a nonwrapped sphere 6 months after enucleation.[14] The sclera does provide an increased barrier early (6 weeks), but it is lost from a combination of inflammation and absorption by 6 months. Also, attachment of the horizontal recti to the conjunctival fornices is preferred because movement of the fornices is the mechanism for movement of the prosthesis. A new integrated implant of hydroxyapapite is under investigation and appears to be a promising advance in enucleation.[15]

Implant size and position are additional factors in migration and extrusion. Too large an implant places tension on anterior supporting tissue layers and may give a proptotic appearance. An implant placed within Tenon's capsule necessarily has less coverage and must be smaller than one placed behind posterior Tenon's capsule (within the muscle cone). Soll[13] first popularized placement of the implant posterior to posterior Tenon's. Securing the implant within the muscle cone in this way decreases the likelihood of migration. The three-layered closure, without undue tension or gaps to allow epithelial ingrowth, minimizes chances of extrusion.

Imbrication of the rectus muscles over spherical implants, regardless of size, often results in the syndrome of superotemporal migration of the implant, ptosis, and difficulty in fitting the prosthesis.[16] It may also displace the socket posteriorly.

Pressure bandages after enucleation help tamponade bleeding and limit edema, which may be massive (Fig. 33-7). If a conformer is also used, it is pressed directly against the suture lines and may erode them. The use of large orbital implants eliminates the need for a conformer.

In the traumatized orbit, tissue loss or damage, especially of Tenon's fascia, may destabilize the implant. Careful repair of Tenon's and use of smaller implants to avoid wound tension are beneficial to minimize migration and extrusion. Homologous scleral patch grafts have been

A

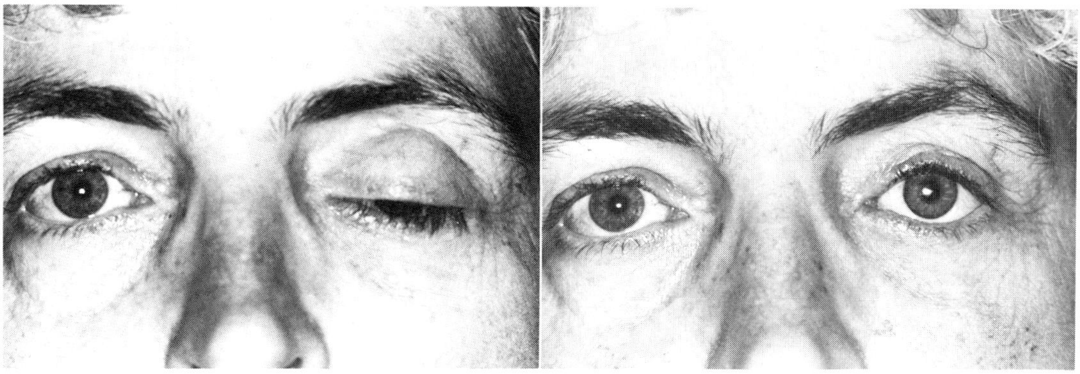

B

Fig. 33-8. **A,** Neurogenic ptosis following enucleation. **B,** After 6 months' observation without recovery, a unilateral fascia frontalis sling was performed.

used successfully following trauma or with early wound dehiscence to prevent migration or extrusion.[17] A large or long-standing wound dehiscence with implant exposure is accompanied by conjunctival epithelial ingrowth, which must be excised or destroyed by swabbing with absolute alcohol before placement of a new implant in a muscle cone.[18] Dermis fat grafting is also useful, especially with a deficit of conjunctiva.

Blepharoptosis

Blepharoptosis following enucleation may be aponeurogenic, myogenic, neurogenic, or from orbital implant migration. Levator aponeurosis dehiscence, levator muscle damage, or paresis of the superior division of the oculomotor nerve may result from excessive manipulation or dissection in the superior orbit or orbital apex. Allen[16] described the syndrome of ptosis from implant migration. It develops when rectus muscles imbricated over a spherical implant slip inferonasally. The sphere is pushed superotemporally, and the superior fornix and upper lid are pulled forward and down.

Prosthetic management of ptosis involves incorporation of a ptosis buckle on the superior pole of the prosthesis to mechanically elevate the lid. Levator surgery, or frontalis suspension if there is poor levator function, is the surgical approach to ptosis correction in the anophthalmic socket (Fig. 33-8). Adjustment of the levator intraoperatively should be done with the prosthesis in place. The ptosis buckle should be removed before surgery if possible. As an alternative approach, a conformer can be placed during levator adjustment to simulate the prosthesis.

Socket Contracture

Enophthalmos due to loss of orbital volume following enucleation may produce a pseudoptosis of the upper lid. Moreover, socket contracture results from shrinkage of some or all of the anophthalmic orbital tissues. Typically, socket contracture causes cicatricial entropion, shallowing of the fornices, and inability to retain a prosthesis (Fig. 33-9). Various processes may lead to socket contracture: fibrosis from trauma with or without tissue loss, implant migration or extrusion, chronic inflammation, infection, and chemical injury. Overzealous dissection or failure to preserve conjunctiva and Tenon's capsule at the time of enucleation may also contribute.

Postoperative socket contracture may be managed with a variety of techniques, including full- or partial-thickness buccal mucosal grafts, secondary orbital implants of silicone or other alloplastic materials, and dermis-fat grafts.[2]

A deep superior sulcus is often a component of the postenucleation socket syndrome.[19] Removal of the globe (with an average volume of 7 ml) and orbital fat atrophy (an estimated 2 to 3 ml) following enucleation with placement of a spherical orbital implant (one with an 18-mm diameter has a volume of approximately 3 ml) results in an orbital volume deficit. That is, an 18-mm orbital implant replaces little more than is lost by orbital fat atrophy, leaving a deficit close to the volume of the enucleated globe. A large and therefore heavy prosthesis is fitted in an attempt to make up the volume loss, and in time this heavy prosthesis will stretch the lower eyelid, which supports it. Drooping of the lower lid and prosthesis, enophthalmos, secondary upper lid ptosis, and a deep superior sulcus make up the full-blown postenucleation socket syn-

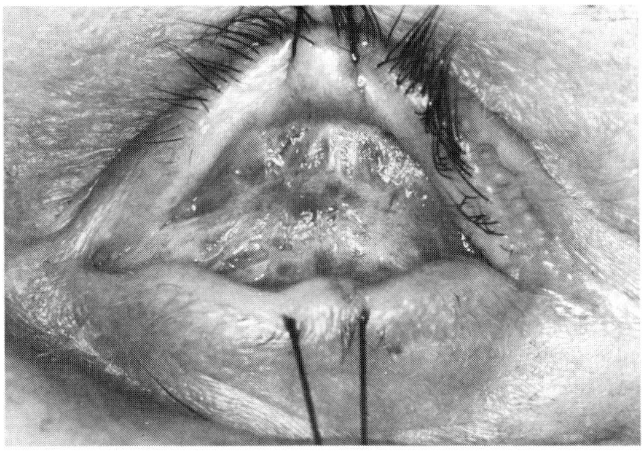

Fig. 33-9. Totally contracted socket.

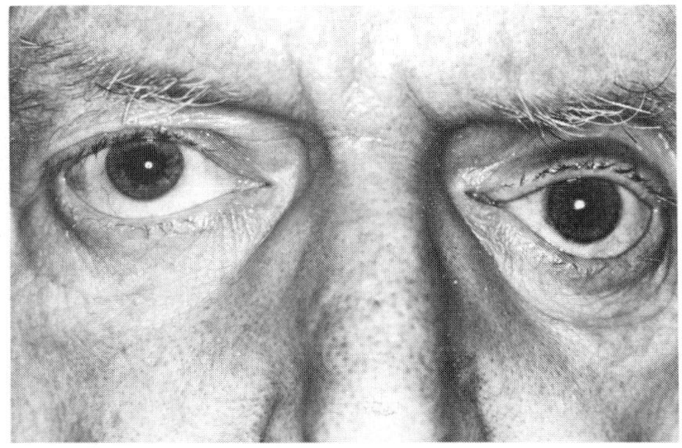

Fig. 33-10. Postenucleation socket syndrome. Note the deep superior sulcus, lax lower lid, and large dystopic prosthesis.

drome (Fig. 33-10). Larger spheres help to offset this syndrome since their increase in volume replacement is proportional to the cube of their radius ($V = 4/3 \pi r^3$). Thus, a sphere of 22-mm diameter replaces approximately 5.5 ml, almost twice the volume of an 18-mm sphere. Treatment of the postenucleation socket syndrome includes volume augmentation with intraorbital and/or subperiosteal implants, horizontal shortening of the lower lid, and fitting of a larger prosthesis.

Conjunctival Cysts

Conjunctival cysts of the orbit may develop at any time after enucleation. They are thought to arise from conjunctival epithelial cell implantation, incarceration, or ingrowth within Tenon's layer; they most often follow enucleation for trauma.[20] Typical symptoms may include progressive difficulty retaining the prosthesis, irritation, pain, and a socket mass. Therapeutic approaches include aspiration of the cyst, combined with injection of absolute alcohol, marsupialization, or excision.

EVISCERATION

Indications and Advantages

As with enucleation, the indications for evisceration are seldom absolute, and the decision must be made by the surgeon and patient only after fully informed consent. Unfortunately, this procedure has become unpopular with many surgeons for fear of sympathetic ophthalmia.

General indications for evisceration include visual loss following endophthalmitis, blind painful eyes not harboring tumors, and certain cases of trauma. When a virulent endophthalmitis is present, evisceration allows debridement of the involved tissues without exposing the orbit to potentially infectious organisms and inflammatory mediators. The implant can be inserted primarily, or the scleral shell may be packed and an implant placed secondarily. The theoretical risk of central nervous system infection via the incised optic nerve meninges after enucleation is avoided, although antibiotics have made this risk minuscule.[10]

Eyes blinded by trauma may also be candidates for this procedure. The potential risk of sympathetic ophthalmia must be accepted by the patient. If an eye is blinded by blunt trauma (cornea and sclera intact), many ophthalmologists consider evisceration. In perforating trauma, with or without uveal prolapse, most ophthalmologists avoid evisceration. As discussed in the enucleation section, such eyes should have primary repair whenever possible, and evisceration or enucleation should be considered only after total blindness has been documented for 2 or 3 consecutive days. Early evisceration (within 10 days) in eyes that are blind after primary repair of perforating trauma is likely safe, but no statistics are available to confirm this. Many patients are unwilling to accept the small risk of sympathetic ophthalmia.

Although the indications for evisceration appear limited, it has advantages, including minimal disruption of orbital anatomy, superior cosmesis, and pain relief. Compared to enucleation, evisceration entails less disruption of orbital anatomy and physiology with fewer attendant complications. The relationships of the lids, conjunctiva, Tenon's fascia, extraocular muscles, and fibromuscular supports of the sclera are relatively well preserved. Being less invasive than enucleation, the procedure is somewhat quicker and is easily performed under local anesthesia, making it appealing for patients in poor general health.

Superior cosmesis with good prosthetic motility results primarily from the less disruptive nature of the operation. Orbital volume loss is less than with enucleation because of the retained sclera or corneoscleral shell and minimal fat atrophy. Motility of the prosthesis is better because the undisturbed rectus muscles impart greater movement to the fornices. All the elements of postenucleation socket syndrome are less likely to develop. Intractable ocular pain is relieved by evisceration as well as by enucleation.[21]

Limitations

The principal limitation of evisceration is the small but real risk of sympathetic ophthalmia. It is impossible to completely remove all uveal tissue by evisceration, especially along the scleral emissaria. Many would argue that should this condition arise, it could be adequately controlled by steroids or other immunosuppressive drugs; others, that the risk is not worth taking just to attain a better cosmetic result. Sympathetic ophthalmia has been reported after evisceration for both trauma and endophthalmitis[4] (see Chapter 24).

Another limitation is the unsuitability of the evisceration specimen for detailed histopathologic examination. Phthisical or microphthalmic eyes are inappropriate for this operation because the size of the intrascleral implant is severely limited.

Surgical Procedure

Patient Preparation and Anesthesia

The same preoperative measures and anesthetic techniques are used as with enucleation surgery. Being less invasive and shorter in duration, evisceration is more commonly done under local anesthesia.

Technique of Evisceration with Retention of the Cornea (Fig. 33-11)

As with enucleation, the surgeon should double-check the chart and consent form and reexamine the patient in the operating room to ensure operating on the correct eye. When possible, the cornea is preserved, allowing a larger implant to be placed.

After a lid speculum is introduced between the lids, an incision is made with Westcott scissors through the conjunctiva and Tenon's capsule, approximately 5 to 6 mm above the superior limbus, just anterior to the superior rectus muscle insertion. The incision is lengthened to 120°, and a limbus-based flap is fashioned. After identifying the superior rectus insertion, the surgeon passes a double-arm 6-0 Vicryl suture through the tendon and disinserts the muscle with scissors.

Next, a 2- to 3-mm sclerotomy parallel to the limbus is made with a blade posterior to the superior rectus insertion. Care is taken to stay external to the plane of the choroid but to expose it. A long cyclodialysis spatula is then inserted through the incision, first directed anteriorly between the sclera and ciliary body to interrupt the firm attachment at the scleral spur, thus allowing the spatula to be seen in the anterior chamber. Wide sweeps are made in all directions to further separate the uvea from the sclera. The scleral incision is opened to 160° to 180° with corneoscleral scissors, and additional dissection with the spatula is done as necessary. If posterior attachments are felt, an evisceration spoon can be used to aid dissection. Care must be taken to avoid scleral perforation.

When freed, the contents of the globe are delivered, intact if possible, with the spoon. Bleeding from the central retinal vessels is controlled by direct pressure with gauze packing for 5 to 10 minutes, supplemented with cautery. Once hemostasis is obtained, the interior of the scleral shell is scraped clear of all residual pigment and tissue with forceps, a Freer elevator, or cotton-tipped applicators. With the intraocular contents removed, the scleral shell will collapse, and a clear test tube can be inserted and used to reexpand the shell and aid inspection in an endoscopic-like manner. The interior of the scleral shell is then swabbed with cotton-tipped applicators soaked in 70% ethanol to denature residual uveal cells. The corneal endothelium is scraped off with a Freer elevator and denatured with alcohol. Irrigation solution containing gentamicin is used to cleanse the scleral shell.

A silicone sphere, usually 16 to 18 mm in diameter for adults, is inserted in the shell. The

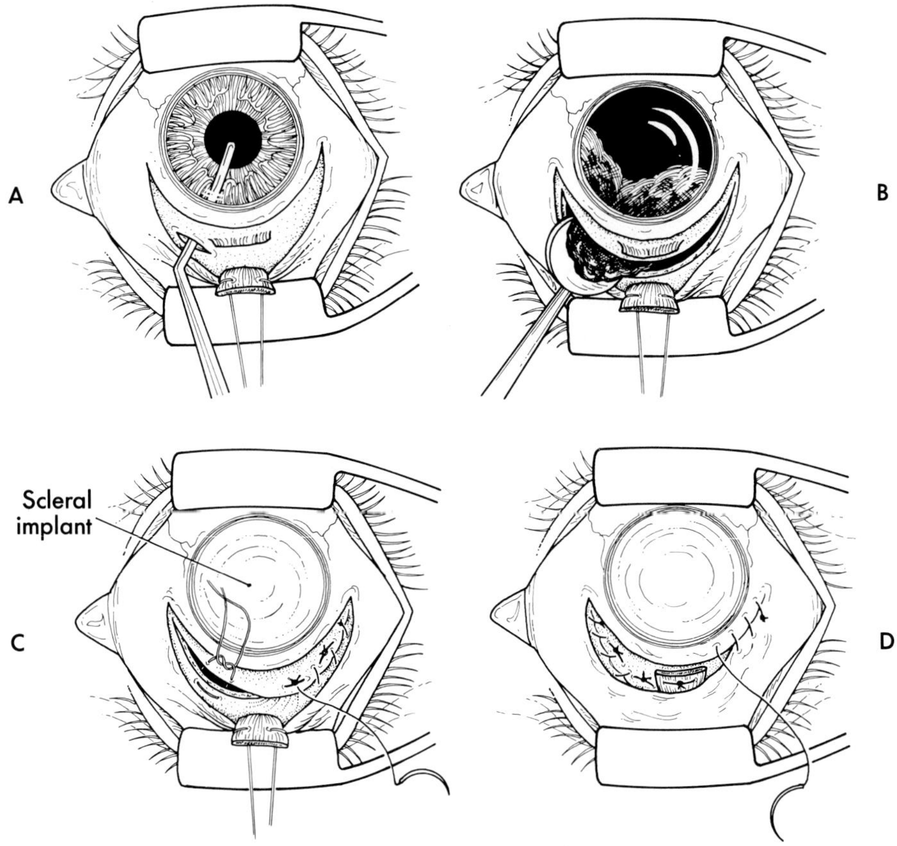

Fig. 33-11. Evisceration with retention of cornea. **A,** A conjunctival incision has been made and the superior rectus disinserted. After incising the sclera, a cyclodialysis spatula is passed through the scleral spur and wide sweeps used to separate the uvea. **B,** The sclera incision is enlarged and the contents of the globe removed. **C,** An intrascleral implant of appropriate size is placed to allow closure of the overlapped wound edges without tension. **D,** The superior rectus is reinserted at its original site and the conjunctiva closed.

appropriate implant will allow overlap of the wound edges by 2 to 3 mm, with a small residual air space around the implant. This space allows shrinkage of the scleral shell without undue tension on the suture lines. Multiple horizontal mattress sutures of 5-0 Vicryl are used to close the scleral incision, overlapping the inferior edge over the superior by approximately 2 to 3 mm. A running 5-0 Vicryl suture is placed to tack down the overlapping scleral edge. The superior rectus is reattached at or near its original insertion, and the conjunctiva is closed with a running 6-0 plain catgut suture. No conformer is inserted.

Broad-spectrum antibiotic ointment is instilled in the socket, and a pressure dressing of two eye pads held in place with tincture of benzoin and 1-inch tape is applied. The dressing is removed in 3 to 4 days and topical antibiotic ointment is begun three times a day. The prosthesis is made in approximately 1 month.

Technique of Evisceration with Keratectomy (Fig. 33-12)

If thinned, traumatized, or diseased, the cornea is removed. After a lid speculum is placed, a 360° limbal peritomy is made with Westcott scissors. A stab incision at the superior limbus is then made and the cornea excised with corneoscleral scissors. The intraocular contents are dissected with a cyclodialysis spatula and removed. The scleral shell is swabbed with 70% ethanol and irrigated with gentamicin. Small scleral triangles are removed at 3 and 9 o'clock to convert the round wound into an ellipse. An appropriate spherical implant is then placed and

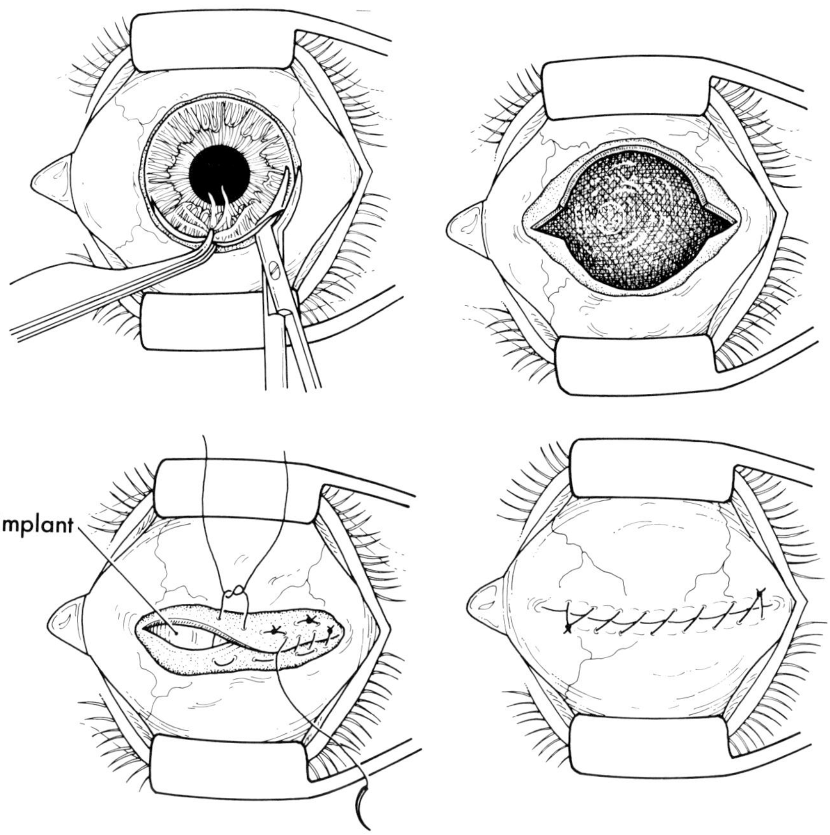

Fig. 33-12. Evisceration with keratectomy. **A,** A 360° limbal peritomy is made and the cornea excised with scissors after a stab incision is made. **B,** Small triangles of sclera are excised at 3 and 9 o'clock converting the wound into an ellipse. **C,** After the implant is placed, the scleral edges are closed with overlapping edges. **D,** The conjunctiva is closed with a running suture.

the scleral edges closed without tension, with the inferior edge overlapping as with retention of the cornea. Usually a 14-mm-diameter sphere is the largest accepted. Multiple interrupted horizontal mattress sutures and a running suture of 5-0 Vicryl are used to close the sclera. The conjunctiva is closed with a running 6-0 plain catgut suture in a horizontal or vertical suture line. Dressing and postoperative care are the same as for evisceration with corneal preservation.

Additional Considerations

Rarely, a blind eye with a corneal or limbal perforation from either traumatic laceration or ulceration undergoes evisceration. In the traumatized eye, primary repair should be undertaken and evisceration considered secondarily. If the corneal defect is small, and has been or is repairable, the usual manner of evisceration with corneal retention may be used. A limbal wound may be reopened and enlarged to 160° to 180° and the evisceration performed through it. However, if there is any question of inadequate corneal integrity, the cornea should be removed.

In cases of endophthalmitis, the scleral cavity may be packed with iodoform-impregnated gauze, which is changed as needed to provide mechanical debridement.[22] Placement of a sphere with delayed primary closure is undertaken when the wound is clean. This technique is postulated to avoid the theoretically increased extrusion rate of the implant in eyes with endophthalmitis.

Complications

Green et al[4] reported four well-documented cases of sympathetic ophthalmia following evisceration. Three cases had undergone evisceration for perforating trauma and one for a perforated corneal ulcer in a long-standing blind eye. In three of the cases, operative notes recorded in detail that great effort was made to remove all uveal tissue. Histopathologic examination of the interior of the scleral shell in all four cases revealed no intact uveal tissue. However, uveal melanocytes were seen within the inner scleral laminae and scleral emissary canals, areas not accessible to evisceration. The greatest inflammatory reaction involved the perioptic sclera and associated canals. Serial section review of the eviscerated specimen in two cases revealed no granulomatous process. Whether the sympathetic uveitis was initiated by the original trauma or by the evisceration operation cannot be answered. It is possible that the trauma was the inciting event and that the clinical and pathologic processes of sympathetic ophthalmia were not yet developed by the time of evisceration (7 to 35 days).

Based on this historic paper, evisceration has fallen into disfavor with many ophthalmologists. No statistics are available for the patient to consider in discussing this possible complication. Nevertheless, a survey completed by 140 members of the American Society of Ophthalmic Plastic and Reconstructive Surgery failed to reveal any cases of sympathetic ophthalmia following evisceration in their patients.[23] In addition, the majority surveyed (70%) preferred evisceration to enucleation in cases of severe endophthalmitis with no chance of preserving vision.

As with enucleation, migration and extrusion of the evisceration implant may occur and are best avoided by precise surgical technique. Early extrusion, before initial wound healing, is usually due to insertion of too large an implant, poor wound closure, or pressure necrosis. Retention of a weakened cornea or traumatized tissues may also play a role. A review of cases over a 10-year period at Wills Eye Hospital in Philadelphia revealed a 22% extrusion rate after evisceration.[24] Analysis of cases with or without keratectomy was not done. Procedures to minimize or repair extrusion have recently been reported.[24,25]

Infection of the scleral shell may occur after evisceration. To minimize this risk, the shell should be irrigated and the alloplastic implants soaked in antibiotic solution. If infection does occur, medical management should be attempted first, and the implant removed if the infection does not resolve.

In an evisceration for endophthalmitis, there is a theoretically increased risk of infection and subsequent implant extrusion. This is the rationale for delayed primary wound closure, as reported by Shore, Dickert, and Levine.[22] Others have never seen an implant extrude under these conditions and argue that if extrusion does occur, there is no greater problem than if the shell was packed initially.[21]

References

1. Brady FB: A singular view, ed 4, Annapolis, 1988, Frank B Brady.
2. Dortzbach RK and Woog JJ: Choice of procedure: enucleation, evisceration or prosthetic fitting over globes, Ophthalmology 92:1249-1255, 1985.
3. Callahan MA and Callahan A: Ophthalmic plastic and orbital surgery, Birmingham, 1979, Aesculapius, 42-54.
4. Green WR et al: Sympathetic uveitis following evisceration, Trans Am Acad Ophthalmol Otolaryngol 76:625-642, 1972.
5. Lubin JR, Albert DM, and Weinstein M: Sixty-five years of sympathetic ophthalmia: a clinicopathologic review of 105 cases (1913-1978), Ophthalmology 87:109-121, 1980.
6. Reynard M, Riffenburg RS, and Maes EF: Effect of corticosteroid treatment and enucleation on the visual prognosis of sympathetic ophthalmia, Am J Ophthalmol 96:290-294, 1983.
7. Kennedy RE: The effect of early enucleation on the orbit in animals and humans, Am J Ophthalmol 60:277-306, 1965.
8. Soll DB: Evolution and current concepts in the surgical treatment of the anophthalmic orbit, Ophthalmic Plast Reconstr Surg 2:163-171, 1986.
9. Soll DB: The anophthalmic socket, Ophthalmology 89:407-423, 1982.
10. Afran SI, Budenz DL, and Albert DM: Does enucleation in the presence of endophthalmitis increase the risk of postoperative meningitis? Ophthalmology 94:235-237, 1987.
11. Birkmann LW and Bennett DR: Meningoencephalitis following enucleation for cryptococcal endophthalmitis, Ann Neurol 4:476-477, 1978.
12. Frueh BR and Felker GV: Baseball implant: a method of secondary insertion of an intraorbital implant, Arch Ophthalmol 94:429-430, 1976.
13. Soll DB: Enucleation surgery, Arch Ophthalmol 87:196-197, 1972.
14. Segrest DR and Dortzbach RK: Barriers to orbital implant migration and extrusion. Paper presented at the American Society of Ophthalmic Plastic and Reconstructive Surgery 14th Annual Scientific Symposium, Chicago, Nov 4, 1983.
15. Perry AC: Clinical update on integrated orbital implants. Paper presented at the American Society of Ophthalmic Plastic and Reconstructive

Surgery 19th Annual Scientific Symposium, Las Vegas, Oct 7, 1988.

16. Allen L: The argument against imbricating the rectus muscles over spherical orbital implants after enucleation, Ophthalmology 90:1116-1120, 1983.
17. McCord CD: The extruding implant, Trans Am Acad Ophthalmol Otolaryngol 81:587-590, 1976.
18. Dryden R and Leibsohn J: Postenucleation orbital implant extrusion, Arch Ophthalmol 96:2064-2065, 1978.
19. Tyers AG and Collin JRO: Orbital implants and post enucleation socket syndrome, Trans Ophthalmol Soc UK 102:90-92, 1982.
20. Hanig CJ and Hornblass A: Treatment of postenucleation orbital cysts, Ann Ophthalmol 81:191-193, 1986.
21. Baylis H et al: Evisceration, enucleation, and exenteration. In McCord DC and Tanenbaum M, editors: Oculoplastic surgery, New York, 1987, Raven Press, 407-424.
22. Shore JW, Dickert JP, and Levine MR: Delayed primary wound closure: use to prevent extrusion following evisceration for endophthalmitis, Arch Ophthalmol 106:1303-1308, 1988.
23. Walter WL: Update on enucleation and evisceration surgery, Ophthalmic Plast Reconstr Surg 1:243-252, 1985.
24. Stephenson CM: Evisceration of the eye with expansion sclerotomies, Ophthalmic Plast Reconstr Surg 3:249-251, 1987.
25. Soll DB: Evisceration with eversion of the scleral shell and muscle cone positioning of the implant, Am J Ophthalmol 104:265-269, 1987.

PART 5

Neuroophthalmic trauma

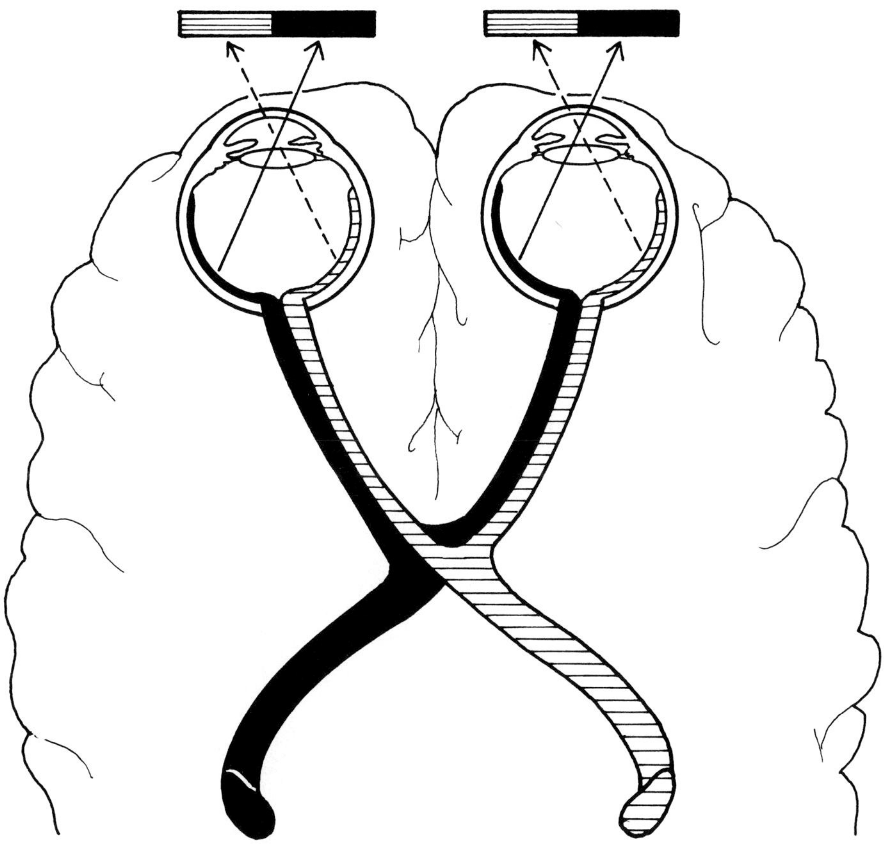

CHAPTER 34

Traumatic optic neuropathy and visual system injury

SIMMONS LESSELL

General principles
Examination
Visual acuity
Color vision
Pupils
Differential diagnosis
Direct optic nerve trauma
Indirect optic nerve trauma
Anterior indirect optic neuropathies
Posterior indirect optic neuropathies
Traumatic aneurysms of the internal carotid artery
Chiasmal trauma
Retrochiasmal visual pathway trauma
Transient cortical blindness after blunt trauma
Visual field defects after penetrating brain wounds
References

Ocular lesions are not the only cause of impaired visual function following trauma. The optic nerve, optic chiasm, and posterior visual pathways are all vulnerable in patients with open or closed head injuries. The ophthalmologist, focused by training and experience on the eye, must nevertheless be prepared to recognize, evaluate, and manage retrobulbar lesions.

GENERAL PRINCIPLES

One of the clinical advantages of ophthalmology is the ability to visualize most of the ocular anatomy by inspecting the globe. Unfortunately, with traumatic optic nerve and chiasmal lesions the abnormalities are apt to be situated beyond the reach of the flashlight, slit-lamp, and ophthalmoscope. In cases of neural trauma, the ophthalmologist must be prepared to substitute inference for observation. Some neural lesions are initially missed because the ophthalmologist simply fails to appreciate the possibility that the visual sensory pathway has been damaged behind the eye. Hence, no assessment of post-traumatic visual impairment can be considered complete unless the nerve and chiasm have been evaluated by the appropriate clinical and laboratory tests.

Ophthalmologists are usually forced to evaluate patients with visual loss immediately after head injuries and under difficult circumstances. The setting is often a general hospital emergency room where special equipment is not available. It is also probable that the patient has other neurological or systemic injuries that complicate evaluation and treatment and may even obscure the presence of visual deficits.

Since the care of head-injured patients with visual impairment is shared between ophthalmologists and nonophthalmologists, it is essential that effective communication be maintained. Communication is accomplished primarily through the medical record. Unfortunately, many ophthalmologists use arcane abbreviations and terms that nonophthalmologists cannot interpret, even if the handwriting is legible! In the interest of good patient care and amity among the various specialties, it makes sense to eschew both abbreviations and jargon and to write simple, legible notes.

EXAMINATION

Injuries to the retrobulbar visual pathways may have a low priority in the trauma scheme, but, when possible, alert, cooperative patients should be transported to a conventional eye examination facility if transport can be accomplished without compromising the care of any nonophthalmic problems. If transport is not immediately feasible, one should conduct a preliminary examination at the bedside but arrange for a more complete evaluation when the patient's condition permits.

Visual Acuity

Accurate measurement of the patient's visual acuity is the single most important part of the examination. In the setting of traumatic visual loss, with social and legal implications added to the medical complexities, the visual acuity examination is too important to delegate. The physician should personally perform such tests.

If the patient is alert, cooperative, ambulatory, and free of external injuries, the examination can be accomplished easily using conventional methods. However, under other circumstances, improvisation may be required. Nevertheless, certain principles apply regardless of the circumstances. First, each eye must be tested individually. If possible, patch the fellow eye to ensure that it is covered. Second, use a clean, well-illuminated standard chart and know the exact distance from the patient's eye to the chart. An acuity fraction means little without an accurate denominator. This is especially apt to be a problem with the reduced Snellen charts (near cards) commonly used to test acuity in general emergency rooms and for patients confined to a bed or stretcher. Some cards have a chain attached that can be used to position the card at the proper distance. If not, one can easily attach an appropriate length of string.

If the patient cannot see the largest Snellen letter, it is better to move the chart closer to the patient and record the reading distance than to use finger-counting. Patients should wear their distance glasses if available. If subnormal acuity is detected, an attempt should be made to improve vision with a pinhole.

Color Vision

Color sense appears to be particularly vulnerable when there is injury to the optic nerve, and tests of color vision are therefore an essential part of the assessment of traumatic visual loss. Ideally one should use the pseudoisochromatic plates designed for detecting congenital dyschromatopsias. Each eye is tested individually, and the score is recorded as the proportion of plates identified correctly. When pseudoisochromatic plates are not available, a color comparison test can be used. The patient is asked to look at a red bottle cap with each eye alternately and to compare the intensity of the color.

Pupils

Pupillary evaluation is a key element in the recognition and differential diagnosis of anterior visual pathway trauma. In patients unable to cooperate, such evaluation may provide the only means of establishing the presence of an anterior visual pathway lesion. Pupillary size should be measured (not estimated), and the direct and consensual reactions to light and near stimulation recorded. The swinging-flashlight test, in which a focused light is swung from one eye to the other, is especially helpful for identifying unilateral or asymmetric afferent defects.[1] A tendency for the pupils to dilate when the light is shone on one eye and to constrict when it is shone on the other indicates an afferent defect on the side that allows the pupil to dilate. If there is mydriasis from traumatic iridoplegia, third nerve paralysis, or other cause, one can still use the swinging-flashlight test; one simply observes the mobile pupil. A positive swinging-flashlight sign in a patient with a normal fundus implies the presence of a retrobulbar lesion or lesion of the anterior visual pathway.

There is a widespread—but erroneous—belief that the pupil will be dilated on the side of a vision-limiting optic neuropathy. In fact, *anisocoria is never the result of a sensory lesion:* Pupils are equal even in patients who have suffered transection of one optic nerve. Anisocoria should never be blamed on a sensory lesion. A patient with uncorrectable reduced acuity in one eye and a dilated pupil has both a sensory and a motor lesion. (See Chapter 35 for a discussion of pupillary signs after trauma.)

The issue of instilling mydriatics for funduscopy inevitably arises in the course of evaluating head-injured patients with visual impairment. Certain simple rules should be scrupulously followed in this regard. Never dilate the pupils of an acutely injured patient with altered consciousness or one who is about to undergo a surgical operation. Never dilate the pupils without the prior approval of the responsible physician. Make and record your observations of the pupils before instilling any drops. Never use a long-acting mydriatic. Atropine, scopolamine, and cyclopentolate are absolutely contraindicated for diagnostic funduscopy in acutely head-injured patients. Instead, use a drug such as 0.5% tropicamide that rapidly produces adequate mydriasis of an acceptably short duration. If you dilate pupils, dilate both. One dilated pupil is apt to cause the medical staff much more confusion and anxiety than two dilated pupils! Make a large, legible entry in the chart indicating the date, time, and name and dose of the drops instilled. Some ophthalmologists also inform the nurse or put a sign on the bed indicating that the pupils were dilated.

DIFFERENTIAL DIAGNOSIS

There are many causes of visual loss after trauma, and neural causes are much less common than ocular causes. Therefore it behooves the ophthalmologist to perform as meticulous a search for an intraocular abnormality as the circumstances permit. However, even if a retinal lesion is identified, for example, one should remain open to the possibility that there is also a retrobulbar lesion.

Missed intraocular lesions are by no means the only source of erroneous diagnoses of traumatic neuropathies. Two other entities deserve consideration: preexisting neuropathies and factitious amblyopia. It should come as no surprise that an injury might call attention to a previously unrecognized visual disorder. In such cases optic atrophy will be evident at the time of injury. Since it takes weeks for optic atrophy to supervene after retrobulbar trauma, the presence of optic atrophy immediately after injury indicates that the optic neuropathy did not result from the recent trauma.

Factitious amblyopia must always be considered in the differential diagnosis of acute retrobulbar neuropathies since the combination of reduced visual function with a normal fundus is common to both (see Chapter 1). Some patients with factitious amblyopia are malingering, whereas others have some psychiatric basis for their alleged visual deficits. Distinguishing between the two is not the ophthalmologist's responsibility. However, the ophthalmologist should be alert to clues from the social and medical history that suggest a psychiatric disorder or potential litigation. Be especially suspicious if the trauma was minor, although seemingly trivial impacts and lacerations have been implicated in bona fide indirect and direct optic nerve injuries, respectively, as described later.

Pupillary reactions may be helpful in differentiating factitious amblyopia from organic visual loss. Monocular or asymmetric visual impairment from a neural lesion should cause a positive swinging-flashlight sign. Factitious visual impairment in contrast does not alter the pupillary reactions. Visual fields may also be useful in diagnosing factitious amblyopia. Concentric field constriction is commonly encountered in these patients. A tubular configuration of the constricted field also strongly supports a diagnosis of factitious amblyopia. Tubular fields are best elicited on a tangent screen.

The diagnosis of factitious amblyopia can be proven only by demonstrating that the patient can see better than he or she alleges. This can be accomplished using one of several techniques that fool the patient (see Chapter 1). Generally, the worse the alleged acuity, the easier it is to establish the diagnosis. Of course, patients may have both an organic visual pathway lesion and factitious amblyopia.

Diagnostic electrophysiology has a limited role in optic nerve and chiasmal injuries. Perhaps the most important is the pattern visual evoked response; well-formed signals with normal latencies in a patient alleging severe visual impairment indicates factitious amblyopia.

DIRECT OPTIC NERVE TRAUMA

Direct optic nerve trauma refers to injuries resulting from objects that penetrate the orbit and impinge on the nerve. These injuries are encountered infrequently, and in virtually all that come to the ophthalmologist's attention the site of injury is the intraorbital segment of the nerve. The intraorbital segment is lax and therefore protected from all but high-velocity impacts. Otherwise it would be hard to explain the paucity of injuries among the thousands of patients who receive retrobulbar anesthetic blocks annually for ophthalmic surgery. On the other hand, high-velocity missiles or any penetrating object that impinges on the nerve in the apex where it is tethered to the optic canal is apt to cause an optic neuropathy. The pathogenesis of the optic neuropathy in direct trauma is often partial or complete transection by the intruding object. Hemorrhages within and around the nerve are also common.

The history usually contains clues that point to direct trauma. Patients typically remain conscious and are aware that they incurred a laceration near the eye or that they were struck by a missile. Most injuries are incurred accidentally, but a significant number are intentional. Gunshot injury to one or both nerves from suicide attempts is not infrequently encountered. Keane,[1] in describing four such cases, emphasizes that self-inflicted gunshots may blind one or both eyes without causing other major damage. None of his patients lost consciousness. Patients (and physicians) may underestimate the depth of the wound, but entry wounds of any size are potentially important. Lid edema and hemorrhage may impede the examination, but every effort should be made to identify rents in the lid or conjunctiva. Lacerations in the brow, near the inner canthus and in the fornices, are particularly apt to be inconspicuous and escape detection if the inspection is casual. The proximal ends of foreign objects that have lodged in the orbit may occasionally be discovered within a laceration. High-velocity missiles such as bullets or shrapnel may reach the optic nerve from entry sites so remote from the orbit that the examining physician may fail to associate the visual loss with the skin wound.

Depending on the nature of the injury, there may be edema and ecchymosis of lid or other cutaneous tissues. In addition to the local changes at the wound site, there is often ptosis, mydriasis, or ophthalmoplegia. There will be proptosis and difficulty repositioning the globe if there is an orbital hematoma, but bruit and ocular pulsation will be absent. There may be any level of visual loss with direct optic nerve trauma. Except in the most minimal injuries, a swinging-flashlight sign will be present. In the acute stage the patient has a normal disc, optic atrophy supervening only after weeks have passed.

Imaging is essential in the diagnosis and management of this and all types of optic nerve trauma (see Chapter 2). Computerized tomographic (CT) scanning is the procedure of choice. With appropriate positioning and technical modifications, one can identify fractures, locate foreign bodies, and appreciate the nature of soft-tissue injuries.

If there is a large orbital hematoma and no local ocular cause of visual impairment is evident, the hematoma should be drained. This is readily accomplished through a canthotomy (see Chapter 26). Foreign bodies easily reached from the wound site can be removed. There is little justification for extracting other foreign bodies since vision is not helped and they are usually well tolerated. However, if infection supervenes, extraction is indicated (see Chapter 31). Decisions about the repair of orbital wall fractures should be made without consideration of the optic neuropathy. Apart from these few considerations, however, there is unfortunately little rational basis for selecting a particular mode of treatment in cases of direct optic nerve trauma. Few publications deal with this topic. Spoor and Mathog,[2] reporting a single case, imply that they manage direct optic nerve trauma

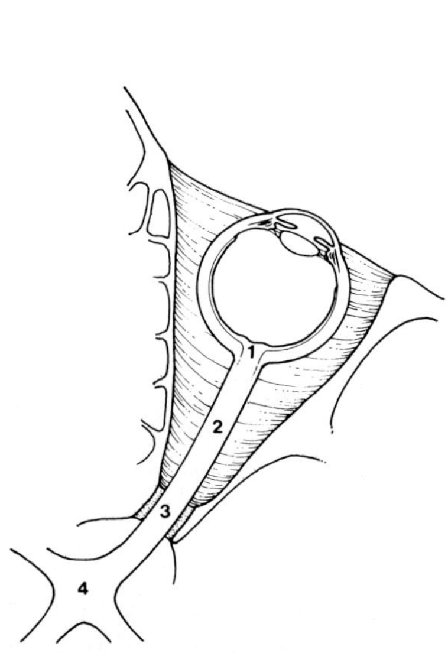

Fig. 34-1. Potential sites of optic nerve trauma. *1*, Intraocular; *2*, intraorbital; *3*, intracanalicular; *4*, chiasmal.

in the same way they manage indirect optic nerve trauma. They treat initially with an intravenous bolus of 500 mg of methylprednisolone followed by 250 mg every 6 hours. Patients who fail to improve after 24 to 36 hours undergo transethmoidal decompression of the optic canal.

INDIRECT OPTIC NERVE TRAUMA

Indirect optic nerve trauma refers to the optic neuropathies that follow closed head trauma. Some experts[3] divide these into an anterior and a posterior variety. Anterior indirect injuries implicate the short (1-mm) intraocular segment of the optic nerve (Fig. 34-1). Not surprisingly, ophthalmoscopic signs are invariably present in these injuries. Posterior indirect injuries refer to "traumatic loss of vision which occurs without external or initial ophthalmoscopic evidence of injury to the eye or its nerve."[4]

Anterior Indirect Optic Neuropathies

Anterior indirect neuropathies are rare and are represented in the literature for the most part by single case reports. Most cases occur when a blunt object intrudes between the globe and the orbital walls. Sometimes seemingly innocent injuries such as getting poked while playing basketball can gouge the eye.[5] At the other extreme are optic nerve avulsions self-inflicted by deranged patients. Anterior indirect optic nerve injuries result when the globe is suddenly rotated or anteriorly displaced. This tears the margins of the lamina cribrosa, the weakest portion of the ocular coat. The central retinal artery may be disrupted in the process. Two reported cases even suggest involvement of the posterior ciliary vessels or their branches.[6,7] Patients with anterior indirect optic neuropathies are typically alert and free of other nonophthalmic injuries. In some cases external evidence of injury is absent, but most patients have lid edema or ecchymosis. There is usually marked impairment of acuity and an obvious defect in the pupillary light response. The disc may be obscured by blood. If the fundus can be visualized, one often finds stigmata of retinal vasoocclusion. If the ciliary vasculature is implicated, the disc will be edematous (Fig. 34-2). A completely avulsed nervehead leaves a deep crater.[8]

The management of these injuries can be summarized succinctly. Patients with signs of central retinal artery occlusion deserve the same measures that are advisable for spontaneous central artery occlusions (see Chapter 26). Otherwise, provided there is no clinical or radiologic evidence of another treatable lesion, special investigations or treatments are unwarranted.

Posterior Indirect Optic Neuropathies

Posterior indirect neuropathies are encountered rather more often than the direct or anterior indirect variety, but they are by no means common. Reported series originating from centers in the United States and Europe are quite small, ranging from 6 to 67 cases. For reasons that are not clear, Japanese series have been larger, ranging up to more than 750 patients.

In contrast to indirect injuries that damage the intraorbital segment of the nerve and an-

A

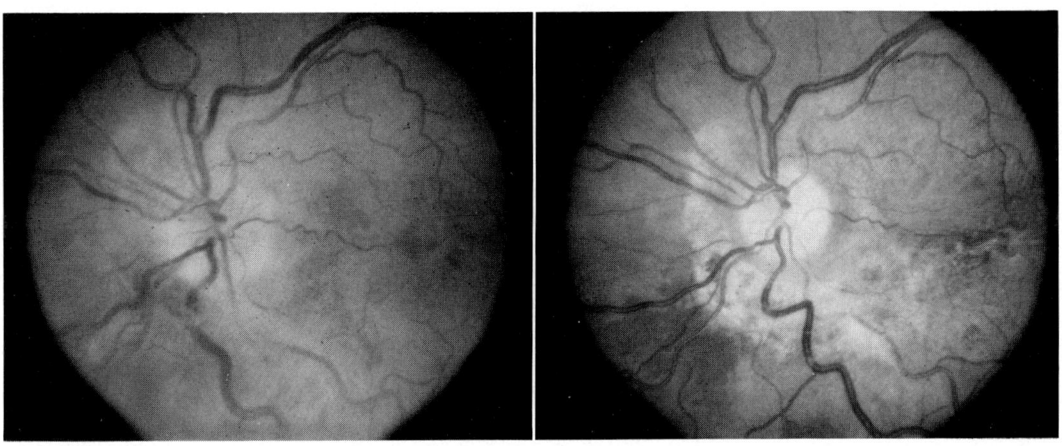

B

Fig. 34-2. **A,** Acute optic nerve avulsion. Optic disc is edematous with retinal vascular compromise. **B,** Optic atrophy is present 1 month later.

terior indirect injuries that damage the intraocular segment, posterior indirect injuries typically damage the intracanalicular segment (Fig. 34-1). The 10-mm intracanalicular portion together with its complement of meninges, the ophthalmic artery, and sympathetic nerves are crowded tightly within the bony canal.

Anderson, Panje, and Gross[9] have demonstrated by holographic studies on human skulls that forces impinging on the face and forehead impact in the region of the canal. These transmitted forces can fracture the sphenoid. If the fracture is displaced, the nerve may be distorted or lacerated. Unlike the tethered intracanalicular segment, the adjacent intraorbital and intracranial segments are free to move. Injury can occur at the ends of the canal if the momentum of the impact displaces the mobile intraorbital and intracranial segments. As one might expect, there are often hemorrhages in or around the nerve.[10] The role of these hemorrhages in causing or contributing to the visual impairment is controversial.

Many posterior indirect injuries, however, appear to involve none of these mechanisms. Instead, they may result from edema and infarction.[11] A particularly instructive autopsy study of a single case[12] indicates that there is a vascular pathogenesis involving the centrifugal vessels in the intracanalicular and perhaps intracranial segments. Since edema is treatable, this particular pathogenesis has important practical implications.

Posterior indirect optic neuropathy occurs predominantly in young males but can occur in both sexes and at all ages. The injury follows blows to the face, forehead, or, less commonly, the temple. In a recent review of 33 civilian cases,[13] the commonest mode of injury was a fall from a bicycle, closely followed by automobile collision. Only 4 injuries occurred in the workplace. Of the 33 patients, 27 suffered loss of consciousness and 8 were unresponsive for at least 24 hours. Nevertheless, as with other traumatic optic neuropathies, the trauma may appear trivial. Nonvisual neurologic deficits are prevalent among patients with prolonged impairment of consciousness and are apt to be permanent. A small proportion of cases are bilateral, and in these cases it may be difficult to rule out injury to the chiasm.

Visual deficits cover the entire spectrum from small Bjerrum scotomas unassociated with

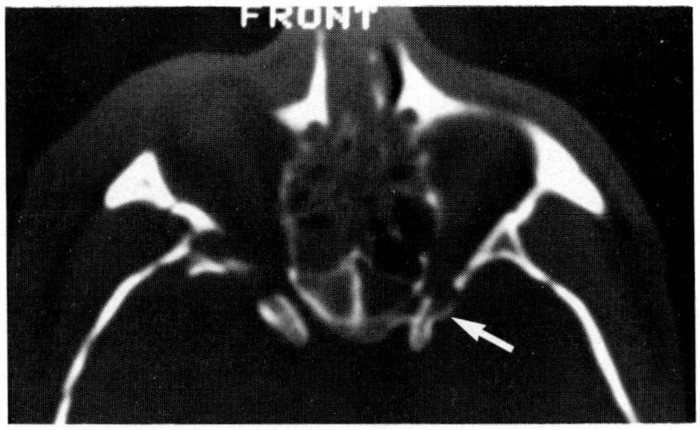

Fig. 34-3. Axial CT scan demonstrating optic canal fracture *(arrow)*.

dyschromatopsia or reduced acuity to complete blindness. A swinging-flashlight sign should be present in all but the most minor injuries. The fundi invariably appear normal because optic atrophy supervenes only after weeks have passed.

Radiologic investigations are imperative whenever an optic neuropathy is considered in the pathogenesis of posttraumatic visual loss. CT scanning of the orbits and head without contrast injection is the initial study of choice (Fig. 34-3). Bone window settings should be used to look for fractures. In Lessell's study, craniofacial fractures were imaged in 17 of 33 cases,[13] but the fracture intersected the optic canal in only 7. Neither the presence nor the location of a fracture correlated with the severity of the optic neuropathy.

Despite an abundance of literature on the subject, controversy remains concerning the proper treatment of patients with posterior indirect optic nerve injuries. Any treatment decision must take into account the fact that some patients improve without surgery or medication. Hughes[11] condemns surgical intervention, having failed to identify any instance in which an operation proved beneficial. Fukado[14-16] wholeheartedly advocates routine optic canal decompression even if there has been a long interval after the injury. Decompression of the optic canal can be accomplished either by craniotomy or through the paranasal sinuses with very little morbidity and mortality. Walsh[17] counsels against surgery in unconscious patients and in cases in which vision and the pupillary response were lost at impact, reserving surgical decompression for patients who suffer delayed loss of vision. Anderson, Panje, and Gross[9] favor the initial use of high-dose corticosteroid treatment and reserve surgery for patients who suffer delayed loss of vision or who achieve improvement with steroid therapy but then relapse. Joseph and colleagues report excellent results with transethmoid-sphenoidal decompression of the optic canal and perioperative steroids.[23]

There has been as yet no controlled study that identifies the best treatment regimen. Considering that cases of posterior indirect trauma are uncommon, it is unlikely that such a study can be conducted. Thus, each hospital should develop guidelines for the management of patients with posterior indirect optic nerve injuries so that treatment can be instituted rapidly but rationally. All too often, therapeutic decisions are made on an ad hoc basis. An interdisciplinary team representing ophthalmology, neurosurgery, and otolaryngology should, therefore, be identified.

No matter how detailed a treatment schema appears to be, it will have to be modified for each individual patient and therefore serves only as a rough guideline. With that caveat, the following general approach to patients with indirect traumatic optic neuropathies is suggested:

- Comatose patients should not undergo decompressive surgery unless it is incidental to another operative procedure.
- If there is no contraindication to the use of systemic high-dose corticosteroids, the patient should be treated with 1 mg/kg/day of dexamethasone in divided doses for 3 days.
- Failure to improve dictates rapid taper and discontinuation of the medication.
- Patients who appear to improve can be switched to a gradually tapering dose of prednisone.
- If the patient relapses when corticosteroids are discontinued, surgical decompression should be considered.
- Although the visual evoked response is used to monitor the visual status of comatose patients in some centers, the swinging-flashlight sign is generally a reliable monitor of clinical response.
- In general, alert patients with 20/40 acuity or worse are candidates for surgical decompression.

The goals, nature, and rationale of transethmoidal decompression under general anesthesia are explained to the patient. The patient is fully informed of the risks of the operation and of the uncertainty of the visual outcome regardless of the mode of therapy. Surgery is performed by the team's otolaryngologist. Systemic corticosteroids are administered if surgery is delayed for any reason.

TRAUMATIC ANEURYSMS OF THE INTERNAL CAROTID ARTERY

Ophthalmologists should be alert to a traumatic lesion that may cause not only blindness but death. Following severe head trauma, a false aneurysm may develop in the cavernous portion of the interal carotid artery.[18,19] Most of these traumatic aneurysms are associated with basal skull fractures. If the aneurysm points into the sphenoid sinus, the patient will have epistaxis and loss of vision. The exact mechanism of visual loss has not been identified, but the loss of vision is typically severe and immediate. Occasionally (5 of 92 patients in one series[18]) the aneurysm is bilateral. The epistaxis is typically delayed for days, and the initial hemorrhage may be slight; however, recurrent epistaxis may occur months or years later and prove fatal. The mortality rate from traumatic aneurysms of the cavernous internal carotid is high, primarily because physicians fail to make the diagnosis.

The role of the ophthalmologist is to alert neurosurgical and otolaryngologic consultants to the possibility of aneurysm in patients who manifest the triad of severe head injury, posterior indirect optic nerve trauma, and epistaxis. Delayed epistaxis in this setting is even more suggestive.

CHIASMAL TRAUMA

The optic chiasm is not immune to the effects of mechanical head trauma (Fig. 34-1).[20] Damage to the chiasm may occur with closed or penetrating trauma. Both varieties are uncommon, but the latter is distinctly rare, since accidental penetration of the cranial cavity that tears the chiasm (direct trauma) is also apt to tear major vessels and lead to death.

The exact mechanism underlying chiasmal neuropathies following closed head trauma has not been identified. Tears or axonal disruption associated with fractures or contusion must occur but probably cannot explain all cases. As with posterior indirect injuries of the nerve, a vascular pathogenesis also may be important. Closed head trauma that causes indirect chiasmal injury is generally severe, and there is usually loss of consciousness and other (nonvisual) neurologic deficits. Anosmia is frequently present, and transient diabetes insipidus develops in many patients. Fractures are often imaged. Although the visual defects are probably incurred at impact or shortly thereafter, there is often a delay before they are recognized. In some cases the delay may reflect the preservation of central acuity. True splitting of the chiasm does not reduce central acuity but produces a bitemporal hemianopia that is inapparent during binocular viewing. The fundus is initially normal in chiasmal trauma, but the discs ultimately become atrophic.

The role of the ophthalmologist is to identify and document the visual deficits. No special treatment has been advocated.

RETROCHIASMAL VISUAL PATHWAY TRAUMA

It is highly unusual for visual symptoms or signs to predominate in patients who have sustained acute trauma to the cerebral hemisphere. Retrochiasmal injuries are apt to be masked by aphasia, confusion, combativeness, or coma, or eclipsed by life-threatening neurologic or nonneurologic problems. In contrast to the situation with acute traumatic optic and chiasmal neuropathies, neuroimaging is usually superior to the clinical examination in detecting, localizing, and characterizing acute intracerebral damage to the visual pathways.

In most cases of acute brain injury, clinical assessment of the integrity of the patient's retrochiasmal visual pathways can be accomplished only by simple bedside tests. Unilateral damage to the tract, geniculate, optic radiations, or visual cortex does not alter Snellen acuity. Acuity remains normal even with absolute, macula-splitting homonymous hemianopias. Snellen acuity is reduced in patients with retrochiasmal lesions only if there is bilateral involvement of the visual pathways.

A relative afferent pupillary defect is sometimes demonstrable in the eye contralateral to an optic tract lesion, but otherwise the pupillary examination is normal. Normal optic discs are the rule in acute injuries, and atrophy supervenes only if the tract or geniculate has been implicated. Opticokinetic nystagmus should be tested in alert cooperative patients since parietal lobe hemianopias will be accompanied by asymmetric responses. Nystagmus is reduced or absent when the stripes are rotated toward the injured parietal lobe. Absent responses to both sides are of no diagnostic value in patients with good acuity.

During acuity testing, some hemianopic patients (and patients with visual hemineglect) ignore one side of the chart. Inattention to people or objects on one side has the same implications. Some hemianopias that encroach upon fixation can be detected with an Amsler grid. However, confrontation testing of the visual fields is the best means of evaluating the function of the retrochiasmal pathways at the bedside.

TRANSIENT CORTICAL BLINDNESS AFTER BLUNT TRAUMA

It has been estimated that transient cortical blindness occurs in 0.4% of patients with head injuries who are evaluated in hospital emergency rooms.[21] Typically the patient has suffered a concussive blow to the occipital region. The patient is either blind on awakening or becomes blind within a few hours. As with all cases of cortical blindness, the pupils respond to light stimulation and the fundi are normal. Amnesia and confusion are commonly present, but there may be no evidence of neurological dysfunction apart from the blindness. Vision recovers spontaneously within hours.

VISUAL FIELD DEFECTS AFTER PENETRATING BRAIN WOUNDS

The medical literature is replete with large case series of patients with hemianopias from missile injuries incurred in battle.[22] Shell fragments are usually responsible. Some of the patients are alert despite the injury and tend to assume that they have suffered an eye injury. Patients may initially be totally blind, the permanent hemianopia becoming apparent when one hemifield clears.

REFERENCES

1. Keane JR: Blindness from self-inflicted gunshot wounds, J Clin Neuroophthalmol 6:247-249, 1986.

2. Spoor TC and Mathog RH: Restoration of vision after optic canal decompression, Arch Ophthalmol 104:804-806, 1986.
3. Kline LB, Morawetz RB, and Swaid SN: Indirect injury of the optic nerve, Neurosurgery 14:756-764, 1984.
4. Walsh FB and Hoyt WF: Clinical neuro-ophthalmology, Baltimore, 1969, Williams & Wilkins, 2375.
5. Park JH et al: Evulsion of the optic nerve, Am J Ophthalmol 72:969-971, 1972.
6. Hedges TR III and Gragoudas ES: Traumatic anterior ischemic optic neuropathy, Ann Ophthalmol 13:625-628, 1981.
7. Wyllie AM, McLeod D, and Cullen JF: Traumatic ischaemic optic neuropathy, Br J Ophthalmol 56:851-853, 1972.
8. Hillman JS, Myska V, and Nissim S: Complete avulsion of the optic nerve: a clinical, angiographic, and electrodiagnostic study, Br J Ophthalmol 59:503-509, 1975.
9. Anderson RL, Panje WR, and Gross CE: Optic nerve blindness following blunt forehead trauma, Ophthalmology 89:445-455, 1982.
10. Pringle JH: Atrophy of the optic nerve following diffused violence to the skull, Br Med J 2:1156-1157, 1922.
11. Hughes B: Indirect injury of the optic nerves and chiasm, Bull Johns Hopkins Hosp 111:98-126, 1962.
12. Ramsay JH: Optic nerve injury in fracture of the skull, Br J Ophthalmol 63:607-610, 1979.
13. Lessell S: Indirect optic nerve trauma, Arch Ophthalmol 107:382-386, 1989.
14. Fukado Y: Results of 350 cases of surgical decompression of the optic nerve, Trans Ophthalmol Soc NZ 25:96-99, 1975.
15. Fukado Y: Results in 400 cases of surgical decompression of the optic nerve, Mod Probl Ophthalmol 14:474-481, 1975.
16. Fukado Y: Microsurgical transethmoidal optic nerve decompression: experience in 700 cases. In Samii M and Jannetta PJ, editors: The cranial nerves, Berlin, 1981, Springer-Verlag, 125-128.
17. Walsh FB: Pathological-clinical correlations. I. Indirect trauma to the optic nerves and chiasm. II. Certain cerebral involvements associated with defective blood supply, Invest Ophthalmol 5:433-449, 1966.
18. Chambers EP et al: Traumatic aneurysms of cavernous internal carotid artery with secondary epistaxis, Am J Neuroradiol 2:405-409, 1981.
19. Keane JR and Talla A: Posttraumatic intracavernous aneurysm: epistaxis with monocular blindness preceded by chromatopsia, Arch Ophthalmol 87:701-705, 1972.
20. Savino PJ, Glaser JS, and Schatz NJ: Traumatic chiasmal syndrome, Neurology 30:963-970, 1980.
21. Grennblatt SH: Posttraumatic transient cerebral blindness, JAMA 225:1073-1076, 1973.
22. Teuber HL, Battersby WS, and Bender MB: Visual field defects after penetrating missile wounds of the brain, Cambridge, Mass, 1960, Harvard University Press.
23. Joseph MP et al: Extracranial optic nerve decompression for traumatic neuropathy, Arch Ophthalmol 108:1091-1093, 1990.

CHAPTER 35

Trauma to the ocular motor system

THOMAS R. HEDGES III

Ocular motor examination in the injured patient
Orbital injury causing ocular motor dysfunction
Ocular motor nerve injuries
Trochlear nerve injury
Abducens nerve injury
Ocular motor nerve injuries
Direct third nerve injury
Third nerve palsy from indirect injury
Ocular motor nerve palsies from minor head trauma
Combined third, fourth, and sixth nerve palsies following trauma
Carotid-cavernous fistula
Pupillary disorders following trauma
Traumatic mydriasis
Traumatic miosis
Trigeminal nerve injury
Seventh nerve injury
Central disorders of eye movements following trauma
Ocular motor findings in coma
Localized central ocular motor effects of trauma
Vertical gaze
Horizontal gaze
Internuclear ophthalmoplegia
Nystagmus
Hypoxic effects on the ocular motor system
References

Virtually any form of ophthalmoplegia can follow head injury. Some ocular motor conditions are more common in trauma, and various types of injury may be more likely to produce specific types of ophthalmoplegia (Fig. 35-1). This chapter approaches trauma to the ocular motor system anatomically, beginning with the extraocular muscles, followed by a discussion of how injury affects each ocular motor nerve, and the pupillary, trigeminal, and facial nerves; the chapter concludes with central ocular motor dysfunction, such as gaze palsy and nystagmus.

OCULAR MOTOR EXAMINATION IN THE INJURED PATIENT

Taking the history of patients with ophthalmoplegia secondary to injury should include determining the types of forces involved. For example, in a patient with a fourth nerve palsy, the likely site of the primary impact is the region of the opposite forehead. Fractures, especially those involving the periorbital areas or the base of the skull, should be identified (see Chapter 27). Shock, coma, or other cause of hypoxia, and the use of narcotic, paralytic, or antiseizure

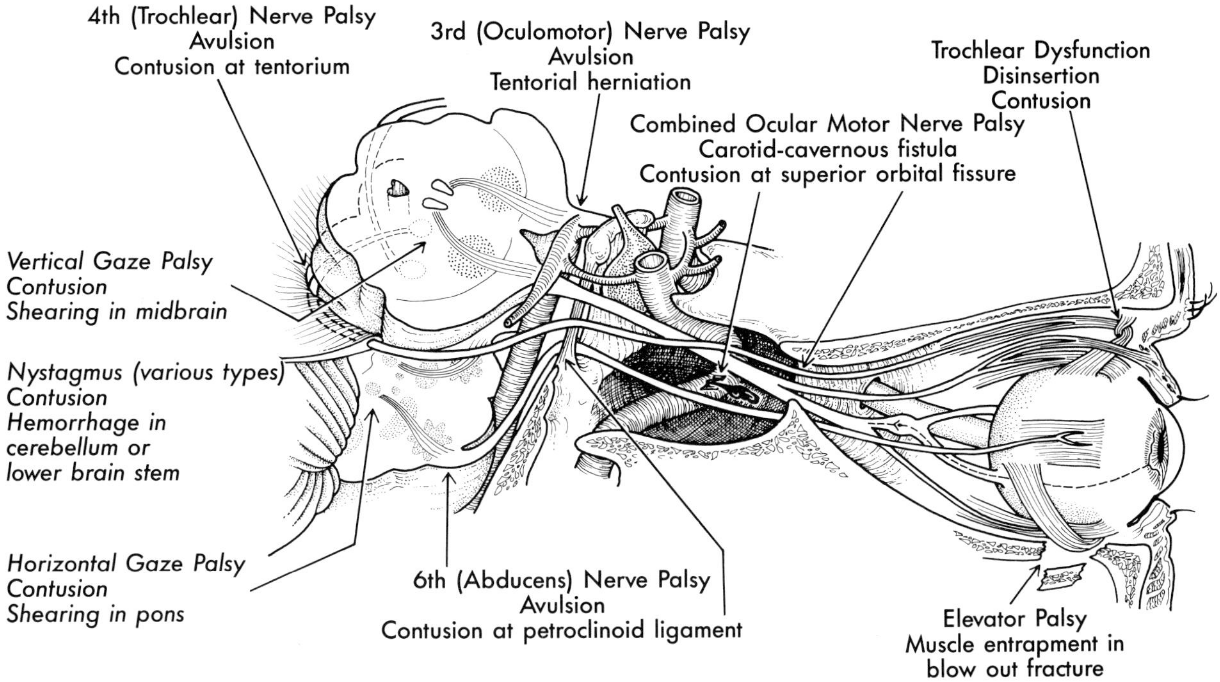

Fig. 35-1. Anatomy of ocular motor system; common sites of injury and associated ocular motor complications.

medications should be noted. It is also important to determine if there have been visual, ocular motor, or neurologic problems before the acute injury.

On examination, the following observations are important,[1] especially in the presence of a complex ocular motor problem:

1. Random eye movements (appropriateness, abnormal head movements)
2. Fixation (steadiness of eyes and head in primary gaze)
3. Lid function (ptosis, lid retraction)
4. Alignment (phoria, tropia)
5. Convergence
6. Ductions (excursions in cardinal positions of gaze)
7. Saccades (speed and accuracy)
8. Pursuit (smoothness at varying velocities)
9. Vestibuloocular reflexes (head turning, chair rotation, suppression)
10. Response to forced eyelid closure (Bell's phenomenon)
11. Optokinetics (OKN)
12. Caloric testing
13. Forced-duction testing

A systematic and inclusive approach to documenting ocular motor findings is useful even if the exact nature of the ocular motor abnormality cannot be readily identified. Complete information collected at this stage may clarify the problem at a later date or in consultation with a colleague.

ORBITAL INJURY CAUSING OCULAR MOTOR DYSFUNCTION

Occasionally, extraocular muscles, particularly the inferior rectus, may be lacerated when there is penetrating orbital trauma.[2,3] Contusion of extraocular muscles causes limited eye movement that is diffuse or that does not coincide with that normally seen with a cranial nerve or gaze palsy. For example, a "double elevator palsy" may be due to entrapment or contusion of the inferior rectus muscle following orbital floor fracture. Traumatic medial orbital wall fracture can cause an apparent Duane's retraction syndrome.[4]

Contused extraocular muscles usually regain normal function within a few days. Forced-duction testing, using forceps or a cotton-tipped applicator, can distinguish restricted from paretic extraocular muscles. Treatment of a restrictive ocular motor problem can be difficult. If the degree of dysfunction remains stable after several months, recession of the restricted muscle may be beneficial.

OCULAR MOTOR NERVE INJURIES

The most common ocular nerve to be affected by trauma is the sixth nerve. The most common cause of fourth nerve palsy is head injury, which may be relatively mild. Traumatic third nerve palsy usually follows severe injury unless there is another underlying cause. Combined ocular motor nerve injuries are relatively rare (Table 35-1).[5] The mechanisms by which these nerves are affected have been the subject of a detailed, but somewhat skewed, study of patients involved in fatal road accidents, in which avulsion of nerve rootlets from the brain stem occurred with surprising frequency.[6]

Trochlear Nerve Injury

The fourth cranial nerve may be affected in mild to moderate closed-head injury, but it may also be injured even when there is no direct blow to the head. Trauma causes one half to one third of all cases of isolated fourth nerve palsies,[5,7,8] and trauma is the assumed cause in many patients with cryptic trochlear nerve palsies.[9]

Direct trauma to the superior oblique tendon may occur following penetrating injury.[10] This may cause restriction of movement of the tendon, resulting in vertical diplopia in upgaze (Brown's syndrome).[11] Patients with superior oblique dysfunction from penetrating injury rarely have trochlear disinsertion.

Most traumatic fourth nerve palsies appear to be due to avulsion of the nerve from the posterior aspect of the midbrain or contusion against the tentorium. It appears that a blow to one side of the forehead will lead to contrecoup forces directed against the contralateral posterior midbrain at the tentorium with consequent injury to CN IV. Pathologic and computed tomographic (CT) evidence of hemorrhage of the brachium conjunctivum favors this explanation.[6,12] As many as one third of traumatic fourth nerve palsies are bilateral,[13] and they are due to the same pathologic factors that cause unilateral trochlear palsies.

Symptoms of fourth nerve palsy are usually those of vertical or oblique diplopia that increases on downgaze and in the direction of gaze contralateral to the affected superior oblique muscle. Many patients have difficulty reading or negotiating stairs. Some notice tilting of the environment, and they may find that tilting the head away from the affected eye reduces the diplopia.

The diagnosis of superior oblique dysfunction is based on the three-step test described by Parks (Fig. 35-2).[14] The presence and degree of excyclotorsion caused by fourth nerve palsy can be determined by using two Maddox rods placed vertically in a trial frame. The Maddox rod is then rotated until both images are parallel and the magnitude of excyclotropia read from the trial frame. Another simple test for ocular torsion is done by asking the patient to view a straightedge. Those with a fourth nerve palsy will indicate that two images join to form an

Table 35-1. Incidence of injury among 1000 cases of ocular motor nerve palsy

Cranial nerve(s)	No.
Isolated VI	55
Isolated III	34
Isolated IV	23
III and IV	9
III and VI	9
III, IV, and VI	8
IV and VI	1

From Rucker CW: The causes of paralysis of the third, fourth, and sixth cranial nerves, Am J Ophthalmol 61:1293, 1966.

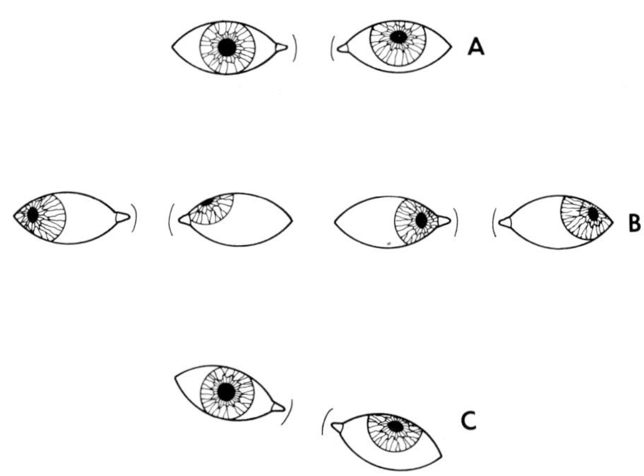

Fig. 35-2. Three-step test for diagnosis of left superior oblique dysfunction. **A,** Left hypertropia in primary gaze. **B,** Left hypertropia increases in right gaze. **C,** Left hypertropia increases on head tilt to left shoulder.

arrow pointing in the direction of the affected fourth nerve. Bilateral fourth nerve injury will cause a straightedge to assume the image of an X, with the point of intersection closer to the side of the more severely injured fourth nerve.

Sixty-five percent of unilateral and 25% of bilateral fourth nerve palsies from trauma require no treatment and resolve spontaneously.[13] Hence, one should wait 6 months before concluding that no further improvement will occur. During this period, patching of either eye will eliminate double vision. A vertical prism may help some individuals, but the dynamic nature of the double vision and the excyclorotation prohibits the use of a prism in most patients.

A variety of surgical procedures have been recommended for fourth nerve palsy. Inferior oblique myectomy is relatively simple and can relieve about 15 prism diopters of vertical deviation. Ipsilateral inferior oblique myectomy (or recession) plus ipsilateral superior rectus resection is useful, especially if the deviation is greater than 15 prism diopters and greater in upgaze. Contralateral inferior rectus weakening in addition to inferior oblique myectomy is more likely to be effective if the deviation is greater in downgaze.[7]

Bilateral fourth nerve paralysis results in right hypertropia in left gaze and left hypertropia in right gaze. V-pattern esotropia in excess of 25 prism diopters and exocyclotorsion greater than 10° indicates bilateral involvement. Bilateral fourth nerve injuries are almost always related to severe head injury, and occasionally a bilateral injury becomes apparent only after surgical correction for an apparently unilateral palsy.[15]

Abducens Nerve Injury

Sixth nerve palsy usually results from more severe head injury than that causing fourth nerve palsy. Loss of consciousness occurs in almost all cases (18 of 21 patients in one series).[16]

Mechanisms of sixth nerve injury include acceleration-deceleration forces exerted on the sixth nerve at the petroclinoid ligament (Dorello's canal), the superior orbital fissure, or where the nerve crosses the anterior inferior cerebellar artery. However, pathologic reports from patients with fatal head injury indicate that the most common point of injury to the sixth nerve is where it exits the pons (Fig. 35-1).[6,17] Crushing injuries of the head are more likely to affect the sixth nerve at the petrous tip, especially if there is simultaneous involvement of the trigeminal nerve.[18] Hyperextension of the cervical spine with or without fracture of cervical vertebrae may be associated with acute or delayed onset of abducens nerve palsy.[19-21] This has been assumed to be due to strangulation of the abducens nerve by branches of the basilar artery, similar to that occurring with increased intracranial pressure.[22]

Sixth nerve palsy causes horizontal double vision that is worse at distance and in the direction of action of the weakened extraocular muscle. One must keep in mind that children can adapt to the double vision quite readily and may not have any complaints, whereas adults may experience discomfort, even when lateral rectus dysfunction is only apparent by cover-uncover or Maddox rod testing.

As with fourth nerve palsies, one should wait 6 months before considering corrective surgery if recovery is incomplete. In mild cases, resection of the weakened lateral rectus muscle combined with recession of the medial rectus muscle can restore a degree of single binocular vision. In most cases, however, overaction of the contralateral medial rectus may require a muscle transposition procedure. Currently, the Jensen procedure is popular.[23,24] Botulinum toxin injection of the ipsilateral medial rectus muscle has been recently shown to help some patients recover more quickly and perhaps more completely from sixth nerve palsy. Apparently the toxin limits contracture of the medial rectus muscle during the period when it remains unopposed following injury.[25]

Ocular Motor Nerve Injuries

Injuries to the third nerve are either direct or the indirect result of transtentorial herniation. In either case, the degree of injury is usually more severe than that causing fourth or sixth nerve injury. In two large series of patients with head injuries, about 1% had third nerve palsies, most from indirect compression associated with subdural or epidural hematomas.[26,27] When third nerve palsy results from relatively minor head injury, an underlying condition, particularly a tumor compressing the third nerve, must be considered.[28]

Direct Third Nerve Injury

Trauma associated with third nerve palsy is usually a severe frontal blow to the head.[27,29] Loss of consciousness occurs in 70% to 100% of patients.[26,29,30] The incidence of skull fracture seen on plain X ray varies from 30% to 70% of patients.[27,29,30] The third nerve may suffer damage to orbital branches, contusion at the superior orbital fissure or at its entry into the cavernous sinus, shearing forces in the midbrain,[31] or avulsion of its rootlets (Fig. 35-1).[6]

Symptoms caused by third nerve palsy include diplopia that is oblique and variable in different positions of gaze. Ptosis of the upper eyelids is common.[29] When the optic nerve is also injured, many patients are bothered more by the cosmetic effects of ptosis and exodeviation of the eye than by double vision. The pupil may be spared in some individuals, but when it is affected in young patients, defective accommodation may also be a problem.[30]

Patients with traumatic third nerve palsy frequently have associated neurologic problems because the injuries are usually severe. Optic nerve, chiasmal, and optic tract damage occurs in up to 75% of cases.[29,30] Other cranial nerves—the fourth and occasionally the fifth, seventh, and eighth—are less commonly affected. Traumatic third nerve palsy may be bilateral.[31] Long tract findings, particularly hemiparesis, occur in about one quarter of cases.[26]

Prognosis for recovery from traumatic oculomotor nerve injury is variable and frequently limited. Furthermore, the complexity of the ophthalmoplegia usually prevents treatment with prisms or surgery.[30] One of the major problems of rehabilitating patients with third nerve injury following trauma is aberrant regeneration (Fig. 35-3). For instance, when the lid paradoxically elevates in downgaze or adduction, ptosis surgery must be done with great caution because of the risk of corneal exposure.[29] It is generally accepted that one should wait about a year to operate on a patient with third nerve palsy.

Third Nerve Palsy from Indirect Injury

Uncal herniation may follow severe head trauma when there is epidural hemorrhage, cerebral hemorrhage, or cerebral edema. The herniation is a complication of subdural hematoma, which, in the elderly, may be caused by relatively minor head injury. When the cerebrum is forced downward by tumor, edema, or hematoma, the uncus of the hippocampal gyrus may be forced past the tentorium, where it compresses the ipsilateral third nerve by forcing it against the posterior clinoid. The distorted and stretched third nerve is also compressed by the posterior cerebral artery as it is also forced downward.[32]

The presence of a third nerve palsy ipsilateral to a suspected subdural hematoma is one of the classic findings in neurology and neurosurgery. It has been the subject of considerable study because of its importance in the era before computed tomographic (CT) scanning.[33] At times the pupil can be spared,[34] and third nerve palsy may be seen contralateral to the side of the cerebral mass. CT scanning has now made this finding less needed clinically, but it should not be forgotten. Epidural hematoma may cause

A

B

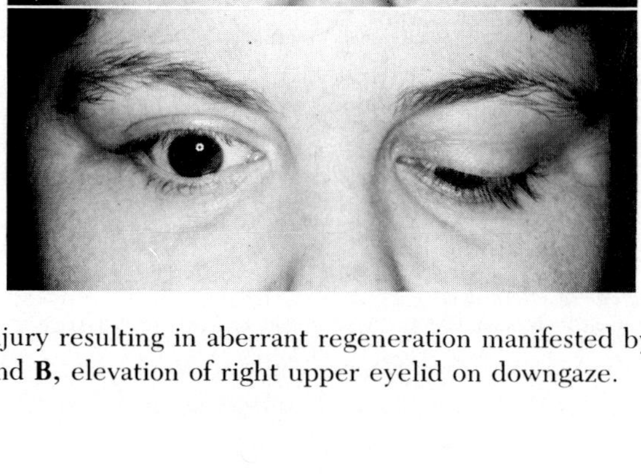

Fig. 35-3. Third nerve injury resulting in aberrant regeneration manifested by **A**, ptosis of right upper eyelid in primary gaze, and **B**, elevation of right upper eyelid on downgaze.

third nerve palsy,[35] even in an awake patient.[36]

Because the pupillary findings in comatose patients are an important indicator of the development of brain herniation, ophthalmologists should refrain from using mydriatric agents except with the permission of the attending neurologist or neurosurgeon. Local injury to the iris should be called to the attention of the attending physicians so that they will not falsely identify the traumatic mydriasis as an indicator of third nerve dysfunction. In a comatose patient, levator function may be determined by sitting the patient upright, whereupon the eyelids will normally elevate unless there is levator dysfunction.[37] Passive head turning or caloric stimulation may assist in determining the presence of external ophthalmoplegia in a patient with a pupillary abnormality. Recovery from third nerve palsy from tentorial herniation may be prolonged, and the palsy may be accompanied by other ocular motor abnormalities, including nystagmus, skew deviation, vertical gaze paresis, and internuclear ophthalmoplegia, because of intrinsic brain stem injury.[38,39]

Ocular Motor Nerve Palsies from Minor Head Trauma

Oculomotor and sixth nerve palsy precipitated by *minor* head injury causing neither skull fracture nor loss of consciousness is so rare that one should almost always investigate such individuals for basal skull tumor, such as meningioma or chordoma.[28] Ocular motor nerves stretched or encased by tumor are especially vulnerable to sudden mechanical stress. This should be kept in mind whenever the effects seem to be out of proportion to the degree of trauma.

Combined Third, Fourth, and Sixth Nerve Palsies Following Trauma

In general, when more than one ocular motor nerve is affected by trauma, the injury is relatively severe. Combined ocular motor nerve injury is much less frequent than isolated injury (Table 35-1).[5] Combined ocular motor nerve palsies may also result from penetrating wounds involving the orbit and superior orbital fissure.

Carotid-Cavernous Fistula

Another cause of combined ocular motor nerve dysfunction following injury is carotid-cavernous fistula. Traumatic fistula should be distinguished from spontaneous dural shunt. However, both may be associated with ophthalmoplegia due to compression or ischemia of one or more of the ocular motor nerves or to congestion of the extraocular muscles. Other symptoms that bring patients to the attention of physicians include asymptomatic bruit, headache, exophthalmos, and ocular congestion.[40,41] Visual loss may be due to exposure of the eye, venous-stasis retinopathy, or optic neuropathy. The optic neuropathy may result from direct injury at the time of the accident, glaucoma from increased episcleral venous pressure, ischemia of the optic nerve, or compression by enlargement of the cavernous sinus or superior ophthalmic vein.[42] The ophthalmoplegia due to carotid-cavernous fistula usually (in 10% to 60% of cases) takes the form of sixth nerve dysfunction (Fig. 35-4).[40,43]

A

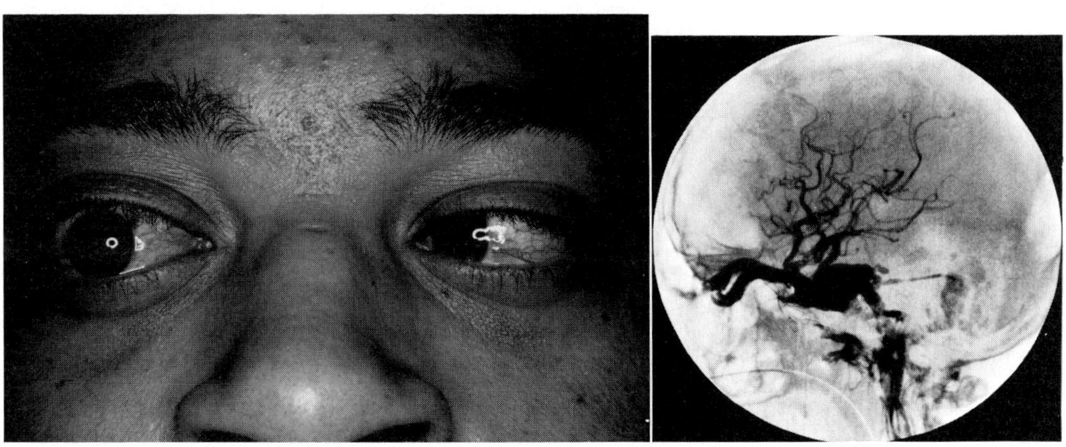

B

Fig. 35-4. **A,** Lateral rectus dysfunction due to sixth nerve injury associated with **B,** carotid-cavernous fistula demonstrated by carotid angiography.

Third nerve palsy is less common, occurring in 0 to 41% of cases, and complete ophthalmoplegia or a combination of ocular motor dysfunction may occur in 10% to 20% of cases.[40,43] The onset of symptoms may be delayed by weeks or months in one third of patients.[40,43]

Current treatment for chronic or vision-threatening carotid-cavernous fistula is by detachable balloon.[41] The prognosis for ocular motor palsy is favorable, but ocular motor nerve dysfunction may also be a complication of balloon treatment, and multiple balloons may be required to close some fistulas.[41]

PUPILLARY DISORDERS FOLLOWING TRAUMA

Traumatic Mydriasis

Pupillary dysfunction in the presence of ocular trauma most often reflects direct injury to the iris sphincter muscle. After contusion of the globe, there may be constriction of the pupil, which may last for hours, followed by iridoplegia. We have seen a patient with a tonic pupil that was supersensitive to weak pilocarpine following blunt orbital trauma. This has been described only rarely in the literature.[44] Spasm of the pupil may also be associated with spasm of accommodation followed by inability to accommodate. Persistent mydriasis and accommodative deficiency may cause functional difficulties, particularly with close visual tasks.[45] On the other hand, an older study showed that the reading difficulty that frequently follows head injury was not associated with accommodative difficulty alone and may be due to other mechanisms.[46]

It is important to document iris injury so that other physicians caring for the patient avoid the false impression that there is third nerve dysfunction, which may indicate tentorial herniation. The patient with pupillary dysfunction following injury should be examined at the slit-lamp, if possible. If cells and flare are visible in the anterior chamber, traumatic injury to the iris muscle is likely, and sphincter muscle tears at the pupillary margin may be apparent. Another indication of iris injury is the observation that the pupil not only lacks normal constriction to light but also does not dilate very well in the dark. Furthermore, such pupils will react less well to various pharmacologic agents including weak pilocarpine, which will cause a parasympathetically denervated pupil to react. A more remote sign of iris injury is transillumination of the iris, particularly in the region of the damaged sphincter muscle. A D-shaped pupillary aperture may reflect iridodialysis.

Mydriasis may also occur from the toxic effects of iron after a penetrating injury is sustained. A fixed dilated pupil may be the initial finding in patients with intraocular foreign bodies that otherwise might go undetected[47] (see Chapter 21).

Traumatic Miosis

Trauma accounts for about 4% of all Horner's syndrome cases.[48] If no other findings are noted, the injury may be to the carotid sympathetic plexus within the neck, important because carotid injury may be associated with dissections or accelerated atherosclerosis. Occasionally, intraoral trauma, as occurs when a child falls on a sharp object, causes Horner's syndrome.[49] The sympathetic chain may also be injured in the chest. Involvement of the first-order neurons descending through the brainstem may be associated with the findings of Wallenberg's lateral medullary syndrome, such as nystagmus, swallowing difficulty, hemiparesis, and alternating analgesia. Cervical spinal cord injuries may cause intermittent oculosympathetic paresis.[50]

TRIGEMINAL NERVE INJURY

In orbital floor fractures the infraorbital nerve is commonly injured; more proximal injury to the trigeminal nerve is relatively infrequent.[51] Penetrating injury (gunshot) can cause facial and ocular anesthesia. Commonly the Gasserian ganglion itself is affected, and when this occurs, there may be associated third, fourth, or sixth nerve injury. Crushing injuries also affect the trigeminal ganglion and its branches. In such cases, the sixth nerve is frequently involved, but complete unilateral ophthalmoplegia may also occur.[52,53]

Despite its relative infrequency,[51] corneal anesthesia is important to recognize in any patient who has been injured, because of the rapidity with which corneal epithelial defects and stromal ulceration can ensue. This is most critical when there is concomitant incomplete closure of one or both eyelids, especially following seventh nerve injury. Patching, lid suturing, or tarsorrhaphy may be urgently required in order to avoid corneal complications (see Chapter 6).

SEVENTH NERVE INJURY

Facial nerve paralysis is a frequent complication of cranial injury. Paralysis central in origin is associated with sixth nerve palsy and hemiplegia. Peripheral facial nerve injury, which has a good prognosis for recovery, results from fracture of the petrous portion of the temporal bone.[54]

Recognition and proper treatment of eye exposure in patients with cranial injuries is of great importance. Incomplete closure of the eyelids during a period of coma or seventh nerve dysfunction requires frequent lubrication of the eye. This must be emphasized to the nurses and other providers of medical care. Tarsorrhaphy may be indicated. It is an easy procedure that is readily reversed if no longer needed. Techniques of tarsorrhaphy are described in Chapter 28.

CENTRAL DISORDERS OF EYE MOVEMENTS FOLLOWING TRAUMA

Almost any type of central gaze dysfunction or nystagmus can follow trauma, but certain ocular motor deficits more commonly follow specific types of injury (Fig. 35-1). In this section, the implications of these disorders in patients with coma will be addressed. Direct injuries from concussion or contusion will be considered from a regional point of view so that when an ophthalmologist confronts a traumatized patient with a central form of ocular motor dysfunction, the abnormality can be localized and appropriate management recommendations made. The ocular motor effects of hypoxia will be reviewed in the last section of this chapter.

Ocular Motor Findings in Coma

According to Fisher,[55] "ocular findings are the most important of the entire examination and their interpretation at the bedside is often the mainstay of diagnosis" in comatose patients. Ophthalmologists should help their neurological and neurosurgical colleagues in interpreting ocular motor function even in the most severely injured patient.

The eyelids tend to be closed during coma when the lower pons is functioning normally. Gradual, slow closure of the eyes after they have been opened is typical in stupor and coma, and this cannot be duplicated voluntarily by hysteric or catatonic patients.[55] One method of determining if the levator muscles function is to sit the patient upright. Even in coma the eyelids will open reflexly for a period of time. Unfortunately this is an awkward procedure if a patient is intubated and attached to other devices.

Transient downgaze deviation, upgaze deviation, and roving eye movements are common in coma. These findings are significant only if they persist. Forced downward deviation of the eyes occurs in thalamic and subthalamic lesions, particularly hemorrhage and infarction. Forced upward deviation is more common in hypoxic conditions (described later). Comatose patients do not make rapid eye movements, and the quick phases of nystagmus may thus be absent.

If an apparently comatose patient makes completely normal ocular responses to caloric stimulation, the possibility of a "locked-in syndrome" must be considered. In this situation, the patient is awake, only appearing unconscious because upper brain-stem injury impedes communication.

Misalignment of the eyes may reflect decompensation of an underlying phoria. This may be horizontal or vertical, but vertical misalignment of the eyes may represent a skew deviation (which may be transient) or paralysis of the third or fourth nerve.

Full conjugate horizontal excursion of the eyes during passive head turning or caloric stimulation of one ear excludes brain-stem lesions at or below the third-nerve nucleus. Brain injury leads to four basic types of abnormal ocular responses: (1) No eye movement, in the absence of drugs and paralytic agents, suggests a major brain-stem lesion. (2) Inability of the eyes to move to one side suggests a unilateral lesion in the pontine gaze center. (3) Lack of adduction of one eye indicates either third nerve palsy or internuclear ophthalmoplegia. (4) Lack of abduction of one eye suggests sixth nerve palsy. Caloric stimulation is thought to be superior to that of passive head turning by some.[56-59] The nystagmus induced by cold water consists of a slow phase toward the direction of the stimulated ear, followed by a contralateral rapid phase. If warm water is used, the opposite reaction is expected. An abnormal labyrinth on one side will cause false responses. Studies relating the overall prognosis for recovery to the type of ocular motor response to caloric stimulation indicate that patients who have a normal response or conjugate horizontal deviation do well. Evidence of an internuclear ophthalmoplegia is associated with a poorer prognosis, and no caloric response with high morbidity and mortality.[56,59]

Localized Central Ocular Motor Effects of Trauma

Vertical Gaze

Impaired vertical gaze is an indicator of upper midbrain or bilateral thalamic damage. Intrinsic brain-stem damage occurring during midline herniation may cause focal areas of ischemia within the tectum and periaqueductal gray matter of the midbrain. This may affect upgaze or downgaze. In some cases, a typical Parinaud's syndrome may occur. This consists of upgaze palsy, paralysis of convergence, midposition pupils that respond to heat but not to light, and convergent movements on attempted upgaze. Downward tonic deviation of the eyes usually occurs in thalamic injuries.

Horizontal Gaze

Conjugate horizontal deviation of the eyes directed away from the hemiparesis with preserved movement of the eyes with passive head-turning or caloric stimuli indicates a lesion above the pontine horizontal gaze center. Conjugate deviation directed toward the side of the hemiparesis ("wrong-way" deviation) indicates unilateral thalamic or ipsilateral frontal hemispheric damage.

Lower pontine hemorrhages from compression may occur when smaller paramedian branches of the basilar artery are compromised as the basilar artery is pressed against the clivus when there is bilateral brain swelling and central herniation. This may cause conjugate or slightly divergent roving eye movements that are not influenced by passive head-turning. With more severe pontine damage, no movements can be elicited with head-turning or caloric stimulation.

Internuclear Ophthalmoplegia

Slowing or limited adduction of one eye and abduction nystagmus of the other eye has been reported to follow trauma.[60-64] It may be mistaken for a partial third nerve palsy. Traumatic internuclear ophthalmoplegia is thought to be due to shearing forces that occur at the junction of the gray and white matter in the medial longitudinal fasciculus as the posterior portion of the brain stem shifts farther than the more anterior portion.[60] Traumatic internuclear ophthalmoplegia is more often bilateral[60-64] than unilateral[61] and may be associated with skew deviation. Prognosis for recovery is good.[61]

Nystagmus

Horizontal nystagmus may be of low frequency and large amplitude if paramedian pontine gaze nuclei are damaged. Higher-frequency, small-amplitude nystagmus is more characteristic of horizontal vestibular nucleus injury. Both types of nystagmus may occur together, with the fast component of "gaze paretic" nystagmus occurring ipsilateral to the lesion and the fast component of the vestibular nystagmus occurring away from the lesion. Cerebellar injury may cause ocular flutter, dysmetria, lateropulsion, rebound nystagmus, and upbeat nystagmus. Pursuit may become saccadic, and there may be inability to suppress vestibuloocular responses to head rotation with visual fixation.

Ocular bobbing, or intermittent downward and upward movements of the eyes, is an important sign in patients with coma.[65,66] Generally this represents lower brain-stem injury, particularly bilateral pontine horizontal gaze center damage. Ocular bobbing, present soon after head injury, may have grave implications. In some patients with pontine injury, the ocular bobbing may occur in a delayed fashion. This may be associated with palatal myoclonus.

Ping-pong gaze consists of horizontal deviation of the eyes that alternates in cycles of a few seconds. This is usually associated with bilateral cerebral hemispheric disease, including hypoxia.

Opsoclonus is a specific type of eye movement consisting of random, rapid, or saccadic movements in many directions. This occurs rarely following severe injury associated with prolonged coma in adults.[67]

See-saw nystagmus can occur when there is injury to subthalamic structures on one side. It has been observed in patients with traumatic chiasmal syndromes[68,69] and following hyperextension head injury with damage to the pontomedullary junction.[70]

Following head trauma, some patients may complain of dizziness despite normal findings on clinical examination. In many such cases, electronystagmography shows abnormal responses.[71] Another cause of persistent vestibular symptoms, especially positional vertigo, is perilymph fistula. Ear, nose, and throat examination is also helpful in such cases, because this condition is treatable.[72]

Latent nystagmus may become manifest after injury to one eye. This leads to visual dysfunction in the remaining eye, even if it is otherwise normal.

HYPOXIC EFFECTS ON THE OCULAR MOTOR SYSTEM

Hypoxic injuries tend to cause more diffuse central nervous system damage than does direct injury. However, certain zones of the brain, including the border areas between the anterior middle cerebral arteries and the middle and posterior cerebral arteries, tend to be more susceptible to hypoxia. In general, permanent brain dysfunction can be expected if there is cardiac standstill for more than 5 minutes. Hypotension and hypovolemia contribute to these effects. Vision is often affected, and severe hypoxia is one cause of cortical blindness. In children, this may lead to strabismus.

Vertical eye movements tend to be affected more prominently following hypoxic injuries. For some reason, the pretectal area of the midbrain is susceptible to metabolic and diffuse hypoxic injuries. In addition to vertical gaze paralysis, sustained vertical deviation has been described following hypoxia. In one study, sustained upgaze in coma followed cardiac arrest in 15 patients, and systemic hypotension in 2 cases, with neuropathologic examination showing diffuse cerebral and cerebellar damage with relative sparing of the brain stem. No focal lesions were found in the upper midbrain or pretectum.[73] Some of the patients demonstrated slow downbeating nystagmus as forced upward gaze resolved. Others developed myoclonic jerks with synchronized upward gaze movements. Sustained downward gaze may also be seen following hypoxia, but this is less common.[74]

Acute bilateral frontal or frontoparietal lesions may produce a form of dyspraxia of ocular motor function termed Balint's syndrome. In this case, voluntary eye movements tend to be inappropriate. Patients direct their eyes to a point away from fixation by performing random searching movements, and they are unable to release fixation. They are inattentive to visual stimuli, even threatening ones. Reflex eye movements appear intact. This syndrome may result from a variety of causes including stroke and multiple sclerosis, as well as hypoxic and penetrating injuries.[75,76]

Rehabilitation of patients with complex ocular motor and visual pathway damage can be extremely frustrating for the ophthalmologist, especially when patients are aphasic and have limited mobility. Every patient with serious head injury is unique and must be approached with patience and extra time. Although the only available treatment may seem rudimentary, such as a trial of reading glasses or the use of an occluder, it may mean much to a person struggling to overcome serious handicaps.

References

1. Hedges TR III: Consultation in ophthalmology, Toronto, 1987 BC Decker, 1-4.
2. Helveston FM and Grossman RD: Extraocular muscle lacerations, Am J Ophthalmol 81:754-757, 1976.
3. Ullman S, Nelson LB, and Martin JJ: Traumatic laceration of the inferior rectus muscle, Am J Ophthalmol 100:855-856, 1985.
4. Miller GR and Glaser JS: The retraction syndrome and trauma, Arch Ophthalmol 76:662-663, 1966.
5. Rucker CW: The causes of paralysis of the third, fourth, and sixth cranial nerves, Am J Ophthalmol 61:1293-1298, 1966.
6. Heinze J: Cranial nerve avulsion and other neural injuries in road accidents, Med J Aust 2:1246-1249, 1969.
7. Khawam E, Scott AB, and Jampolsky A: Acquired superior oblique palsy, Arch Ophthalmol 77:761-768, 1967.
8. Burber LJ, Kalvin NH, and Smith JL: Acquired lesions of the fourth cranial nerve, Brain 93:567-574, 1970.
9. Coppeto JM and Lessell S: Cryptogenic unilateral paralysis of the superior oblique muscle, Arch Ophthalmol 96:275-277, 1978.
10. Bachynski BN and Flynn JT: Direct trauma to the superior oblique tendon following penetrating injuries of the upper eyelid, Arch Ophthalmol 103:1510-1514, 1985.
11. Blanchard CL and Young LA: Acquired inflammatory superior oblique tendon sheath (Brown's) syndrome: report of a case following frontal sinus surgery, Arch Otolaryngol 110:120-122, 1984.
12. Lavin PJM and Troost BT: Traumatic fourth nerve palsy: Clinicoanatomic correlations with computer tomographic scan, Arch Neurol 41:679-680, 1984.
13. Sydnor CF, Seaber JH, and Buckley EG: Traumatic superior oblique palsies, Ophthalmology 89:134-138, 1982.

14. Parks MM: Isolated cyclovertical muscle palsy, Arch Ophthalmol 60:1027-1035, 1958.
15. Kushner BJ: The diagnosis and treatment of bilateral masked superior oblique palsy, Am J Ophthalmol 105:186-194, 1988.
16. Crouch ER and Urist MJ: Lateral rectus muscle paralysis associated with closed-head trauma, Am J Ophthalmol 79:990-996, 1975.
17. Lindenberg R: Significance of the tentorium in head injuries from blunt forces, Clin Neurosurg 12:129-142, 1966.
18. Summers CG and Wirtschafter JD: Bilateral trigeminal and abducens neuropathies following low-velocity, crushing head injury, J Neurosurg 50:508-511, 1979.
19. Rosa L et al: Multiple cranial nerve palsies due to a hyperextension injury to the cervical spine, J Neurosurg 61:172-173, 1984.
20. Schneider RC and Johnson FD: Bilateral traumatic abducens palsy: a mechanism of injury suggested by the study of associated cervical spine fractures, J Neurosurg 34:33-37, 1971.
21. Nabors MW et al: Delayed abducens nerve palsies associated with cervical spine fractures, Neurology 37:1565, 1987.
22. Cushing H: Strangulation of the nervi abducentes by lateral branches of the basilar artery in cases of brain tumor, Brain 33:204-235, 1910.
23. Lee DA et al: Surgical treatment of lateral rectus muscle paralysis, Am J Ophthalmol 97:511-518, 1984.
24. Helveston EM, Merriam W, and Ellis FD: Extraocular muscle-tendon transfer with scleral augmentation, Am J Ophthalmol 89:819-823, 1980.
25. Scott AB and Kraft SP: Botulinum toxin injection in the management of lateral rectus paresis, Ophthalmology 92:676-683, 1985.
26. Solomons NB, Solomon DJ, and DeVilliers JC: Direct traumatic third nerve palsy, S Afr Med J 58:109-111, 1980.
27. Memon MY and Paine KWE: Direct injury of the oculomotor nerve in craniocerebral trauma, J Neurosurg 35:461-464, 1971.
28. Eyster EF, Hoyt WF, and Wilson CB: Oculomotor palsy from minor head trauma: an initial sign of basal intracranial tumor, JAMA 220:1083-1086, 1972.
29. Krohel GB: Blepharoptosis after traumatic third-nerve palsies, Am J Ophthalmol 88:598-601, 1979.
30. Elston JS: Traumatic third nerve palsy, Br J Ophthalmol 68:538-543, 1984.
31. Tognetti F, Godano U, and Galassi E: Bilateral traumatic third nerve palsy, Surg Neurol 29:120-124, 1988.
32. Walsh FB and Hoyt WF: Clinical Neuro-ophthalmology, Baltimore, 1969, Williams & Wilkins, 2402-2404.
33. Pevehouse BC, Bloom WH, and McKissock W: Ophthalmologic aspects of diagnosis and localization of subdural hematoma: an analysis of 389 cases and review of the literature, Neurology 10:1037-1041, 1960.
34. Keane JR: Oculomotor palsy with pupillary sparing in subdural hematoma: two cases with documented tentorial herniation, Mount Sinai J Med 41:161-165, 1974.
35. Sunderland S and Bradley KC: Disturbances of oculomotor function accompanying extradural haemorrhage, J Neurol Neurosurg Psychiatry 16:35-46, 1953.
36. DiTullio MV: Epidural hematoma with complete third nerve paralysis in an awake patient, Surg Neurol 7:193-194, 1977.
37. Lessell S: Personal communication, 1974.
38. Keane JR. Bilateral ocular motor signs after tentorial herniation in 25 patients, Arch Neurol 43:806-807, 1986.
39. Caplan LR and Zervas NT: Survival with permanent midbrain dysfunction after surgical treatment of traumatic subdural hematoma: the clinical picture of a Duret hemorrhage? Ann Neurol 1:587-589, 1988.
40. Henderson JW and Schneider RC: The ocular findings in carotid-cavernous fistula in a series of 17 cases, Am J Ophthalmol 48:585-597, 1959.
41. Debrun G et al: Treatment of 54 traumatic carotid-cavernous fistulas, J Neurosurg 55:678-692, 1981.
42. Hedges TR III, Debrun G, and Sokol S: Reversible optic neuropathy due to carotid-cavernous fistula, J Clin Neuroophthalmol 5:37-40, 1985.
43. Walker AE and Allegre GE: Carotid-cavernous fistulas, Surgery 39:411-422, 1956.
44. Hornblass A: Pupillary dilatation in fractures of the floor of the orbit, Ophthalmic Surg 10:44-46, 1979.
45. Peli E: Functional difficulties resulting from traumatic anisocoria, Am J Optom Physiol Opt 61:548-550, 1984.
46. Wescott V: Concerning accommodative asthenopia following head injury, Am J Ophthalmol 19:385-391, 1932.
47. Monteiro MLR et al: Iron mydriasis, Am J Ophthalmol 97:795, 1984.
48. Maloney WF, Younge BR, and Moyer NJ: Evaluation of the causes and accuracy of the pharmacologic localization in Horner's syndrome, Am J Ophthalmol 90:394-402, 1980.
49. Pruett RC: Horner's syndrome following intraoral trauma, Arch Ophthalmol 78:420-421, 1967.
50. Ben Jur PH: Intermittent Horner's syndrome: recurrent alternate Horner's syndrome in cervical cord injury, Ann Ophthalmol 7:955-962, 1975.
51. Walsh FB and Hoyt WF: Clinical neuro-ophthalmology, Baltimore, 1969, Williams & Wilkins, 2359-2360.

52. Jefferson G and Schorstein J: Injuries of the trigeminal nerve, its ganglion and its divisions, Br J Surg 42:561-581, 1955.
53. Summers CG and Wirtschafter JD: Bilateral trigeminal and abducens neuropathies following low-velocity, crushing head injury, J Neurosurg 50:508-519, 1979.
54. Walsh FB and Hoyt WF: Clinical neuro-ophthalmology, Baltimore, 1969, Williams & Wilkins, 2359-2360.
55. Fisher CM: The neurological examination in the comatose patient, Acta Neurol Scand Suppl 45:1-56, 1969.
56. Barrios RR, Bottinelli MD, and Medoc J: The study of ocular motility in the comatose patient, J Neurol Sci 3:183-206, 1966.
57. Mueller-Jensen A, Neunzig H-P, and Emskotter T: Outcome prediction in comatose patients: significance of reflex eye movement analysis, J Neurol Neurosurg Psychiatry 50:392, 1987.
58. Van Den Berge JH et al: Interobserver agreement in assessment of ocular signs in coma, J Neurol Neurosurg Psychiatry 42:1163-1168, 1979.
59. Poulsen J and Zilstorff K: Prognostic value of the caloric-vestibular test in the unconscious patient with cranial trauma, Acta Neurol Scand 48:282-292, 1972.
60. Rich JR, Gregorius FK, and Hepler RS: Bilateral internuclear ophthalmoplegia after trauma, Arch Ophthalmol 92:66-68, 1974.
61. Beck RW and Meckler RJ: Internuclear ophthalmoplegia after head trauma, Ann Ophthalmol 13:671-675, 1981.
62. Rosati G et al: Reversible bilateral internuclear ophthalmoplegia due to head trauma: a case report, Eur Neurol 20:80-83, 1981.
63. Baker RS: Internuclear ophthalmoplegia following head injury, J Neurosurg 51:552-555, 1979.
64. Jammes JL: Bilateral internuclear ophthalmoplegia due to acute cervical hyperextension without head trauma, J Clin Neuroophthalmol 9:112-115, 1989.
65. Susac JO et al: Clinical spectrum of ocular bobbing, J Neurol Neurosurg Psychiatry 33:771-775, 1970.
66. Rosenberg ML: Spontaneous vertical eye movements in coma, Ann Neurol 20:635-637, 1986.
67. Digre KB: Opsoclonus in adults: report of three cases and review of the literature, Arch Neurol 43:1165-1175, 1986.
68. Sabin TD and Poche JA: Pure torsional nystagmus as a consequence of head trauma, J Neurol Neurosurg Psychiatry 32:265-267, 1969.
69. Keane JR: Intermittent see-saw eye movements: report of a patient in coma after hyperextension head injury, Arch Neurol 35:173-174, 1978.
70. Frisen L and Wikkelso C: Posttraumatic seesaw nystagmus abolished by ethanol ingestion, Neurology 36:841-844, 1986.
71. Toglia JU: Acute flexion-extension injury of the neck, Neurology 26:808-814, 1976.
72. Singleton GT et al: Perilymph fistulas: diagnostic criteria and therapy, Ann Otolaryngol 87:797-806, 1978.
73. Keane JR: Sustained upgaze in coma, Ann Neurol 9:409-412, 1981.
74. Keane JR, Rawlinson DG, and Lu AT: Sustained downgaze deviation: two cases without structural pretectal lesions, Neurology 26:594-595, 1976.
75. Waltz AG: Dyspraxias of gaze, Arch Neurol 5:74-83, 1961.
76. Holmes G: Disturbances of visual orientation, Br J Ophthalmol 2:449-458, 1918.

PART 6

Injury prevention and medicolegal aspects of eye trauma

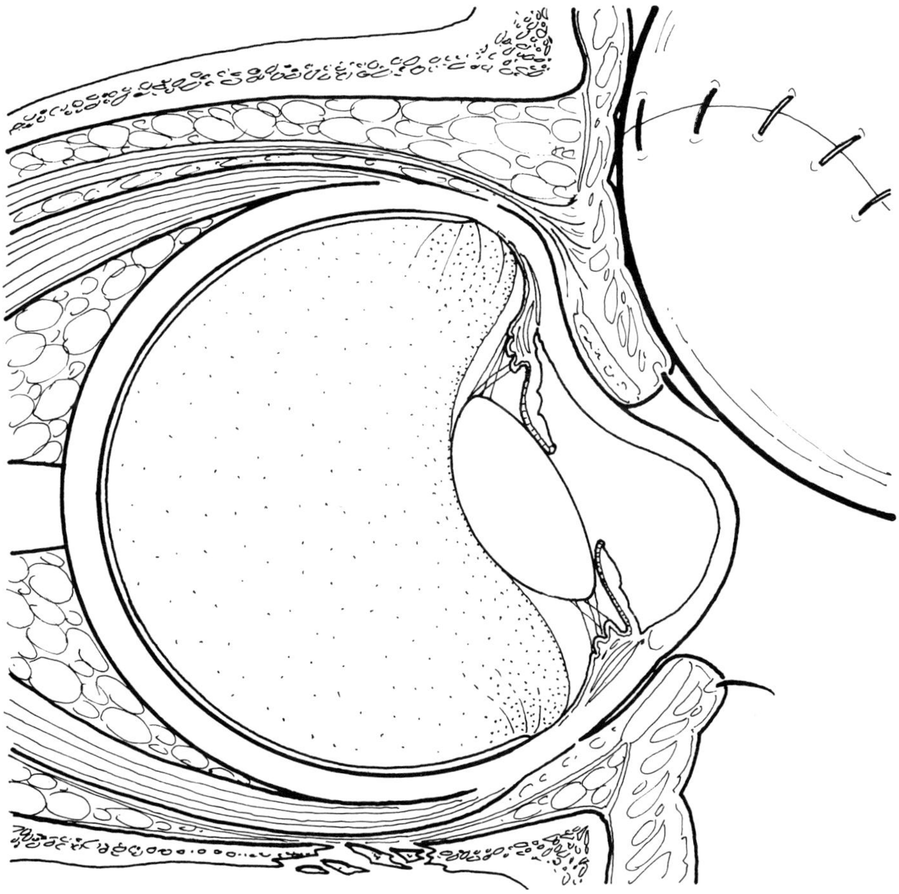

CHAPTER 36

Epidemiology and prevention

OLIVER D. SCHEIN
PAUL F. VINGER

General epidemiology of ocular injury
Work-related trauma
Recreation-related trauma
Prevention
Patients at risk
Available protection
 Streetwear frames with 2-mm polycarbonate lenses
 Sports frames with 3-mm polycarbonate lenses
 Polycarbonate sports eye protectors
 Face mask/helmet combinations
 Industrial eye protectors
References

Despite great strides in the diagnosis and treatment of ocular injuries during the last decade, until very recently there has been only limited progress toward understanding the epidemiology and prevention of eye trauma. This is, in part, because of the difficulties in obtaining meaningful data. One can easily collect case series of specific diagnostic or therapeutic situations and make extrapolations from them, but defining general rates and risk factors for ocular injury from the specific study population is problematic.

Epidemiology studies of ocular injury have generally taken one of several forms. The first is a hospital-based survey of ocular injury over specific time periods.[1-3] Such data are valuable because diagnoses are verified by ophthalmologists and details of the injuries can be described. These studies, however, are limited in that the results may reflect geographic or demographic bias inherent in the referral patterns of specific hospitals and so may not be generalizable. A related form of survey is the voluntary registry, such as the Eye Injury Registry of Alabama[4] and the National Eye Trauma system.[5] These registries can provide detailed information about specific clinical cases. However, it is impossible to estimate rates or risk factors for injury, since the percentage and types of unreported injury are not known. A third approach has been directed toward measuring the incidence of eye injury in defined populations.[6-11] This approach yields important data about rates of disease but rarely elucidates clinical details or risk factors. Finally, some information is available from philanthropic organizations (e.g., the National Society to Prevent Blindness),[12] consumer product surveys (e.g., the National Electronic Injury Surveillance System), medical organizations and private practices.[13]

Although each of these epidemiologic strategies has both weaknesses and strengths, there have been a number of significant findings and consistent themes in the eye trauma literature.

GENERAL EPIDEMIOLOGY OF OCULAR INJURY

Estimates of the incidence of ocular injury (number of new injuries occurring in a known population over a specified time interval) have varied somewhat by location and research strategy. The National Society to Prevent Blindness has estimated that more than 2.4 million eye injuries occur each year in the United States.[12] In one population-based study in Wisconsin in 1979, Karlson and Klein[7] found that the incidence of acute, hospital-treated eye injuries was 423 per 100,000 residents. In this predominantly rural population, assaults, work-related events, sports, motor vehicle accidents, and falls accounted for most of the injuries. The highest rates were for men aged 20 to 24 years (940 per 100,000). In comparison, Glynn, Seddon, and Berlin[9] found a high rate of eye injury in New England. This study, which relied on telephone interviews after random digit dialing, yielded a rate of 9.75 eye injuries per 1000 adults; 59 percent of the injuries occurred at work, the rate was 5.5 times greater for men than women, and injury rates declined linearly with age.

Tielsch, Parver, and Shankar[6] used hospital discharge summaries to examine the incidence of hospitalized ocular trauma cases in Maryland from 1979 through 1986 and found the annual incidence to be 13.2 per 100,000. Age and sex strongly affected the incidence. Males were at significantly greater risk in all age groups except the most elderly. A bimodal age pattern of risk had peaks at 15 to 29 years and over 70 years, the peak in the older group being secondary to falls. Nonwhites had a greater risk than whites. Extrapolating from the Maryland data, these authors estimated about 30,000 admissions for ocular trauma as a primary diagnosis and about 60,000 as a primary or secondary diagnosis in the United States per year.

Comparative data are available from Sweden, where a more manageable population and a tradition of medical and population registries facilitate epidemiologic surveys. In Stockholm county, with a population of 1.5 million, Blomdahl and Norell[8] found perforating ocular injury to be approximately six times more common in men than women, and rates of injury peaked in young men aged 10 to 19 (94.3 perforating eye injures per 1,000,000 person-years). Most injuries occurred during daylight hours; the most

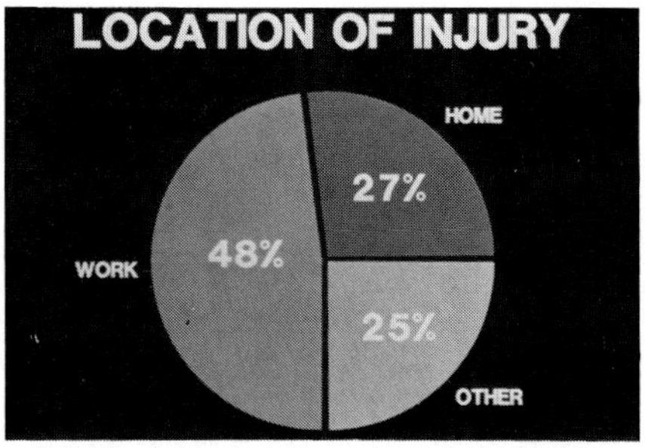

Fig. 36-1. Location of eye injuries in a New England population. (Published courtesy of Ophthalmology [95:300-305, 1988]).

common concurrent activity was paid work (27%), followed by play or sports (23%). Studies have also been undertaken to examine specific types of eye injury. For instance, in Olmstead County, Minnesota, the mean annual incidence rate for traumatic hyphema was 20.2 per 100,000 among males and 4.1 per 100,000 among females.[10]

Hospital and registry-based data sets have provided more detailed information on the specific nature of the eye injuries and the context in which they occur. Schein et al[1] studied over 3000 patients with eye trauma seen in a single eye emergency department in Boston. In addition to the ubiquitous finding of a preponderance of injuries in young males, they found that 8% of the patients suffered injuries to both eyes and 15% had a history of prior eye injury. Approximately 5% of injuries were considered severe (e.g., ruptured globe, intraocular foreign body, hyphema, orbital/facial fracture), and a disproportionate number of these occurred in those under 15 years of age. Approximately one half of the injuries occurred at the workplace (Fig. 36-1). Ruptured globes were associated with workplace injuries and children at play. Although only about 3% of all injuries were sports related, 11% of the severe injuries and 60% of hyphemas occurred in this group. In addition to work, sports, and play, the home is a common site for ocular injury.[4] Assault plays a variable role but appears to be most important in eye injuries among young urban males.

WORK-RELATED TRAUMA

Work-related injuries account for a substantial percentage of ocular injuries in virtually all reported surveys. The actual incidence of occupational injury is difficult to estimate, however. Similarly, it is difficult to compare studies, since the classification of occupations may vary. Although it is tempting to associate specific occupations with eye injuries, the overlap in work tasks makes definitive classification impossible. For example, if a plumber injures an eye while removing a nail, is this a carpentry or a plumbing accident?

The National Institute for Occupational Safety and Health (NIOSH) estimated that approximately 900,000 occupational eye injuries occurred in 1982.[14] Physician visits for ocular complaints ranked second only to those for dermatologic conditions in the workplace. In a survey of over 1000 occupational eye injuries in 1979,[15] the construction and manufacturing industries together accounted for 70% of cases, chemical injuries for 18%, and metal manufacturing for 52%. Schein et al[1] reported 63% of occupational injuries as construction related and 18% associated with the auto repair industry. The findings related to automobile workers were especially interesting since the injuries were not only more frequent than expected in relation to the size of the working population but included a disproportionate number of ruptured globes.

Only two thirds of subjects injured at the work site reported that protective eye wear was available. Moreover, in settings where severe injury was recorded, only one third claimed that such eye protection was available. Only 10 percent of those injured at work were wearing some kind of protective eye wear at the time of injury; none of these had a severe injury. Of those with penetrating ocular injuries at the work site, 40% were pursuing legal action against employers.

More precise epidemiologic information is available from Scandinavia. In 1973, approximately 12% of all industrial accidents in Finland were eye injuries.[16] Eye injuries accounted for approximately one third of all industrial accidents that needed only ambulatory treatment and about one fifth of accidents causing an absence from work of one or two days.

In addition to the broad areas of construction-related work and automobile repair–related tasks, agriculture has also been specifically related to ocular injury.[16] In all kinds of work-related injury, hand tools play an important role, accounting for approximately the same number of injuries as machine tools. This may explain the frequency of ocular injuries occurring in the home, where many are caused by unprotected use of hammers, nails, and drills. Such injuries are not classified as occupational, but the context, risk factors, and potential preventive strategies are similar.

RECREATION-RELATED TRAUMA

Sports and play account for a large proportion of eye injuries. In the Boston survey,[1] sports and play accounted for 34% of the ruptured globes and 70% of hyphemas. In the Stockholm study,[8] 23% of perforating eye injuries were caused by play or sports, and recreation accounted for 25% of the severe injuries recorded in the Alabama registry.[4] Sports-related injury has been specifically associated with the occurrence of hyphema.[1,10] Particular sports associated with ocular injury vary by season and location.[40] However, in the United States several patterns are clear. Baseball and softball account for more than 10,000 ocular injuries per year, and racket sports over 7000.[17] Football, basketball, and golf have also been frequently associated with ocular injury. The widespread use of ocular and facial protection in school and amateur ice hockey has dramatically reduced the frequency and severity of these injuries.[18,19] For racket sport injuries, increasing experience and age have not been associated with reduced frequency.[20,21]

Other sports and recreational activities deserving specific mention include war games, boxing, and air guns. Easterbrook and Pashby[22] reported on 26 cases of severe eye injury suffered during war games. Eye guards were provided, and none of the injuries occurred while they were being worn. Competitive boxing is associated with a high rate of eye injury. Among 74 boxers in the New York area, Giovinazzo et al[23] found at least one demonstrable sign of ocular injury in two thirds. The injuries included damage to the angle, lens, macula, and peripheral retina. Although the actual incidence of eye injuries from BB or air guns is unknown, such trauma may cause devastating ocular damage. All BB guns possess the muzzle velocity to penetrate the globe. Some high-powered air rifles may, furthermore, penetrate bone and deeper tissue.[24] Air gun–related injuries accounted for 235 of recreation-related perforating injuries reported to the National Eye Trauma System.[25]

The childhood ocular injury rate in Massachusetts has been estimated as approximately 84 per 10,000, suggesting that in a given year 1 of 119 children will suffer an eye injury requiring hospital treatment.[26] The incidence of pediatric (up to age 15) eye trauma requiring hospitalization in Maryland was estimated at 15.2 per 100,000 in 1982.[27] Males outnumbered females 4 to 1, and the incidence was highest (23.7 per 100,000) among the 11- to 15-year-olds. Sports-related injuries accounted for a significant portion of eye injuries in this age group, while blows and falls were common in younger children. A Canadian survey stressed the prevalence of projectiles, especially rocks and sticks, in child-related injuries.[28] Injuries from household objects and hazardous toys (e.g., nails, glass, darts) accounted for fewer but more severe injuries. As with BB injuries, eye trauma associated with fireworks tends to affect the young with severe injury.[29]

Motor vehicle accidents also contribute to the spectrum of ocular injury. Although these injuries are not as frequent as sports- and industry-related occurrences, eye trauma in the context of a motor vehicle accident is often severe and associated with other facial trauma. Several European studies have linked a reduced incidence of ocular injury to the mandatory use of seat belts.[30,31]

PREVENTION

The vast majority of eye injuries are preventable with existing, relatively inexpensive protective devices. Provision of the proper protection requires a knowledge of the patient's work, hobby, and sports history, an explanation of the potential eye injury risks in these activities, and a prescription for protective eyewear. Most patients require only a brief discussion with the ophthalmologist or technician, possibly supplemented by written material, to be adequately informed about the risks of eye injury from their activities and the suggested means of minimizing the frequency or severity of potential eye injuries.[32] Once the ophthalmologist has made recommendations, it is up to the patient to choose whether or not to make the hobby/work/home/sports environment safer (using seat belts while driving, placing adequate protective guards on machinery, engaging in safer sports and recreational activities, wearing protective eyewear, and so on).

Although most ophthalmologists support the prevention of eye injuries as a laudable clinical goal, too few have incorporated an injury-prevention program into their practices. This is true despite the fact that a legal claim could be made against the ophthalmologist for negligence or failure to prescribe the lens material or eyewear of choice if a preventable injury occurs.[33]

Society bears a great burden from ocular injury, from both the direct costs of hospitalization and follow-up care and the indirect costs of days lost from work. Both types of cost are enormous, and the effect of a severe eye injury is felt personally and economically for many years because of the young population that is at highest risk. Studies of ocular injury do not support the belief that victims of eye trauma suffer accidents that are sudden "twists of fate." Most ocular injuries occur in predictable situations and hence are potentially preventable. As the primary provider of eye care, it is imperative that the ophthalmologist encourage the patient to avoid needless eye injuries by recognizing hazardous situations and adopting appropriate preventive measures and protective devices.

PATIENTS AT RISK

Some patients, such as the functionally one-eyed, would suffer severe morbidity as a consequence of eye injury and, thus, deserve great emphasis on prevention. A person is functionally one-eyed if loss of the better eye would result in a significant change in life-style due to poor vision in the remaining eye. This concept is useful when discussing injury prevention with a patient. When one eye has been removed or has no light perception, it is obvious that loss of the remaining eye would be a disaster. But what if the "worse" eye has some useful vision? A surgeon would be hindered by loss of stereopsis if a 20/20 eye were lost even if the remaining eye were 20/20. A bus driver who loses the better eye and is left with a 20/50 best-corrected amblyopic eye can no longer legally drive and so is severely compromised.

In general, a best-corrected visual acuity of less than 20/40 in one eye of any patient, especially a child, indicates the need for greater emphasis on prevention, especially since loss of the better-seeing eye makes driving illegal in many states.

With proper protection, the potential risk to a functionally one-eyed person can be reduced to such a low level by adequate protective devices that full participation in most occupations and sports is possible (with the exception of boxing, full-contact martial arts, and wrestling, for which adequate protection is not yet available).

Another group at greater risk of severe injury are patients who have had previous eye surgery. Since corneal and limbal incisions never regain full strength, cataract and keratoplasty wound dehiscence may occur following blunt trauma, often many years after surgery.[34] Radial keratotomy incisions, similarly, have demonstrated suboptimal healing for many years after surgery.[35,36] Since a blow from a fist can rupture a globe after radial keratotomy, similar energy delivered from a tennis ball, baseball, or body collision in sport could be expected to have a similar result.[37] Therefore, every postsurgical patient, especially those at high risk (e.g., police, fire fighters, automotive and construction workers, professional and amateur athletes), should be advised that the eye is in a permanently weakened state, and appropriate protective eyewear should be prescribed.

The risk of traumatically induced retinal detachment after successful retinal detachment surgery has not been documented. The potential risk varies greatly with the individual patient, depending on the condition of the vitreous and retinal anatomy, so that the retinal surgeon must individualize recommendations. Preexisting ocular conditions such as myopic retinal thinning, lattice degeneration, sickle cell anemia, subluxated lens, diabetic neovascularization, and scleromalacia may make the eye more prone to severe injury from relatively minor trauma.

AVAILABLE PROTECTION (FIG. 36-2)

Table 36-1 lists the various eye protectors and their uses. Eye protectors are needed for (1) one-eyed people (i.e., if the best corrected visual acuity in the poorer eye is worse than 20/40, since loss of the better eye would result in significant impairment such as inability to drive), (2) those with eye conditions that could be made worse if the eye were hit (e.g., thin retina, bleeding tendency, weak sclera), (3) those whose work activities involve a risk of flying particles,

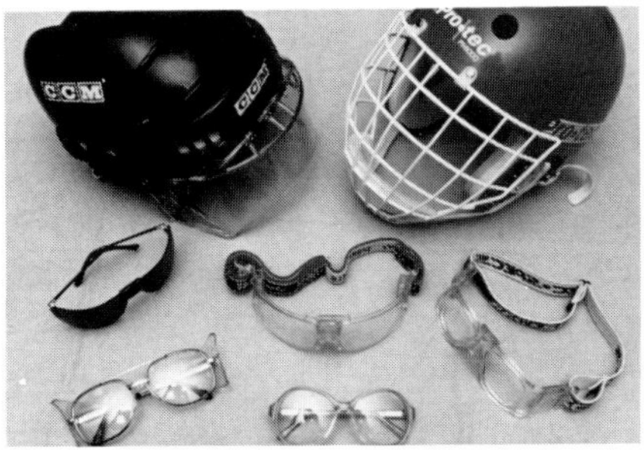

Fig. 36-2. Examples of eye protection available for recreation and work.

Table 36-1. Eye protectors

Type	Uses
Polycarbonate lenses (2-mm center thickness)	In streetwear frames; usually give adequate, cosmetically acceptable protection in day-to-day use for active people. *Constant wear suggested for the functionally one-eyed.*
Polycarbonate lenses (3-mm center thickness)	In sports frames (e.g., Action Eyes, Rec Specs), for sports that use a ball or have contact potential.
Polycarbonate sports eye protectors	With no prescription, for use by contact lens wearers or those who usually do not wear glasses; protectors should pass the racket sport protector standard (e.g., Sports Goggle, Liberty; New Yorker, Leader; Albany, Leader).
Industrial safety glasses with polycarbonate lenses and side shields	For use around machinery, storage batteries, and flying particles.
Industrial safety goggles with polycarbonate lenses	Give better protection than safety glasses; may be worn over regular streetwear spectacles.
Face mask/helmet combinations	For collision sports (e.g., hockey, football, lacrosse). Functionally one-eyed people should wear sports eye protectors under the face mask for added protection.

NOTE: Glass lenses, ordinary plastic lenses, open (lensless) eyeguards, and contact lenses do not give adequate eye protection for active people.

and (4) those who engage in sports in which there is a risk of eye injury.

Glass and allyl resin (CR-39) spectacle lenses have relatively little impact resistance; will shatter on impacts commonly encountered in sports, industry, and falls; and have caused ocular injury by breaking on impact. Polycarbonate spectacle lenses have many times the impact resistance to missiles of all types, are thinner and lighter, have good ultraviolet blocking and ghost-image-reduction capabilities, and are as scratch resistant as coated allyl resin lenses.[38] Thus, polycarbonate is the lens material of choice for all patients, since no age group is free from ocular trauma risk. The games of children are replaced by the games, hobbies, and work of adults, and then by the falls of the elderly.

Polycarbonate, however, has some disadvantages that may lead the patient to opt for the decreased impact resistance of glass or CR-39 lenses. Polycarbonate is more expensive and adds at least $10 to the spectacle cost; it is not available in all prescriptions; it has some degree of chromatic aberration at the lens periphery in high minus lenses (i.e., patients sometimes notice colored fringes at black-edged borders); it is not available in blended or progressive bifocals, some special occupational bifocals, or as a photochromic lens; and it is not as scratch resistant as glass. However, even if impact resistance is ignored, the vast majority of patients with moderate refractive errors prefer the thinness and light weight of polycarbonate.

Streetwear Frames with 2-mm Polycarbonate Lenses

Whenever ophthalmologists write a spectacle prescription, they have the opportunity to give the patient added protection from eye injury. Although many streetwear frames have relatively little resistance to impact, the great strength of a polycarbonate lens greatly reduces the globe-lacerating potential of broken glass or CR-39 spectacle lenses.

This frame/lens combination is satisfactory for general daily wear by all patients, including the one-eyed; for athletes who wear spectacles and are involved in "eye-safe" sports (those that do not involve a thrown or hit ball, use of a bat or stick, or close aggressive play with body contact); and for use under a face mask (except for the one-eyed) in sports such as hockey, football, and lacrosse.[39] Although a racket sport eye protector is advisable for tennis and badminton, this streetwear frame-lens combination is certainly safer than going "bare-eyed."[20]

Sports Frames with 3-mm Polycarbonate Lenses

Sports frames must pass the racket sport eye protector standards of either the Canadian Standards Association or the American Society for Testing and Materials.[21] This frame/lens combination is indicated for spectacle wearers who participate in high eye-risk, noncollision sports (e.g., racket sports, baseball, basketball, soccer) and for functionally one-eyed players of all sports. The impact requirements of the racket sport eye protector standards are significantly higher than those of the ANSI Z87 industrial standard. Industrial safety glasses are not a substitute for sports eyewear.

At this time there are no standards for noncollision sports such as soccer and basketball. Standards are available only for racket sports; thus, these are the best available guidelines for protective wear in other sports, although they remain to be definitively demonstrated as fully satisfactory in these other activities.

Polycarbonate Sports Eye Protectors

These protectors must pass either the Canadian Standards Association or the American Society for Testing and Materials racket sports eye protector standards. They are indicated for contact lens wearers or athletes who ordinarily do not wear glasses, especially those with weakened corneas due to previous surgery, who are playing a high eye-risk sport. These protectors can also be worn by emmetropes beneath a face mask for added protection.

Face Mask/Helmet Combinations

Face mask/helmet combinations are suggested for high-energy impact sports including hockey, football, baseball, lacrosse, fencing, downhill skiing, motorcycling, and snowmobiling. Adequate face mask/helmet combinations (such as the hockey face/head protector system) have essentially eliminated eye and face injuries to protected players.[19] For instance, it is far safer, from an eye injury standpoint, to play hockey with a face mask/helmet combination than to play tennis without eye protection.

Industrial Eye Protectors

These eye protectors must meet the ANSI Z87 standards. Goggles offer more protection than spectacles. For activities that pose a hazard to the face and the eyes, a face shield should be worn. Since face shields are often removed to inspect work or do small touch-up grinding or finish chipping, safety glasses with sideshields must always be worn under a face shield. Sideshields are always indicated on spectacles since protection is decreased by approximately 25% when these are removed.

References

1. Schein OD et al: The spectrum and burden of ocular injury, Ophthalmology 95:300-305, 1988.
2. Wykes WN: A 10-year survey of penetrating eye injuries in Gwent, 1976-85, Br J Ophthalmol 72:607-611, 1988.
3. Chiapella AP and Rosenthal AR: One year in an eye casualty clinic, Br J Ophthalmol 69:865-870, 1985.
4. Morris RE et al: Eye injury registry of Alabama (preliminary report) demographics and prognosis of severe eye injury, South Med J 80:810-816, 1987.
5. Parver LM: Eye trauma: the neglected disorder, Arch Ophthalmol 104:1452-1453, 1986.
6. Tielsch JM, Parver L, and Shankar B: Time trends in the incidence of hospitalized ocular trauma, Arch Ophthalmol 107:519-523, 1989.
7. Karlson TA and Klein BEK: The incidence of acute hospital-treated eye injuries, Arch Ophthalmol 104:1473-1476, 1986.
8. Blomdahl S and Norell S: Perforating eye injury in the Stockholm population: an epidemiological study, Acta Ophthalmol 62:378-390, 1984.
9. Glynn RJ, Seddon JM, and Berlin BM: The incidence of eye injuries in New England adults, Arch Ophthalmol 106:785-789, 1988.
10. Kennedy RH and Brubaker RF: Traumatic hyphema in a defined population, Am J Ophthalmol 106:123-130, 1988.
11. Powell JW: National athletic injury/illness reporting system: eye injuries in college wrestling, Int Ophthalmol Clin 21(4):47-58, 1981.
12. National Society to Prevent Blindness: Fact sheet, New York, 1980, The Society.
13. Vinger PF: The incidence of eye injuries in sports, Int Ophthalmol Clin 21(4):21-46, 1981.
14. Leads from the MMWR: Leading work related diseases and injuries—United States, JAMA 251:2503-2504, 1984.
15. US Department of Labor Statistics: Accidents involving eye injuries, Report 557, April 1980.
16. Saari M and Parvi V: Occupational eye injuries in Finland, Acta Ophthalmol Suppl 161:17-28, 1984.
17. Strahlman E and Sommer A: The epidemiology of sports-related ocular trauma, Int Ophthalmol Clin 28:199-202, 1988.
18. Vinger PF: Sports eye injuries: a preventable disease, Ophthalmology 88:108-112, 1981.
19. Pashby TJ: Eye injuries in Canadian amateur hockey, Can J Ophthalmol 20:2-4, 1985.
20. Vinger PF and Tolpin DW: Racquet sports: an ocular hazard, JAMA 239:2575-2577, 1978.
21. Easterbrook M: Ocular injuries in racquet sports, Int Ophthalmol Clin 28:232-237, 1988.
22. Easterbrook M and Pashby TJ: Eye injuries associated with war games, Can Med Assoc J 133:415-418, 1985.
23. Giovinazzo VJ et al: The ocular complications of boxing, Ophthalmology 94:587-595, 1987.
24. Sheets W and Vinger P: Ocular injuries from air guns, Int Ophthalmol Clin 28:225-227, 1988.
25. Parver LM: The national eye trauma system, Int Ophthalmol Clin 28:203-205, 1988.
26. Gallagher S: Massachusetts Statewide Comprehensive Injury Prevention Program: Personal communication, 1989.
27. Strahlman E, Elman M, and Baker S: The incidence and causes of pediatric ocular trauma: a population-based study, Invest Ophthalmol Vis Sci 29(ARVO suppl):63, 1988.
28. LaRoche GR, McIntyre L, and Schertzer RM: Epidemiology of severe eye injuries in childhood, Ophthalmology 95:1603-1607, 1988.
29. Wilson RS: Fireworks, blindness: a cooperative study, South Med J 73:728-731, 1980.
30. Vernon SA and Yorsten DB: Incidence of ocular injuries from road traffic accidents after introduction of seat belt legislation, J Roy Soc Med 77:98-200, 1984.
31. Cole MD, Clearkin L, and Dabbs T: The seat belt law and after, Br J Ophthalmol 71:436-440, 1987.
32. Vinger PF: The eye and sports medicine. In Duane TD and Jaeger EA, editors: Clinical ophthalmology, vol 5, Philadelphia, 1985, Harper & Row.
33. Classé JG: Legal aspects of sports-related ocular injuries, Int Ophthalmol Clin 28:211-214, 1988.
34. Farley MK and Pettit TH: Traumatic wound dehiscence after penetrating keratoplasty, Am J Ophthalmol 104:44-49, 1987.
35. Glasgow BJ et al: Traumatic dehiscence of incisions seven years after radial keratotomy, Am J Ophthalmol 106:703-707, 1988.
36. Binder PS et al: Histopathology of traumatic corneal rupture after radial keratotomy, Arch Ophthalmol 106:1584-1590, 1988.

37. Pearlstein ES et al: Ruptured globe after radial keratotomy, Am J Ophthalmol 106:755-756, 1988.
38. Davis JK: Perspectives on impact resistance and polycarbonate lenses, Int Ophthalmol Clin 28: 215-218, 1988.
39. International Federation of Sports Medicine: Position statement: eye injuries and eye protection in sports, The Physician & Sportsmedicine 16:49-51, 1988.
40. Larrison WI, Hersh PS, and Shingleton BJ: Sports-related ocular trauma, Ophthalmology 97:1265, 1990.

CHAPTER 37

Medicolegal considerations

PHILIP A. SHELTON

Basic malpractice issues
- Requirements for litigation to proceed

Specific applications to eye trauma and emergency care
- Duty
  - Emergency department care and coverage
  - Follow-up to and from other emergency room physicians
  - Physician-patient relationship
  - Abandonment
  - Good Samaritan
- Standard of care
  - State of the art versus standard of care in the community
  - Record keeping
  - Consent
- Proximate cause—if problems develop
- Damages

General guidelines to avoid malpractice litigation

References

BASIC MALPRACTICE ISSUES

The ultimate dispute mechanism in our civilized society is the adversary proceeding, or court trial. The historical roots may lie in the selection of individual or tribal champions who fought in mortal combat for an idea, land, or principle in contention. The mechanism, now highly stylized and more complex, still consists of a referee (judge), two or more adversaries (parties), their champions (attorneys), and a finder of facts (jury). The rationale for this system is that it is thought to be the best way to discover the truth.

Unfortunately, the abrasive aspects of the adversary system often evoke angry, confused, and indignant responses from the physician who is not trained in the rules of the system or familiar with its mechanisms. These responses are uniformly counterproductive. It is important, therefore, to maintain a posture of equanimity when confronted by the unexpected or unfamiliar.

Requirements for Litigation to Proceed

To prevail in a malpractice suit, the plaintiff must prove each of four elements:

1. The physician had a duty to the patient.
2. The physician breached the applicable standard of care (negligence).
3. The negligent act or omission was the cause of damage.
4. There was, in fact, damage.

SPECIFIC APPLICATIONS TO EYE TRAUMA AND EMERGENCY CARE

Duty

Emergency Department Care and Coverage

Trauma is often first treated in the emergency department of a general hospital. The clear duty of the initial examiner (the emergency room physician or nurse) is to triage, or sort, the various problems presented. In general, there is a three-category system.

Emergency—injuries that threaten life or limb if not treated immediately. Typically, eye injuries are not in this group unless associated with a multiple trauma involving other head or chest injuries with immediate threat to the respiratory or cardiovascular system.

Urgent—injuries that require prompt but not immediate care. Eye injuries are typically in this group.

Nonurgent—injuries whose care can be delayed for some period of time without adverse effect. These include (1) chronic conditions that have been tolerated for some time, have typically developed slowly, and need to be treated but for which time is not a critical factor (e.g., chronic headaches, sprains, arthritis) and (2) conditions that do not need medical care.

It is the responsibility of the hospital or institution to set the standards and guidelines for the person acting as triage officer.

Follow-up to and from Other Emergency Room Physicians

If the rules or regulations of the hospital or its department of ophthalmology require referral to a specialist under specific circumstances and such referral is not made, the violation of such rules, regulations, and standards may be introduced as evidence of negligence *(Darling v. Charleston Community Memorial Hospital)*.[1]

Even in the absence of specific written guidelines, rules, or regulations, the emergency room physician or any physician is duty bound to refer a patient to a specialist if the patient's condition requires a degree of knowledge, skill, or training that is not commensurate with the physician's *(Lewis v. Soriano)*.[2]

The 1985 case of *Marles v. Mandel*[3] held that the national and local standard for on-call systems is to have a specialist able to see the patient within 30 minutes of the time called in the case of a thoracic surgeon. The defendant hospital had a published policy adopting this standard. The attending thoracic surgeon could not be found for over 1 hour and arrived 20 minutes after notification. The patient died despite immediate surgery. The court held that the jury should have been allowed to determine whether the hospital or the physician should be held responsible for the failure of the on-call system.

Judgmental errors may be the basis for liability only where there is failure to comply with recognized medical standards that would be exercised by similar physicians under similar circumstances. Such liability may be founded upon failure to visit the patient promptly when called *(Riggs v. Christie)*.[4] An incorrect diagnosis may lead to failure to properly attend the patient *(Willard v. Hutson)*.[5]

Physician-Patient Relationship

The duty of the physician to treat the patient arises most commonly from a voluntary agreement based on the implied promise by the physician to care for the patient and a promise by the patient to pay for the services rendered.

In an emergency situation, however, the physician's duty may arise from undertaking to provide treatment even though there may be no intent ever to charge for the services and no consensual promise by the patient ever to pay. Hence the courts often find the existence of a physician-patient relationship where the physician merely undertakes or begins treatment to or on behalf of the patient.

An example of such minimal undertaking is found in the case of *Giallanz v. Sands*.[6] The defendant physician, who was sick and on the inactive staff of a hospital, was contacted by the director of a drug rehabilitation center a few blocks from the hospital and told that the center had a female client with a high fever and signs of overdose. Dr. Strack (the defendant physician) told the director to take the woman to the hospital emergency room and tell them he had "recommended" that she be seen. The physician went to the hospital the next day and wrote on the chart the information he had received from the clinic director. He never met the patient, examined her, made any diagnosis, or suggested any therapy. She subsequently died of meningitis, allegedly because of negligent misdiagnosis and treatment. Despite the absence of contact between the doctor and the patient, the appellate court refused to dismiss Dr. Strack from the case, holding that he did not use good judgment in allowing his name to be used to admit a patient he never met or intended to meet.

From this case and others it is clear that if a specialist physician is contacted by an emergency room physician and gives any advice or the appearance of any advice (including suggesting a follow-up in the morning) a physician-patient relationship has been undertaken.

The Virginia case of *Lyons v. Graether*[7]

seems to outline the minimum contact necessary to establish the duty, or doctor-patient, relationship. A new patient with a specific complaint (vaginal infection) made an appointment to see the doctor. When she arrived at the physician's office, he refused to see her because she was accompanied by her seeing-eye dog. He made no effort to recommend another physician. She delayed finding another gynecologist and suffered harm thereby. The court stated that the physician, through his employee, had made an appointment to see the patient at a specific time for a specific problem and that at the least he was duty bound to refer her elsewhere for care that he had not provided. Thus, your staff can make you liable without your having seen or even spoken to the patient.

Abandonment

Once initiated, the physician-patient relationship continues until it is dissolved by mutual consent of the parties or by the patient's unilateral dismissal of the physician.

The physician can unilaterally terminate the relationship only by giving the patient adequate notice or arranging for suitable care by another physician. Failure to do this when there is an existing need for medical services may allow the physician to be held liable for abandonment. It is necessary that the act of abandonment be the proximate (legal) cause of the damages suffered by the patient, or there will be no liability.

Good Samaritan

The first Good Samaritan statute was enacted in California in 1959. The objective of this and all subsequent statutes was to encourage the physician to render emergency aid on highways and other public places. The various state laws are all different except for their brevity. They all generally hold that the physician (or in some cases any volunteer) shall not be liable for injuries alleged to have been suffered as a result of an act or omission of an act in rendering first aid unless the volunteer was grossly negligent or rendered less than "ordinary care." Most statutes require that the aid be rendered gratuitously.

Some Good Samaritans have been held liable to the victim if the volunteer's actions worsened the victim's condition by increasing the danger, leading the victim to believe incorrectly that the danger was past, or inducing the victim to forgo help from others.[8]

Standard of Care

State of the Art versus Standard of Care in the Community

The standard of care typically quoted is, "that degree of skill and learning ordinarily used under the same or similar circumstances by members of the profession." For ophthalmology, all jurisdictions use at least a statewide, and most now use a national, standard. In *McCormack v. Linberg*[9] and *Logan v. Greenwich Hospital Association*,[10] the court specifically held that the standard of care for a specialist is national, not local, and that a specialist must be held to the same standard of care as other specialists in the field. It also generally required that expert testimony be called to establish a breach of this standard since such matters are beyond the competence of the lay jury. The major exception is called *res ipsa loquitur*, or "the thing speaks for itself." This doctrine, if applicable, allows the case to go to the jury without expert medical testimony to support it. The general rule is that the circumstances must be of such a character that a layperson is able to say as a matter of common knowledge and observation, that the consequences of professional treatment were not such as ordinarily would have followed had due care been exercised. Thus the *res ipsa* doctrine generally applies to sponges left in operative sites. *Res ipsa* has specifically been ruled inapplicable in ophthalmology cases of viral corneal infection occurring postthyroidectomy (*Merrit v. Deaconess Hospital et al*[11]), of endophthalmitis occurring during cataract surgery (*Adams v. EENT Hospital et al*[12] and *Schofield v. Idaho Falls Latter Day Saints Hospital*[13]), and of retinal detachment following a cataract extraction with vitreous loss (*Stundon v. Stadnick*[14]).

In the area of ophthalmic plastic and reconstructive surgery, *res ipsa* has also been ruled inapplicable in cases of infection following scar excision (*Pink v. Slater*[15]), corneal scarring due to lagophthalmos following rhizotomy (*Wagner v. Olmedo*[16]), and ptosis following lid block anesthesia for pterygium excision (*Charlton v. Montefiore*[17]).

By far the most important change in the standard of care is represented in a trilogy of Washington state cases: *Helling v. Carey*[18] (1974), *Gates v. Jensen*[19] (1979), and *Harris v. Groth*[20] (1983).

The Helling court concluded that the failure to test for glaucoma in patients under 40 was negligent in spite of uncontradicted expert testimony that this was not the standard of care. The court invoked a judicially determined standard of care based on a 1932 T. J. Hooper[21] decision, in which a tugboat had damaged its barges in tow in stormy seas because of failure to have a radio receiver that would have given an updated weather report. Tugs did not usually carry radio receivers, but Judge Learned Hand said in the opinion, "Courts must in the end say what is required; there are precautions so imperative that even their universal disregard will not excuse their omission."

Following the Helling case, the Washington State legislature redefined the standard of care as the exercising of that degree of skill, care, and learning *possessed* by other persons in the same profession. The court in *Gates v. Jensen* held that this is a much broader standard than exercising the degree of skilled care and learning *practiced* by other persons in the same profession. This "reasonable prudence" test may therefore require a standard of practice higher than that exercised by the medical profession. Thus the court found for the plaintiff against the defendant ophthalmologist, who failed to do visual fields and a dilated fundus examination in a patient whose tension was in the glaucoma suspect range and who subsequently suffered damage to her optic nerves.

The most recent case in this trilogy, *Harris v. Groth*, was won by the ophthalmologist because the jury instruction requested by the plaintiff was overly broad and did not correctly state the law. It is questionable at best if angle closure glaucoma in this case could have been detected by measuring intraocular pressure. However, the court reiterated its view that a "reasonable prudence" standard is applicable in the state of Washington rather than an "average practitioner" standard. No other state has yet followed this "reasonable prudence," or court-imposed, standard, but the trend seems to be in that direction.

In summary, there seems to be a tendency to extend the required standard of care beyond that ordinarily *used* by members of the profession locally to that level of skill, care, and learning *possessed* by other professionals, often on a national level. In making this decision, the court will balance ability, impact, and cost. This tends to accelerate the speed by which the standard of care approaches the state of the art.[22]

Record Keeping

Medical records are essential to the defense against medical malpractice actions. The records are admitted as evidence under the Hearsay Rule's Business Record exception. This means that they are presumed to be accurate and truthful. This exception states that contemporaneously recorded data made in the usual course of business for business purposes may be admitted without the usual safeguards of truth such as an oath, cross examination, and viewing by the jury. However, the opposing party can challenge the presumption that the records are accurate and truthful and attempt to show that they are biased, prejudiced, or untrue. Therefore, any alteration or even well-meaning changes made in these records can be disastrous to the defense.

Since malpractice suits may often be litigated 2 to 5 years after the treatment in question, the office or hospital medical record is often the only detailed record of what actually occurred. Negligent failure to maintain these records for the statutory required period of time, or intentional destruction of medical records needed by a plaintiff to proceed with a claim, has led to court rulings that shifted the burden of proof so that defendants had to attempt to prove themselves nonnegligent rather than leave the proof to the plaintiff.

Consent

In early malpractice cases the touching of a person's body without consent was a "battery." The modern view is that the standard of care requires the physician to inform the patient of the nature of the proposed treatment, alternative therapies (including none), and the risks and reasonably expected benefits of each therapy, and only then to secure consent. A growing minority of states have ruled that the disclosure should be such that a reasonable patient could make an intelligent choice based on its contents. This standard does not require expert witness testimony as to the usual actions of physicians in the specialty.

In the majority of states, however, the standard of disclosure required is "measured by those communications a reasonable practitioner in the same branch of medicine would make under the same or similar circumstances." In addition, these states require expert medical evidence to establish this standard.

The 1984 case of *Welch v. Whitaker*[23] concurred in the directed verdict in favor of the ophthalmologist who allegedly failed to warn the patient of the possibility of corneal scarring subsequent to the removal of a corneal foreign body and rust ring. No expert medical evidence was presented by the patient-plaintiff on the issues of the standard of disclosure, the standard of care of removal of the foreign body, and the proximate cause of the corneal scarring.

In the vast majority of states, the patient-plaintiff must then prove that a reasonable patient, as well as the individual plaintiff, would not have given consent having been informed of the risk or outcome that actually transpired.

Some exceptions to the informed consent doctrine relieve the physician of the duty to fully disclose. Medical emergencies and patient incompetency (which may require guardian consent) are clear examples. Voluntary waiver, where the patient knowingly and intelligently declines to be informed in order to reduce the anxiety upon disclosure, is a rarely used but available exception. The most controversial exception is the therapeutic one, where it is *clearly* poor medical practice and potentially harmful to the patient's health to fully disclose the risks. The problem with the therapeutic exception is to balance the individual patient's right to make informed decisions against society's policy, which encourages procedures needed to maintain a healthy populace.

The trend seems to be toward the reasonable patient standard of disclosure, with physicians having almost no relief from the requirement of an exhaustive recitation of all possible alternatives and complications, even those they may never have encountered. This pendulum has swung to the extreme, and the hope that some counterforce is due may be apparent in *Hook v. Rothstein*.[24] In this case the court pointed out that the physician should be concerned with the patient's best interests and not what a lay jury, untrained in medicine and employing perfect hindsight, might later conclude should have been disclosed (Referral to dissent in *Scaria v. St. Paul Fire and Marine Insurance Company*[25]). However, if a state-of-the-art alternative is safe, effective, and of reasonable cost and availability, it should be disclosed, even if not recommended.

Proximate Cause—If Problems Develop

Once plaintiffs have demonstrated a breach (negligence) in the applicable standard of care, they must connect the negligent act or omission with the damage suffered. The standard for proving causation requires expert testimony.

In most jurisdictions the defendant-physician may be called by the plaintiff as a fact witness, but jurisdictions vary as to whether the defendant-physician may be used by the plaintiff as a medical expert. In most states defendants are subject only to questions about facts and are not required to give their expert medical opinion. Local legal guidance on this point is essential (*McDermott v. Manhattan Eye and Ear Hospital*[26]).

In *Hall v. Bacon*[27] the plaintiff was not entitled to recover against his physicians even if they were negligent in failing to diagnose and notify him of his injury. No expert evidence was offered that the 36-day delay in diagnosis of a fractured orbit caused fat atrophy and enophthalmos. In fact, the plaintiff's expert said that a delay in surgery was indicated in the presence of excessive facial swelling, which was present in this case. In addition, the prolongation of pain and suffering was not actionable in the absence of expert testimony that the cause of pain and suffering was the failure to diagnose the orbital fracture earlier.

Damages

Damages in ophthalmology cases are usually clearly evident and measurable by such yardsticks as loss of visual acuity or field, diplopia, cosmetic defects, and lost wages. Pain and suffering, although subjective, can be objectively valued by the jury upon persuasive evidence.

One interesting case held that a patient does *not* have a duty to submit to cataract surgery in order to reduce the damages caused by malpractice (*Frisnegger v. Gibson*[28]). The patient sustained a cataract subsequent to the perforation of his eye by the defendant ophthalmologist, who was injecting the eyelid preparatory to chalazion removal. The patient suffered severe depression and refused removal of the cataract, which had incapacitated him. This trial approved a reasonable person test for the jury to determine if damages should be reduced rather than the mandatory test requested by the defendant.

GENERAL GUIDELINES TO AVOID MALPRACTICE LITIGATION

It is often a traumatic and frightening experience for an ophthalmologist to be involved as a defendant in a medical malpractice suit. The initial shock should not precipitate irrational or angry behavior, which is counterproductive to the physician's interests. Cooperation with one's attorney is essential to securing the best possible defense. Although even a careful and competent ophthalmologist may be subject to nonmeritorious claims, avoidance of malpractice litigation is enhanced by following a few simple rules.

1. Be kind to your patients. Nothing breeds litigation like hostility.
2. Keep good records. They are essential to your defense and unparalleled as the best available evidence.
3. Inform your patients of all the possibilities. Only the physician can ask, "Do you understand what you have read or been told? If not, what are your questions?"
4. Don't be afraid of second opinions. They increase your stature in the patient's view.[29]
5. Write letters. Document your records with return-receipt-requested letters discharging patients, following up on significant no-shows, explaining complex points to patients, and so on.
6. Be careful what you say about others. Careless words may entrap another physician in a needless malpractice suit. If your remark was malicious (that "butcher," "quack," etc.), you may be sued for slander. Be wary of violating patient privacy and confidentiality by remarks over the phone that may be overheard.
7. Train, monitor, and control your employees. They are your agents when acting within the scope of their employment. Have written job descriptions and protocols to be followed in all phases of the work. From telephone manners and questions to the technical aspects of fundus photography and other procedures, your staff's negligence will usually be viewed as your own.[30]

References

1. *Darling v Charleston Community Memorial Hospital*, 33 Ill 2d 326, 50 Ill App 2 253, 86 Sup Ct 1204 Cert den.
2. *Lewis v Soriano*, 374 So2d 829, Miss, 1979.
3. *Marles v Mandel*, 477 So2d 1036, Florida District Court App, 1985.
4. *Riggs v Christie*, 342 Mass 402 173 NE2d 610, 1961.
5. *Willard v Hutson*, 234 Ore 148 378 P2d 966, 1963.
6. *Giallanz v Sands*, 316 So2d 77, Florida District Court App 1975.
7. *Lyons v Graether*, 239 SE2d 103, Va, 1977.
8. Annot 64ALR 2d 1181.
9. *McCormack v Linberg*, 352 NW2d 30 Minn App, 1984.
10. *Logan v Greenwich Hospital Association*, 465 A2d 294, Conn, 1983.
11. *Merritt v Deaconess Hospital et al*, 357 NE2d 65, Ohio, 1975.
12. *Adams v EENT Hospital et al*, La App, 346 SO2d 327, La, 1977.
13. *Schofield v Idaho Falls Latter Day Saints Hospital*, 409 P2d 107, Idaho, 1975.
14. *Stundon v Stadnick*, 469 P2d 16, Wyo, 1981.
15. *Pink v Slater*, 218 P2d 272, Calif, 1955.
16. *Wagner v Olmedo*, 365 A2d 643, Del, 1976.
17. *Charlton v Montefiore*, 45 Misc Rep 2d 153, Sup Ct, Queens, NY, 1/15/65.
18. *Helling v Carey*, 519, P2d981, Wash, 1974.
19. *Gates v Jensen*, 595 P2d, 919, Wash, 1979.
20. *Harris v Groth*, 663 P2d 113, Wash, 1983.
21. The TJ Hooper, 60 F2d 737, 2nd Cir, 1932.
22. Shelton PA: Start of the art v. the standard of care, Int J Cataract Surg 1:7-16, 1984.
23. *Welch v Whitaker*, 317 SE2d 758, SC App, 1984.
24. *Hook v Rothstein*, 16 SE2d 690, SC App, 1984.
25. Referral to dissent in *Scaria v St Paul Fire and Marine Insurance Company*, 227 NW2d 647, 659, 1975.
26. *McDermott v Manhattan Eye and Ear Hospital*, 16 App Div Rep 2d 374, NY, 1962.
27. *Hall v Bacon*, 453 P2d 816, Idaho, 1969.
28. *Frisnegger v Gibson*, 598 P2d 574 Mont, 1979.
29. Shelton PA: Second opinions—a guide to the perplexed, Int J Cataract Surg 2:3-34, 1985.
30. Shelton PA: Vicarious liability and the employer/employee relationship, Int J Cataract Surg 1:2-20, 1984.

APPENDIX

Guidelines for tetanus prophylaxis

TERESA P. KUNZWILER

Primary immunization
Tetanus prophylaxis

Tetanus is a serious disease with a fatality rate of 26% (52% for patients over age 60). Although preventable with appropriate immunization, the average number of cases reported annually remains stable at 90 per year.[1-5]

Clostridium tetani, the causative bacteria, are anaerobes with a generalized distribution. They have been recovered from soil, feces, fresh and salt water, and household dirt. In reported cases from 1982 to 1984, 41% followed indoor injuries, 39% followed gardening and other outdoor injuries, 4% followed animal-related injuries, 4% followed major trauma, and 12% arose from other and unknown circumstances.[1] Approximately two thirds of patients were 50 years of age or older. Universal primary immunization, with subsequent maintenance of adequate antitoxin levels through appropriately timed boosters, is necessary to protect persons in all age groups.

PRIMARY IMMUNIZATION

Primary immunization[2,3] for tetanus consists of a series of three injections given at timed intervals. A routine diphtheria, pertussis, and tetanus immunization (DPT) is recommended for children under age 7. The initial dose is given at age 6 weeks or older, the second dose 4 to 8 weeks later, and the third dose 4 to 8 weeks later. A tetanus, diphtheria (Td) injection is recommended for adults every 10 years to maintain active immunization. Adults with an uncertain history of a completed primary series should receive the primary series. Recent serologic surveys have shown that half of all persons over 60 years of age lack the protective antibody against tetanus toxoid.

TETANUS PROPHYLAXIS

When prophylaxis is indicated in children under age 7, the use of DPT is advised. After age 7 the use of Td is indicated for prophylaxis. The standard dose is 0.5 ml given intramuscularly.

Patients with an unknown or negative history of tetanus vaccination should be considered nonimmunized and for prophylaxis may require passive immunization with tetanus immune globulin (TIG). The recommended dose is 250 units given intramuscularly. Passive immunization provides protection for approximately 4 weeks. Td and TIG administered at the same session are given in different syringes at separate sites. Arrangement of appropriate follow-up to complete the immunization series is recommended.

Although there have been no documented cases of tetanus secondary to eye injuries, pa-

Table A-1. Tetanus prophylaxis for various patient histories and wounds

Immunization history	Type of wound	Prophylaxis
Complete immunization (3 or more doses)	Clean, minor	Less than 10 years since immunization, no booster necessary More than 10 years since immunization, 1 dose Td
	Tetanus-prone	More than 5 years since immunization, 1 dose Td (more frequent boosters are not needed and can exacerbate side effects)
Uncertain immunization or less than 3 doses	Clean, minor	1 dose Td (DPT for under age 7); complete immunization series as appropriate
	Tetanus-prone	1 dose Td (DPT for children under age 7) and 1 dose TIG; separate syringes and injection sites; complete immunization series as appropriate

Explanation of abbreviations: Td, tetanus, diphtheria immunization; DPT, diphtheria, pertussis, and tetanus immunization; TIG, tetanus immune globulin.

tients with severe injuries should have their immunization status evaluated and appropriate immunization instituted (Table A-1).

Because the tetanus organism is a spore-forming anaerobe, it is unlikely to be a risk in minor, superficial corneal injuries. Clean injuries, such as ruptured globes caused by blunt trauma and simple lacerations without prolapsed tissue or retained foreign body, are probably at very low risk for tetanus. Eye injuries considered tetanus-prone include, but are not limited to, untreated lacerations and ruptures more than 6 hours old, wounds contaminated with soil or manure, lacerations incarcerated with retained prolapsed devitalized tissue, puncture wounds, and any wound with a retained foreign body.

In summary, the need for tetanus toxoid (active immunization) with or without TIG (passive immunization) depends on the nature of the wound, the interval since injury, and the patient's immunization history.

References

1. Tetanus—United States, 1982-1984, MMWR 34:602-611, 1985.
2. Advisory Committee on Immunization Practices: Diphtheria, tetanus, and pertussis: guidelines for vaccine prophylaxis and other preventive measures, MMWR 34:405-426, 1985.
3. LaForce FM: Immunizations, immunoprophylaxis, and chemoprophylaxis to prevent selected infections, JAMA 257:2464-2470, 1987.
4. Beeson P, McDermott W, and Wyngaarden J: Cecil textbook of medicine, Philadelphia, 1979, WB Saunders, 436-441.
5. Braunwald E et al: Harrison's principles of internal medicine, ed 11, New York, 1987, McGraw-Hill, 558-561.

Index

A

Abandonment, 405
Abducens nerve, 283
  injury to, 383
Abrasions, of orbital soft tissue, 287-288
Acanthamoeba keratitis, 76-77
Acid burns
  clinical course and therapy for, 89-90
  etiology, 89
  pathophysiology, 89
Afferent pupillary defect (APD), 12
  with penetrating ocular trauma, 239-240
Aircraft, cabin pressure and humidity in, 23
Air embolization, 190
Airway obstruction, with maxillofacial injuries, 53
Alkali burns
  anterior chamber and lens in, 82-83
  clinical course and evaluation, 83
    in acute phase, 83
    in early reparative phase, 83-84
    in immediate phase, 83
  endothelium in, 82
  epithelium in, 80-81
  etiology of, 80
  history for, 5-6
  Hughes classification of, 83
  medical therapy for, 84-86
  pathophysiology of, 80-83
  pH effect in, 80
  stroma in, 81-82
  surgical therapy for, 86-89
Allen picture cards, 58
Allyl resin lenses, 400
Alveolar nerves, 279
Amblyopia
  anisometropic, 56
  critical period in, 58
  detection of, 58-59
  factitious, 373
  minimization of, 134
  occlusion therapy for, 59
Amikacin, for endophthalmitis, 250
Aminoglycoside, 43
  for corneoscleral lacerations, 158
Amniocentesis, trauma from, 56
Amyloidosis, 289
Anesthesia
  complications and contraindications for, 49
  with enucleation, 355
  in eyelid laceration repair, 327
  for lacrimal system injuries, 336
  for lid injuries, 51-53
  management of, 50-51
  for ocular injuries, 47-51
  in open eye–full stomach patient, 50
  for orbital injuries, 53
  retrobulbar, 49-50
  risk of, 44
  subconjunctival, 48-49
  topical, 47-48
Aneurysms, internal carotid artery, 377
Animal bites
  affecting lacrimal system, 334
  epidemiology of, 347-348
  examination of, 348-349
  history of victim in, 8, 348
  incidence of, 347
  therapy for, 349-352
Anisocoria, 372-373
Antacid aspiration prophylaxis, 50
Anterior chamber
  alkali burns of, 82-83
  in chalcosis, 229
  examination of after injury, 16
  inflammatory process in, 16, 139-141
Anterior chamber angle
  changes in after trauma, 139-141
  fibrosis of, 139-141
  tissue damage of, 140*f*
Anterior chamber washout, 110-111
Anterior ciliary body, 117
Anterior rings of tissue, 117-118

Anterior segment
examination of, 12-17
intraocular foreign bodies in, 169-173
pathophysiology of wound healing in, 136-141
reconstruction of following ocular trauma, 175-183
reconstruction techniques for, 176-183
removal of membranes in, 180
results of reconstruction of, 183
tears in, 118*f*
Anterior segment trauma. *See also specific injuries*
associated with tissue disruption, 118-120
bleeding with, 120, 121*f*
response to, 120
Anterior stromal puncture technique, 72-73
Antibiotic ointment, 77
Antibiotics
for alkali burns, 84
for chemical injury, 91
for corneal epithelial defect, 76-77
for corneoscleral laceration management, 144
for dog bite prophylaxis, 351
for endophthalmitis prophylaxis, 246-248
for lid burn prophylaxis, 317
prophylactic, 43
systemic, 43
topical, 43
Antibodies, topical, for microbial keratitis, 68
Antifibrinolytic agents
side effects of, 109
for traumatic hyphema, 108-109
Antiglaucoma medications, for alkali burns, 84
Applanation tonometry, 18
Aqueous leakage, 16
Argon laser endophotocoagulation, 223*f*
Arteriography, for intraocular foreign bodies, 343
Artificial tears, 317
Ascorbate
for alkali burns, 85
for chemical injury, 91
Astigmatism
with dislocated lens, 129
effects of corneal injury on, 159-160
suture placement effects on, 160-164
"with-the-rule," 56
Autograft transplantation, 87
Autoimmune disease, in sympathetic ophthalmia etiology, 256
Avulsive injuries, repair of, 332

B

Bacillus cereus, in endophthalmitis, 243, 244
Bacillus infections, antibiotic prophylaxis for, 43
Bacterial infections, 242-243, 248
Balint's syndrome, 389
Bandage lens, 144-145
Bandage soft contact lens
for alkali burns, 84
for corneal lacerations, 144-145
for corneoscleral lacerations, 158
for intraocular foreign bodies, 171-172
for lid burn, 317
Barbiturates, 50-51
Bare light perception vision, 11
Basement membrane complex, regeneration of, 81
Battle signs, 53
Belle indifference, la, 21
Bell's phenomenon, 315, 316
quality of, 318
Berlin's edema. *See* Commotio retinae
Birth trauma, 56
Bjerrum scotomas, 376
Blepharoptosis, 361
Blindness
from eye injuries in childhood, 55
fear of, 44
optic nerve, 290-292
tests for total, 21-22
transient cortical, 378
Blood. *See also* Hemorrhage
aspiration of from eye, 216, 218*f*
in healing response, 208-209
pools of old, 216-217
subretinal, 219-221
Blowout fractures, 309
surgery for, 310
Blunt trauma
anterior tears with, 118*f*
conjunctival, 63-64
corneal, 65
glaucoma associated with, 120-122
history for, 7-8
lens injury with, 126
maculopathies with, 187
to orbital soft tissues, 287-293
to peripheral retina, 195-202
to posterior segment, 204-205
transient cortical blindness after, 378
treatment of, 122-124
to vitreous base, 198-199
Bone-free localization, 28
Bone grafts, autologous, 312-313
Bowman's layer, elastic qualities of, 137-138
Brain-stem injury, 388
Brain wounds, visual field defects with, 378
Bupivacaine (Marcaine), 48-49
as lid block, 51-52
Burns
acid, 89-90
alkali, 5-6, 80-89
eyelid, 315-322
thermal, 8

C

Caldwell projection, 25, 300, 302*f*
Caloric stimulation, 387
Canalicular repair, 335, 336
Canthotomy, lateral, 292
Canthus
  lateral, 293*f*
  medial, 275
Capillary microapplicator, 145
Capsular rupture, 151-152
  with lensectomy, 214
Care standards, 405-407
  state of the art versus standard in community, 405-406
Carotid artery, 262
  traumatic aneurysms of, 377
Carotid-cavernous fistulas, 276, 288-289, 385-386
Cataracts, 100*f*
  anterior surgical approach to, 130-132
  contusion, 126
    management of, 128-129
  extracapsular extraction and phacoemulsification of, 151
  extraction of, 215*f*
  intraocular lenses for, 134
  with traumatic hyphema, 106
Cautery, surface, 73
Cefazolin, 43
  for corneoscleral laceration management, 143-144
Cellulitis
  orbital, 291
  postoperative, 359
Cephalosporin, 43
  for corneoscleral lacerations, 158
Cerebellar injury, 388
Cerebrospinal fluid leakage, 53
Chalcosis, 229
  clinical findings for, 229
  clinical setting of, 228-229
  explanation of damage in, 229
  outcome of, 229
Charlton v. Montefiore, 405
Chemical injuries, 79-80
  acid, 89-90
  alkali, 80-89
  history for, 5-6
  incidence of, 315
  specific therapy for, 90-92
Chemosis, 106
  underlying injury with, 13
Chiasmal trauma, 377-378
Child abuse, 57-58
  historical and physical features in, 57
  laws mandating reporting of, 57-58
  ocular manifestations of, 57
  ophthalmic findings in, 57
Children
  amblyopia in, 58-59
  epidemiology of eye injury in, 55-56
  examination of, 56
  ocular injury rate in, 397-398
  traumatic hyphema with, 114
  unique forms of eye trauma in, 56-58
Chorioretinal adhesion, for giant retinal tears, 201
Choroidal injuries, 19
Choroidal neovascularization, 192
Choroidal rupture, 190-192
  treatment of, 192
Cicatrization, 320-321
Ciliary arteries, 281-282
Ciliary body
  attachment to scleral spur, 117
  exposure of face of, 139
  separation of from scleral spur, 119
  tear of, 119
Ciliary ganglion, 283
Cinematography, high-speed, 196
Citrate
  for alkali burns, 85
  for chemical injury, 91
Clindamycin, 43
  for corneoscleral lacerations, 158
Clinical evaluation, of injured eye and ocular adnexa, 3-23
Clostridium tetani infection, 44, 409
Clot formation, 106, 111
Cocaine, 48
Collagen, 136
  in healing response, 209
Collagenase
  in cornea, 81
  inhibitors of for alkali burns, 86
Collagen fibers, 136-137
Collagenolysis, with alkali burns of stroma, 81-82
Collagen shield, 74
Color confusion test, 22
Color vision testing, 372
Coma, ocular motor findings in, 387-388
Commotio retinae, 188-189, 205
Compression cyanosis, 190
Computed tomography (CT), 25
  drawback of in localization, 29
  image resolution in, 28-29
  in injured eye and orbit, 28-32
  for intraocular foreign bodies, 170, 343
  for lacrimal system evaluation, 335
  for optic nerve trauma, 374
  for orbital fracture, 305-307
  of orbits, 30, 284-286
  scans of, 29-31*f*
Concussion, edema with, 188-189
Concussive endotheliopathy, 15

Confounding factors, identification of, 4
Conjunctiva, 274
  edema of, 63
  evaluation of for injury, 11
  examination of after injury, 13
  persistent prolapse of, 293
  postoperative cysts of, 362
  transplantation, 74-75
Conjunctival adhesions, lysis of, 91
Conjunctival injury
  blunt trauma, 63-64
  foreign body, 64
  laceration, 64-65
Conjunctival peritomy, 292
Conjunctivodacryocystorhinostomy, 339
Connective tissue, wound healing of, 323-324
Contrecoup, 126
  mechanism of, 187
Contusion injury, 205
  histopathology of in animal models, 208
  ocular motor dysfunction with, 381-382
  to orbital soft tissue, 288
Cornea. *See also* Corneal epithelium; Corneal injuries; Corneal lacerations
  abrasion of, 64*f*, 68
    multiple, 13*f*
    with traumatic hyphema, 106
    treatment for, 68
  acid burns of, 89
  bloodstaining of, 110, 113
  in chalcosis, 229
  contents of, 136-137
  discontinuities of, 14
  edema and supporation of, 14-15
  effects of penetrating injury on, 159-160
  effects of suture placement on, 160-164
  endothelial healing in, 138
  epithelial healing in, 138
  examination of after injury, 14-16
  foreign bodies in, 14
  functional component of, 136
  healing anomalies in, 138
  mechanism of ulceration and repair with alkali injury, 82*f*
  normal and flattened contours of, 165*f*
  pathophysiology of wound healing in, 137-139
  penetration of, 95
  rupure of, 65
  stromal healing in, 138
  sutures used on, 146-148
  swelling of, 15
  symmetrical contours of, 160*f*
  thinning of after chemical burn, 91-92
  vascularization of, 167
Corneal collagen fibers, 136-137
Corneal epithelium
  defect, erosion and ulceration of, 68-70
  healing of, 138
  infected ulceration of, 75-76
    treatment of, 76-77
  morphology of defect, erosion and ulceration of, 69*f*
  persistent defect and noninfected stromal ulceration of, 73
    therapy for, 73-75
  recurrent erosion of, 70-73
  ultraviolet radiation and electrical injury of, 77
Corneal injury, 68
  blunt trauma, 65
  foreign body, 65-67
  infected ulceration, 75-77
  pathogenesis in, 68-70
  persistent epithelial defect and noninfected stromal ulceration, 73-75
  recurrent erosion of, 70-73
  ultraviolet radiation and electrical, 77
Corneal lacerations, 14
  with iris incarceration, 149-151
  with lens involvement, 151-152
  nonperforating, 144-145
  repair of, 95-96
  simple full-thickness, 145-149
  stellate, suturing of, 166-167
  suture placement in, 164-167
  suture removal from, 167-168
  suture tightening in, 167
  suturing techniques for, 164-168
    topographic considerations and, 159-168
  with vitreous involvement, 152
Corneoscleral injury
  anterior segment sequelae of, 175
  rupture, 106
Corneoscleral lacerations
  injury hierarchy and repair technique for, 144-157
  irreparable penetrating, 157
  management of, 143-158
  postoperative management of, 157-158
  preoperative management of, 143-144
  simple, 152-153
  with tissue loss, 155-157
  with uveal and vitreous prolapse, 154-155
Corneoscopy, 168
Corrugator muscle, 265
  superciliaris, 267-268
Cortical blindness, transient, 378
Corticosteroids
  for alkali burns, 85
  for chemical injury, 91
  for corneoscleral lacerations, 158
  for endophthalmitis, 249-250
  for periorbital swelling, 292

Corticosteroids—cont'd
  for sympathetic ophthalmia, 257
Coup injury, 126, 187
Cranial nerves, 261-262
  five, 278
  seventh
    injury to, 387
      superficial, 266*f*
Crawford hook, 337
Crawford intubation, 336, 337*f*
Crushing injury, 288
Cryotherapy, 221
Cyanoacrylate tissue adhesive, 44, 67, 178
  for corneal lacertions, 145-146
Cyclodialysis cleft, 117
Cyclodialysis spatula, 96
Cycloplegia, 76
  for iris injury, 97
  topical, 77
Cycloplegics
  for alkali burns, 85
  for chemical injury, 91
  for traumatic hyphema, 108
Cyclosporin A, 257
Cytotoxic drugs, 257

D

Dacryocystorhinostomy, 336, 339
Dalen-Fuchs nodules, 254, 256*f*
  histology of, 255
Deprivation amblyopia, 59
Descemet's membrane
  elastic qualities of, 137-138
  rupture of, 56, 65
Dexamethasone, 249
  ointment, 70
Diagnostic imaging, 25-38. *See also specific techniques*
Diathermy, 73
  bimanual bipolar, 150-151, 173
  for giant retinal tears, 201
Dilation, 18
Documentation, 45
Dog bites, 347
  adjunct medical therapy for, 350-351
  decontamination of, 349, 350
  epidemiology of, 347-348
  examination of, 348-349
  incidence of, 347
  postoperative care of, 351-352
  surgical repair of, 350
  therapy for, 349-352
  victim history in, 348
Double elevator palsy, 381
Duane's retraction syndrome, 381
Dysgonic Fermenter-2, 348
Dyspraxia, 389

E

Edema, soft tissue, 288-289
Electrical burns
  to cornea, 77
  effects of, 315-316
Electrocautery, 359
Electromagnets, 230
  case selection for, 230
  extractions with, 231*f*
  surgical technique with, 230-232
Electrophysiologic testing, 22
Electrophysiology, 373
Electroretinogram (ERG)
  in acute setting, 20-21
  in siderosis, 228
Elschnig's pearls, 141
Emergency department, care and coverage in, 403-404
Emergency room, physicians' duty in, 404
Emphysema, orbital, 290, 299
Endodiathermy, 219, 221*f*
  unimanual bipolar, 222
Endolaser photocoagulation, 221
  for retinal tears, 234
Endophthalmitis, 365
  infectious, 17
  posttraumatic, 43, 242
    antibiotic prophylaxis and therapy for, 246-248
    diagnosis of, 243-246
    fungal, 246, 248
    guidelines for management of, 247
    management of, 250
    microbiology of, 242-243
    prevention of, 158
    prognosis for, 250-251
    recommended drug therapy for, 245-246
    steroids for, 249-250
    vitrectomy for, 248-249
Endothelium, alkali burns of, 82
Enucleation, 354
  advantages of, 355
  blepharoptosis with, 361
  complications of, 359-362
  conjunctival cysts with, 362
  deferral of, 44
  globe perforation with, 359
  hemorrhage with, 359
  implant migration in, 360-361
  indications for, 354-355
  infection with, 359
  limitations of, 355
  orbit injury with, 359

Enucleation—cont'd
procedure of, 355-359
socket contracture with, 361-362
for sympathetic ophthalmia, 257-258
Epidemiology studies, 395
Epidermal growth factor (EGF)
for alkali burns, 86
for corneal wounds, 138
Epiphora, 298
Epithelium. *See also* Corneal epithelium
alkaline burns of, 80-81
wound healing of, 323
Ethmoidal wall fracture, 308
Ethmoid sinuses, 279-280
fracture of, 63-64
Etidocaine (Duranest), 48, 49
Evisceration, 354
advantages of, 362-363
complications of, 365-366
indications for, 354, 362-363
with kertectomy, 364-365
limitations of, 363
with retention of cornea, 363-364
surgical procedure for, 363-365
Examination
anterior segment, 12-17
approach to patient in, 8
in children, 56
ERG and VEP in acute setting, 20-21
external, 9-11
of extraocular motility, 12
goal of, 8
of intraocular pressure, 18
of optic nerve, 19-20
of pupils, 11-12
technique of, 8-9
for visual acuity, 11
of visual fields, 12
of vitreous body and retina, 18-19
Excimer laser, 73
Exophthalmos, posttraumatic, 296
Extraocular motility testing, 12
Extraocular muscles, 284
Eye. *See also specific parts*
clinical evaluation of, 3-23
drainage from, 342
evulsion of, 56
injuries to
epidemiology of in children, 55-56
history for, 4-8
infectious risk factors to, 43
initial evaluation of, 3-4
instability of, 41
management problems with, 41
mechanical risk factors to, 42-43
occult or unsuspected, 8-9
self-inflicted in children, 56-57
Eye. *See also specific parts*—cont'd
injuries to—cont'd
with systemic injury, 41
time limitation in, 41
Eyebrow
anatomy of, 266-268
skin, 267
Eye-injured patient
decreasing risk to health of, 44
evaluation of, 23
maximizing surgical success for, 43-44
minimizing psychic trauma of, 44-45
minimizing risk of further injury to, 42-44
minimizing risk of legal involvement with, 45
pediatric, 55-59
preoperative check list for, 45
preparation of for surgery, 41-45
pretransport therapy for, 22-23
Eye Injury Registry of Alabama, 395
Eyelid. *See* Lids
Eye movement
central disorders of, 387-398
hypoxic effects on, 389
Eye protectors, 399-401
Eye shield protection, 9
for preoperative patient, 42
Eye-trauma patient. *See* Eye-injured patient
Eye trauma surgeons, risk of liability in, 41
Eye trauma surgery. *See also* Surgery; *specific procedures and techniques*
goals of preparation for, 41-42
management problems in, 41
maximizing success of, 43-44
minimizing risk of legal involvement with, 45
preparation of patient for, 41-45

F

Face
areas of step-off in, 11
arterial supply to, 262
evaluation of injuries to, 10
examination of in eye trauma, 9-11
lymphatic supply to, 262-265
motor nerves in, 266
muscles of expression in, 265-266
sensory innervation of, 261-262
soft tissues of, 261-266
venous supply to, 262
Face mask/helmet, 400
Facial muscles, 265-266
Facial nerve akinesia, 49-50
Facial nerve block, 42
Facial symmetry, 261
Facial veins, 262
Fibrinolytic agents, 109

Fibroblast growth factor, 138
Fibroblasts
  with nonpenetrating injury, 122
  with posterior segment injury, 206-207
Fibronectin, 86
Fibrous ingrowth, 122, 123*f*, 205-206
Fires, residental, 315
Flieringa ring, 177
Fluorescein angiography, 188
  for choroidal rupture, 191-192
  of macular holes, 193
  for sympathetic ophthalmia, 254
Fluorescein staining, 65
Forced-choice preferential looking tests, 58
Forced-duction testing, 12, 299-300
Foreign bodies. *See also* Intraocular foreign bodies (IOFBs)
  anterior segment intraocular, 169-173
  in cornea, 14
  CT scan of, 29*f*
  culturing of, 67
  deeply embedded in cornea, 67
  intraorbital, 341-346
  in lacrimal system injuries, 334-335
  perforating eye, 226
  plain film localization of, 25-26, 28
  in posterior segment, 19
  posterior segment intraocular, 44, 226-235
  removal of from cornea, 66-67
  retained, 5
  traction bands in track of, 205
  ultrasound localization of, 35
  vitreous, 19
Foreign-body injury
  checklist for, 6-7
  conjunctival, 13, 64
  corneal, 65-67
  history for, 6-7
Frontalis muscle, 267
Frontal sinuses, 280
Fundus
  lesions of, 190, 193
    intervention for, 187
  retroillumination from, 15*f*
  traumatic macular hole in, 191*f*
Funduscopy, 373
Fungal infections, in endophthalmitis, 242-243, 248

G

Galea aponeurotica, 268
Gates v. Jensen, 406
Gavaris monocanalicular tube, 339
Gaze paretic nystagmus, 388
Gentamicin, 43
Ghost cell glaucoma, 124
Giallanz v. Sands, 404
Glare, 97-98
Glass spectacle lenses, 400
Glaucoma
  acute without hemorrhage, 120-121
  angle recession, 122
    chronic, 121-122
  associated with blunt injury to angle, 120-122
  borderline open-angle, 122
  ghost cell, 124
  histopathologic changes with, 122
  from inflammation of anterior segment, 128
  with optic nerve injury, 20
  pupillary block, 112
  in siderosis, 228
  with trabecular meshwork healing, 119
  traumatic, 117-124
  with traumatic hyphema, 112-113
  treatment of, 122-124
Glaucoma medications, 91
Globe
  abnormal position of, 9, 324
  asymmetry of, 296
  compression of, 195
  displacement of with orbital fracture, 295-296
  perforation of, 210, 359
  phases of deformation of, 196*f*
  posterior view of, 285*f*
  ptosis of, 311
  ruptured, 56
    management of, 213
    precautions for, 9
  traumatic deformation of, 197*f*
  unstable with corneoscleral lacerations, 153
Goggles, 401
Gonioscopy, 16, 120
  with chronic glaucoma, 121
  for intraocular foreign bodies, 170
Goniosynechialysis, 179-180
  results of, 183
Good Samaritan statute, 405
Guibor-type probe, 336
Gunshot wounds, 7

H

Hall v. Bacon, 407
Harris v. Groth, 406
Head injury
  oculomotor nerve palsy from, 385
  principles of treatment of, 371-372
Helling v. Carey, 405-406
Helmets, 400
Hemidesmosomes, 68
Hemoglobin electrophoresis, 107

Hemorrhage
with enucleation, 359
"flame," 19
MRI of, 37
soft tissue, 289
subretinal, 219-221
High-risk groups, 398-399
History
importance of, 4
past ocular and medical, 5
of prior treatment, 5
of specific injuries, 5-8
of trauma event, 4-5
Hook v. Rothstein, 407
Horizontal gaze, 388
Horner's muscle, 275
Horner's syndrome, 386
Hospital-based epidemiological data, 396
Hounsfield artifacts, 29
Hull burr, 313
Hydrochloric acid, 89
Hydrofluoric acid, 89
Hydroxymethyl cellulose (Celluvisc), 74
Hypersideremia, 228
Hyperventilation, to reduce intracranial hypertension, 53
Hyphema, traumatic, 104
associated ocular findings, 105-106
causes and demographics of, 104
in children, 114
classification of, 105
clinical outcomes and prognosis for, 114
clot formation and dissolution in, 106
complications of, 112-113
evaluation of, 107
mechanism of injury in, 105
pathophysiology of, 105-106
with sickle cell disease, 113-114
special considerations in, 113-114
surgical intervention for, 109-112
treatment of, 107-109
Hyphemectomy, automated, 111-112
Hypoxia, 389
in eye-injured patient, 23
Hysteria
following eye trauma, 21
testing for, 21-22

I

Ice packs, 291
Immersion waterbath technique, 32
Industrial eye protectors, 401
Infection, with enucleation, 359
Informed consent, 45, 406-407
Infraorbital artery, 283
Infraorbital nerve
branches, 52
sensation in, 298-299
Infratrochlear nerve block, 52-53
Infusion port, permanent, 214*f*
Injuries. *See also specific sites*
chemical, 79-92
history for specific types of, 5-8
history of event, 4-5
Intercanthal distance, 298
Intracapsular surgery, 172-173
Intraocular foreign bodies (IOFBs), 169
complications of, 173
composition of, 171, 227
diagnosis and localization of, 227
in endophthalmitis, 244, 248
intraretinal and subretinal, 232-233
with lens injury, 172-173
without lens involvement, 171-172
magnetic characteristics of, 169-170
management of, 229-235
mechanisms of damage caused by, 226-227
pathophysiology of damage by, 227-229
in posterior segment, 226-235
preoperative evaluation of, 169-171
prognosis with presence of, 241
removal of large, 233-234
treatment of, 171-173
Intraocular foreign body films, 244
Intraocular implant, extrusion of, 17
Intraocular inflammation, management of, 129
Intraocular infusion, port location in, 213-214
Intraocular lens
benefits of, 181
in corneal repair surgery, 152
for lens trauma, 134
placement of, 180-182
suturing of, 177
Intraocular pressure (IOP), 18
in decreased atmospheric pressure, 23
elevated, 20, 128
with blunt injury, 122-124
prevention of during surgery, 50
management of, 291-292
Intraorbital foreign bodies, 341
fundamentals of management of, 341-343
imaging modalities of, 343
initial management of, 343-344
late effects of, 345-346
surgical treatment of, 344-345
Iridectomy
peripheral, 112
unintentional, 216
Iridodialyses, 117
with intraocular foreign body, 173
repair, 102*f*
Iridodonesis, 129

Iridoplasty, 182-183
Iris
  blunt trauma to, 97
  in chalcosis, 229
  changes in after trauma, 139-141
  deformities of, 97
  examination of after injury, 16-17
  incarcerated, 149-151
    but nonprolapsing, 95-96
  injury to, 95-102, 386
    penetrating, 95-97
  laser and surgical repair of, 97-102
  peripheral edge of, 117
  peripheral tear of, 118-119
  prolapsed, 153
  retroillumination of, 15*f*, 16-17
  in siderosis, 228
  stromal tears of, 97
  surgical reconstruction of, 99
  surgical repair of, 97
Iris root, stretching at, 97
Iritis, traumatic, 105
Irrigation, for chemical injury, 90-91
Isobutyl cyanoacrylate (Histoacryl), 87
Israeli Ocular Injuries Study, 55

J

Jackson intubation, 336
Johnson rod, 337

K

Kayser-Fleiser ring, 229
Keratectomy
  with evisceration, 364-365
  superficial, 176, 177*f*
  superficial epithelial, 71-73
Keratitis
  Acanthamoeba, 76-77
  antibodies for, 68
  exposure, 77
  fungal, 76-77
  infectious microbial, 75-76
Keratoconjunctivitis sicca, unsuspected, 73
Keratoepithelioplasty
  for alkali burns, 87-88
  allogenic, 75
Keratometry, 168
Keratopathy
  bullous, 73
  exposure, 317
  toxic epithelial, 77
Keratoplasty, 44, 65
  for alkali burns, 88
Keratoplasty—cont'd
  for chemical burn, 90, 92
  lamellar, 176
  penetrating, 75, 156-157, 176-178
Keratoprosthesis
  for alkali burns, 89
  temporary, 224
Koeppe lens, 16

L

Lacerations
  conjunctival, 64-65
  corneoscleral, 143-158
  location of and outcome, 240
  size of and outcome, 240
Lacrimal artery, 282
Lacrimal gland, 280
  resuspension of, 332
Lacrimal nerve, 52, 283-284
Lacrimal pump, 276
  problems with, 339
Lacrimal sac trauma, 339
Lacrimal system
  anatomy of, 335*f*
  excretory, 275-276
    evaluation of injuries to, 10
  injuries to, 334-339
    anesthesia for, 336
    complications of, 339
    from dog bite, 349
    evaluation of, 334-336
    instrumentation for repair of, 336-337
    surgery for, 337-339
  intubation of, 337-338
Lamellae
  anterior and posterior, 270-275
  inlay grafting of, 156
    preparation of donor tissue for, 157*f*
Lamellar keratoplasty
  for alkali burns, 88
  for chemical injury, 90
Lamina papyracea, fracture of, 63-64
Landers-Foulks keratoprosthesis, 224*f*
Landers-Foulks lens, 178
Laser photocoagulation, 193-194, 221, 223*f*
  for choroidal neovascularization, 192
  for retinal dialysis, 198
  for retinal tears, 234
    giant, 201
Laser surgery, for iris injury, 97-99
Lateral canthal structures, 271*f*
Lateral canthal tendon reconstruction, 332
Lateral retinaculum, 270
LeFort fractures, 307-308

Lens. *See also* Lens injury
alkali burns of, 82-83
capsular breaks in, 17
in chalcosis, 229
changes in after trauma, 141
dislocated into anterior chamber, surgical repair of, 132
fibrous plaque in, 141
involvement of in corneal laceration, 151-152
irregularities in, 18*f*
irregular light transmission through, 17
management of dislocated or subluxed, 129-130
position of, 17
removal of, 178-179
in siderosis, 228
Lens capsule, 215*f*
Lensectomy, 214-216, 234
open-sky, 178*f*
Lens injuries, 126
equatorial expansion theory of, 126-127
evaluation of, 127-128
examination of, 17
with intraocular foreign bodies, 172-173
management approaches to, 128-130
pathophysiology of, 126-127
surgical treatment of, 130-134
Levator aponeurotic complex, 274
Levator dihiscence, 290
Levator muscles, 281*f*
Lid akinesia, 9
Lid blocks
indications for, 51
techniques for, 51-53
Lid burns
classification of, 316
early management of, 317
epidemiology of, 315-316
examination of, 316-317
intermediate management of, 318-322
tarsorrhaphy for, 317-318
Lidocaine (Xylocaine), 48-49
Lids. *See also* Lid block; Lid burns
abnormal positioning of, 10
anesthesia for injured, 51-53
anatomy of, 335*f*
dog bite injury of, 348
edema of, 290
ecchymosis of, 10-11, 289
examination of in eye trauma, 9-11
hemorrhage of, 289-290
hygiene for, 317
lacerations of, 325
full-thickness, 330-332
partial-thickness, 330
late reconstruction of, 322
margin of, 275
muscles of, 265
Lids. *See also* Lid block—cont'd
penetrating injury of, 323-332
clinical evaluation of, 324-325
presurgical management of, 325-326
surgical repair of, 326-332
topography of, 268-269
wound healing in, 323-324
Limbal autograft transplantation, 74-75
for alkali burns, 88*f*
Limbal stab incision, 147
Limbal wound healing, 139
Lockwood's ligament, 274
Logan v. Greenwich Hospital Association, 405
Lymphatic drainage system, 262-265
Lyons v. Graither, 404-405

M

Macular hole, traumatic, 191*f*, 193-194
Maculopathies, traumatic, 187-194
Maddox rods, 382
Magnetic resonance imaging (MRI), 25
evaluation of, 36
of hemorrhage, 37
in injured eye and orbit, 36-38
for intraocular foreign bodies, 171
T1-weighted images in, 36-38
T2-weighted images in, 37-38
Malingering
definition of, 21
testing for, 21-22
Malpractice suits
applications of to eye trauma and emergency care, 403-407
basic issues of, 403
damages in, 407
guidelines for avoiding, 408
and informed consent, 406-407
minimizing risk of, 45
record keeping and, 406
requirements for litigation in, 403
Mandibular fracture, pharyngeal obstruction with, 53
Maxilla, free-floating, 307
Maxillary artery, 262
Maxillary bone, 276
Maxillary vein, 262
Maxillofacial injuries, airway obstruction with, 53
McCannel suture technique, 99, 100*f*, 101*f*
McCormack v. Linberg, 405
McDermott v. Manhattan Eye and Ear Hospital, 407
Medial canthal injuries, repair of, 332
Medial wall fractures, 308
Medical history, 5
Medical records, importance of checking, 45

Medicolegal considerations, 403-408
  in eyelid laceration, 326
Medroxyprogesterone (Provera)
  for alkali burns, 85
  for chemical burns, 91
Meningitis, 53
Merrit v. Deaconess Hospital et al, 405
Metal locators, 227
Metoclopramide, 50
Microscopic hyphema, 105
Microvitrectomy, automated, 152
Miosis, traumatic, 386
Miotics, 108
Mirror test, 22
Monocanalicular intubation, 336, 338
Monocular blindness, tests for, 22
Motility restriction, 12
Motor nerves, 266
Motor vehicle accidents, 398
Mucocele formation, 345-346
Mucous membrane grafts, 87
Muller's muscle, 274
Multiplanar reconstruction, 28
MVR blade, 218-219
Mydriasis, traumatic, 106, 385, 386
Mydriatics, 373
Myopia, induced, 129

N

Nasal intubations, 53
Nasociliary nerve, 284
  course of, 282*f*
Nasolacrimal drainage system, 298
Nasoorbital fractures, 308
National Eye Trauma system, 395
National Institute for Occupational Safety and Health data, 397
Nd-YAG laser, 98
Negligence, 407
Neurectomy, 357
Neurologic testing, 343
Nocturnal lagophthalmos, 77
No light perception (NLP), 11
Nuclear sclerosis, removal of, 131
Nystagmus, 388-389
  latent, 389

O

Oblique muscles, 284
Oblique plane reconstruction, 28-29
Occlusion therapy
  guidelines for, 59
  methods of, 59
Occult trauma, ruling out, 9-10
Ocular adnexa, anatomy of, 261-280
Ocular bobbing, 388
Ocular history, 4
Ocular injuries
  available protection from, 399-401
  epidemiology of, 395-396
  general anesthesia for, 50-51
  patients at risk for, 398-399
  prevention of, 398
  with recreation-related trauma, 397-398
  retrobulbar anesthesia and facial nerve akinesia for, 49-50
  subconjunctival anesthesia injections for, 48-49
  topical anesthesia for
    agents, 47-48
    indications for, 47
  with work-related trauma, 396-397
Ocular motility, 299
Ocular motor nerve
  injuries to, 382-386
  palsy, 382, 385-386
Ocular motor system
  hypoxic effects on, 389
  orbital injury causing dysfunction of, 381-382
  trauma to, 380-389
    examination for, 380-381
Ocular region arteries, 263*f*
Ocular region veins, 264*f*
Ocular surface replacement, 87
Ocular surface stabilization, 176
Ocular trauma
  anterior segment reconstruction following, 175-183
  diagnostic imaging of, 25-38
  penetrating
    historical perspective on outcomes of, 238-239
    prognosis of, 239-241
Oculomotor nerve, 283
  injury to, 383-385
Oculomotor nerve palsy, 385
Ophthalmia, sympathetic, 253-258, 355
Ophthalmic artery, 281, 282
  palpebral brances of, 283
Ophthalmic evaluation, goals of initial, 3-4
Ophthalmic veins, 283
Ophthalmological principles, 371-372
Ophthalmoplegia, 290, 380
  internuclear, 387-388
Opsconclonus, 388
Optic canal, 276
  decompression, 376-377
Optic chiasm trauma, 377-378
Optic foramen, 276-277
Optic nerve, 282, 283
  CT scan of, 306
  direct trauma to, 373-375
  examination of after injury, 19-20

Optic nerve—cont'd
  indirect trauma to, 375-377
  injury to, 20
Optic nerve blindness, 290-292
  therapy for, 292
Optic neuropathies
  anterior indirect, 375
  differential diagnosis of, 373
  direct, 373-375
  examination for, 372-373
  indirect, 375-377
  posterior indirect, 375-377
  principles of, 371-372
Orbicularis oculi muscle, 265, 269-270
Orbicularis spasm, 9
Orbit. *See also* Orbital fractures; Orbital soft tissues
  anatomy of, 280-286
  anesthesia for injuries to, 53
  anterior structures of, 273*f*
  blood vessles of, 281-283
  blunt trauma to soft tissues of, 287-293
  detecting soft-tissue changes in, 37
  diagnostic imaging of, 25-38
  dimensions of, 276
  extraocular muscles of, 284
  floor of, 278-279
    fractures of, 308-309
    repair of fracture of, 311-313
  imaging of, 284-286
  injury of with enucleation, 359
  nerves of, 283-284
  ocular motor dysfunction with injury to, 381-382
  osteology of, 276-280
  penetrating injury of, 343
  roof, 278
    fractures of, 308
  walls of, 276-279
Orbital cellulitis, 291
Orbital decompression, 292-293
Orbital emphysema, 299
Orbital fascia, 280-281
Orbital fat, 270, 272*f*
Orbital fractures, 56, 295
  classification of, 307-309
  CT scan of, 297*f*
  diagnosis of, 30
  examination of, 295-300
  management of, 310-313
  photographic documentation of, 300
  radiographic evaluation of, 300-307
Orbital hematomas, 53
Orbital implant
  migration of, 360-361
  placement of, 357, 358*f*
Orbital rim, 276
  fractures of, 296, 309
  palpation of, 296
Orbital septum, 270, 272*f*
Orbital soft tissues
  abrasions of, 287-288
  contusion injuries to, 288
  crush injury to, 288
  edema of, 288-289
  emphysema of, 290
  examination of, 287
  hemorrahge of, 289
  ophthalmoplegia of, 290
  ptosis of, 290
  surgery of, 292-293
  therapy for trauma to, 291-292
Oropharyngeal airway insertion, 53
Osteology, 276
  orbital dimensions of, 276

P

Paracentesis
  for alkali burns, 86
  for traumatic hyphema, 110-111
Paranasal sinuses, 279
Paraorbital sinuses, 279-280
Patch grafting, 155-156, 176
  full-thickness, 157, 157*f*
Patching, for corneal epithelial defect, 76
Paton's method, 166
Pediatric eye-trauma patient, evaluation and management strategies for, 55-59
Penetrating injuries
  eyelid, 323-332
  histopathology of in animal models, 207-208
  to posterior segment, 205-206
  prognosis and outcomes for, 238-241
  in sympathetic ophthalmia, 255
Penetrating keratoplasty, 88
Penlight examination, 13
Periorbita, 280
Periorbital echymosis, 10-11
Periorbital sinuses, fracture of, 63
Periosteal elevator, 312
Peripheral anterior synechiae, 122
Peritomy, 292, 356
Phacodonesis, 129
Phacoemulsifiers, 214
Pharyngeal obstruction, 53
pH effect, in alkali burns, 80
Phoroptor, 22
Photophobia, 77, 97
Photoreceptor cells, 221
Photoreceptor fragmentation, 189
Physician-patient relationship, 404-405
Pink v. Slater, 405
Placido disk imagery, 168

Plain film radiography
  advantages of, 25
  Caldwell projection of, 25, 300, 302*f*
  cranial base view of, 304*f*
  of dog bite, 348
  graphic examples of, 26-27*f*
  of injured eye and orbit, 25-28
  lateral projection of, 302
  for orbital fracture, 300-305
  Rhese projection of, 302, 303*f*
  specialized applications of, 304-305
  Water projection of, 25, 300, 301*f*
Platelet-derived growth factor (PDGF)
  for corneal wounds, 138
  in healing response, 209
Pneumocranium, 53
Pneumotonometry, 18
Poison Control Center, 6
Polycarbonate lenses, 400
Polycarbonate sports eye protectors, 400
Polymorphonuclear neutrophils (PMNs), accumulation of with alkali burns, 80, 81
Postenulceation socket syndrome, 361, 363
  treatment of, 362
Posterior segment
  animal models of trauma to, 206-208
  blunt trauma to, 204-205
  factors influencing healing of traumatic injury, 208-209
  intraocular foreign bodies in, 226-235
  management of nonpenetrating injuries without rupture, 212-213
  management of penetrating injuries and globe rupture, 213
  pathophysiology of trauma to, 204-210
  penetrating trauma to, 205-206
  surgical management of injuries to, 209-210, 212-224
  surgical methods used in, 213-224
  trauma. *See specific sites of*
Prednisone, 257
Prenatal trauma, 56
Preoperative check list, 45
Preretinal membranes, 218-219
Prevention, 398
Procaine (Novocaine), 48
Prolene mattress sutures, 320
Proparacaine (Ophthaine), 48
Protective devices, 399-401
Proximate cause, 407
Pseudoguttata, 15
Psychic trauma, minimizing of, 44-45
Ptosis, 290, 311
  postoperative, 357
  prosthetic management of, 361
Punctal occlusion, 86
Pupillary margin tearing, 118
Pupillary reflexes, as indicator of visual-system function, 12
Pupils
  disorders of following trauma, 388
  evaluation of, 372-373
  examination of after trauma, 11-12
  reactivity, 300
Purtscher's retinopathy, 189-190

Q

Quickert-Dryden tubing, 336, 337*f*

R

Rabies
  prophylaxis for dog bites, 350-351
  vaccination, 347-348
Raccoon's eye sign, 289
Radial keratotomy, 65
Radiography
  for intraocular foreign bodies, 170-171
  methods, 25-38. *See also specific types*
  for orbital fracture, 300-307
  plain film, 25-28
Radiologic studies, 227
Record keeping, 406
Recreation-related trauma, 397-398
Rectus muscles, 284
  entrapment of, 299
Recurrent erosion syndrome, 69
  diagnosis of therapy for, 70
  medical therapy for, 70-71
  pathogenesis of, 68-70
  surgical therapy for, 71-73
  symptoms of, 70
  therapy of, 70
Red-green glasses, 22
Reepithelialization, 80, 81
  with alkali burn, 83-84
  after chemical burns, 91
Reflex blepharospasm, elimination of, 342
Retina
  attachment of to ora serrata, 117
  blunt trauma to peripheral, 195-202
  in chalcosis, 229
  contusion of, 188-189
  detachment of, 18, 205
    dialysis and, 117, 198-199
    with giant tears, 201-202
    mechanism of, 207*f*
    rhegmatogenous, 195, 196*f*, 198-199
    with traumatic tears, 200
    ultrasound of, 33-35
  dialysis of, 117, 196*f*

Retina—cont'd
  dialysis of—cont'd
    without detachment, 198
    with rhegmatogenous detachment, 117, 198-199
  edema of, 19
  examination of after injury, 18-19
  hemorrhage of, 19
    in newborn, 56
  incarcertion of, 221
  lacerations of in healing response, 209
  reattachment of, 221-223
  in siderosis, 228
  tears in, 120, 195
    clinical setting for, 197
    pathophysiology of from blunt trauma, 195-197
    without detachment, 200
    with detachment, 200
    giant with detachment, 201-202
    giant without detachment, 200-201
  treatment of breaks in, 234
Retinal artery, central, 281
Retinal pigment epithelium (RPE), 188, 219
  alteration of, 189
  in healing response, 209
  hyperplastic, 256*f*
  nodules at, 254, 255
Retinitis sclopetaria, 192-193
Retinoic acid, 86
Retinopathies, Purtscher's, 189-190
Retinotomy, 222*f*
Retroaural hematomas, 53
Retrochiasmal visual pathway trauma, 378
Retroillumination, 15*f*, 127*f*
  of iris, 16-17, 227
Retromandibular vein, 262
Riolan, muscle of, 275

S

Saliclylates, 108
S-antigen, 256
Schiotz tonometry, 18
Schmidt-Rimpler test, 21-22
Sclera
  contents of, 137
  evaluation of after injury, 13
  exposure of, 65
  healing of, 139
  posterior lacerations of, 155
  ruptures or discontinuities of, 18-19
Scleral buckling, 223-224
Scleral closure, zippering technique of, 154-155
Scleral flap, 99
Sclerotomies, 133*f*, 363
Sclerotomy knife, 215
See-saw nystagmus, 388
Seidel fluorescein test, 14, 67
Self-mutilation, 56-57
Sensory nerves, facial, 261-262
Serum-derived proteins, in healing response, 209
Seventh nerve injury, 387
Sickle cell disease, complications of traumatic hyphema with, 113-114
Sickle prep, 107
Siderosis, 227-228
Silastic tubing, 339
Silicone oil, 224
Sinsky hook, 173
Sinuses, risk of mucocele formation with injury to, 345-346
Sixth nerve palsy, 383
Skin grafting
  for lid burns, 318, 320-321
  lysis of adhesions and, 318-321
  lysis of contracture and, 318
Slit-lamp examination, 18
  key to successful, 13
Snellen letters, 58
Socket contracture, postoperative, 361-362
Soft tissue
  anatomy of, 261-276
  localization, 28
Sphenoid bone, 280
Sphenoid sinuses, 280
Sphincter muscle
  injury of, 97
  radial tears in, 139
Sphincteroton lysis, 98
Sphincter pupillae, 117
Sports injuries, 397, 398
Staphylococcus epidermidis, 242
Staphylococcus infections, antibiotic prophylaxis for, 43
Stents, 336-337
Steroids
  for endophthalmitis, 249-250
  for sympathetic ophthalmia, 257
  for traumatic hyphema, 108
Strabismus
  surgery, 346
  traumatic, 58
Streetwear frames, 400
Streptococcus infections, antibiotic prophylaxis for, 43
Stroma
  alkali burns of, 81-82
  breakdown of with chemical burn, 92
Stryker burr, 313
Stundon v. Standnick, 405
Subconjunctival emphysema, 63
Subconjunctival hemorrhage, 65

Subconjunctival infections, 43
Subdural hematomas, 289
Subfoveal hemorrhage, 193
Subperiosteal hematomas, 289
  CT scan of, 306
Subretinal blood, 219-221
Subretinal clot removal, 220*f*, 221
Subretinal fluid drainage, 222
Sulfuric acid, 89
Sulfurous acid, 89
Superior orbital vein, 283
Superoxide scavengers, 86
Suprachoroidal hemorrhage, increased intraocular volume with, 42
Supraorbital artery, 282
Supratrochlear, regional blocks of, 52-53
Supratrochlear vein, 262
Surgery. *See also* Eye trauma surgery; *specific techniques*
  for alkali burns, 86-89
  for corneal epithelial defect and noninfected ulceration, 74-75
  preparation of patient for, 41-45
  timing of, 212
Suture knot, 149*f*
Suture placement
  compression factors in, 161
  effects of on cornea, 160-164
  eversion and inversion effects of, 161-163
  for linear corneal lacerations, 164-166
  splinting and torquing effects of, 163
  for tissue loss and stellate lacerations, 166-167
  wound override of, 163-164
Sutures
  buried subcutaneous, 328-329
  corneal, 146-148
  for enucleation, 357
  in eyelid laceration repair, 327
  eyelid marginal, 331-332
  horizontal mattress, 329
  intermarginal, 319*f*
  interrupted, 328
  for lacrimal system repair, 337, 339
  placement of, 331*f*
  removal of, 167-168
  running, 328
    shoelace, 165-166
    subcuticular, 329
  tightening of, 167
  types used in lid repair, 329*f*
  vertical mattress, 329-330, 331*f*
Sweet's triangulation methods, 28
Swinging-flashlight test, 372
Sympathetic ophthalmia, 253
  clinical features of, 254
  differential diagnosis of, 256-257
Sympathetic ophthalmia—cont'd
  with enucleation, 355
  etiology of, 255-256
  histological features of, 255
  incidence of, 253-254
  penetrating wound in, 255
  treatment and prognosis of, 257-258

T

Tarsorrhaphy, 319*f*
  for alkali burns, 86-87
  for lid burn, 317-318
Tarsus, 274
  plates of, 274-275
Tearing injuries, response to, 120
Tear substitutes, 84
Teeth, sensory abnormalities of, 279
Temporal fossa, 276
Tenon's space hematoma, 289*f*
Tenon's tissue, prolapse of, 65
Testing, identifying areas requiring, 4
Tetanus, 409
  guidelines for, 325*t*
  primary immunization for, 409
  prophylaxis, 44
    for dog bites, 350
    guidelines for, 409-410
Tetanus immune globulin (TIG), 409
Tetanus toxoid, 325-326
Tetracaine (Pontocaine), 47-48
Therapeutic plan, 4
Thermal burn injury, 8
Third nerve injury
  direct, 383-384
  indirect, 384-385
Tight lens syndrome, 70
Tissue adhesive, 176
  for alkali burns, 97
  application of, 145-146
  for corneal lacertions, 145-146
Tomograpic sections, 28
Tonometry, 18
Trabecular meshwork, 117
  bleeding around, 120
  tear of, 119-120
Trabeculectomy, 112
Transconjunctival advancement, 321-322
Transconjunctival flap, 321*f*
Transillumination, 227
Transportation, of eye-injured patient, 22-23
Transvitreous bands, 219*f*
Transvitreous drainage, 222*f*
Treatment, prior history of, 5
Trephination, 178

Trigeminal nerve, 279, 284
  injury to, 386
Tripod fractures, 308-309
Trochlear nerve, 283
  injury to, 382-383

U

Ultrasound, 25, 227
  A-scan, 35*f*
  B-scan, 33-34*f*, 35*f*
    showing posterior capsular disruption, 128*f*
  with ERG, 20
  in foreign body localization, 35
  in injured eye and orbit, 32-36
  for intraocular foreign bodies, 170-171
Ultraviolet radiation injury, 77
Uveal melanin, 256
Uveal tract, rupture of, 139
Uvea prolapse, 154-155
Uveitis, phacoanaphylactic, 127-128

V

Vancomycin, 43
van Lint technique, 51
Vannas scissors, 149
Venography, orbital, 304-305
Vertical gaze, 388
Vibration, of eye-injured patient, 23
Viscoelastic, 67, 147
  for intraocular foreign bodies, 172
  for iris repair, 96
Visual acuity
  with orbital hemorrhage, 289
  with penetrating ocular trauma, 239
  testing, 11, 372
Visual electrical evoked potentials (VEEP), 21
Visual evoked potential (VEP), in acute setting, 20-21
Visual field defects
  with choroidal rupture, 191
  after penetrating brain wounds, 378
Visual field testing, 12
  for malingering or hysteria, 22
Visual pathway trauma, retrochiasmal, 378
Visual system injury
  differential diagnosis of, 373
  principles of, 371-372
Vitamin A analogs, 74
Vitrectomy, 194
  anterior, 132, 179
  case selection for, 232
  efficacy of, 209-210
  for endophthalmitis, 248-249
Vitrectomy—cont'd
  intraocular lens with, 152
  pars plana, 134, 224, 232
  in posterior segment injury, 216-217
  special situations in, 232-234
  surgical techniques with, 232
  timing of, 210
  in treatment of retinal breaks, 234
Vitreoretinal surgery, 178
Vitreoretinal traction, 201
  acute, 205
Vitreoretinopathy, proliferative, 201-202
Vitreous
  hemorrhage of
    prognosis with, 240
    ultrasound of, 33
  herniation, 129
  incarceration of, 153*f*
  involvement of in corneal laceration, 152
  opacities of, 18
  prolapsed, 154*f*
    with corneoscleral lacerations, 154-155
  removal of opaque, 216*f*
  traction of, 193
  ultrasound in planning surgery of, 32-33
Vitreous bands, 217-218
Vitreous base
  avulsion, 198
  blunt trauma to, 198-199
  traction from blunt trauma, 195-196
Vitreous body, examination of after injury, 18-19
Vitreous cutting device, 215-216
Vitreous-lens admixture, in healing response, 209
Vogt-Koyanagi-Harada syndrome, 254-257

W

Wagner v. Olmedo, 405
Water's projection, 25, 300, 301*f*
Welch v. Whitaker, 407
Wessely-Comberg-Pfeiffer procedure, 28
Whitnall's ligament, 274
Whitnall's tubercle, 280
Work-related trauma, 396-397
Wound care
  for eyelid laceration, 326
  in lid repair surgery, 330
Wound healing
  of anterior segment, 136-141
  of cornea, 137-139
  of iris or angle, 139-141
  of lens, 141
  local factors affecting, 324

Wound healing—cont'd
  of penetrating eyelid trauma, 323-324
  primary, 323-324
  of sclera or limbal injury, 139
  secondary, 324
  systemic factors affecting, 324
Wound infection, from dog bites, 351

X

X-ray film. *See* Plain film radiography

Z

Ziegler blade, 173
Zinn's annulus, 278*f*, 281
Zonules, 117
  disruption of, 129
  injury to, 120
Zygoma, 276
  fractures of, 308-309
Zygomaticomaxillary suture, 276
Zygomaticotemporal nerve, 284
Zygomaticus muscles, 265-266